Clinical Medicine and the Nervous System
Series Editors: John P. Conomy and Michael Swash

Titles in the series already published

Headache
Richard Peatfield

Epilepsy: Electroclinical Syndromes
Edited by Hans Lüders and Ronald P. Lesser

Forthcoming titles in the series

Electrophysiological Diagnosis
E. M. Sedgewick

Hydrocephalus and the Cerebrospinal Fluid
Edited by J. D. Pickard and R. O. Weller

Neurological Emergencies
Michael Swash and John P. Conomy

The Heart and Stroke

Exploring Mutual Cerebrovascular and Cardiovascular Issues

Edited by Anthony J. Furlan

With 52 Figures

Springer-Verlag
London Berlin Heidelberg New York
Paris Tokyo

Anthony J. Furlan, MD
Director, Cerebrovascular Program, The Cleveland Clinic Foundation, Cleveland, Ohio, USA

Series Editors:

John P. Conomy, MD, Head, Department of Neurology,
The Cleveland Clinic Foundation, Cleveland, Ohio, USA

Michael Swash, MD, FRCP, MRCPath, Consultant Neurologist,
The London Hospital, Whitechapel, London, UK

ISBN-13: 978-1-4471-3131-1 e-ISBN-13: 978-1-4471-3129-8
DOI: 10.1007/978-1-4471-3129-8

British Library Cataloguing in Publication Data
The Heart and Stroke: exploring mutual cerebrovascular and cardiovascular issues.
– (Clinical medicine and the nervous system).
1. Heart – Diseases 2. Cerebrovascular disease
I. Furlan, A.J. II. Series
616.1'207 RC682

Library of Congress Cataloging-in-Publication Data
The Heart and stroke.
(Clinical medicine and the nervous system)
Includes bibliographies and index.
1. Cerebrovascular disease. 2. Heart – Diseases. 3. Cerebrovascular Disease – Complications and sequelae. 4. Heart – Diseases – Complications and sequelae. 5. Embolism. I. Furlan, A.J. (Anthony John), 1947– . II. Series. [DNLM: 1. Cerebrovascular Disorders – complications. 2. Heart Diseases – complications. WG 200 H4363] RC 388.5.H424 1987 616.8'1 87-4340

Softcover reprint of the hardcover first edition 1987

Typeset by Wilmaset, Birkenhead, Wirral

2128/3916-543210

In Memory of
Anthony J. Furlan, Sr.

ON

DISORDERS

OF THE

CEREBRAL CIRCULATION;

AND

ON THE CONNECTION

BETWEEN

AFFECTIONS OF THE BRAIN

AND

DISEASES OF THE HEART.

BY

GEORGE BURROWS, M. D.,

Late Fellow of Caius College, Cambridge; Fellow of the Royal College of Physicians, London; Physician and Lecturer on the Principles and Practice of Medicine, at St. Bartholomew's Hospital.

WITH COLOURED PLATES.

PHILADELPHIA:
LEA & BLANCHARD.
1848.

Title page from editor's (AJF) copy of the first American edition of Burrows' monograph (1848). First published in London, 1846.

Preface

In recent years there has been a resurgence of interest in heart/brain interactions. Traditional concerns regarding cerebral embolism have been flip-flopped to address the effects of brain lesions on the heart. Hybrid terms such as "neurocardiology" and "cardiovascular neurobiology" have not only been coined but deemed the "interdisciplinary area of the 1980s" with the bold suggestion that communication between neurologists and cardiologists must be increased. Cardioembolism itself is being reassessed with more sources and more strokes being uncovered daily. Risk factors are shared and stroke victims usually die from heart attacks. Cardiopulmonary resuscitation (CPR) classes abound, even though CPR may restart the heart but not the brain. This has given rise to the less familiar but vital concept of cardiopulmonary *cerebral* resuscitation (CPCR). Most recently, the intimate relationship between cardiovascular and cerebrovascular disease was called to public attention when artificial heart recipients sustained debilitating strokes.

Although the first monograph dealing with the relationship between heart disease and stroke was published by Sir George Burrows in 1846 (frontispiece), few recent texts are devoted exclusively to the subject. Being mindful of the book explosion, it nonetheless seemed appropriate to gather some of the recent information on heart/brain relationships in one place. Thankfully, I was able to get some others to agree and the substance of this book is the result of their efforts. The physical book, the typing, the binding, the encouragement to proceed owe much to many including my secretary, Tee Roberts, my publisher, Michael Jackson, and my friend, Jack Conomy. The inspiration ultimately came from my patients and my father, whose asymptomatic carotid bruit I listened to until the day he died suddenly of a myocardial infarction.

Cleveland, Ohio
January 1987

Anthony J. Furlan

Series Editors' Foreword

In 1965, both Series Editors were first-year house officers in neurology and fledgling students of the nervous system. We learned in the laboratory of Professor David Cohen, then at Cleveland's Case Western Reserve University, that the nervous system of a pigeon could, through techniques of operant conditioning, be trained to control cardiac rate upon cue. David Cohen introduced us to a new term as well: "cardiovascular neurobiology." A few hundred yards to the west in Cleveland, Irvine Page at the Cleveland Clinic Foundation was nailing down 20 years of painstaking physiologic and biochemical work on what he termed "the mosaic of hypertension." He introduced a then extraordinary concept: that no matter what the cause of hypertension may be, in the end, the chronic vascular hypertensive state is sustained by the central nervous system. The thought that an important and often lethal cardiovascular disease was bound up somehow with the nervous system was exciting and revolutionary. In the ensuing two decades, concepts like those espoused by Irvine Page and David Cohen, along with their historic conceptual precursors and more revealing subsequent scientific elaborations, have taken root in clinical medicine. The interdependence of heart and brain in health and their pathologic effects, one organ upon the other, are becoming increasingly well understood. With that better understanding have come new methods of dealing with problems in humans in which the heart and brain are simultaneously or sequentially affected by a common disruptive cause. The most common and most morbid of these clinical settings is stroke.

Anthony Furlan has assembled an outstanding panel of contributors to this volume. Many are readily recognized as leaders and founders of an emerging branch of medicine which links heart and brain together in the context of stroke and other cardiovascular disorders. That linkage and its illumination has an important bearing on a combination of illnesses – heart attack and stroke –

which together are by far the leading causes of death in much of the world.

The text of *The Heart and Stroke* is clear and fundamental. We feel it has much to say to students and generalists regarding problems encountered in hospital wards, emergency centers, and outpatient departments every day. The volume can serve also as a benchmark text for more advanced clinicians and investigators in cardiac and cerebrovascular illnesses. *The Heart and Stroke* is pleasurable reading and a most welcome addition to the Clinical Medicine and the Nervous System series.

Cleveland, Ohio
London
March 1987

John P. Conomy
Michael Swash

Contents

Section B CARDIOVASCULAR NEUROBIOLOGY

Contributors

F. M. Abi-Samra, MD
Director, Electrophysiology Laboratory, Cardiology Division, The Ochsner Clinic, 1514 Jefferson Highway, New Orleans, Louisiana 70121, USA

N. S. Abramson, MD
Coordinator for Clinical Research, Resuscitation Research Center, University of Pittsburgh, 3434 Fifth Avenue, Pittsburgh, Pennsylvania 15260, USA

R. D. Adams, MD
Chief, Neurology Service Emeritus Massachusetts General Hospital, 55 Fruit Street, Boston, Massachusetts 02114, USA
Bullard Professor of Neuropathology Emeritus, Harvard University, 25 Shattuck Street, Boston, Massachusetts 02115, USA
Director, Eunice Kennedy Shriver Laboratory Emeritus, 200 Trapelo Road, Waltham, Massachusetts 02254, USA

K. L. Barnes, PhD
Head, Section of Research, Department of Brain and Vascular Research, The Cleveland Clinic Foundation, 9500 Euclid Avenue, Cleveland, Ohio 44106, USA

H. J. M. Barnett, MD
Scientific Director, John P. Robarts Research Institute, PO Box 5015, London, Ontario N6A 5K8, Canada
Professor of Neurology, Department of Clinical Neurological Sciences, University of Western Ontario, 7th Floor, University Hospital, PO Box 5339, London, Ontario N6A 5A5, Canada

E. G. Beven, MD
Chairman, Department of Vascular Surgery, The Cleveland Clinic Foundation, 9500 Euclid Avenue, Cleveland, Ohio 44106, USA

J. P. Conomy, MD
Chairman, Department of Neurology, The Cleveland Clinic Foundation, 9500 Euclid Avenue, Cleveland, Ohio 44106, USA

L. A. Cupples, PhD
Associate Professor of Public Health, Epidemiology and Biostatistics, School of Public Health, Boston University School of Medicine, 80 East Concord Street, Boston, Massachusetts 02118, USA

R. B. D. D'Agnostino, PhD
Chairman, Mathematics and Statistics, Department of Mathematics, Boston University, 111 Cummington Street, Boston, Massachusetts 02118, USA

J. D. Easton, MD
Chairman, Department of Neurology, Brown University, 110 Lockwood Street, Providence, Rhode Island 02903, USA

C. M. Ferrario, MD
Chairman, Department of Brain and Vascular Research, The Cleveland Clinic Foundation, 9500 Euclid Avenue, Cleveland, Ohio 44106, USA

C. M. Fisher, MD
Professor of Neurology Emeritus, Harvard Medical School, Neurologic Service, Massachusetts General Hospital, 55 Fruit Street, Boston, Massachusetts 02114, USA

F. M. Fouad, MD
Clinical Science Department, Research Division, The Cleveland Clinic Foundation, 9500 Euclid Avenue, Cleveland, Ohio 44106, USA

A. J. Furlan, MD
Director, Cerebrovascular Program, The Cleveland Clinic Foundation, 9500 Euclid Avenue, Cleveland, Ohio 44106, USA

V. C. Hachinski, MD
Professor, Department of Clinical Neurological Sciences, University of Western Ontario, 339 Windermere Road, London, Ontario N6G 2N9, Canada

R. G. Hart, MD
Assistant Professor, Division of Neurology, Department of Medicine, University of Texas, 7703 Floyd Curl Drive, San Antonio, Texas 78284, USA

N. R. Hertzer, MD
Head, Section of Cerebrovascular Surgery, Department of Vascular Surgery, The Cleveland Clinic Foundation, 9500 Euclid Avenue, Ohio 44106, USA

R. E. Hobbs, MD
Codirector, Cardiovascular Training Program, Department of Cardiology, The Cleveland Clinic Foundation, 9500 Euclid Avenue, Cleveland, Ohio 44106, USA

R. E. Jackson, MD
Assistant Residency Director, Emergency Medicine, William Beaumont Hospital, 3535 13 Mile, Royal Oak, Michigan 48072, USA

S. C. Jones, PhD
Director, Cerebrovascular Research Laboratory, The Cleveland Clinic Foundation, 9500 Euclid Avenue, Cleveland, Ohio 44106, USA

W. B. Kannel, MD
Professor of Medicine and Chairman, Section of Preventive Medicine and Epidemiology, The Evans Memorial Department of Clinical Research and Department of Medicine, University Hospital, Boston University School of Medicine, 80 East Concord Street, Boston, Massachusetts 02118, USA

S. Lauzier, MD
Clinical Research Fellow, Cerebrovascular Disease, Department of Clinical Neurological Sciences, University Hospital, 339 Windermere Road, London, Ontario N6A 5A5, Canada

S. R. Levine, MD
Cerebrovascular Fellow, Henry Ford Hospital, 2799 West Boulevard, Detroit, Michigan 48202, USA

J. R. Little, MD
Head, Section of Cerebrovascular Surgery, Department of Neurosurgery, The Cleveland Clinic Foundation, 9500 Euclid Avenue, Cleveland Ohio 44106, USA

F. D. Loop, MD
Chairman, Department of Thoracic and Cardiovascular Surgery, The Cleveland Clinic Foundation, 9500 Euclid Avenue, Cleveland, Ohio 44106, USA

J. D. Maloney, MD
Director, Electrophysiology Laboratory, Department of Cardiology, The Cleveland Clinic Foundation, 9500 Euclid Avenue, Cleveland, Ohio 44106, USA

J. P. Mohr, MD
Sciarra Professor of Clinical Neurology, Columbia University, Director of Cerebrovascular Research, Neurological Institute, 710 West 168th Street, New York, NY 10032, USA

J. W. Norris, MD
Associate Professor of Medicine, Sunnybrook Medical Center, Department of Neuroscience, 2075 Bayview Avenue, Ontario M4N 3M5, Canada

V. M. Patel, MD
Instructor, Section of Neurophysiology, Department of Neurology and Neuroscience Program, Baylor College of Medicine, 1 Baylor Plaza, Houston, Texas 77030, USA

E. D. Salgado, MD
Cerebrovascular Stroke Fellow, The Cleveland Clinic Foundation, 9500 Euclid Avenue, Cleveland, Ohio 44106, USA

P. Safar, MD
Director, Resuscitation Research Center, University of Pittsburgh, 3434 Fifth Avenue, Pittsburgh, PA 15260, USA

B. A. Sandok, MD
Chairman, Department of Neurology, Mayo Clinic, 200 First Street, SW, Rochester, Minnesota 55901, USA

J. E. Skinner, PhD
Professor, Section of Neurophysiology, Department of Neurology and Neuroscience Program, Baylor College of Medicine, 1 Baylor Plaza, Houston, Texas 77030, USA

P. J. Sweeney, MD
Department of Neurology, The Cleveland Clinic Foundation, 9500 Euclid Avenue, Cleveland, Ohio 44106, USA

K. M. A. Welch, MD
Chairman, Department of Neurology, Henry Ford Hospital, 2799 West Boulevard, Detroit, Michigan 48202, USA

P. A. Wolf, MD
Professor of Neurology, Section of Preventive Medicine and Epidemiology, Boston University School of Medicine, 89 East Concord Street, Boston, Massachusetts 02118, USA

Introduction

An Example of Research on Heart-Brain Interactions: Cardiopulmonary-Cerebral Resuscitation*

P. Safar and N. S. Abramson

Congratulations to Dr. Anthony Furlan, initiator and editor of this book *The Heart and Stroke*, for this novel multidisciplinary approach to teaching medical knowledge about the most prevalent cripplers and killers in the industrialized world—ischemic-anoxic emergencies of heart and brain.

The similarities and pathophysiologic interactions between ischemic events in the heart and brain have been explored by researchers since the early 1970s for focal ischemia (Zuelch 1977) and global ischemia (Safar 1963, 1986; Safar and Vaagenes 1986). Recognition of these relationships has evolved during the past 2 decades, as cardiopulmonary resuscitation (CPR) has evolved into cardiopulmonary-cerebral resuscitation (CPCR) (Safar 1987). Research in this area is currently growing at a rapid rate. The importance of CPCR is illustrated by the fact that among the 2 million people who die each year in the United States, about one-fourth die prematurely, i.e., before senility and without incurable disease. Many of these deaths occur in "hearts too good to die," a concept introduced by Claude Beck (1960), and with "brains too good to die" (Safar 1963, 1977, 1978).

At present only about one-half of prehospital CPR attempts result in restored spontaneous circulation. One-half of these subsequently die in the hospital (the majority from combined secondary cardiovascular and cerebral deterioration). Among long-term survivors (at best one-fourth of all CPR attempts), 10%–40% suffer permanent brain damage. Considering the fact that, before the 1950s, prehospital apnea and pulselessness meant certain death, the present results are encouraging. They are, however, far from what might be possible. The arrested heart can be restarted (with emergency cardiopulmonary bypass) after over 20 min of normothermic and over 60 min of hypothermic cardiac arrest (Safar et al. 1987). Some cerebral neurons can survive up to 60 min of normothermic ischemic anoxia (Hossmann 1982). Our animal experiments and human data have shown that cardiac arrest of over 5 min followed by CPR and special

* Supported in part by the Asmund S. Laerdal Foundation and the National Institutes of Health (NINCDS) Grant NS-15295.

intensive care can occasionally be survived without brain damage (Breivik et al. 1978; Abramson et al. 1985; Safar 1986).

Dr. Furlan asked us to illustrate the importance of multidisciplinary research into heart-brain interactions by the example of our *personal* history on CPCR.

In the 1950s, stimulated by Elam's demonstration that mouth-to-tube (or mask) ventilation can maintain adequate blood gas values in apneic adults (1954), Safar performed experiments on curarized (but not intubated) human adult volunteers (1958). These experiments demonstrated for the first time the failure of the then taught chest-pressure arm-lift methods of artificial respiration (Safar 1959) and established steps A and B of the ABCs of modern CPR, i.e., airway control (head-tilt, mouth-open, jaw-thrust) (Safar et al. 1959) and breathing support (direct mouth-to-mouth or nose ventilation) (Safar et al. 1958). Gordon demonstrated the superiority of mouth-to-mouth ventilation over manual methods in children (1958). Kouwenhoven at the Johns Hopkins Hospital observed some of Safar's experiments in the late 1950s. In 1960, Kouwenhoven, who had researched ventricular fibrillation and defibrillation since the 1930s, published, together with Knickerbocker and Jude, their results in dogs and patients of artificial circulation by intermittent chest compressions, i.e. step C of CPR—circulation support (1960). Prior to the 1950s, artificial ventilation by mouth-to-mouth was practiced only occasionally in newborns, and artificial circulation by chest compressions was practiced widely only in research laboratories.

In 1960, Safar showed that sternal compressions alone in man cannot adequately ventilate the lungs (Safar et al. 1961a). Starting in 1960, he combined steps A, B, and C into phase I (basic life support) of a CPR system (Harris et al. 1967) and added phase II (advanced life support for restoration of adequate spontaneous circulation)—steps D (drugs and fluids), E (electrocardiography), and F (fibrillation treatment, defibrillation); and phase III (prolonged life support)—steps G (gauging salvageability), H (humanizing the result by restoring consciousness), and I (intensive care) (Safar 1964, 1968–1987). Steps D, E, F had existed since the turn of this century, but were used primarily in laboratory animals. Multiorgan systems-oriented intensive care (long-term resuscitation), introduced in the United States in the late 1950s (Safar 1961b), was expanded in the 1970s to "brain-oriented extracerebral life support" for patients in coma or with multiple organ failure (Safar 1977).

Implementation of modern resuscitation called for education research (Winchell 1966) and the organization of community-wide emergency medical services (EMS) systems (Safar 1968), to provide a life support chain from the prehospital scene, via transportation with life support, to hospital special care units.

Since the inception of modern CPR we have considered the brain as its main target organ and restoration of human mentation as the principle goal of resuscitation (Safar 1963). Only when effective methods for reversing airway obstruction, apnea, and pulselessness were developed did research into brain resuscitation after cardiac arrest become a priority.

Starting in 1970, the laboratory research initiatives of the Pittsburgh group included: demonstration of postcardiac arrest global cerebral hypoperfusion (Snyder et al. 1975); the first demonstration of a brain damage ameliorating effect of a treatment (reflow promotion) directed at secondary postcardiac arrest changes (Safar et al. 1976); development of a neck tourniquet monkey model for studying global brain ischemia without cardiac ischemia (Nemoto et al. 1977); and the extension of short-term animal models of cardiac arrest into long-term outcome models with development of an animal ICU (Safar 1985b). This permits long-term continuous control of postischemic arterial pressure, blood gases, and other vital parameters to allow secondary derangements to mature and to give experimental treatments time to act.

During the past decade, we have learned that head ischemia alone leads to less neurological damage than total body circulatory arrest of the same duration. This suggests that, in addition to the secondary cerebral changes originating in the brain itself, there are secondary extracerebral changes that might hamper recovery of brain function—the postresuscitation syndrome (Negovsky et al. 1983; Safar 1985a). After normothermic cardiac arrest of 10–20 min, followed by restoration of spontaneous normotension, the hyperemia-hypoperfusion sequence of cerebral blood flow was paralleled by similar patterns of cardiac output (Safar and Vaagenes 1986). Many factors other than the insult and the experimental treatment to be tested influence outcome (Safar 1985b). We learned to control many of these factors, but are far from identifying and controlling them all. A key factor, of course, is prompt restoration of normotensive perfusion pressures, which open-chest CPR or emergency cardiopulmonary bypass are more likely to provide than any form of presently available external CPR (Bircher 1984; Safar et al. 1987).

The postischemic-anoxic encephalopathy has an extremely complex pathogenesis. The expensive and difficult long-term animal experiments of severe heart and brain ischemia have been rewarding. They have thus far shown statistically significant, but clinically still suboptimal and inconsistent, mitigation of postglobal brain ischemic damage, by each of the following six special postarrest treatments: (1) protocol-defined brain-oriented life support (Safar 1977, 1986; Breivik et al. 1978; Abramson et al. 1986); (2) intraarterial hemodilution, hypertension, and heparinization (Safar et al. 1976), best delivered by emergency cardiopulmonary bypass (Safar et al. 1987); (3) barbiturate loading (Bleyaert et al. 1978); (4) calcium entry blocker (Vaagenes et al. 1984); (5) a free radical scavenger solution (Vaagenes et al. 1986); and (6) a multifaceted treatment protocol designed to promote cerebral blood flow and depress cerebral metabolism (Gisvold et al. 1984). At present, the limit of tolerance of normothermic temporary global ischemia (cardiac arrest) seems to be the same for heart and brain, namely between 10 and 20 min of no blood flow. Our animal experiments provide cautious optimism that it will ultimately be possible to achieve maximal reversibility of clinical death.

Our present research *goals* on clinical death are threefold (Safar 1986): (1) to determine the biological *limits* to the reversibility of clinical death, (2) to maximize therapeutic *potentials* with presently available technology, and (3) to develop reliable *predictions* of outcome with severe brain damage.

Our *hypotheses* concerning the obstacles to achieving maximal reversibility of clinical death focus on four secondary processes (Safar 1986): (1) cerebral as well as overall reperfusion failure, (2) cerebral as well as overall reoxygenation injury (cell-necrotizing cascades of biochemical reactions), (3) cerebral intoxication from postischemic derangements of extracerebral organs—ranging from cardiac pump failure and general microcirculatory obstruction to gastrointestinal-hepatic failure, causing "self-intoxication," and (4) alterations of blood by stasis and reoxygenation (with toxic plasma and malfunctioning and obstructing blood cells) interacting in deleterious ways with endothelium and tissues.

We have learned so far from over 500 long-term monkey and dog experiments: that postcardiac arrest cardiovascular and brain failure worsen each other; that postcardiac arrest pulmonary failure is preventable by modern respiratory intensive care; that postcardiac arrest renal failure is transient and not a major problem; and that secondary postcardiac arrest cardiovascular-microcirculatory derangements hamper recovery and need extensive investigation. The multiple-organ failure of this "postresuscitation syndrome," described by Negovsky in experiments without intensive care, also occurs in experiments with intensive care (Safar 1985a, 1986). We conclude that the multifactorial pathogenesis of the postresuscitation syndrome calls for etiology-specific multifaceted combination therapies.

We have developed a broad-scope mechanism for the systematic study of sudden clinical death. This mechanism ranges from bench research to human trials. It includes a perfused rat heart preparation, a rat cardiac arrest model, short-term mechanisms-oriented animal experiments, and long-term outcome-oriented animal models (Safar 1985b); and it culminates in a randomized clinical study of CPCR, to test and prove the "final answers" (Kelsey et al. 1986; Abramson et al. 1986a–c).

The latter is a multicenter international clinical trial of CPCR after cardiac arrest—the Brain Resuscitation Clinical Trial (BRCT). This study, difficult to conduct, was initiated in 1979 (Safar 1977) and is the first and still the only one of its kind. Its main objective was to establish a reliable mechanism for the study of clinical cardiac arrest. The severity of the insult is estimated, resuscitation and intensive care are controlled, and outcome variables are measured. The specific objective of the first phase of this study (BRCT I, 1979–1984) was to determine the brain damage ameliorating effect of high-dose thiopental loading (Abramson et al. 1986a,b; Kelsey et al. 1986). The second and currently ongoing phase (BRCT II, 1984–1988) is testing the efficacy of a calcium entry blocker (lidoflazine) in ameliorating postischemic brain damage in comatose cardiac arrest survivors (Abramson et al. 1986c). At present, 23 hospitals are collaborating, 15 in the United States and 8 in Europe. Preliminary results from this extensive data base suggest considerable interactions between postischemic heart and brain failure. Final analyses of BRCT I data provide no evidence to support the use of high-dose thiopental loading after cardiac arrest. The results of BRCT II are expected to be available in late 1987. BRCT III (1989–) may well test experimental therapies aimed at preventing or reversing the free radical and calcium-shift triggered reoxygenation injury to heart and brain, believed to occur and to damage cells after restoration of perfusion.

The goal of these clinical trials is primarily to scientifically and definitively test promising therapeutic approaches developed in the laboratory. Each phase then has the potential to develop an additional component of the therapeutic armamentarium for the restoration of meaningful recovery after severe ischemic insults. Its large data base teaches much new knowledge about the natural course of cardiac arrest and the postresuscitation syndrome, about treatment modalities, and about outcome predictions concerning heart, brain, and the entire organism.

Since the early 1960s (Safar 1963) research into the reversibility of terminal states and clinical death inevitably has made us aware of the importance of the quality of survival, of brain death determination and certification (Grenvik and Safar 1981), of letting die patients in a persistent vegetative state (Grenvik and

Safar 1981), and of "the right to die" (Wanzer et al. 1984; Safar 1968–1987). The resuscitability of brain function with normal human mentation must be the determining factor.

This Introduction summarizes our own experiences as an example. Many other investigators have contributed to our knowledge of heart-brain interactions in resuscitation medicine. These have been reviewed elsewhere (Safar 1968–1987; 1986). Studies on acute dying and resuscitation are needed and lend themselves to a systematic approach. Joint planning of laboratory and clinical research by active investigative groups is necessary—to cross-fertilize ideas, to avoid wasteful duplication, to agree on models, and to more fully utilize each group's greatest potentials. The same applies to *The Heart and Stroke*. Severe focal cerebral insults also deserve a resuscitative approach. Focal and global heart-brain pathologies deserve multidisciplinary approaches for resuscitation and research.

This book by Furlan et al. considers heart-brain interactions in various insults and diseases, and goes beyond research by including clinical and epidemiological issues. This book will thereby help build bridges between several disciplines and technologies, which we consider essential for future progress in acute medicine.

References

Abramson NS, Meisel A, Safar P (1986a) Informed consent in resuscitation research. JAMA 246: 2828–2830

Abramson NS, Safar P, Detre K, et al., Brain Resuscitation Clinical Trial (BRCT) I Study Group (1986b) Randomized clinical study of cardiopulmonary-cerebral resuscitation: thiopental loading in comatose cardiac arrest survivors. N Engl J Med 3: 397–403

Abramson NS, Detre K, Hedstrand U, Mullie A, The BRCT II Study Group (1986c) Methodology of the brain resuscitation clinical trial (BRCT) II: post-cardiac arrest calcium entry blocker (lidoflazine) administration. In: Bergmann H, Kramer H, Steinbereithner K (eds) Beitraege zur Anaesthesiologie und Intensivmedizin. Proc. VII European Congress of Anaesthesiology, Vienna, September 7–13, 1986. Maudrich, Vienna, vol. 18, pp 135–136

Beck CF., Leighninger DS (1960) Death after a clean bill of health. JAMA 174: 133–135

Bircher N, Safar P (1985) Cerebral preservation during cardiopulmonary resuscitation. Crit Care Med 13: 185–190

Bleyaert AL, Nemoto EM, Safar P, et al. (1978) Thiopental amelioration of brain damage after global ischemia in monkeys. Anesthesiology 49: 390–398

Breivik H, Safar P, Sands P, et al (1978) Clinical feasibility trials of barbiturate therapy after cardiac arrest. Crit Car Med 6: 228–244

Elam JO, Brown ES, Elder JD, Jr (1954) Artificial respiration by mouth-to-mask method. A study of the respiratory gas exchange of paralyzed patients ventilated by operator's expired air. N Engl J Med 250: 749–754

Gisvold SE, Safar P, Saito R, et al. (1984) Multifaceted therapy after global brain ischemia in monkeys. Stroke 15: 803–812

Gordon AS, Frye CW, Gittelson L, et al. (1958) Mouth-to-mouth versus manual artificial respiration for children and adults. JAMA 167: 320

Grenvik A, Safar P (eds) (1981) Brain failure and resuscitation. Clinics in critical care medicine. Churchill Livingstone, New York

Harris LC, Kirimli B, Safar P (1967) Ventilation-cardiac compression rates and ratios in cardiopulmonary resuscitation. Anesthesiology 28: 806–813

Hossmann KA (1982) Review: treatment of experimental cerebral ischemia. J Cereb Blood Flow Metab 2: 275–297

Kelsey SK, Abramson NS, Detre K, et al. (1986) Randomized clinical study of cardiopulmonary resuscitation: design, methods and patient characteristics. Am J Emerg Med 4: 72–86

Kouwenhoven WB, Jude JR, Knickerbocker GG (1960) Close-chest cardiac massage. JAMA 173: 1064–1067
Negovsky VA, Gurvitch AM, Zolotokrylina ES (1983) Postresuscitation disease. Elsevier, Amsteram
Nemoto EM, Bleyaert AL, Stezoski SW, et al. (1977) Global brain ischemia: a reproducible monkey model. Stroke 8: 558–564
Safar P, Escarraga L, Elam J (1958) A comparison of the mouth-to-mouth and mouth-to-airway methods of artificial respiration with the chest-pressure arm-lift methods. N Engl J Med 258: 671–677
Safar P, Aguto-Escarraga L, Chang F (1959a) A study of upper airway obstruction in the unconscious patient. J Appl Physiol 14: 760
Safar P (1959b) The failure of manual artificial respiration. J Appl Physiol 14: 84–88
Safar P, Brown TC, Holtey WH, et al. (1961a) Ventilation and circulation with closed chest cardiac massage in man. JAMA 176: 574–576
Safar P, DeKornfeld TJ, Pearson JW, et al. (1961b) Intensive care unit. Anaesthesia 16: 275–284
Safar P (Chm) (1963) International Symposium (1962) on "Resuscitation: controversial aspects." Anesthesiology Monograph and Resuscitation Series, vol. 1. Springer, Berlin Heidelberg New York
Safar P (1964) Community-wide cardiopulmonary resuscitation. J Iowa Med Soc Nov: 629–635
Safar P (Chairman, Committee on Acute Medicine, American Society of Anesthesiologists) (1968) Community-wide emergency medical services. JAMA 204: 595
Safar P (1968–1987) Cardiopulmonary-cerebral resuscitation. World Federation of Societies of Anaesthesiologists. A. Laerdal, Stavanger; W. B. Saunders, London. 1st edn 1968, 2nd edn 1981, 3rd edn 1987 (in press)
Safar P, Stezoski SW, Nemoto EM (1976) Amelioration of brain damage after 12 minutes cardiac arrest in dogs. Arch Neurol 33: 91–95
Safar P (1977) Cardiopulmonary-cerebral resuscitation (CPCR). In: Safar P (ed) Advances in cardiopulmonary resuscitation. Springer, Berlin Heidelberg New York, pp 195–207
Safar P (ed) (1978) Brain resuscitation. Special symposium issue. Crit Care Med 6: 199–291
Safar P (1985a) Effects of postresuscitation syndrome on cerebral recovery from cardiac arrest. Review and hypotheses. Crit Care Med 13: 932–935
Safar P (1985b) Long-term animal outcome models for cardiopulmonary-cerebral resuscitation research. Crit Care Med 13: 936–940
Safar P (1986) Cerebral resuscitation after cardiac arrest. A review. Circulation 74 (Suppl IV): 138–153
Safar P, Vaagenes P (1986) Systematic search for brain resuscitation potentials after total circulatory arrest. In: Baethmann A, Go KG, Unterberg A (eds) Mechanisms of secondary brain damage. Plenum, New York, pp 349–375
Safar P, Abramson NS, Bircher N, Levine R, Pretto E (1987) Open-chest cardiopulmonary resuscitation for cardiopulmonary bypass for prolonged cardiac arrest resistant to cardiopulmonary resuscitation. JAMA (in preparation)
Snyder JV, Nemoto EM, Carroll RG, et al, (1975) Global ischemia in dogs: intracranial pressures, brain blood flow and metabolism. Stroke 6: 21–27
Vaagenes P, Cantadore R, Safar P, et al. (1984) Amelioration of brain damage by lidoflazine after prolonged ventricular fibrillation cardiac arrest in dogs. Crit Care Med 12: 846–855
Vaagenes P, Safar P, Cantadore R, et al. (1986) Outcome trials of free radical scavengers and calcium entry blockers after cardiac arrest in 2 dog models. Ann Emerg Med 15: 665 (abstract)
Winchell SW, Safar P, (1966) Teaching and testing lay and paramedical personnel in cardiopulmonary resuscitation. Anesth Analg 45: 441–449
Zuelch KJ, Kaufmann W, Hossmann K-A, Hossmann V (eds) (1977, vol I; 1979, vol II) Brain and heart infarct. Springer, Berlin Heidelberg New York

Section A

CARDIOEMBOLIC STROKE

Chapter 1

The History of Cerebral Embolism and Hemorrhagic Infarction*

C. M. Fisher

This chapter traces the evolution of the basic ideas about vascular disease particularly as they relate to embolism and especially cerebral embolism. Included is a description of the early hypotheses concerning pale and hemorrhagic infarcts which have been directly linked to embolism.

Embolism and Thrombosis

There can be no doubt that Virchow (1847) discovered the process of embolism and by his observations on human pathological material laid the basis of much of the knowledge of both embolism and thrombosis. In 1 month in 1846 he performed 76 postmortem examinations and found blood clots in the veins of the extremities in 18 and in the pulmonary arteries in 11. He deduced from this that the venous bloodstream might transport intravascular coagula for considerable distances to points where the venous channels narrowed sufficiently to obstruct further advance. He immediately undertook a series of experiments to test the capacity of the venous blood current to carry foreign bodies. Pieces of rubber, muscle, and blood clot inserted into the internal jugular vein were carried to the lungs. In the following year he reported evidence of the same phenomenon on the arterial side of the vascular system and described seven cases of obstruction of cerebral, splenic, renal, hepatic, and limb arteries by clots which appeared to have arisen in the left auricle or upon the valves of the heart. At the same time he presented experimental data which proved that coagula and foreign bodies could be transported by the arterial bloodstream. Thus, within the space of 2 years it was established that blood clots need not form at sites where they are found at autopsy but may be carried from peripheral and cerebral veins to the pulmonary arteries and from the left auricle and heart valves to the peripheral arteries.

* This study was supported in part by the Freed Foundation, Washington, DC

Although Virchow is properly credited with the discovery of embolism as a process distinct from thrombosis, the idea did not entirely originate with him. Vesalius (reference from Virchow) knew of the frequency with which gangrene of an extremity was associated with unnatural depositions in the left auricle and Lancisi had recorded a case of heart disease in which the right hand suddenly had been deprived of blood and turned gangrenous. The chief cause of delay in recognizing the principle of embolism was the failure to differentiate between antemortem and postmortem intravascular clots. In the latter part of the sixteenth and early seventeenth century the large coagula found in the heart at autopsy were believed to have formed during life and these "cardiac polyps" were offered as the explanation for all manner of symptoms. Kerkring (1670) stated that such clots were cadaveric but his opinion went unheeded. After almost 200 years of this doctrine the pendulum swung the other way; not only was the interpretation of Kerkring accepted but the Pastas (1786) argued that all intravascular clots were postmortem. Finally, Haller and Morgagni in the late 1700s took the more correct intermediate position, that most clots were postmortem but that intravascular clotting could take place during life. Matthew Baillie (1793) said that it was "known to every person acquainted with the animal economy that the blood coagulated in the vessels of the living body." As examples of the latter process he called attention to the clotting that follows ligature or develops within an arterial dilation.

At about the same time, John Hunter (1793) noted the frequency of inflammation of veins after surgery and phlebotomy and in association with inflammatory lesions of all kinds. There began a period of speculation concerning the mechanism of formation of intravascular thrombi. Hunter believed the venous clots formed as an "exudate" from the wall of the blood vessel and, if adhesions did not form, the clots could be swept into the general circulation and carried to distant parts. This was one of the first suggestions of the possibility of embolism. Hunter's paper stimulated widespread interest in the whole subject of vascular disease and soon his ideas concerning the part played by the veins in inflammation were adopted by Cruveilhier (1829), who became deeply impressed with the importance of phlebitis, stating, "*La phlebite domine toute la pathologie.*" He maintained that all inflammation was basically a capillary phlebitis. Noting that thrombosis occurred in veins whose walls were apparently normal, he concluded the coagulation within veins was the earliest sign of phlebitis. Similarly, clotting within arteries or within the chambers of the heart was attributed to an arteritis whose earliest manifestation was blood coagulation. At times, however, the clot within the vessel was formed from a mixture of exudate and the formed elements of the blood. Bochdalek (1846) while studying hemorrhagic infarcts of the lung found blood clots within the pulmonary arteries. He pursued the above line of reasoning that if clotting of venous blood meant inflammation of vein, clotting of arterial blood signified inflammation of arteries. Hemorrhagic infarction was therefore attributed to an inflammation of the pulmonary arteries.

In 1846 and 1847 Virchow presented his evidence for the principle of embolism. His recognition that a blood clot need not have formed where it was found at autopsy was a giant step forward in the study of intravascular clotting. Virchow also showed experimentally that the lining of an artery was very resistant to irritants and that the arterial wall never poured an exudate into the lumen. He also demonstrated that clotting within an artery required damage to the intima. This was the death blow to the doctrine of phlebitis and arteritis which had sidetracked pathological thought for almost 50 years. Virchow clearly laid down rules for the mechanical clotting of blood within vessels and divided clots into three types: (1) *mural*, as in aneurysms, on atheromatous ulcers, and in dilated cardiac chambers; (2) *general occluding*, a widespread intracapillary clotting no longer recognized except as disseminated intravascular clotting; and (3) *local occluding*, which was of two kinds: (a) associated with disease of the vessel wall (inflammation, compression by tumor) and (b) associated with an intact vessel wall. The latter two types of clot are thrombotic and embolic respectively, but not until 1854, 7 years later, did Virchow introduce the terms embolus, embolism, thrombus, and thrombosis.

Other events may also have determined Virchow's important advance. For many years it had been recognized that tumors and abscesses must metastasize by way of the circulation. This phenomenon engrossed many workers and all kinds of materials were injected experimentally into veins and arteries. Worms and their cysts were widely distributed through the body and were probably transported by the bloodstream. In addition, an extensive clinical and experimental literatre on air embolism had accumulated. In 1828 Allibert reported a case of gangrene of an extremity and blockage of its artery by a clot that was similar to one in the left auricular appendage. Victor Francois (1832) suggested that gangrene due to a sudden arterial blockage could be caused by a clot that was dislodged and carried to the artery by the bloodstream. He attributed the final blockage to an arteritis produced by the arrival of the fragment of clot. Virchow did not know of these two French reports and Tiedemann (1843) in his classic work on vascular disease did not mention embolism, further evidence of Virchow's claim to originality. In 1846 Hasse described several cases of brain softening due to occlusion of cerebral arteries and included cases of embolism without recognizing them as such. Virchow in his summary of the medical literature found 11 examples of embolic disease although in none was the fundamental process appreciated, the embolic plugs usually being attributed to arterial inflammation. It is evident that to Virchow must go the credit for the precise elaboration of the doctrine of embolism.

Similarly, Virchow's views on intravascular clotting had been preceded by many observations in the first half of the nineteenth century. As already mentioned, Cruveilhier's theory of phlebitis and arteritis dominated the other theories of clotting such as the presence of a chemical principle or the mechanical theory later to be developed by Virchow. It was widely known that a clot formed in the vicinity of a ligature and on the walls of an aneurysm. Laennec (1835) knew that stasis alone could produce coagulation. Carswell (1838) had demonstrated clotting around sutures passed through the lumen of a vessel. Clots within varicose veins, in dilated cardiac auricles, and in the dilated venous plexuses of the pelvis were well recognized. That a blood clot could completely block an artery was scarcely appreciated. Dupuytren (referred to in Virchow 1847) found arterial obliteration in cases of peripheral gangrene but attributed it to an inflammation of the artery. Cruveilhier and Carswell had also found arterial obliteration in cases of peripheral gangrene but gangrene occurred so frequently without blockage of the vessel at autopsy there was no agreement whether the clot was the cause or effect of the gangrene, or at one time was the cause and at another time, effect. Moreover there was disagreement as to the changes which take place in organs following interruption of their blood supply.

In this confusion concerning the relation of arterial obstruction to gangrene and necrosis, the brain became the first organ in which necrosis was clearly attributed to arterial occlusion. Cerebral softening had been recognized since postmortem examinations were first practiced and was always held to be inflammatory in nature. Ligature of the carotid artery often produced paralysis on the opposite side of the body and even death, but it was claimed that in these cases brain softening was never seen. Rostan (1820) first suggested that in some patients, particularly the elderly, softening of the brain might be a form of gangrene or necrosis due to calcification and gradual closure of the cerebral arteries. He met strong opposition from many pathologists who maintained that such softening was always inflammatory. Rostan did not furnish pathological evidence for his theory. Carswell (1838) was the first to state definitely that softening of the brain was a form of necrosis resulting from obliteration of cerebral arteries. He described softening consequent to fibrous thickening in the middle cerebral and basilar arteries. In 1846 Hasse presented a series of cases of brain softening due to plugged arteries, the site of the vessel blockage clearly corresponding with the location of the softening. Several of Virchow's cases of embolic disease exhibited brain softening due to arterial occlusion. Following Virchow's paper many authors soon reported similar cases: Rühle (1853) described three cases and Cohn (1860) reported several more. It was not long before cerebral embolism was firmly established clinically and pathologically.

Infarction

The concept of "infarction" had an interesting origin. Laennec (1835) first used the term to refer to the process in the lungs which had up to that time been called pulmonary apoplexy. He observed that the veins were engorged and the tissues were filled with solidified, half-dried blood, "*une sorte d'infarctus*." Later he referred to this condition as "*hemoptoique infarctus*," which Virchow translated as "*hemoptoischen infarkt*" and "*hemorrhagischen infarkt*." Later Litten (1880), disregarding the original meaning of the word infarctus (*infarcire*—to stuff), termed a pale softening a white infarct. The practice of designating any necrotic or softened focus an infarct has continued.

The mechanism of infarction particularly *hemorrhagic infarction* has been elusive. Bouillaud (1826) first noted that the arterial branches adjacent to a pulmonary infarct contained blood clots. He did not consider these clots as etiologically important but recommended that other pathologists examine the arteries more closely. Bochdalek (1846) was aware that in pulmonary infarcts the nutrient artery was not always obstructed by clot but ignored this, attributing the infarct to an inflammation of the capillaries of arteries with secondary intravascular clotting. This idea was consistent with the teaching of the time.

Virchow was uncertain of the mechanism, and in his original paper on embolism did not clearly attribute hemorrhagic infarction to embolic occlusion. His hesitancy in drawing such a conclusion was probably the result of his failure so often to find the responsible clot. He postulated that an unexplained extravasation took place into the parenchyma and this extravasation caused the necrosis and sometimes also resulted in arterial obliteration. Virchow, however, appreciated the fact that pulmonary infarction was similar to infarction of the spleen and kidneys. In 1854, 7 years after his original paper, he wrote, "The relation of hemorrhagic infarction in the lungs, kidneys, and spleen to blockage of vessels is not clear as yet. Often the blockage appears to be secondary. However, the multiplicity of the foci, the age of the clot, and the presence of other obstructive clots seems to favor their being embolic." In his experimental study of venous embolism in which bits of rubber, muscle, fat, and blood clot were injected into the jugular veins, hemorrhagic infarcts of the lungs could not be produced. Further, he demonstrated that after ligature of the pulmonary arteries injected dye could still reach all parts of the lungs through the bronchial arteries. Although he did not clearly present any theory of hemorrhagic infarction, he suggested that blockage of an artery, incomplete at first, might be responsible. He also surmised that capillaries could be injured by temporary ischemia and that blood entering through collateral channels might extravasate through the damaged walls. Kirkes (1852) was the first to state with certainty that hemorrhagic infarcts were embolic in origin, and this view was soon widely accepted.

In 1860 Cohn published his extensive treatise on embolic disease. Not clearly recognizing hemorrhagic infarction of the brain he did not consider its pathogenesis. He closely studied the process in other organs, both in experimental animals and in humans at autopsy. He remarked that hemorrhagic infarcts of the lung were never related to obstruction of the larger pulmonary arteries but were a manifestation of capillary embolism with superimposed or secondary spreading capillary thrombosis. This latter process resulted in increasing pressure within the nonobstructed capillaries and finally extravasation of red cells. If the capillary walls were more resistant, a focal area of inflammation resulted, the gross picture being one of mixed inflammation and infarction. Cohn attempted to produce pulmonary embolism experimentally using rubber, paper, cork, wax, degenerating muscle, particles of pus and gangrenous lungs, mercury, glue mixture, indigo oil, pigment emulsion, and pulverized indigo. He too failed to create hemorrhagic pulmonary infarction by these methods. He concluded, from postmortem observations, that in the spleen hemorrhagic infarction could result from embolic occlusion of both the large arteries and the capillaries. In the former case the hemorrhages were attributed to a collateral influx of blood which distended and ruptured capillaries. This postulated mechanism received support from experiments in which ligature of the celiac artery resulted in swelling and hemorrhagic infarction of the upper half of the spleen. The influx of blood was traced to collaterals from the stomach, diaphragm, and abdominal wall. Experimental embolism of the celiac and splenic arteries produced circumscribed hemorrhagic foci in the spleen, something achieved in no other organ. Cohn also studied the process of infarction in the kidney. Unsuccessful in directing experimental emboli into the renal artery from the aorta, he resorted to the method of simple ligature. This resulted in the surprising discovery that obstruction of the renal artery in animals caused a striking hyperemia, the medulla being markedly engorged, the cortex less so. Small hemorrhages into the parenchyma occurred in some cases. If the vein was also ligated, the hyperemia was increased. This was evidence that venous reflux was not responsible. Cohn, who had originated the theory of venous reflux to explain red infarction, was therefore forced to abandon it as his experiments proceeded. His explanation for the hyperemia and extravasation after ligature was that a failure of the *vis a tergo* caused the blood to stagnate on the venous side and the influx of collateral blood from the spermatic, adrenal, and capsular arteries resulted in engorgement and disruption of the capillaries. That the blood came from collateral channels was evident, for if in addition to ligature of the main artery all collaterals were tied, no hemorrhage occurred. Cohn invoked a similar mechanism to explain hemorrhagic infarction, although his experiment did not duplicate the conditions of clinical embolism. He was the first to emphasize that renal infarcts differed from those of lung and spleen in often having a pale center and a surrounding zone of hyperemia or extravasation. In other experiments, he studied the effect of ligating the superior mesenteric artery and found that the bowel also became greatly engorged due to the influx of collateral blood. In summary Cohn discarded the theory of venous reflux. He regarded the process of infarction in the lung as different from that in kidney, spleen, and gastrointestinal tract, holding that in the former it was a capillary phenomenon, while in the latter it was due to collateral blood entering an ischemic territory whose venous drainage was stagnant.

Following Cohn many workers tried further to elucidate the mechanism of hemorrhagic infarction. Beckmann (1858) concluded that venous regurgitation was the cause of hemorrhagic infarction of the intestine following embolism of the superior mesenteric artery. He argued that such blood could come only from two sources, collateral arteries or veins, but excluded the first source on the grounds that collateral vessels would not produce such a uniform extravasation over so great a length of intestine. Beckman was the first to point out that all renal "infarcts" were not hemorrhagic and that actually the majority were pale from the beginning. Blessig (1859) repeated Cohn's experiments on the kidney and obtained the same results.

Cohnheim's monograph on embolism was published in 1872 and presented in detail the hypothesis that hemorrhagic infarction results from a combination of two events: (1) The blockage of an "end artery" by an embolus with ischemic damage of the vascular endothelium and (2) a venous reflux into this tissue due to the local fall of pressure resulting from arterial obstruction, extravasation taking place through the damaged capillaries. His theory rested on experimental evidence derived largely from studying the tongue of the curarized frog. When wax emboli lodged in its vessels capillary diapedetic hemorrhages occurred and blood was seen flowing backwards in veins. When the tongue was temporarily ligatured at the base, the vascular endothelium underwent ischemic changes and on release of the ligature extravasation occurred. He repeated these studies in other organs, using several different species of animals, and obtained the same results. He concluded that the organs in which hemorrhagic infarction occurred (lung, spleen, kidney, gastrointestinal tract, brain, and retina) are those supplied by a system of terminal or end arteries. Differences in the extent of hemorrhagic effusion from case to case in humans were attributable to variations in the venous reflux as determined by the presence or absence of venous valves, the degree of thrombosis in veins, the presence of raised venous pressure due to cardiac failure, and cardiac hypertrophy. Cohnheim's theory soon became widely accepted although it did not remain unchallenged for long.

In the following year von Zielonko (1873) reported, after microscopic studies of the web of a frog's foot, that the hemorrhages occurring after arterial obstruction were due to a collateral influx from neighboring arteries and not to venous reflux. In his opinion arterial obstruction caused capillary and venous stasis and increased capillary pressure (capillaries sometimes pulsated) and extravasation due to the increased pressure. In 1875, Cohnheim and Litten, by injecting dyes after experimental pulmonary embolism in dogs, showed that, contrary to the statement of Virchow, the tissue distal to an obstruction was stained much less than normal, indicating that the collateral supply did not fully compensate although it seemed sufficient to prevent parenchymal changes. From this paper it is evident that Cohnheim did not intend that the term "end artery" be so restricted as to exclude even terminal capillary anastomoses but rather to indicate an artery with no important arterial anastomoses. Kossuchin (1876) repeated Cohnheim's experiments on the frog's tongue and disagreed with him, concluding that diapedetic hemorrhages resulted from raised capillary pressure following influx of blood from collateral capillaries and not from veins. Litten in 1880 repeated Cohn's renal studies in detail and satisfied himself that infarcts in no way depended on venous reflux but that blood entering from collateral vessels by way of the capillaries was responsible. He tied off every arterial channel leading to the kidneys leaving the renal vein open and found no hyperemia or bloody extravasation. Collateral blood supply was necessary for the production of hemorrhages. Having refuted the basis for Cohnheim's theory of venous reflux he conducted further experiments which showed that in the kidney at least the vascular endothelium was not as sensitive to anoxia as Cohnheim had assumed. Temporary ligature up to 4 h did not result in altered increased permeability to methylene blue. Since experimental infarction could be produced within an hour or so, other factors must have been at work. He explained the extravasation of infarction as being mechanical in origin, i.e., collateral channels carry blood to the ischemic territory and due to the lack of *vis a tergo* the blood accumulates in the veins and the capillaries dilate with resulting diapedesis and rupture. Evidence in support of this idea is the fact that ligature of the renal vein produces hemorrhagic extravasation more readily than any other method. Litten, moreover, withdrew the conclusions made jointly by Cohnheim and himself, that the arterial branches in the lungs were "end arteries." The change in theory, however, was not as great as it seemed for he found that any anastomosis between the lung and adjacent structures or of the arteries of one territory of the lung with a neighboring territory was always through capillaries and no larger collateral channels could be demonstrated. In his opinion the same was true of the kidney. He concluded that such collateral flow was never sufficient to maintain the integrity of tissue whose main artery was blocked. In other words, the vessels were, in fact, functional end arteries. Litten again emphasized that hemorrhagic infarcts in the kidney were not as uniformly red as infarcts of the lung and spleen. He found, as had Beckmann, that renal infarcts usually consisted of a central pale area (coagulation necrosis) surrounded by a hemorrhagic zone which in some cases was relatively slight. Litten called these pale areas "white infarcts," thus giving a new meaning to the term infarction. He concluded that this pale infarct was the primary process and not a decolorized red infarct, as was the current belief. These pale areas occurred so early after arterial obstruction that removal of extravasated blood would have been impossible.

Von Recklinghausen (1881) reviewed the literature on thrombosis and embolism up to 1883, and decided that the hemorrhages following embolism were due to the influx of collateral blood with resultant stasis and extravasation. He introduced evidence which Knapp had collected while closely following the development of retinal hemorrhages after embolism of the central retinal artery. Hemorrhages first became apparent within a day or two after embolic occlusion and were much more prominent when only a small branch was occluded than when a larger artery was affected. He assumed that the collateral blood flow was probably greater when a small rather than a large branch was occluded. Von Recklinghausen also noted partial hyaline thrombi within the capillaries of fresh red infarcts and suggested they probably added to the capillary obstruction and extravasation. He offered another speculation that afterwards became popular, namely that dilatation of the capillary bed occurs in the territory distal to an arterial obstruction due to paralysis of the vasomotor nerves.

In 1887 Welch, working with Mall, reinvestigated some of these problems. They used the small intestine in their experiments and were able to settle once and for all that the blood which produces hemorrhagic infarction comes from the collateral circulation and not by reflux from veins. Having demonstrated that the blood pressure was very low in the vessels within the hemorrhagic infarct, they found they could produce such infarction by clamping and gradually compressing the superior mesenteric artery until a critical level was reached, whereupon the bowel suddenly became hemorrhagic. There were no demonstrable changes in the vascular wall in this experiment and it was concluded that hemorrhage occurred by diapedesis from small veins and capillaries in which the circulation was sluggish and irregular.

Fujinami writing in 1898 included several references to original papers that have not been reviewed here. Among these was the monograph of Perl (1874), which reported the production of typical hemorrhagic infarcts in the lung by the use of wax emboli in animals weakened by repeated bleeding. This is probably the first time that hemorrhagic infarcts were produced by experimental embolism. Another paper (Grawitz 1891) expressed the opinion that an embolus was found so infrequently in cases of pulmonary infarction that it was questionable if this condition was related to embolism at all; rather it was the result of brown induration, infection, pleural effusion, etc. Willgerodt (1893) is quoted as having rejected Grawitz's conclusions contending that infarcts were definitely related to embolism and, further, that hemorrhagic infarction of the lung occurred only if there was some preexisting disorder of circulation. Fujinami himself was able to produce pulmonary infarcts in experimental animals by injecting wax into the jugular veins. He also carefully examined many human pulmonary infarcts and was always able to find an embolus if he searched diligently enough. He could not be sure that it was always in the proper place in the vessel to account for the zone of ischemic necrosis. He felt that experimental and human pulmonary infarcts were the same but that animals required more emboli and more secure blockage because their lungs were healthy whereas human lungs were frequently the site of additional disease processes, circulatory and inflammatory. He declared that experimental hemorrhagic infarction required two obstructions, one in the main vessel and another directly proximal to the infarction.

The work of Forbes in 1901 was presented in detail in Beattie and Dickson's textbook (1925). In one set of experiments in rabbits and dogs either the main renal artery or one of its branches was ligated and the changes in the kidney followed minutely. It was found that the infarcted area was red initially, even in its center, while later, within 4 or 5 h the central part became pale. It was concluded that infarcts, at least in the kidneys and spleen, were always red.

Microscopically the initial redness was shown to be due to capillary congestion and not to extravasation, so that Forbes' disagreement with other observers (Beckmann, Litten) is merely a matter of definition of "red." This work is largely responsible for the former belief among pathologists that all infarcts are at first red.

Karsner and Austen (1911) carried out an extensive investigation of experimental renal and splenic infarcts and concluded from this that all infarcts were first "hyperemic," then hemorrhagic, and finally pale due to coagulation necrosis. The blood pigment was, in their opinion, removed by plasmatic diffusion. Extravasation, which is our chief interest here, occurred as early as 4 h in the spleen, but in the kidney did not reach significant proportions for 24–48 h. Karsner and Ash (1912–1913) used radish and turnip seeds as emboli and showed in experimental animals that interference with pulmonary circulation (ligation of pulmonary venous branches or partial collapse of lung (intrapleural injections of oil) usually resulted in typical hemorrhagic infarcts. Since these emboli produced no infarction when the lung was healthy, it was inferred that human pulmonary infarcts are determined by preexisting disease of the lung.

McCallum (1940) in his textbook stated that the two deciding factors as to whether an infarct shall remain anemic or assume a deep red color were (1) the arrangement of the circulation and (2) the density of the tissue. He regarded all infarcts as originally pale and remarked on the fact that in some cases the embolic plug may lie at such a distance from the pulmonary infarct as to raise doubt as to whether the two are directly related. Karsner (1949) classed infarcts as hemorrhagic if the naked eye examination showed a rich blood content. He held that all infarcts are hyperemic at first and in those tissues with a rich blood supply and a loose arrangement of tissues, hyperemia passes over into the hemorrhagic type. White or anemic infarcts are pallid because of decolorization of the blood in the original region of infarction. The less the hemorrhage, the earlier the infarct becomes pale. Hence the higher incidence of pallid infarcts in kidney, heart, and brain whose blood supply is not so rich. Reactionary hyperemia is common at the edges. He also stated that tying off collaterals only influences slightly the degree of hemorrhage in experimental infarction and rejected any relation of the process to the degree to which a vessel is an end artery.

In summary there appeared to be general agreement that the extravasation in hemorrhagic infarction of lung, spleen, kidney, intestine, and, perhaps, retina was a matter of collateral influx via capillaries from the surrounding tissue. Many of the details, however, remained controversial and statements in textbooks concerning the process often lacked clarity.

Hemorrhagic Infarcts of the Brain

Prior to 1900, hemorrhagic infarcts of the brain were scarcely mentioned in textbooks of pathology. Thereafter they were often described, particularly in the German literature. Schwartz in 1930 concluded from his studies of apoplexy that hemorrhagic infarction and massive cerebral hemorrhage were fundamentally the same process, any difference being quantitative. He attributed the hemorrhagic extravasation in both cases to functional vascular changes which result in partial stasis and capillary diapedesis of red blood cells, in the manner described by Ricker. In 1927 Ricker had presented a theory ascribing to stimulation or paralysis of vasomotor nerves almost every pathological process of blood vessels. He argued that the walls of the smaller blood vessels reacted in several different ways to efferent impulses, depending on the strength and duration of the nervous discharge. Mild stimulation caused dilatation whereas stronger stimulation resulted in vasoconstriction. However, when fatique set in, the capillary relaxed and dilated when the arteriole was still partially constricted, a state which the author called "peristasis." If the arteriole constricted and closed completely, "stasis" ensued. Between these two stages there were many intermediate states in which the various elements of the blood escaped, e.g., plasma, white blood cells, and red blood cells. Ricker named the intermediate processes liquor diapedesis, leukodiapedesis, and erythrodiapedesis respectively. His theory was challenged by many workers but nonetheless persisted for many years as the explanation of vascular phenomena. Perhaps there were sufficient grounds for some of his conclusions, but it must be recalled that his ideas were largely based on the effects produced in the pancreatic vessels of laboratory animals by such agents as sodium iodide solution, silver nitrate, ammonia, tannin, camphor, and heat (131°F). There is no evidence that his findings apply to clinical events.

Schwartz's view that hemorrhagic infarction and cerebral hemorrhage were the same process was immediately disputed by Böhne (1931), who pointed out the obvious pathological differences. He felt that a red infarct was at first pale, becoming secondarily hemorrhagic, but did not suggest any mechanism for its production. Hiller (1935) was of the opinion that blood reached the infarcted tissue via collateral arterial channels. He attributed the greater extravasation in gray matter to the greater abundance of capillaries there. He rejected venous reflux and incomplete arterial occlusion as factors in the etiology of red infarction and claimed that red infarcts occurred distal to atherosclerotic thombotic occlusion as readily as distal to embolic occlusion. Fazio (1949) pointed out that red softenings are not uniform but rather hemorrhagic areas are interspersed with pale areas. He tentatively attributed the redness to partial occlusion of the vessel of supply which in conjunction with many other factors affecting cerebral circulation such as venous congestion, vasospasm, etc. determines a nonuniform stasis and intense vasodilatation in which cells, WBC, then RBC, diapedese into the gray matter of the area, *following which* necrosis may occur.

Fisher and Adams (1951) in a study of 66 cases of cerebral hemorrhagic infarction (excluding infarction secondary to compression of the posterior cerebral artery at the tentorium) found evidence of embolism in all except three. Hemorrhagic infarction was often part of a larger infarct, the rest of which was pale. The hemorrhagic part usually lay proximal to the pale portion and was confined exactly to an arterial vascular territory. Dissection of the vessels showed that in many cases of combined hemorrhagic and pale infarction, there was no embolic plug. Or if one was present it was not found at the appropriate sites to account for the hemorrhagic portion, but lay farther distally in the arterial tree, often at the proximal boundary of the *pale* part of the infarct. It was postulated that brain embolism is a dynamic process in which embolic material may be arrested temporarily, causing ischemic infarction, and then migrate distally exposing the damaged endothelium to arterial blood pressure with resultant diapedetic capillary and vascular hemorrhages. Eventually emboli undergo lysis and disappear.

Hain et al. (1952) produced unusually bloody hemorrhagic infarcts in dogs if a clip was placed on the middle cerebral artery (MCA) in the zone of the perforating branches but not when the clip lay distal to all the perforating vessels. In monkeys for unknown reasons a similar procedure produced only pale infarction. Harvey and Rasmussen (1951) noted hemorrhagic infarction in two monkeys after 50 min of temporary occlusion of the MCA. Zülch (1955) concluded that infarcts are hemorrhagic when the obstruction is intermittent, when collateral flow is present but insufficient or when the infarct involves the distal territories of two arteries. Faris et al. (1963) found that ligation of the middle cerebral artery in dogs made hypertensive by surgical coarctation produced hemorrhagic infarction whereas in normotensive controls the infarction was pale. The lesion in the basal ganglia in their illustration resembled a hemorrhage rather than a hemorrhagic infarct. Ligation of the anterior and posterior cerebral arteries at the time of ligation of the MCA resulted in pale infarction presumably due to prevention of collateral flow. Prophylactic low molecular weight dextran also prevented the hemorrhagic extravasation (Hardin et al. 1963). Waltz (1966) after applying a clip to the MCA of animals observed the following changes: darkening and reddening of the venous blood, slowing of venous and arterial streams, constriction of arteries, cortical pallor, sludging, stasis and platelet emboli in veins, emptying of the column of blood from the vessels, and perivenous hemorrhages. These hemorrhages were associated with a slight increase in blood pressure and the appearance of thrombi in veins and it was postulated that similar changes were operative in human hemorrhagic infarction.

An important contribution is that of Seki et al. (1983). Using their model of thalamic infarction in dogs, they demonstrated that recirculation after 6–12 h of vascular occlusion regularly produced hemorrhagic infarction. In these animals rCBF fell to less than 50% with vascular occlusion, recirculation resulted in a transient increase in rCBF followed by a fall to preocclusion levels, electrical activity became almost flat, and recovery did not occur following reflow. Their results indicate that hemorrhagic extravasation occurs early after restoration of flow.

As a prototype of the process of hemorrhagic infarction one might adopt that which occurs regularly in the posterior cerebral artery (PCA) territory with advanced herniation of the temporal lobe. As it runs from below to above the tentorium, the PCA is compressed against the firm edge of the tentorium with compromise of the lumen. The indentation on the artery persists and can be seen on gross pathological examination. The hemorrhagic infarct involves all PCA territory distal to that point. The process of compression could be gradual or intermittent and thus parallel Welch's experiment in which the mesenteric artery was slowly compressed to a critical degree. By analogy it might be inferred that at times in cerebral embolism the arterial lumen does not become totally occluded immediately, but rather a critical flow continues.

A pathological finding so characteristic of the process of hemorrhagic infarction in the vertebral-basilar system that it demands consideration when a mechanism is proposed is the occurrence of regions of hemorrhagic infarction scattered at various levels of the brain stem and cerebellum in the wake of a migrating embolic mass which at postmortem is found at its final place of arrest at the upper bifurcation of the basilar artery or in the PCA on one or both sides. Each area of hemorrhagic infarction produced by this embolism-in-transit conforms to the territory of a basilar branch which is free of embolic particles. As the major embolus advances along the basilar artery (BA), a crucial reduction in flow could be operative or temporary blockage of the mouth of a branch followed by exposure to full arterial pressure could be a factor. The same considerations apply to infarction in the deep territory of the penetrating branches of the MCA territory in embolus to that artery. On the other hand if it were only a matter of capillary-venous stagnation followed by steady or intermittent restoration of pressure and flow that causes the petechial extravasation of blood, it would be anticipated that all embolic infarcts would be hemorrhagic in view of the abundance of collateral blood flow across the border zone anastomotic networks. But hemorrhagic infarcts are not found in this circumstance. A favorite site of hemorrhagic infarction is the basal ganglia in the territory of the MCA, an area in which collateral flow is actually poor.

Hemorrhagic infarction is prone to occur when local cerebral ischemia occurs distal to an arterial atherosclerotic stenosis as the result of a severe transient fall of systemic blood pressure. During surgical anesthesia infarction is particularly likely to be hemorrhagic whether it occurs as a result of transient hypotension or is due to embolism. There are often small areas a few millimeters wide of hemorrhagic infarction at the outlying borders of large pale infarcts but this is not the type under discussion here. Their small size and localization suggests they are related to collateral capillary flow. In carefully mapping out typical large hemorrhagic infarcts of the cortical convolutions it was often found that the hemorrhagic border was exactly coextensive with the most distal twigs of the arterial territory involved, clearly indicating that the cause of the hemorrhagic infarct lay on the arterial side of the vascular system. It is remarkable that hemorrhagic infarction is not observed in central retinal artery branch embolism.

It should be emphasized that venous occlusion regularly causes hemorrhagic infarction and must always be considered in the differential diagnosis. In this type, venous engorgement is probably the main factor. The hemorrhagic infarcts of arterial and venous origins resemble each other to some extent with the difference that in those resulting from venous occlusion the white matter and gray matter are equally hemorrhagic while arterial hemorrhagic infarction is largely limited to gray matter. The cause of this sparing of white matter is not understood. Gray matter is much more vascular than white but how this translates into a specific hemorrhagic alteration is obscure. Possibly venous drainage of white matter has a greater margin of safety and is sufficient to prevent engorgement to the point of extravasation. The hemorrhagic aspect of arterial hemorrhagic infarction is always superimposed on an underlying ischemic process whereas in hemorrhagic infarction of venous origin the ischemic insult may be less severe.

Clinically, there have been several significant developments in the past 25 years. The great frequency of cerebral embolism as the cause of stroke came to be appreciated. From the point of view of therapy especially the prevention of cerebral embolism from the heart the introduction of anticoagulants was a major advance (Foley and Wright 1950; Owren 1963; Fisher 1979). Whether the administration of prophylactic heparin and/or sodium warfarin in the days immediately after a major cerebral embolus carries with it an unacceptable risk of precipitating fatal hemorrhage into a hemorrhagic infarct is still under discussion and the subject will be dealt with in another chapter (Furlan et al. 1982; Cerebral Embolism Study Group 1984).

The concept derived from pathological studies that emboli often migrate, undergo lysis, and disappear received support from serial angiographic studies (Fisher 1960, unpublished material; Dalal et al. 1965). Angiography also confirmed the principle of artery-to-artery embolism which had been inferred from pathological studies. The exact role of such embolism in the causation of transient ischemic attacks (TIAs) has yet to be determined. Finally the range of possible sources of cerebral embolism was expanded by the discovery that mitral valve prolapse can serve as a source (Kostuk et al. 1977).

References

Allibert PC (1828) Recherches sur une occlusion peu connue des vaisseaux arteriels consideréé comme cause de gangrène. Paris

Baillie M (1793) Trans. Soc. for the Improvement of Medical and Chirurgical Knowledge (London) 1: 119–137

Beattie JM, Dickson WEC (1925) General pathology, 3rd edn, Heinemann, London

Beckmann O (1858) Embolie der arteria mesenterica superior. Virchows Arch Path Anat 13: 501–505

Blessig R (1859) Ueber die Veranderungen der Niere Nach Unterbindung der Nierenarterie. Virchows Arch Path Anat 16: 120–136

Bochdalek VA (1846) Einiges über den sogennanten Infarctus haemoptoicus Laennecii Vierteljahrschrift fur die Praktische Heilkunde (Prag) 9: 1–6

Böhne C (1931) Kompakte Hirnblutung und hämorrhagische Hirnerweichung Z Klin Med 117: 30–54

Bouillaud J (1826) Observations pour servir à l'Histoire de l'Apoplexie pulmonaire. Arch Gén Méd 12: 392–406

Carswell R (1838) Pathological anatomy, London

Cerebral Embolism Study Group (1984) Immediate anti-coagulation of embolic stroke: brain hemorrhage and management options. Stroke 15: 779–789

Cohn B (1860) Klinik der Embolischer Gefässkrankheiten. Hirschwald, Berlin

Cohnheim J (1872) Untersuchungen ueber die Embolische Processe. Hirschwald, Berlin

Cohnheim J, Litten M (1875) Ueber die Folgen der Embolie der Lungenarterien Virchows Arch Path Anat 65: 99–115

Cruveilhier J (1829) Anatomie pathologique du Corps humain, Paris, vol 1, Chap 11, p 7

Dalal PM, Shah PM, Aiyar RR (1965) Arteriographic study of cerebral embolism. Lancet 2: 358–361.

Faris, AA, Hardin CA, Poser CM (1963) Pathogenesis of hemorrhagic infarction of the brain. I. Experimental investigation of role of hypertension and of collateral circulation. Arch Neurol 9: 468–472.

Fazio C (1949) Red softening of the brain. J Neuropath Exp Neurol 8: 43–60

Fisher CM (1979) Reducing risks of cerebral embolism. Geriatrics 34: 59–66

Fisher CM, Adams RD (1951) Observations on brain embolism. J Neuropath Exp Neurol 10: 92–94

Foley WT, Wright IS (1950) The treatment of cerebral thrombosis and embolism with anticoagulant drugs; preliminary observations. Med Clin North America 34: 909–924

Francois V (1832) Essaie sur les Gangrènes spontanées, Paris

Fujinami A (1898) Beiträge zur Entstehung der Hämorrhagischen Infarkte der Lunge. Virchows Arch Path Anat 152: 61–106

Furlan AS, Cavalier SJ, Hobbs RE, Weinstein MA, Modic MT (1982) Hemorrhage and anticoagulation after non-septic embolic brain infarction. Neurology 32: 280–282
Hain RF, Westhaysen PV, Swank RL (1952) Hemorrhagic cerebral infarction by arterial occlusion; experimental study. J Neuropath Exp Neurol 11: 34–43
Hardin C, Hendren, TH, Faris AA, Poser CM (1963) Pathogenesis of hemorrhagic infarction of the brain. II. Protective effect of low molecular weight dextran. Arch Neurol 9: 473–476
Harvey J, Rasmussen T (1951) Occlusion of middle cerebral artery; experimental study. Arch Neurol Psychiatr 66: 20–29
Hasse KE (1846) Ueber die Verschliessung der Hirn arterien als nächste Ursache einer Form der Hirnerweichung. Z Rat Med 4: 91–111
Hiller F (1935–1937) In: Bumke O, Foerster O (eds) Handbuch der Neurologie, vol 11. Springer, Berlin, p 311
Hunter J (1793) Observations on the inflammation of the internal coats of veins. Trans Soc Improv Med Chirurg Knowl (London) 1: 18–29
Karsner HT (1949) Human pathology, 7th edn, Lippincott, Philadelphia
Karsner HT, Ash JE (1912–1913) Studies in infarction. II. Experimental bland infarction of the lung. J Med Res 27: 205–224
Karsner HT, Austin JH (1911) Studies in infarction. JAMA 57: 951–958
Kirkes WS (1852) On some of the principal effects resulting from the detachment of fibrinous deposits. Med Chir Tr 35: 281–324
Kossuchin A (1876) Zur Lehre von dem embolischen Infarcte. Virchows Arch Path Anat 67: 449–491
Kostuk WJ, Boughner DR, Barnett HJM, Silver MD (1977) Strokes: a complication of mitral-leaflet prolapse? Lancet 2: 313–316
Laennec RTH (1835) A treatise on the disease of the chest and on mediate auscultation (Translated by John Forbes), 4th edn, London
Litten M (1880) Untersuchungen über dem haemorrhagischen Infarct and über die Einwirkung arterieller Anaemie auf das Lebende Gewebe, Z Klin Med 1: 131–227
MacCallum WG (1940) A textbook of pathology, 7th edn. Saunders, Philadelphia
Owren PA (1963) The results of anticoagulant therapy in Norway. Arch Int Med 111: 240–247
Ricker G (1927) Sclerose und Hypertonie der innervierten Arterien. Springer, Berlin
Rostan L (1820) Recherhes sur une Maladie encore peu connue qui a recu le nom de Ramollissement du Cerveau, Paris
Rühle (1853) Drei Falle halbseitiger Lähmung verursacht durch Verstopfung einer Gehirnarterie. Virchows Arch Path Anat 5: 189–198
Schwartz P (1930) Die Arten der Schlaganfälle des Gehirns and Ihre Enstehung. Monographien aus dem Gesamtgebiete der Neurologie und Psychiatrie, vol 58
Seki H, Ogawa A, Yoshimoto T, Sato H, Suzuki J (1983) Hemodynamics in hemorrhagic infarction—an experimental study. No To Shinkei 35: 460–464
Tiedemann F (1843) Von der Verengung und Schliessung der Pulsadern in Krankheiten. Heidelberg
Virchow R (1847) Ueber die akut Entzündung der Arterien. Virchows Arch Path Anat 1: 272–378
von Recklinghausen F (1883) Handbuch der Allgemeinen Pathologie. Ferdinand Enke, Stuttgart
von Zielonko JV (1873) Ueber Entstehung der Hämorrhagien nach Verschluss der Gefässe, Virchows Arch Path Anat 57: 436–455
Waltz AG (1966) Cerebral vascular disease, In: Siekert RG, Whisnant JP (eds) 5th Princeton Conference. Grune and Stratton, New York, pp 177–183
Welch WH (1887) Hemorrhagic infarction. Trans Assoc Amer Physicians 2: 121–132
Zülch KJ (1955) Proc 2nd Internat Congr Neurol 2: 613

Chapter 2

Observations on Brain Embolism with Special Reference to Hemorrhagic Infarction*

C. M. Fisher and R. D. Adams

The embolic process, i.e., the morbid changes which develop in an organ whose blood supply has been impoverished by the embolic occlusion of nutrient arteries, constitutes an important chapter in neuropathology and one to which little thought appears to have been given in recent years. The belief is widely held that this subject was fully elucidated by the pioneers of pathology and that further investigation of it would yield little additional information. Our recent neuropathological experience has convinced us that such a view is by no means justified. There are many problems awaiting solution in this field of cerebrovascular disease, not the least of which are the cause and mechanism of hemorrhagic infarction. The paradoxical phenomenon of an occluded artery causing not only ischemic necrosis, but also vascular engorgement and hemorrhage in the region of its distribution, has been a controversial topic for at least a century, and many aspects of it are still disputed. Based on the casual observation that often in cases of hemorrhagic infarction of the brain at autopsy no arterial obstruction could be found at the appropriate site although the clinical setting suggested embolism (e.g., atrial fibrillation), we undertook a systematic assessment of our neuropathological material to investigate the relation of hemorrhagic infarction to embolism and the mechanism of hemorrhagic infarction. From these studies we were able to draw inferences concerning the dynamics of embolism.

The brain is a very satisfactory organ in which to study these problems, for the vessels are thin walled, are easily seen as they lie on the surface, and their territories of supply are well known. Thus, the relation of a given area of ischemic necrosis to the occlusion of a vessel can often be determined with more exactness than in any other organ.

---

* *Editors' Note.* This paper by C. M. Fisher and R. D. Adams was prepared in 1950 and was presented at the Annual Meeting of the American Association of Neuropathologists, 11 June 1950. An abstract was published in the *Journal of Neuropathology and Experimental Neurology* (1951) 10: 92–94. The full paper was never published and the authors were invited to have it included in this volume in its original form of 35 years ago. Some of the original illustrations could not be found, but those included here are quite representative.

This study was supported in part by the Multiple Sclerosis Society of Canada.

Historical Background

The study of hemorrhagic infarction in lung, spleen, kidney, and intestine has gone on sporadically during the past century. Opinions as to its pathogenesis have often differed sharply and even in the textbooks of today there is a vagueness which underlines the fact that more precise ideas as to the pathogenesis of hemorrhagic infarction are still awaited. Following the introduction of Cohnheim's theory of venous reflux, a series of papers was presented which clearly refuted this hypothesis and pointed rather to the importance of collateral arterial influx, at least in the case of the kidney and the intestine. Forbes (1901) was largely responsible for the belief among pathologists that all infarcts are at first red.

MacCallum (1940), in his textbook, stated that the deciding factors as to whether an infarct shall remain anemic or assume a deep red color were: (1) the arrangement of the circulation and (2) the density of the tissue. He regarded all infarcts as originally pale and remarked on the fact that in some cases the embolic plug lay at such a distance from the pulmonary infarct as to raise doubt as to whether the two were directly related. Karsner (1949) classed infarcts as hemorrhagic if the naked eye examination disclosed a rich blood content. He reiterated the same view presented 35 years previously, that all infarcts are at first congested and in those tissues with a rich blood supply and a loose arrangement this hyperemia gives way to a hemorrhagic state. White infarcts are said to be pallid because of decolorization of blood in the region of the infarction. According to the author, the infarct becomes pale earlier if there is little hemorrhage; hence the higher incidence of pallid infarcts in kidney, heart, and brain whose blood supply is not so rich.

Prior to 1900, hemorrhagic infarcts of the brain were scarcely mentioned in textbooks of pathology. In more recent years, they have been described frequently, particularly in the German literature. Schwartz, in 1930, concluded from his studies of apoplexy that hemorrhagic infarction and massive cerebral hemorrhage were fundamentally the same process, any difference being a quantitative one. He attributed the hemorrhagic extravasation in both cases to functional vascular changes which result in partial stasis and capillary diapedesis of red blood cells, in the manner described by Ricker. In 1927 Ricker had presented a theory ascribing to stimulation or paralysis of vasomotor nerves almost every known pathological process of blood vessels. He held that the walls of the smaller blood vessels reacted in several different ways to efferent impulses, depending on the strength and duration of the nervous discharge. Mild stimulation caused dilatation whereas stronger stimulation resulted in vasoconstriction. However, when fatigue set in, the capillary relaxed or dilated at a time when the arteriole was still partially constricted, a state which the author called "peristasis." If the arteriole should constrict and close completely, "stasis" ensued. Between these two states, there were many intermediate stages characterized by escape of the various elements of the blood, i.e., plasma, white blood cells, and red blood cells. Ricker named the intermediate processes liquordiapedesis, leukodiapedesis, and erythrodiapedesis, respectively. His theory was challenged by many workers in the field of vascular disease, but, nonetheless, it is still frequently used to explain many vascular phenomena.

There are perhaps sufficient grounds for some of his conclusions, but it must be recalled that his evidence is largely based on the effects produced in the pancreatic vessels of laboratory animals by such agents as sodium iodide solution, silver nitrate, ammonia, tannin, camphor, and heat (131°F). There is no proof that his results apply to human pathology.

Schwartz's view that hemorrhagic infarction and cerebral hemorrhage were the same process was immediately disputed by Böhne (1931), who pointed out the obvious pathological differences. He felt that a red infarct was at first pale, becoming secondarily hemorrhagic, but he did not suggest any mechanism for its production. Hiller (1935) was of the opinion that blood reached the infarcted tissue via collateral arterial channels. He attributed the more marked extravasation in the gray matter to the greater abundance of capillaries there. The author rejected venous reflux and incomplete arterial occlusion as possible factors in the etiology of red infarction and felt that red infarcts occurred just as readily distal to embolic occlusions as distal to atherosclerotic, thrombotic ones. Fazio (1949) has written the most recent review of the subject and pointed out that red softening is usually accompanied by a pale area of softening. He tentatively attributed the redness to partial occlusion of the vessel of supply, which in conjunction with many other factors affecting cerebral circulation such as venous congestion and vasospasm, determines a nonuniform diapedesis of red blood cells within the gray matter of that area.

From this brief review it becomes fairly obvious that we possess only a very limited knowledge of the process of hemorrhagic infarction in the brain. In the first place, there is no agreement as to the type of vascular disease of the brain with which it is associated. Secondly, the topography of the hemorrhages within the infarct has not been described fully, nor the relationship of the infarct to the intravascular clots. Finally, the mechanism of this type of softening has not been clearly formulated.

Analysis of the Pathological Material at the Boston City Hospital in 1949

During the year 1949 an attempt was made to examine the brain of every fatal case of cerebrovascular disease. Exclusive of cases referred from other hospitals there were 925 autopsies during that year and the brain was removed in 740 cases, that is in all cases in which there were no autopsy restrictions. As shown in Table 2.1, some form of vascular disease was discovered in 179 or 24% of these cases. This high percentage of vascular disease of the brain is probably due in part to the large number of aged patients in general hospitals today. Fifty-four percent of our cases were over 60 years of age and 13% were over 70 years at the time of death.

In the examination of the brain in these cases of suspected vascular occlusion the following method was adopted. The brain was removed carefully, and immediately suspended in formalin. Formalin was injected into the third ventricle through the tuber cinereum, but never into the carotid arteries because of the risk of dislodging an intravascular clot. In many cases fluid was injected

Table 2.1. Incidence of vascular disease of brain proven by autopsy at Boston City Hospital 1949

Total number of autopsies		925
Total number of brains examined		740
Number of cases of cerebrovascular disease		179 (24%)
Embolism	57	
Thrombosis	20	
Atherosclerosis with multiple small infarcts	34	
Hemmorrhage	29	
Indeterminate	17	
Hypertensive encephalopathy	7	
Ruptured saccular aneurysm	5	
Cerebral vein thrombosis	5	
Tuberculous meningitis and arterial thrombosis	4	
Vascular syphilis	1	

into the carotid and vertebral arteries in the neck to determine their patency. After fixation, a horizontal section was made through the cerebral hemispheres at approximately the level of the globus pallidus, to expose any major softenings. The brain arteries were then carefully dissected, often with the aid of a loupe or a dissecting microscope. The position of all intravascular clots that completely filled the lumen of the vessel was charted as was also the general form and location of the softened brain tissue. The occluded vessels were then cut transversely with a razor blade and microscopic sections were prepared. Success in locating the vascular clots depended to a great extent on the patience of the examiner.

Table 2.1 shows the relative frequency of the different types of vascular disease. Some of these pathological diagnoses are self-explanatory, but others require further comment. Under thrombosis we have included only cases in which there was demonstrable occlusion of large arteries by a clot which had formed in situ. In every case atherosclerosis was pronounced. The thrombus, if recent, was red and laminated; if time permitted, there was organization and endothelialization of the thrombotic material. The tissue supplied by the thrombosed vessel was usually in a state of infarct necrosis. The softened tissue varied in appearance according to the length of the interval between the vascular occlusion and death. In every instance the necrotic tissue was pale and at most only a moderate congestion of vessels and a few petechial hemorrhages could be found in gray matter at the junction of healthy and damaged tissue.

By atherosclerosis with multiple small infarcts we refer to the numerous small foci of ischemic necrosis which are so often found in the basal ganglia, cerebral white matter, and pons of brains with pronounced atherosclerosis. These small infarcts varied in appearance from foci of softening to small fenestrated cavities and patches of grayish discoloration according to their age and size. No attempt was made to find the occlusion because usually the vessel was a small artery or pre-arteriole and time-consuming serial sections would have been required. It is of interest that in our material the sum of these last two groups, thrombosis of large arteries and atherosclerosis with multiple small infarcts, was less than that of brain embolism. Moreover, large brain arteries were occluded by embolus three times as often as by thrombus.

Under the diagnosis of "indeterminate" we have included those cases in which there was an obvious large or moderate-sized focus of infarct necrosis of unknown cause. Frequently the softening was old, so that it was impossible to decide upon the nature of the vascular occlusion if it was found. Sometimes it was impossible to decide whether a fresh intravascular clot was a thrombus or embolus. There was little or no atherosclerosis in most of these cases and no demonstrable source for embolism or evidence of embolism in other viscera. Probably more of these cases belong in the embolic than the thrombotic group.

Under hypertensive encephalopathy we have included only cases in which malignant hypertension, hypertensive retinopathy, and malignant nephrosclerosis or acute glomerulonephritis were associated with neurological symptoms during life. Some of these cases, especially those in the 6th decade of life, had atherosclerosis and infarction of brain tissue. The characteristic pathological changes were brain swelling, multiple petechial hemorrhages in gray matter and pons, hyperplastic and necrotizing arteriolar lesions, and microscopic foci of tissue necrosis with glial proliferation.

Brain embolism, which comprises the largest group, was established in 26 of 57 cases by the macroscopic demonstration of a vascular occlusion and confirmation by microscopic examination. In the remaining 31 cases the embolus was not found and the diagnosis was based on three types of evidence: (1) the existence of a source of embolism or the presence of atrial fibrillation; (2) the finding of recent infarcts in other viscera where thrombotic occlusion of vessels is rare, i.e., spleen and kidney; and (3) the finding of multiple recent infarcts in the brain and the absence of significant atherosclerosis. The various combinations of these three factors are tabulated in Table 2.2.

Table 2.2. Evidence for brain embolism: 57 cases

Anemic infarcts		19
Embolus found proximal to infarct	14	
Embolus not found but assumed	5	
Source demonstrated in four		
Multiple visceral		
Multiple brain infarcts in one		
Hemorrhagic infarcts		38
Embolus found	12	
Embolus not found but assumed	26	
Source+multiple visceral—multiple brain infarcts	5	
Source+multiple visceral infarcts	7	
Source+multiple brain infarcts	3	
Source only	3	
Multiple visceral infarcts	1	
Multiple visceral—multiple brain infarcts	1	
Multiple brain infarcts without atherosclerosis	6	

The source of the emboli in the 26 cases where the embolus was demonstrated in a brain artery was: thrombotic material in the left atrial appendage in 4 cases, a mural thrombus in the left ventricle attached to infarcted myocardial tissue in 3 cases, a clot adhering to an atheromatous ulcer in the ascending aorta in 1 case, and atrial fibrillation without demonstrable clot or valvular disease in the left side of the heart or in the aorta in 13 cases. In five cases no source could be determined clinically or pathologically, though some form of heart disease was present in each instance. In none of these cases could atheromatous material be seen within the embolus.

The character of the infarcts produced by embolic occlusion deserves careful consideration. Unlike thrombotic infarcts, which were almost invariably pale or nonhemorrhagic, many of the infarcts due to embolism were in part hemorrhagic. To be more exact, in one-third of the 57 cases the infarct was pale, while in two-thirds it was partly hemorrhagic (cf. Table 2.2). As stated above, by hemorrhagic softening we refer not to a mere congestion or suffusion of blood vessels or a few petechial hemorrhages along the margin of the infarct, but to myriad petechial hemorrhages in a large portion of it. These hemorrhages were usually small, 0.2–2.0 mm in diameter, of irregular shape, and confined to the more vascular gray matter, either ganglia or cerebral cortex. Exceptionally the white matter was also involved. Rarely one or two larger hemorrhages had formed in the softened tissue yet the multiple and confluent small hemorrhages all through the softened tissue permitted easy differentiation from a primary brain hemorrhage.

In 14 of the 19 cases of nonhemorrhagic infarction due to the occlusion of a brain artery it was possible to find an embolus lodged securely at a point in an artery immediately proximal to the infarct. In four of the remaining cases the infarct was either small or several weeks old and the embolus was not identified; and in only one case with a large, fresh, pale infarct did we fail to demonstrate the embolus. In these cases of nonhemorrhagic brain infarction the embolus had obviously caused a virtually complete ischemia of the brain tissue.

In the 38 cases of partly hemorrhagic infarction, however, the embolus was found in only 12 instances. Moreover, in 10 of these 12 cases the embolus was found distal to the place in the artery where it should have been to account for the whole area of infarction, and often it lay distally well within the softened area, at the apex of the pale portion of the infarct. In the other two cases the diagrams of the location of the arterial emboli, made at the time of the gross examination, were not sufficiently exact to be sure of the relation of the embolus to the infarct. In two brains with multiple recent infarcts embolic material was detected in arteries proximal to pale infarcts, but was never found proximal to the hemorrhagic infarcts. Some of these relationships of embolus to infarct will be illustrated in the cases cited below.

Table 2.3. Analysis of hemorrhagic infarcts: 47 cases

Proven embolism in brain arteries	12 cases
Probable arterial embolism	26
Thrombosis of cerebral veins	5
Cause indeterminate	4
	47

Table 2.3 summarizes all of the hemorrhagic infarcts in our 1949 series of cases. Of the 47 cases of hemorrhagic infarction 5 were due to venous thrombosis, 12 to proven embolism, 26 to probable embolism (cf. Table 2.2), and in 4 the cause and mechanism could not be determined. Thus, it appears that embolism is the most frequent cause of hemorrhagic infarction.

Illustrative Cases

(*Note*: The original paper contained ten cases, five of which have been omitted to conserve space.)

Case 1: Hemorrhagic Infarct in the Peripheral Territory of the Right Middle Cerebral Artery. A hypertensive woman, aged 54, with atrial filbrillation was found on the floor with a left hemiplegia and died 24 h later. Pathological examination showed a softening in the right cerebral hemisphere part of which was hemorrhagic and part nonhemorrhagic (Fig. 2.1a). An embolus was found lodged at the parietal bifurcation of the right middle cerebral artery at the apex of the anemic portion of the infarct. This was definitely embolic in microscopic sections. The embolus lay distal to the Rolandic branch which supplied the hemorrhagic portion of the infarct and which was free of embolic material (Fig. 2.1b).

It is postulated that the embolus in the right middle cerebral artery had caused the infarct in the central region by blocking the Rolandic branch and then had moved distally to the point where it was found at autopsy. The circulation in the more proximal part of the infarct was restored and the tissue was rendered hemorrhagic.

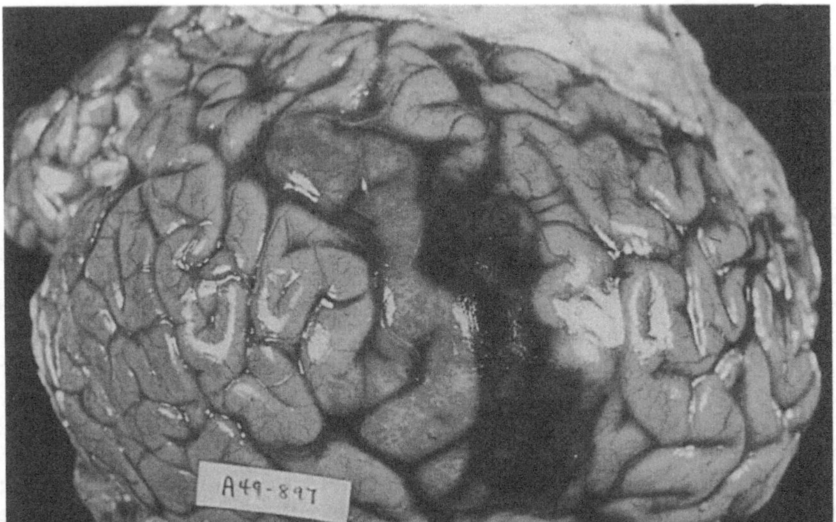

a

Fig. 2.1. a Case 1. Hemorrhagic infarct in pre-Rolandic region and pale infarct in post-Rolandic area.

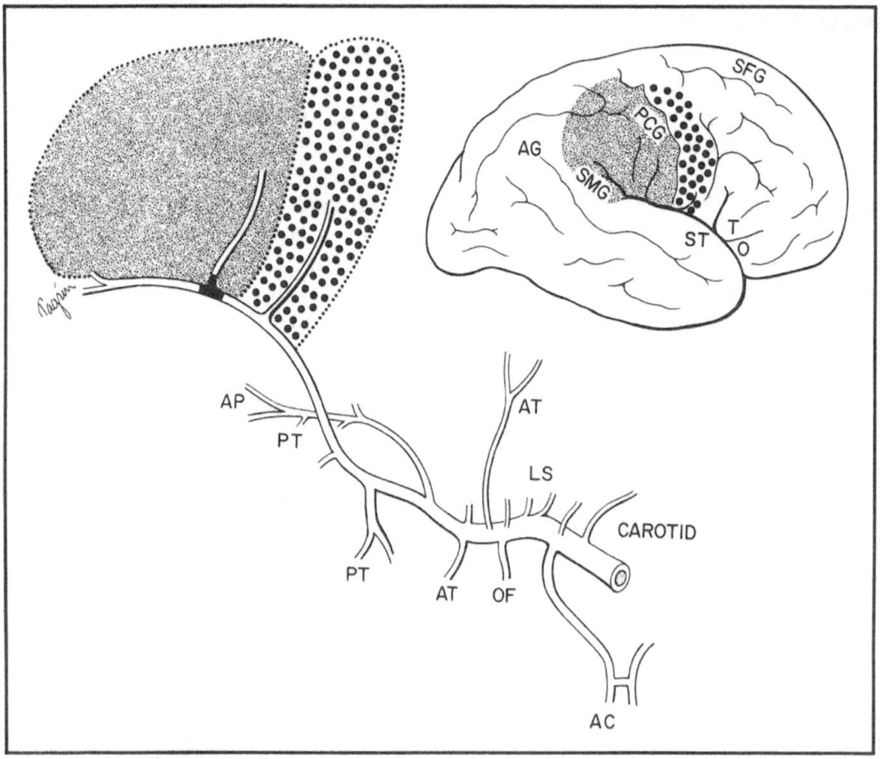

b

Fig. 2.1. b Case 1. Diagram of hemorrhagic and pale infarcts and arteries of supply. The embolic plug blocks the branches to the pale infarct.

Case 2. Hemorrhagic and Pale Infarction in the Territory of the Middle Cerebral Artery. A woman, aged 66, with atrial fibrillation suddenly developed a left hemiplegia from which she died 16 days later. Pathologically there was hemorrhagic infarction of part of the head of the left caudate nucleus and putamen and anemic softening of the left frontal, temporal, and parietal lobes and the insula (Fig. 2.2a). Reddish gray material obstructed the left middle cerebral artery at the first major bifurcation beyond the origin of the penetrating arteries (Fig. 2.2b). Microscopic sections of the occluding material showed amorphous thrombotic material with red blood cells. The clot was not attached to the vessel wall. Fibroblasts and histiocytes were seen in the clot. The left atrium was filled with red antemortem thrombus adherent to the wall of the atrium. There were recent and old renal infarcts.

The source of the emboli in this case was in all probability the clot in the left atrium. The embolus in the left middle cerebral artery lay distal to the penetrating branches which supplied the territory of hemorrhagic infarction and immediately proximal to the pale areas of infarction. In this case the embolus must have lodged in the first portion of the middle cerebral artery long enough to have infarcted the caudate and lenticular nuclei, as well as the cortical mantle, and then moved distally to the major bifurcation.

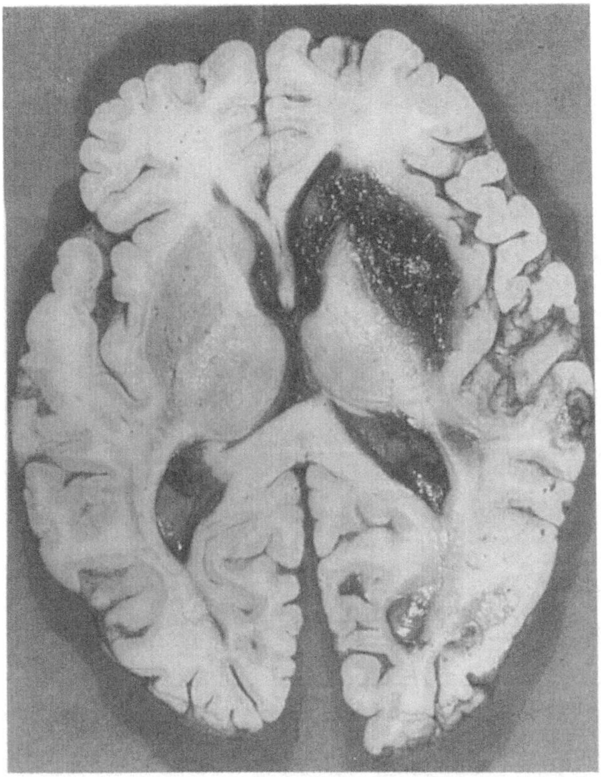

a

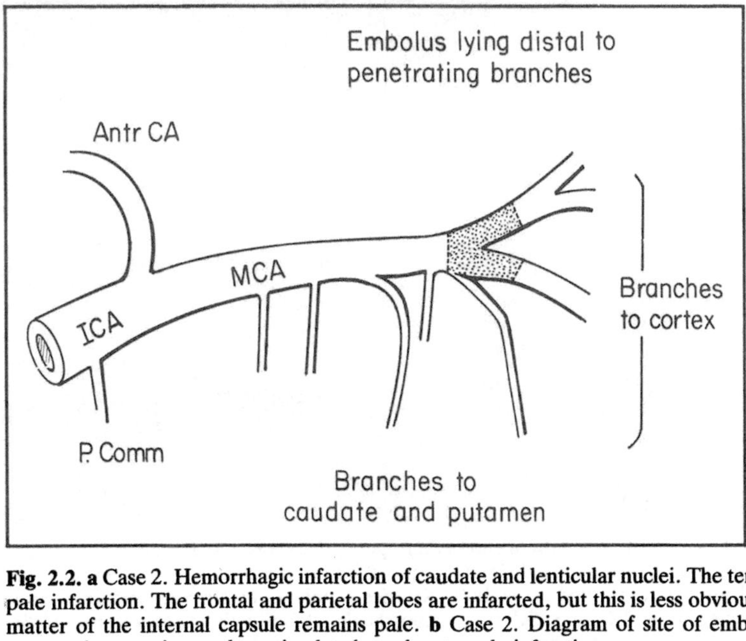

b

Fig. 2.2. a Case 2. Hemorrhagic infarction of caudate and lenticular nuclei. The temporal lobe shows pale infarction. The frontal and parietal lobes are infarcted, but this is less obvious. Note that white matter of the internal capsule remains pale. **b** Case 2. Diagram of site of embolic plug distal to penetrating arteries, and proximal to branches to pale infarction.

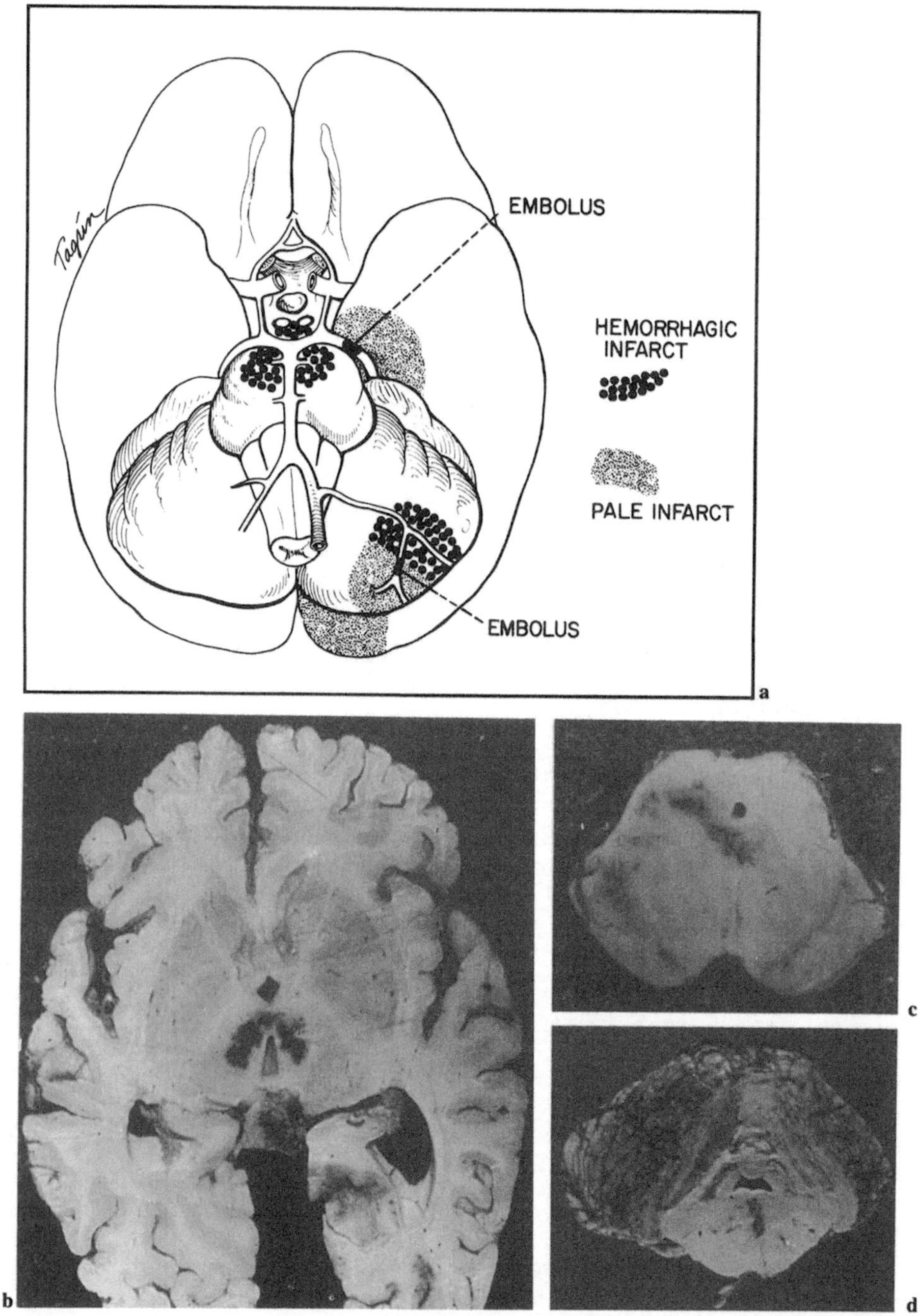

Fig. 2.3. a Case 3. Diagram of infarction in cerebellum, pons, thalamus, and left posterior cerebral artery territory. Arteries supplying the pale infarcts—posterior inferior cerebellar artery branch and posterior cerebral artery are blocked by emboli. Arteries supplying hemorrhagic infarcts (*heavy dots*) are unobstructed. **b, c, d** Case 3. Selective hemorrhagic infarction in territory of penetrating arteries of thalamus, midbrain, and pons.

Case 3. Extensive Hemorrhagic and Pale Infarction Within the Basilar System. A woman, aged 65, with a history of rheumatic heart disease and more recently cardiac failure collapsed on the street and was brought to the hospital comatose. The pupils were dilated and unreactive to light and the limbs did not move. Atrial fibrillation was present. Death occurred 20 h after hospital admission.

Pathological examination showed severe mitral stenosis and a large left atrial mural thrombus. There were old splenic and renal infarcts. There was extensive infarction in the territory of the vertebral basilar system: (1) recent hemorrhagic and anemic infarction of the left inferior cerebellar hemisphere; (2) hemorrhagic infarction in the pons, midbrain, and medial portions of each thalamus; and (3) a large pale softening in the left inferior temporo-occipital region (Fig. 2.3a).

Embolic material similar microscopically to the atrial thrombus was found in the branch of the left posterior inferior cerebellar artery leading to the pale portion of the infarct and in the left posterior cerebral artery just proximal to the pale infarct. No clot was found in the basilar artery or in vessels leading to hemorrhagic areas.

It would appear that embolic material was carried up the left vertebral artery. A piece of it lodged in the left posterior inferior cerebellar artery. That part of the cerebellar infarct whose vessels of supply did not remain obstructed became hemorrhagic whereas the portion distal to the embolic plug remained pale. The main part of the embolus entered the basilar artery and moved into the left posterior cerebral artery. The pons, midbrain, and thalamic became infarcted and as the embolus migrated they became hemorrhagic. The left occipital lobe became infarcted, but remained nonhemorrhagic because its arterial supply was still blocked by the embolus. This case provides one of the best examples of the dynamics of cerebral embolism as deduced from our studies.

Case 4. Example of the Process in the Territory of the Left Posterior Cerebral Artery. A hypertensive man, aged 55, known to have paroxysmal atrial fibrillation, suddenly went blind and became apprehensive. Three hours later vision had improved; next morning he was irrational. Examination showed a right upper quadrantanopia. The patient was disoriented, vague in his memory, and unable to name common objects. The blood pressure was 240/140. Transient atrial fibrillation was documented in the hospital. The patient died unexpectedly on the eighth hospital day.

Pathological examination showed hemorrhagic and anemic infarction of the left occipital and inferior temporal regions in the territory of the posterior cerebral artery (Fig. 2.4). The more medial and anterior portion of the infarct was hemorrhagic, whereas the lateral parts were pale. A careful search of the posterior cerebral arteries and their branches, as well as the basilar artery, revealed no definite occlusion. The large arteries were moderately atherosclerotic. There were the usual cellular changes of recent infarct necrosis and red blood corpuscles and disintegrating neutrophil leukocytes had escaped from the small vessels whose walls were necrotic. There was a recent splenic infarct.

Despite the failure to demonstrate a source for embolism or emboli in either the brain or splenic arteries, there was presumptive evidence of the embolic process, i.e., paroxysmal atrial fibrillation, infarcts of approximately the same age in the brain and spleen, the sudden onset of the stroke, and no atherothrombotic obstruction of the left posterior cerebral artery. Failure to find

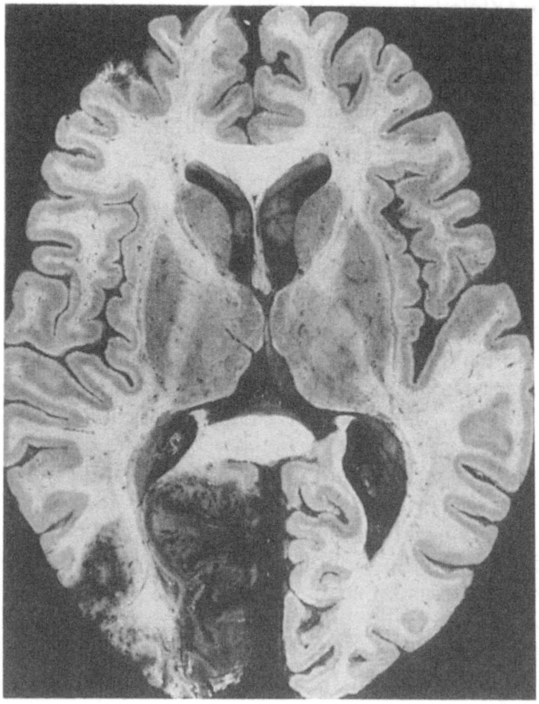

Fig. 2.4. Case 4. Hemorrhagic infarction in the territory of the left posterior cerebral artery.

embolic material in the appropriate vessels in cases of presumed embolism is common.

Case 5. Hemorrhagic Infarction in the Territory of the Right Anterior Choroidal Artery. A woman, aged 66, suddenly collapsed with a left hemiplegia. She moved the right limbs, but responded by groaning. Atrial fibrillation was present and the blood pressure was 220/140. She died 3 days after the onset of neurological symptoms. Pathological examination showed recent infarction of the right cerebral hemisphere in the distribution of the middle cerebral artery. On horizontal section the softening involved the upper part of the caudate nucleus, the lenticular nucleus, the anterior and posterior limbs of the internal capsule, the insula, the cerebral mantle, and the central white matter. The softened tissue was generally pale except the inner two-thirds of the globus pallidus and the most posterior portion of the putamen, which were speckled with small hemorrhages. The right middle cerebral artery was tightly occluded by a dark clot which extended from its first bifurcation back to the origin of the anterior choroidal artery, whose orifice was not blocked. The clot in the middle cerebral artery had the typical microscopic appearance of embolus and was not attached to the vessel wall.

Presumably, the embolus at one time blocked the anterior choroidal artery, causing infarction. Distal migration restored circulation with the production of a hemorrhagic alteration.

Discussion

The Pathology of Hemorrhagic Infarction

The general aspects of brain softening and infarction are well known and a detailed description of this process is beyond the purpose of this communication. It should suffice to point out those features that are characteristic of hemorrhagic infarction and provide some clue as to its pathogenesis.

From a study of our cases it can readily be determined that the form and distribution of a brain softening which was hemorrhagic did not differ from that usually seen in a pale infarct. In each instance the softened brain tissue corresponded to the distribution of one or more brain arteries. This alone usually distinguished it from the hemorrhagic softening of venous thrombosis. As would be expected, the tissue at the extreme margin of the territory supplied by the occluded artery usually remained firm owing to collateral supply from neighboring vessels. The abundance and efficiency of this collateral supply appeared to vary from one case to another, probably accounting for the slightly different size and form of the infarcts. The range in size of hemorrhagic softenings was as great as that of nonhemorrhagic ones. Furthermore, there was usually little difference between the two as regards the intensity of the destructive process. In only a few cases was the destruction of tissue by a hemorrhagic softening less complete than in a pale one of comparable size.

The outstanding feature of the hemorrhagic infarcts in this series was the fact that in nearly every case some part of the total infarct remained nonhemorrhagic. Most often it could be seen at a glance that a large part of the softening was pale. Invariably the hemorrhagic part was proximal to the pale portion. Usually the full extent of the hemorrhages could not be determined by inspection of the external surface of the brain, because in some cases they did not reach the pial surfaces at any point or in only a few convolutions. Parts which were externally pale and soft were found hemorrhagic when the brain was sectioned. Moreover, the degree of hemorrhagic change within the hemorrhagic part of the infarct was variable. In some cases the hemorrhages were so numerous that it was impossible to see normal tissue between them and in others the congestion of vessels and extravasation of red corpuscles was relatively slight. Occasionally, it was difficult to decide whether to call one of the latter type hemorrhagic or pale, but for the purposes of this study we have chosen only unquestionable cases.

The most common sites of hemorrhagic softening were the putamen, part of the head of the caudate nucleus, the orbital-frontal, posterolateral frontal, and anterior temporal convolutions, and the insula. These parts are supplied by the lenticulostriate, orbital-frontal, ascending frontal, and temporal branches of the middle cerebral artery. Hemorrhagic infarction also involved the cerebellar cortex, base of pons, and midbrain, thalamus, or cerebral structures situated within the territory of the posterior cerebral arteries. It should be stressed that the hemorrhagic part of the infarct usually corresponds to the entire territory of one or more branches of a major brain artery. It is not unusual in a massive pale infarction to find a few petechial hemorrhages at its margin, i.e., in the watershed between two major cerebral arteries. But we are not referring whatsoever to that process.

The number, size, and exact distribution of the hemorrhages varied from case to case. In nearly all cases the cerebral cortex and the gray matter of the lenticular and caudate nuclei and of the thalamus were more hemorrhagic than the corresponding white matter, and often the latter remained pale or at most was hemorrhagic only near the corticomedullary junction. The hemorrhages ranged in size from 0.2 to 5.0 mm; rarely one or several hemorrhages measuring up to 2.0 cm or more could be found. There was considerable uniformity in the size and pattern of the hemorrhages. In most cases the affected gray matter was speckled with myriad hemorrhages so that little gray tissue could be seen between them. Yet, the general architecture of the cortex or the nuclear mass was preserved and there was no difficulty in distinguishing between a hemorrhagic infarct and a brain hemorrhage. Within a red infarct small nonhemorrhagic zones were often seen. In the cerebral cortex the hemorrhages were round or linear and tended to be perpendicular to the pial surface. They extended in some instances under the pia for a short distance. In the cerebellar cortex the hemorrhages were more numerous in the granular than the molecular layer, resulting in a striking laminated appearance macroscopically. The borders of the red infarct were quite sharply defined in many cases. For example, the cerebral cortex on one side of a sulcus could be hemorrhagic whereas that on the other side remained pale.

The color and consistency of the brain tissue varied according to the age of the lesions. Dark or reddish-black coloration characterized the recent hemorrhagic infarct of only a few hours' or days' duration. In lesions 2–3 weeks old the color had become a lighter brick-red. With the ultimate solution of the red blood corpuscles the whole lesion took on a yellow-brown color and was eventually converted from a softening to an orange-brown trabeculated cavity. In this latter stage the lesion was still distinguishable from an old hemorrhage by the existence of a mesh of fibrous and vascular trabeculae and the relative lack of fibrous tissue encapsulation. The orange-brown color which was due to hematoidin and hemosiderin granules was retained for some years.

The relationship of the embolus to the softened tissue was of the greatest importance. As stated above, the embolic plug was found in only 12 of the 38 cases of hemorrhagic infarction. In 10 of these 12 cases no embolus was found in the artery running to the hemorrhagic portion of the infarct, the embolic plug usually lying just proximal to the pale portion of the infarct. *In the 26 cases where no embolic material could be found, the pathological picture was otherwise completely similar or analagous to that seen in cases where the embolus was present.* This finding strongly favored our belief that emboli often break up or "dissolve." *In three of the cases where we failed on gross examination to demonstrate an embolus, one or more embolic fragments were found in random microscopic sections of the more peripheral parts of the pale portion of the infarct, almost certain proof that emboli do shatter.*

The appearance of the emboli varied from case to case. In contrast to an arterial thrombus, which is of red color, the emboli were red, white, gray, or mottled. Sometimes they filled the vessel for a distance of 1 or 2 cm. The occluded portion of the vessel was larger than the adjacent part. The occluded blood vessel was often of healthy appearance without atheroma or other disease. There were, however, numerous exceptions in which the vessels were atherosclerotic. The most frequent site for lodgement of the embolus was at a bifurcation or any abrupt narrowing of the artery. Secondary, dark red thrombus was sometimes found either proximal or distal to the embolus.

Our practice in the examination of the obstructed vessels was to obtain at least one, and if in doubt several, transverse sections for microscopic examination. At times it was impossible to decide whether a recent clot was an embolus or thrombus. The histologic criteria which we have employed are those which are considered valid by most pathologists, namely that the clot be composed of interlacing bands of fibrin, red corpuscles, and white cells, that there be indications that the clot has formed some days before death as shown by disintegration of nuclei and invasion by fibroblasts, endothelial cells, or macrophages and that it fill the vessel lumen, preventing the usual scalloping or waviness of the internal elastic lamina, but not be attached to the vessel wall. If the intravascular clot was of considerable length, an attempt was made to examine at least two sections from different parts of it so as not to overlook a point of attachment and thrombus formation. All of the cases reported above satisfied these criteria.

Several additional characteristics of the red infarct became apparent in microscopic sections. The hemorrhages surrounded or were in relation to small blood vessels, probably capillaries, venules, and small arterioles. Occasionally, blood cells were seen around a small artery or vein. It was sometimes possible in cases several days old to determine that some of the cells in the walls of these vessels were necrotic, but seldom to the degree usually seen in large nonhemorrhagic infarcts. The earliest hemorrhagic infarct in our material occurred in a patient who survived only 6 h and indicates that the hemorrhages may occur early in the development of the softening. In this case there had been insufficient time for the migration of neutrophilic leukocytes. The nerve cells were shrunken and darkly stained and the nuclei were barely visible. The glia-cell nuclei were dark and granular. Some of the endothelial cells of the small vessels within the hemorrhages stained poorly, already tending toward eosinophilia and irregular nuclear borders. In hematoxylin and eosin stains a pinkish precipitate, possibly of blood plasma, had diffused around the vessels between the red corpuscles or in some places where no hemorrhage had occurred. The cells in the walls of the larger arteries and veins and the overlying meninges stained normally.

In cases where the infarct was 24–48 h old neutrophilic leukocytes had migrated into the damaged tissue. They formed collars around small blood vessels being mixed with red corpuscles but also invaded nonhemorrhagic necrotic tissue. These cells were increasingly abundant in cases which had survived the vascular occlusion for 2–5 days, giving the well-known pseudo-inflammatory reaction of infarcted tissue. Fragmentation of the neutrophilic leukocytes occurred during the 3rd, 4th, and 5th days, often leaving multiple foci of nuclear debris among the altered nerve and glia cells. The latter cells were still visible in hematoxylin and eosin stains in infarcts 7–10 days old. Macrophages were found in increasing numbers after 48 h and phagocytosis of red corpuscles could be detected. Blood pigment was found in macrophages after the 7th or 8th day. Myelin stains disclosed an altered staining reaction of the white matter within the first 48 h; the medullated fibers were pale, and those along the margins of the infarct were irregularly swollen, with many end bulbs. The red blood corpuscles stained well in most of the myelin stains, providing the clearest pictures of the pattern of the hemorrhages and the congested blood vessels.

The later reparative processes, by abundant macrophages and by astrocytic and fibroblastic connective tissue, were the same as those of nonhemorrhagic infarction. The only differences between the two was the large number of pigment-filled macrophages seen in the hemorrhagic infarct.

The Mechanism of Hemorrhagic Infarction as Deduced from our Studies

From an analysis of the pathologic findings in the above cases the following points emerge: (1) Hemorrhagic infarcts due to arterial occlusion are nearly always embolic. (2) Hemorrhagic infarcts almost always occur in combination with pale infarcts. (3) The hemorrhagic portion is always proximal to the pale portion. (4) The embolus is found in only a minority of cases, but when it is present, it is so placed as to leave open the vessels supplying the hemorrhagic portion of the infarct and block those to the pale portion, i.e., it lies just distal to the arteries supplying the hemorrhagic portion and proximal to arteries leading to the pale portion. (5) The hemorrhagic portion is always the site of definite ischemic necrosis in addition to the congestion and petechial hemorrhages. (6) The pathologic features in the 28 cases of hemorrhagic infarction in which the embolus was not seen grossly were the same as in the 12 where the embolus was found. This is an important finding. (7) The red or hemorrhagic parts of the infarct usually correspond closely to the territory of one or more arteries or their branches and do not correspond to the distribution of veins. (8) An infarct distal to an embolus found in situ is always pale (there were no exceptions to this in our material). It is unusual in a *recent* case of purely pale necrosis not to find the embolus. (9) The gray matter of the basal ganglia and the cerebral cortex are the usual sites of congestion and hemorrhage, the white matter remaining pale. Red infarcts may be found in any part of the brain and brain stem. (10) Occasionally, the pale zones of the infarct are of small extent while the hemorrhagic infarction is very extensive (case 4). Gross embolic material may not be seen in the larger arteries and the embolus will seem to have disappeared. If such infarcts were studied in microscopic serial sections, we believe that small fragments of embolic material would be found in the majority of recent cases. In older cases traces of the embolus will no longer be found. (11) Minor hemorrhagic infarction of an entirely different dimension from that herein discussed may be found at the periphery of large areas of pale necrosis due either to embolism or thrombosis. These border hemorrhages are probably due to collateral circulation.

From these facts the following theory of hemorrhagic infarction of the brain is formulated. *An embolus upon reaching a brain artery becomes slowed up or arrested in a narrowed part of the vessel, usually at a bifurcation, and causes ischemic necrosis of the tissue supplied by that vessel. The embolic material then undergoes a change; it may become more compact, assume a different shape, shatter, or fragment and the pieces are then carried into the outlying peripheral branches or arterial twigs where they are difficult to find postmortem. Or instead of fragmenting the entire embolus may move distally for a short distance and then become securely lodged in one or two large branches. Proximal branches, which were previously occluded, are now exposed to the force of arterial blood pressure, and the capillary bed which they supply becomes congested with blood. Extravasation occurs through the distended capillaries and other small vessels. Parts of the brain supplied by vessels which are still occluded by emboli remain pale except at the extreme margins between normal and ischemic brain where collateral vessels permit some limited influx of blood into the damaged capillary bed.*

A strong point of evidence in support of this concept is the fact that the red infarct is always proximal to the pale portion so that the responsible mechanism must be active in that region alone. This hypothesis accounts for the great frequency of mixed infarcts, that is, partially red and partially white. The notable absence of embolus in vessels leading to the hemorrhagic parts of the infarct, and the lack of extravasation of blood in nearly all cases of thrombosis and in those cases of embolus where the clot is attached or tightly lodged within the vessels so that it cannot move, are also explained.

A slight modification of this theory may be necessary to explain certain cases in which hemorrhagic infarcts in the cerebellum, pons, and thalamus occur in association with pale infarcts in the territory of the posterior cerebral arteries, as in case 3. Small pieces of embolus may have entered several branches of the vertebral and basilar arteries, with the resulting infarcts being pale or hemorrhagic depending on whether the embolus was securely and permanently lodged or was movable. Another possible explanation would be that the embolus was of great length, and as it passed upwards in the basilar system one branch after another became temporarily occluded long enough to produce ischemic necrosis of the tissues. Our knowledge of the range in shape, size, and consistency of emboli as they are carried along in the bloodstream is very limited. In case 1 the territory of a branch coming off at right angles from the main vessel was strikingly hemorrhagic; yet no embolus could be found in the arterial trunk at the origin of, or anywhere along, that arterial branch. A branch arising at right angles should be particularly prone to temporary occlusion as an embolus moves slowly past its mouth.

A mechanical theory of this type may seem excessively simple, but close scrutiny of cases of embolic disease for 2 years has failed to disclose a single case in which this explanation could not apply. Whether ischemic damage to the capillary endothelium plays a small or an important part in the production of the hemorrhages cannot be answered with finality. Litten (1880), Welch (1887), and others were not impressed with the importance of endothelial damage whereas Broman (1940), studying experimental fat embolism, concluded that the petechial hemorrhages could only be accounted for in this way. The experiments of Litten and Welch, who found that temporary ligation of the renal and superior mesenteric arteries, respectively, even for several hours did not result in hemorrhagic infarction when the ligature was released and the patency of the lumen restored, must be cited in opposition to our hypothesis. Welch, working with Mall, on the other hand, was able to produce hemorrhagic infarction in the small intestine by gradually occluding the superior mesenteric artery by means of a special clamp, hemorrhages occurring when the pressure in the vessel fell to one-fifth of normal. All collateral channels had been ligated in their experiment, thus reproducing the situation within the brain where collaterals are relatively few.

It is a distinct possibility that such a mechanism is sometimes operative in red infarction of the brain, for an arrested embolus could partially obstruct the mouths of adjacent side branches, reducing the blood flow in them below a certain critical level. This would explain the relative lack of ischemic necrosis in some cases of hemorrhagic infarction, but is not in keeping with our failure to find any obstruction whatsoever in vessels leading to the red portions of infarcts. Experimental occlusion of cerebral vessels for varying periods and to varying degrees is clearly indicated to settle this rather important point.

The possible role of vasospasm proximal to the embolus is more difficult to assess. Fazio (1949) has recently suggested that vasospastic phenomena precipitated by an embolus are important factors in the production of hemorrhagic infarction. Our data do not allow a definite opinion on this point though there is considerable evidence against it. For example, in cases 1 and 5, the hemorrhages were exactly limited to the area supplied by one arterial branch. It is unlikely that vasospasm could evoke such complete and uniform effects in a single branch and leave completely unaffected other neighboring branches. Also, the complete absence of hemorrhagic infarction in many cases of brain embolism would be difficult to explain, for one would hardly expect pronounced vasospastic effects in one case of embolic occlusion and none in another. Villaret and Cachera (1939) and Broman (1940) have described temporary vasoconstriction or vasospasm both near to and distant from the site of lodgement of embolic material within the pial vessels of experimental animals. Villaret and Cachera, using the cranial window technique of Forbes, were able to photograph local vascular spasms lasting 3–6 min after embolization. From the examination of animals after various periods of survival the authors were led to believe that fluctuating spasm producing a moniliform appearance of vessels could persist for as long as 30 days after acute embolization. This chronic spasm involved vessels of approximately 15 μm and could result in arrest or stagnation of the circulation in the "very small vessels." These vascular changes were observed in only 5 of 19 animals and the authors were unable to decide whether such vasospasm caused either a functional derangement of the brain or infarct necrosis. Indeed, as it turned out, the cases in which vasospasm was seen usually showed no infarct necrosis. Broman, who observed emboli in pial vessels by means of a microscope and later studied the permeability of the vessels to trypan blue, concluded that the circulation in spastic, contracted vessels was not arrested, even with the simultaneous intravenous administration of adrenaline; nor was the permeability of a vessel distal to a point of vasospasm ever altered. Therefore, even if the possibility of vasospasm is conceded, there is very little experimental evidence that it produces drastic circulatory effects. In regard to experimental cerebral embolism, great caution must be exercised in transferring such data to human cases, for the embolic material in these experiments is often of most unnatural type (starch granules, fat, glass, bits of stone, glass beads) and, secondly, the pial vessels under observation are but a fraction of the size of some of those which must be involved in human cases of hemorrhagic infarction. Lastly, there is good evidence that human cerebral vessels when touched, rubbed, or electrically stimulated are not as easily excited to spasm as those of rabbits, cats, and dogs (Echlin 1942).

It appears to be improbable that the hemorrhagic extravasation is due to collateral influx as has been demonstrated in the lung, spleen, kidney, and intestine because the brain infarct distal to an arrested embolus or thrombus is always more or less pale, and yet gradual thrombosis should provide optimal conditions for the development of a collateral circulation. At times small areas of extravasation are found in the periphery of an infarct, involving a part of a single gyrus, and these we would attribute to collateral influx. But as has been stated previously, these tiny, outlying red areas are not presently under discussion. Although collateral influx will carry blood to the occluded vessels (the vessels distal to either an embolus or thrombus always contain fluid blood), it seems almost certain that such an influx never discolors large areas of a pale infarct. If collateral influx were a factor, it should not spare one area and affect a neighboring one whose pattern of blood supply is for all purposes the same. We have not observed any relationship between the hemorrhagic infarct and the large surface anastomotic loops that connect the cerebral arteries and cerebellar arteries, respectively. Cohnheim's (1872) theory of venous influx must play no part in cerebral red infarcts. Careful dissection of the brain will usually show the hemorrhage to be exactly limited to the territory of an artery and not to that of any vein. Venous congestion due to cardiac failure or repeated convulsions may influence the degree of congestion and extravasation of blood, but probably does not otherwise alter the picture.

Another possibility that deserves a word of comment concerns the behavior of the circulation just proximal to an occlusion. Microscopically, Cohnheim (1872), von Zielonko (1873), and Kossuchin (1876) have each described a greatly increased blood flow along the side branches immediately proximal to the embolic obstruction. This at times is said to reach such proportions as to lead to hemorrhagic extravasation. As previously shown, the red part of a brain infarct lies in the territory of the artery or arteries just proximal to the occlusion, and this mechanism must, therefore, be considered. The most certain refutation of this idea, however, comes from the fact that the region of hemorrhagic discoloration is invariably necrotic. The increased collateral flow, as described by Cohnheim and others, not only does not cause necrosis, but in fact is probably contrived by nature to protect neighboring tissue from necrosis.

There is another rather uncommon, but striking, type of hemorrhagic infarction, namely that occurring with space-occupying hemispheric lesions and transtentorial herniation of the temporal lobe. The hemorrhagic softening of the occipital lobe due to compression of the posterior cerebral artery should shed some light on the mechanism of this lesion. In these cases it is often difficult to be sure what has happened to the artery, but there is good reason to assume that it was caught between the brain hernia and the free edge of the tentorium. At death, the artery is usually patent; therefore, the obstruction must have been due either to compression, or compression and local spasm. It is likely that some release of the vascular obstruction occurs after infarct necrosis has been produced and the lesion then becomes hemorrhagic for the same reason as in the migration of embolic material. On the other hand, Welch's results in reducing the blood flow by four-fifths and producing hemorrhagic infarction might find application in such cases.

It seems to us that the theory of *migratory embolism* provides the most plausible explanation for all the peculiar properties of hemorrhagic infarction in the human brain. We are as yet unprepared to say whether or not this theory can be applied to other organs such as the intestine, kidney, spleen, and retina.

A few further points require comment. That all brain infarcts are at first red is clearly impossible if by red we mean true hemorrhagic infarction, for the extravasated blood is known to persist for months or years in the form of hemosiderin pigment. Whether or not all brain infarcts are hyperemic at first, we cannot say, but a mild degree of congestion of vessels is not improbable. The explanation for the selective congestion and hemorrhages of the cortex and basal ganglia and the relative sparing of the white matter has been attributed to the relative abundance of capillaries in the former. Capillaries are several times more abundant in gray than in white matter. Evidence that this explanation is correct is found in the fact that in the cerebellum the hemorrhagic extravasation occurs in the granular layer and not the molecular layer, whose capillary density is much less. Rarely one observes a pale infarct, probably due to an embolus, in which no embolus can be found. This is difficult to explain unless the circulation of the patent arteries within an infarct was not restored or there is a certain critical period beyond which movement of the embolus and opening up of the vessels does not result in extravasation of blood.

The clinical implications of this theory of embolic occlusion are of interest. Presumably, if embolic material can fragment and move distally after causing necrosis of the tissue within the territory of a vessel, it could do so before the tissue is totally and irreversibly destroyed. Thus, it is possible for embolic material to render certain parts of the brain ischemic with resultant paralysis of nervous function and then move distally in the vessel, permitting complete restitution of the circulation and recovery of function. This appears to have happened in one of our cases where despite a transient aphasia, right hemiplegia and hemianesthesia, which lasted several days, the only brain lesion demonstrated at autopsy 3 weeks later was a small infarct in the posterior parietal lobe. In all probability an embolus temporarily obstructed the blood supply to the posterior frontal, anterior parietal, and superior parts of the temporal lobes and had then migrated to a small terminal branch in the parietal lobe before ischemic necrosis was produced. The efficiency of collateral circulation is a variable factor in such cases and may at times account for the lack of either hemorrhage or necrosis. Migratory embolism is therefore one of the causes of transient apoplectic phenomena.

References

Böhne C (1931) Kompakte Hirnblutung und hämorrhagische Hirnerweichung, Z Klin Med 117: 30–54

Broman T (1940) Über cerebrale Zirkulationsstörungen. Acta Path Microbiol Scand [Suppl] 42

Cohnheim J (1872) Untersuchungen ueber die Embolische Processe, Hirschwald, Berlin

Echlin FA (1942) Vasospasm and focal cerebral ischemia, experimental study. Arch Neurol Psychiatr 47: 77–96

Fazio C (1949) Red softening of the brain. J Neuropathol Exp Neurol 8: 43–60

Forbes (1901) cited in Beattie JM, Dickson WEC (1925) General pathology, 3rd edn, Heinemann, London

Hiller F (1935–1937) In: Bumke O, Foerster O (eds) Handbuch der Neurologie Berlin, vol 11. Springer, Berlin, p 311

Karsner HT (1949) Human pathology. 7th edn, Lippincott, Philadelphia

Kossuchin A (1876) Zur Lehre von dem embolischen Infarcte. Virchows Arch Path Anat 67: 449–491

Litten M (1880) Untersuchungen über dem haemorrhagischen Infarct and über die Einwirkung arterieller Anaemie auf das Lebende Gewebe. Z Klin Med 1: 131–227

MacCallum WG (1940) A textbook of pathology, 7th edn, Saunders, Philadelphia

Ricker G (1927) Sclerose und Hypertonie der innervierten Arterien. Springer, Berlin

Schwartz P (1930) Die Arten der Schlaganfälle des Gehirns and Ihre Entstehung. Monographien aus dem Gesamtgebiete der Neurologie und Psychiatrie, vol. 58

Villaret M, Cachera R (1939) Les Embolie cérébrales, Masson, Paris

von Zielonko JV (1873) Ueber Entstehung der Hämorrhagien nach Verschluss der Gefässe. Virchows Arch Path Anat 57: 436–455

Welch WH (1887) Hemorrhagic infarction. Trans Assoc Am Physicians 2: 121–132

Chapter 3

Evaluation of Patients with Suspected Cardioembolic Brain Infarction

B. A. Sandok

Introduction

Cardioembolic mechanisms have been implicated with increasing frequency as a cause of brain ischemia (Mohr et al. 1978). Increased understanding of heart-brain relationships and more sophisticated diagnostic studies have heightened our awareness of heart disease as an important mechanism underlying cerebrovascular disease (Easton et al. 1980).

Establishing cardiac disease as a cause of brain infarction may, at times, appear deceptively simple. However, in the majority of instances it is a diagnosis of inference, suggested only after considering both the neurologic and cardiologic aspects of the clinical presentation, and upon review of the diagnostic studies which have been judiciously selected to reduce the likelihood of the other causative mechanisms of brain ischemia. Additional studies are available which are capable of identifying pathologic cardiac physiology and anatomy associated with the development of intracardiac thrombi. In spite of improved technology, the diagnosis of cardioembolic brain ischemia (CEBI) continues to be based primarily upon the judgment and experience of the examining physician. The diagnostic approach shown in Table 3.1 will serve as an outline for the discussion to follow.

Clinical Presentation

Given a patient with brain infarction, one is obliged to attempt to identify the underlying pathophysiologic mechanism responsible for the deficit. In most instances the mechanism will be related to large-vessel atherosclerosis, but other large-vessel arteriopathies as well as smaller-vessel disease and hematologic and cardiac mechanisms must be considered. The neurologic and cardiologic features of the clinical presentation provide clues for a potential cardioembolic mechanism.

Table 3.1. Diagnostic approach to suspected cardioembolic stroke

CLINICAL PRESENTATION
Cerebral infarction

Neurologic:	Are there features which suggest a cardioembolic mechanism? Other mechanism?
Cardiologic:	Is there a cardiac condition present which will predispose to systemic embolization?

DIAGNOSTIC EVALUATION: Designed to identify mechanism of infarction.
Consider: diagnostic value (risk/benefit/cost).
Will it alter management?

General medical studies
Neurodiagnostic studies
Cardiologic studies

MANAGEMENT PLAN

Neurologic Aspects

A number of clinical features have been traditionally mentioned as being characteristic of cardioembolic brain ischemia. These are listed in Table 3.2. Taken as a group these symptoms are indeed suggestive of CEBI, but they are nonspecific, are nondiagnostic, are infrequent in patients with CEBI, or may be encountered in patients with other mechanisms of infarction, and therefore have proven less than infallible indicators.

Table 3.2. Clinical features of cardioembolic brain infarction (Mohr et al. 1978; Easton et al. 1980)

Sudden onset (nonsudden in 21%)
Lack of antecedent TIA (11% had TIA)
Alteration in level of consciousness (infrequent, nondiscriminating)
Seizures at onset (infrequent, nondiscriminating)
Headache at onset (nondescriminating)
Wernicke type of aphasia (also seen with other mechanisms)

Additional clinical factors are useful in suggesting a cardioembolic mechanism:

1. *Distribution of the infarction*: The middle cerebral artery distribution is the most common site of embolization (±75%), with the posterior cerebral artery and basilar artery accounting for an additional 10% each. The anterior cerebral artery distribution is a very *uncommon* site for embolization;

infarction in this distribution is therefore unlikely to be cardioembolic in origin.

2. *Age of the patient*: In the younger (i.e., <45 years) patient there is a lesser likelihood that an atherosclerotic mechanism is playing a role; cardiac mechanisms are more frequently identified.
3. *Other evidence of systemic embolization*: Although an uncommon occurrence in the group of patients presenting with cerebrovascular disease, evidence of prior embolization to brain or elsewhere in the body, when present in the clinical profile, is highly suggestive of a cardioembolic mechanism.
4. *Absence of symptoms/signs of extracranial carotid occlusive disease* ipsilateral to the ischemic event does not definitely implicate a cardiac source, but increases its likelihood. Conversely, the presence of such findings does not eliminate a cardioembolic mechanism.
5. *The presence of general cardiac symptoms* coincident with the cerebral ischemic event (i.e., chest pain, palpitations, tachybradydysrhythmias, etc.), when present, should suggest a cardiac mechanism.
6. *The presence of a cardiac condition known to be associated with systemic embolism* makes the possibility of CEBI a strong consideration. One must be cautious as multiple mechanisms may coexist in a given patient.

Cardiologic Aspects

As indicated above, the neurologic aspects of the cerebrovascular event may provide inferential data to suggest a cardioembolic mechanism. More often, it is not the neurologic presentation but the presence of a cardiac disorder known to produce systemic embolization that suggests the causative mechanism. Table 3.3

Table 3.3. Cardiac conditions associated with systemic-cerebral embolism

I. *Disorders affecting the heart wall*
   A. Acute myocardial infarction
   B. Remote myocardial infarction—akinetic segments, aneurysms
   C. Congestive heart failure
   D. Cardiomyopathy
   E. Atrial myxoma
   F. Congenital heart disease—paradoxical embolism

II. *Disease of the heart valves*
   A. Mitral stenosis/regurgitation (rheumatic heart disease)
   B. Mitral valve prolapse
   C. Prosthetic heart valves
   D. Infective endocarditis
   E. Nonbacterial thrombotic endocarditis

III. *Heart rhythm dysfunction*
   A. Atrial fibrillation
   B. Bradytachydysrhythmias

IV. *Complications of heart manipulation*
   A. Cardiac catheterization
   B. Cardiac surgery

(modified after Breuer 1983) provides a partial listing of cardiac disorders associated with systemic-cerebral embolism. Brief clinical comments will be made about each.

Acute Myocardial Infarction (Bean 1938; Thompson et al. 1978). Cerebral ischemic events occur in less than 2% of patients. Mural thrombi with systemic/cerebral embolization occur most frequently in the first 2 weeks postinfarction. There is increased risk of embolization with increased size of infarct (increased CPK), congestive heart failure, and septal involvement.

Remote Myocardial Infarction. Damage to cardiac muscle may result in akinetic segments and ventricular aneurysms which may then be a source of thrombus formation and subsequent embolization. As many as 75% of patients with ventricular aneurysm postmyocardial infarction (MI) have thrombi in the aneurysm (Juergens et al. 1960). Therefore, identification of such a lesion in a patient with brain infarction without other cause would strongly suggest a cardioembolic source. Patients post MI with brain ischemia without evidence of occlusive cerebrovascular disease should be evaluated for abnormalities of the ventricular wall.

Congestive Heart Failure. Regardless of cause, congestive heart failure predisposes to intracardiac and pulmonary venous thrombi and is associated with a ninefold increase in brain infarction (Wolf et al. 1978).

Cardiomyopathies (Segal et al. 1978). Both idiopathic and secondary varieties may be associated with congestive heart failure and rhythm disorders (atrial fibrillation is the most common) and a high incidence of intracardiac thrombi. Cerebral/systemic embolization may be the presenting symptom of the cardiomyopathy.

Atrial Myxoma (Sandok et al. 1980). This is a rare tumor and thus a rare but treatable cause of cerebral ischemia to be considered in the differential diagnosis of patients without other identifiable cause presenting with: (1) recent progressive cardiac symptoms, (2) general systemic symptoms resembling polymyalgia rheumatica or subacute bacterial endocarditis, or (3) evidence of systemic and/or cerebral embolization.

Congenital Heart Disease—Parodoxical Embolization (Jones et al. 1981). The appearance of a focal brain lesion in the face of overt congenital heart disease with right-to-left shunting leads one to suspect a cardioembolic ischemic event (or abscess or hemorrhage). Embolization may also occur in patients with a patent foramen ovale and nonovert heart disease. This mechanism should be considered when there is evidence of deep vein thrombosis, a history of recent pulmonary embolism, and perhaps the onset of a cerebral event coincident with performing a Valsalva maneuver.

Rheumatic Heart Disease (Mitral Stenosis/Mitral Regurgitation). The frequency of systemic emboli in mitral stenosis has been reported to be 10%–75% (Adams et al. 1974). About half involve the brain, with about two-thirds occurring within 1 year after the onset of atrial fibrillation (Szekely 1964). Mitral regurgitation alone (with or without atrial fibrillation) may also be associated with systemic embolization.

Mitral Valve Prolapse. The occurrence of cerebral and retinal ischemic events as a consequence of myxomatous degeneration of the mitral valve has been suggested by clinical (Barnett 1982), pathologic (Donaldson et al. 1981), and epidemiologic (Sandok et al. 1982) observations. Other causes of brain infarction should always be sought even when the typical findings of mitral valve prolapse (MVP) are in evidence. Cardiac evaluation searching for MVP is indicated in younger patients with cerebral ischemic symptoms and perhaps in all patients when no cause is identified.

Prosthetic Valves. The replacement of defective valves clearly improves cardiac output, but whether overall survival free of emboli is improved is subject to question. Thromboembolic rates differ depending upon valve type and anticoagulation regimen. Mechanical valves have higher complication rates than tissue valves (Kloster 1979). Thromboembolism may be increased in patients with shortened platelet survival (Weily et al. 1974).

Infective Endocarditis (Jones et al. 1969; Greenlee and Mandell 1973; Pruitt et al. 1978). As many as one-third of patients will have cerebral ischemic events or other focal neurologic symptoms, and of these 6%–15% may present with neurologic disease. Streptococci and staphylococci account for 90% of the offending organisms, but unusual bacteria as well as fungi must be considered in drug abuse or immunosuppressed patients, or those on intravenous hyperalimentation. Secondary neurologic complications which may enter into the differential diagnosis include: meningoencephalitis or multiple embolic events causing an encephalopathic picture; arteritis; intracerebral hemorrhage or mycotic aneurysm formation (5%); and brain abscess (5%). It is important to recall that 95% of patients with infectious endocarditis present with "nonspecific" symptoms of fever, heart murmur, anemia, arthralgia, myalgia, and elevated sedimentation rate. The presence of these symptoms in a patient with cerebral ischemia should alert the clinician to the possibility of endocarditis.

Nonbacterial Thrombotic ("Marantic") Endocarditis (Reagan and Okazaki 1974; Kookier et al. 1976). This should be suspected as a cause of cerebral ischemia in patients with cancer (particularly adenocarcinoma), either known or occult (also: uremia, lupus, and acute rheumatic fever). The vegetations are small (frequently not seen on two-dimensional echocardiography) and consist of platelet-fibrin depositions which may give rise to multiple small emboli. Disseminated intravascular coagulation may coexist.

Atrial Fibrillation. Patients with atrial fibrillation (AF) are at increased risk for cerebral ischemia (Hinton et al. 1977). This risk is 5× for patients with chronic nonrheumatic AF and increased 17× in patients with rheumatic heart disease (Wolf et al. 1978). In the latter group the association is clear and direct. In the former the clinician must be aware that many of the same factors which predispose to chronic nonrheumatic AF are also associated with the presence of extracranial atherosclerosis, and AF may merely be an incidental finding.

Bradytachydysrhythmias. Although relatively common in elderly patients, they are most often associated with nonfocal symptoms due to reduced cardiac output (giddiness, syncope, etc.). Focal CNS symptoms may occur but appear to be rare (Reed et al. 1973; McHenry et al. 1976).

Cardiac Catheterization. Focal ischemic events are uncommon (less than 1%) and may predominate in the posterior circulation. The differential diagnosis includes encephalopathy and seizures secondary to the contrast agents (Dawson and Fischer 1977).

Cardiac Surgery. Extensively and prospectively studied (Breuer 1980) the frequency of occurrence of cerebral ischemic events in cardiac surgery is approximately 5%, with major disability being present in only 2%. Many factors may contribute to the production of cerebral infarction. The frequency of occurrence may be higher for valvular surgery than myocardial revascularization.

Diagnostic Evaluation

The probability of a cardioembolic mechanism for stroke and the extent and nature of any subsequent evaluation is based upon the clinical neurologic and cardiologic assessments. The potential risk, benefit, and cost to the patient must be considered in planning a diagnostic evaluation. The studies selected should be those which are likely to yield diagnostic information and reduce the likelihood of more common or specifically treatable causes of brain ischemia. Diagnostic studies which involve some degree of risk or expense should not be performed routinely but should be selected for those patients in relatively good clinical condition in whom a management plan has not yet been established. In many patients, the findings obtained (either positive or negative) from performing additional diagnostic studies serve to demonstrate or document known or suspected cardiac pathology and will not alter management plans. Under these circumstances such studies appear to be marginally indicated.

General Medical Studies

Abnormalities found on initial studies including the ECG, chest X-ray, and hematologic/chemical studies may alert one to the underlying stroke mechanism, while normal results provide information about the patient's general health status. When appropriate, serial ECGs, cardiac enzymes, blood cultures, etc. should be obtained.

Neurodiagnostic Studies

Computed tomographic scanning (CT) is usually performed in patients with suspected CEBI. CT may suggest cardioembolism when multiple areas of infarction are demonstrated, especially when concentrated in the middle cerebral artery distribution. Hemorrhagic infarction on CT, although suggestive of an embolic cause, is uncommon and not specific; the majority of infarcts on CT are nonhemorrhagic and appear as regions of reduced attenuation.

The decision to proceed with cerebral angiography is an individual one which has been made even more difficult with the introduction of intravenous digital subtraction angiography (DSA). This relatively safe procedure usually affords satisfactory visualization of extracranial vessels and is capable of identifying atherosclerotic stenosis and occlusion. However, its ability to visualize and resolve details in the intracranial vessels is quite inferior to conventional angiography. The advantages provided by DSA must be balanced against the disadvantages of incomplete visualization of the intracranial vessels where two observations are of relevance: (1) studies performed 1 or 2 days postinfarction may show evidence of intraluminal clot, whereas angiography performed several days later may be normal, and (2) the majority of intracranial vascular occlusions, especially when seen in the middle cerebral artery distribution, are felt to be of embolic origin and their visualization should raise the suspicion of this mechanism (Gacs et al. 1982).

Cardiologic Studies

Several tests are now available which may afford information about altered cardiac anatomy and physiology and thereby provide additional inferential information about a potential cardioembolic mechanism.

Radionuclide angiocardiography (Kostuk et al. 1978) is a noninvasive method for visualizing and evaluating left ventricular wall function. Akinetic segments and aneurysms which may be associated with CEBI can be seen. It has been suggested that any patient with a past history of myocardial infarction who is experiencing cerebral or retinal ischemic events and on angiography lacks convincing evidence of significant cerebral vascular disease should be considered for radionuclide angiocardiography.

Long-term electrocardiographic (Holter) monitoring has been advocated as an additional procedure to be performed in patients with focal cerebral ischemia. Although there is still some disagreement about which types of cardiac arrhythmias are associated with systemic embolization, a recent study (Abdon et al. 1982) of 86 patients with focal cerebral ischemic events has shown that on long-term monitoring 44% (38/86) had permanent or episodic atrial arrhythmias of the type known to cause cerebral embolism, only 45% of which (17/38) were present in the resting ECG.

Two-dimensional echocardiography (2DE) is capable of demonstrating some cardiac lesions with embolic potential as well as the presence of intracardiac thrombus, and has been used extensively in the evaluation of patients with cerebral ischemia to detect occult cardiac sources of emboli in patients without evident heart disease and to verify anatomically an embolic source in those with known heart disease. Identification of thrombus is infrequent and the failure of 2DE to image thrombus does not rule out a cardioembolic source. A number of studies have shown that the yield of clinically useful information is low (Greenland et al. 1981; Larson et al. 1981; Bergerson and Shah 1981; Lovett et al. 1981) and that 2DE findings often are not influential in management decisions (Knopman 1982). 2DE is a useful procedure in patients with cerebral ischemia under the age of 45 when another diagnosis is not evident. In older patients 2DE is indicated only when there is no other cause for stroke evident and either the cardiac or neurologic features suggest a possible cardioembolic mechanism, and the information obtained confirming this suspicion will alter management plans.

Conclusions

The diagnosis of cardioembolic brain infarction is difficult. Clinical information and ancillary laboratory studies which serve to reduce the likelihood of other causative mechanisms and which demonstrate altered cardiac pathophysiology known to be associated with embolism increase the level of confidence with which such a diagnosis is made. Unfortunately in many cases, neither the clinical evaluation nor the available technology are sufficiently sensitive or specific to establish a certain diagnosis. Multiple mechanisms frequently coexist and the diagnosis of cardioembolic brain infarction continues to be based primarily upon the judgment and experience of the physician.

References

Abdon N, Zettervall O, Carlson J, Berglund S, Sterner G, Tejler L, Turesson I (1982) Is occult atrial disorder a frequent cause of non-hemorrhagic stroke? Long-term ECG in 86 patients. Stroke 13: 832–837

Adams GF, Merrett JD, Hutchinson WM, Pollack AM (1974) Cerebral embolism and mitral stenosis: survival with and without anticoagulants. J Neurol Neurosurg Psychiatr 37: 378–383

Barnett HJM (1982) Embolism in mitral valve prolapse. Ann Rev Med 33: 489–507

Bean WB (1938) Infarction of the heart. III. Clinical course and morphological findings. Ann Intern Med 12: 71–94

Bergerson GA, Shah PM (1981) Echocardiography unwarranted in patients with cerebral ishemic events. NEJM 304: 489

Breuer A (1982) Neurologic complications of heart disease. ANA Special Courses, Washington DC (syllabus)

Breuer AC, Furlan AJ, Hanson M, Lederman RJ, Loop FD, Cosgrove DU, Estafanous FG (1980) Central nervous system complications of myocardial revascularization: a prospective analysis of 400 patients. Stroke 11: 136

Dawson DM, Fischer EG (1977) Neurologic complications of cardiac catheterization. Neurology 27: 496–497

Donaldson RM, Emanuel RW, Earl CJ (1981) The role of two-dimensional echocardiography in the detection of potentially embolic intracardiac masses in patients with cerebral ischemia. J Neurol Neurosurg Psychiatr 44: 803–809

Easton JD, Sherman DG (1980) Management of cerebral embolism of cardiac origin. Stroke 11: 433–442

Gacs G, Merei FT, Bodosi M (1982) Balloon catheter as a model of cerebral emboli in humans. Stroke 13: 39–42

Greenland P, Knopman DS, Mikell FL (1981) Echocardiography in the diagnostic assessment of stroke. Ann Int Med 95: 51–53

Greenlee JE, Mandell GL (1973) Neurological manifestations of infective endocarditis: a review. Stroke 4: 948–963

Hinton RC, Kistler JP, Fallon JT, Friedlich AL, Fisher CM (1977) Influence of atrial fibrillation on incidence of systemic embolism. Am J Cardiol 40: 509–513

Jones HR, Siekert RG, Geraci JE (1969) Neurologic manifestations of bacterial endocarditis. Ann Int Med 71: 21–28

Jones HR, Caplan LR, Come PC, Swinton NR, Breslin D (1981) Paradoxical cerebral emboli: an occult cause of stroke. Ann Neurol 10: 105

Juergens JL, Edwards JE, Achor RWP, Burchell HB (1960) Prognosis of patients surviving first clinically diagnosed myocardial infarction. Arch Int Med 105: 444–450

Kloster FE (1979) Complications of artificial heart valves. JAMA 241: 2201–2203

Knopman DS, Anderson DC, Asinger RW, Greenland P, Mikell F, Good DC (1982) Indication for echocardiography in patients with ischemic stroke. Neurology 32: 1005–1011

Kookier JC, MacLean JM, Sumi SM (1976) Cerebral embolism, marantic endocarditis and cancer. Arch Neurol 33: 260–264

Kostuk WJ, Chamberlain MJ, Chin Sang H (1978) Radionuclide angiocardiography, a non-invasive method for evaluating left ventricular ejection fraction and regional wall motion; comparison with contrast left ventricular angiography. Can Med Ass J 119: 887–893

Larson EB, Stratton JR, Pearlman AS (1981) Selective use of two-dimensional echocardiography in stroke syndromes. Ann Int Med 95: 112–114

Lovett JR, Sandok BA, Giuliani ER, Nasser FN (1981) Two-dimensional echocardiography in patients with focal cerebral ischemia. Ann Int Med 95: 1–4

McHenry LC, Toole, JF, Miller HS (1976) Long-term ECG monitoring in patients with cerebrovascular insufficiency. Stroke 7: 264–269

Mohr J, Caplan LR, Melski JW, Goldstein RJ, Duncan GW, Kistler JP, Pessin MS, Bleich HL (1978) The Harvard Cooperative Stroke Registry: a prospective registry. Neurology 28: 754–762

Pruitt AA, Rubin RH, Karchmer AW, Duncan GW (1978) Neurologic complication of bacterial endocarditis. Medicine 57: 329–343

Reagan TJ, Okazaki H (1974) The thrombotic syndrome associated with carcinoma: a clinical and neuropathological study. Arch Neurol 31: 390–395

Reed RL, Siekert RG, Meredith J (1973) Rarity of transient focal cerebral ischemia in cardiac dysrhythmia. JAMA 223: 893–895

Sandok BA, Giuliani ER (1982) Cerebral ischemic events in patients with mitral valve prolapse. Stroke 13: 448–450

Sandok BA, von Estoroff I, Giuliani ER (1980) CNS embolism due to atrial myxoma: clinical features and diagnosis. Arch Neurol 37: 485–488

Segal JP, Stapleton FF, McClellan JR, et al. (1978) Idiopathic cardiomyopathy: clinical features, prognosis and therapy. In: Harvey WP (ed) Current problems in cardiology. Yearbook Medical Publishers, Chicago, pp 1–49

Szekely P (1964) Systemic embolism and anticoagulant prophylaxis in rheumatic heart disease. Br Med J 1: 1208–1212

Thompson PL, Robinson JS (1978) Stroke after acute myocardial infarction: relation to infarct size. Br Med J 2: 457–459

Weily HS, Steele PP, Davies H, Pappas G, Genton E (1974) Platelet survival in patients with substitute heart valves. NEJM 290: 534–537

Wolf PA, Dawber TR, Kannel WB (1978) Heart disease as a precursor of stroke. Adv Neurol 19: 567–577, Raven, New York

Wolf PA, Dawber TJ, Thomas HE Jr, Kannel WB (1978) Epidemiologic assessment of chronic atrial fibrillation and stroke. The Framingham Study. Neurology 28: 973–977

Chapter 4

Cardioembolic Sources of Stroke

E. D. Salgado, A. J. Furlan, and J. P. Conomy

Although the incidence of ischemic stroke has been declining in recent years, the proportion of such events attributed to cardiogenic causes has increased. This is in part due to the introduction and development of noninvasive diagnostic modalities (e.g., echocardiography, prolonged cardiac monitoring, radionuclide left ventricular cardiography, and magnetic resonance imaging) which have allowed us to better detect cardioembolic sources. Although there are obvious difficulties in attribution, it is estimated that 20% of ischemic strokes are related to cardiac emboli (Mohr et al. 1978).

Generally speaking, factors that promote stasis, turbulence, and low flow in the left side of the heart will lead to thrombosis and embolism. Disorders of cardiac rhythm, valves, and walls may either singly or in combination give rise to brain emboli.

Disorders of Cardiac Rhythm

Nonvalvular Atrial Fibrillation

The prevalence of nonvalvular atrial fibrillation (NVAF) increases with age. Population studies have estimated the prevalence to be 2%–5% over age 60 (Hart et al. 1983; Kannel et al. 1982). Fifteen percent of ischemic strokes occur in patients with atrial fibrillation (Mohr et al. 1978) and perhaps 70% of these are cardioembolic (Hart et al. 1983a; Wolf et al 1978). High prevalence and emboligenic potential make atrial fibrillation the leading cardioembolic source of stroke.

Most patients with NVAF have intrinsic heart disease (e.g., hypertensive, ischemic, rheumatic, cardiomyopathic). While all NVAF patients have a sixfold increase in stroke risk as compared with the general population (Wolf et al. 1978), even the smaller subgroup with "isolated" atrial fibrillation has a fourfold increased risk of stroke as compared with similar age and sex-matched controls (Brand et al. 1985).

Blood stasis within the left atrium results from decreased ability to pump blood into the ventricle combined with increased atrial pressure, both of which promote thrombus formation. Damage to the atrial endocardium from ischemic or rheumatic valve disease may also be a contributing factor.

Echocardiography may fail to detect smaller clots, particularly those in the auricular appendage where they are most frequently found at autopsy. Intracardiac thrombi may not be detected even at autopsy for a variety of reasons including autopsy technique, previous embolization, and spontaneous dissolution of clot.

Embolism tends to be more frequent in the first weeks or months following the onset of the dysrhythmia (Wolf et al. 1983). Recurrent embolism tends to occur early as well (Kelley et al. 1984; Hart et al. 1983a; Wolf et al. 1983). Chronic atrial fibrillation is frequently preceded by paroxysmal atrial fibrillation, which may further increase stroke risk due to the abrupt change in rhythm leading to dislodgment of left atrial thrombus. Clinical evidence to support this hypothesis comes from the known 3%–6% risk of stroke following electrical cardioversion in patients with atrial fibrillation (Turner et al. 1965; Bjerkelund et al. 1969). Furthermore, initial thrombus is more friable and disorganized, which may further enhance embolic potential.

Recent evidence suggests that embolism from atrial fibrillation is more likely to produce strokes and prolonged transient ischemic attacks (TIAs) (greater than 60 min) than embolism from atherosclerotic carotid lesions (Harrison et al. 1984).

Sick Sinus Syndrome

Sinoatrial dysfunction may lead to episodes of sinus bradycardia, atrial fibrillation, or alternating episodes of bradycardia and supraventricular tachycardia ("bradytachy" syndrome). Ischemic, hypertensive, and rheumatic heart disease are the most common causes of sick sinus syndrome (SSS). Less common causes include limb-girdle dystrophy, myotonic dystrophy, and Friedrich's ataxia.

The clinical manifestations are most commonly the result of decreased cardiac output leading to global brain hypoperfusion and complaints of dizziness and syncope (Fairfax et al. 1976; Rubinstein et al. 1976; Wan et al. 1972). Focal neurological deficits are rare and more likely to result from the concomitant occurrence of atherosclerosis than from embolism (Samarasinghe et al. 1973; Fairfax et al. 1976a). Whether embolism in SSS is a result of transient atrial fibrillation, abrupt changes of rhythm, or other mechanism remains to be clarified.

"Benign" Cardiac Dysrhythmias

We suspect that "benign" dysrhythmias in the presence of a thrombogenic valve surface may help to unleash embolic material. For example, nearly half of our patients with prolapsed mitral valve and an ischemic event had a dysrhythmia on prolonged monitoring (multiple premature contractions, short runs of supraventricular tachycardia).

Disorders of Cardiac Valves

Rheumatic Heart Disease

Approximately 1% of the adult population in the United States has rheumatic heart disease (RHD). The incidence and mortality rates of RHD have dramatically declined over the past century largely due to the development and use of antimicrobial agents as well as general improvement in socioeconomic conditions.

Rheumatic heart disease probably results from hypersensitization of cardiac tissue following group A streptoccocal infection. While a pancarditis typically occurs, valvulitis has the greatest clinical importance. The mitral valve is most commonly involved and appears fibrosed and deformed. Verrucae are common along cusp borders and calcification may be superimposed. Mitral stenosis with various degrees of regurgitation, increased left atrial pressure, atrial dilatation, atrial fibrillation, and heart failure are the pathophysiological consequences.

Embolism is a significant cause of morbidity and mortality. At least 20% of RHD patients will suffer systemic emboli, most involving the brain (Abernathy et al. 1973). Most emboli originate from clot in the left atrium, although clot and calcific material from the mitral valve itself may also embolize. The aortic valve may also be diseased but it is much less likely to cause embolism. Rheumatic mitral stenosis carries a 3%–4%/year incidence of embolism (Coulshed et al. 1970).

Several factors have been associated with the formation of left atrial thrombus in RHD: atrial fibrillation, age, severity of mitral stenosis, and heart failure (Abernathy et al. 1973). However, the risk of embolism is not as clearly related to the severity of mitral stenosis, perhaps because a significantly decreased mitral aperture cross-sectional area limits clot from traversing through. Other factors mentioned above are better associated with embolism (Abernathy et al. 1973; Coulshed et al. 1970). Atrial fibrillation, in particular, enhances stroke risk 17-fold (Wolf et al. 1978).

The sensitivity of two-dimensional echocardiography for detecting left atrial thrombus in RHD is about 60% while specificity is close to 100% (Shrestha et al. 1983). Many undetectable thrombi may be found within the atrial appendage at autopsy or during open heart surgery.

Infective Endocarditis

Infectious endocarditis is relatively rare in the general population. However, the proportion of cases due to virulent pathogens has increased in recent years, and nervous system complications are more common in this group. Indeed, neurological complaints not uncommonly prompt the patient to seek medical attention early in the course of the illness.

The common substrates associated with bacterial endocarditis are rheumatic valvular heart disease and congenital cardiac and valvular abnormalities. The mitral valve is affected most often, the aortic valve next, and a combination of the two is third. In the recent era, nosocomial infections, prosthetic heart valves

(Fig. 4.1), drug abuse, and intravenous hyperalimentation have all been associated with infective endocarditis particularly when superimposed upon normal cardiac valves.

Valvular vegetations consist of platelets and fibrin or fibrinoid material attached to damaged endothelium or prosthetic valves and harbor infecting organisms which cause further endocardial destruction (Fig. 4.2). The more virulent organisms (i.e., *Staphylococus aureus*, enteric gram-negative bacilli, fungi) tend to produce larger and more friable vegetations.

Embolic cerebral infarction is the most common neurological complication of infectious endocarditis, occurring in approximately 15% of patients (Pruitt et al. 1978; Jones et al. 1969). Another embolic complication is mycotic aneurysm formation, which occurs in approximately 5% of patients (Roach et al. 1965). Mycotic aneurysms are thought to result from vasa vasorum involvement with infective organisms (Molinari et al. 1973). Mycotic aneurysms are frequently multiple and tend to occur in distal branches of the middle cerebral artery; their most feared consequence is a fatal intracranial hemorrhage.

Embolism occurs more frequently in patients with clinical evidence of mitral valve disease (Pruitt et al. 1978). The more virulent organisms increase the risk of embolism, which also tends to occur earlier in the course of the illness. Late embolism (after 3 months) is relatively rare. Brain embolism may carry a mortality rate as high as 80% (Pruitt et al. 1978).

Two-dimensional echocardiography is more sensitive than M-mode in detecting vegetations (Martin et al. 1980). Sensitivity approaches 90% (Stafford et al. 1965). Morbidity and mortality have been related to the presence of vegetations on echocardiography (Stafford et al. 1985; Come et al. 1982).

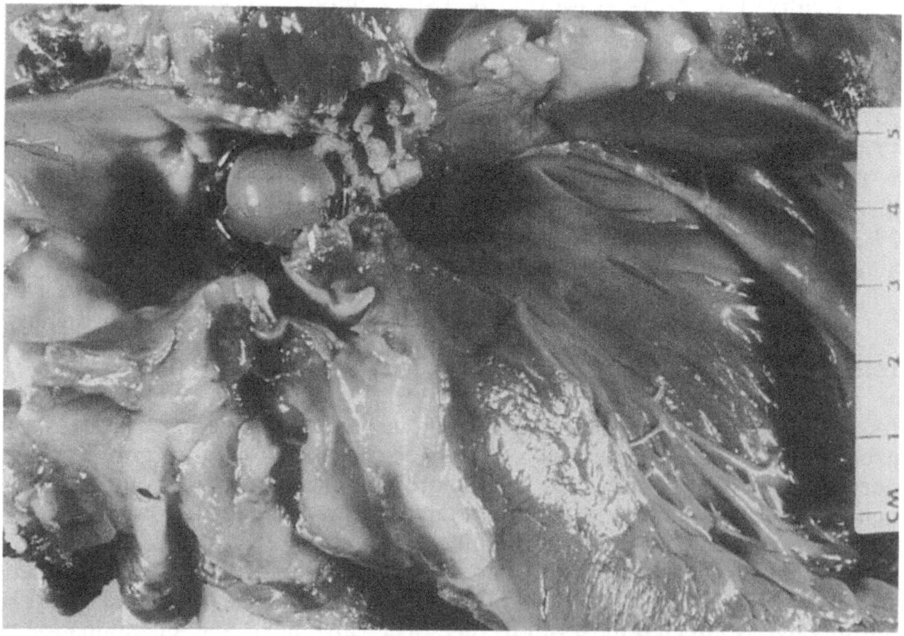

Fig. 4.1. Prosthetic valve endocarditis. (Courtesy of Dr. N. B. Ratliff, Jr.)

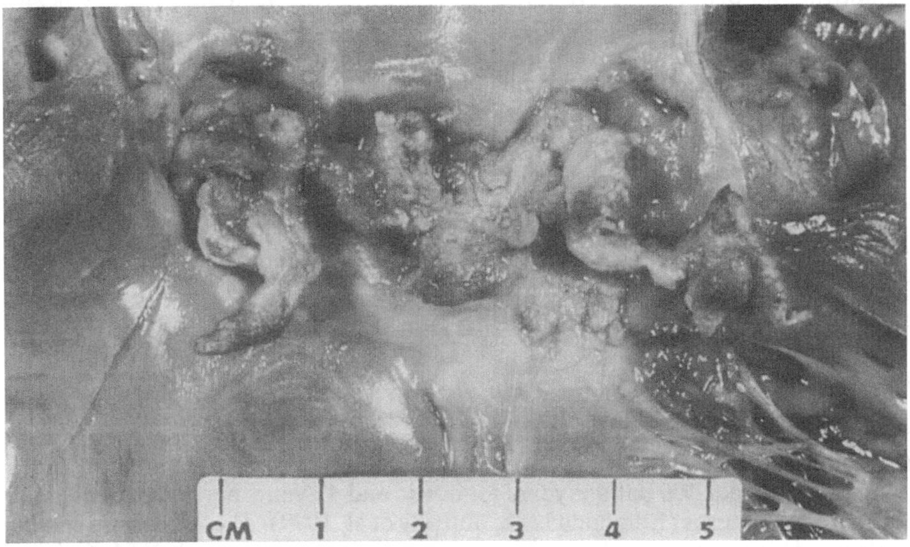

Fig. 4.2. Native aortic valve endocarditis. (Courtesy of Dr N. B. Ratliff, Jr.)

Nonbacterial Thrombotic Endocarditis

Nonbacterial thrombotic endocarditis (NBTE) is found in about 1.5% of all autopsies (Deppioch et al. 1976). NBTE is most common in patients with debilitating diseases, particularly those with adenocarcinomas of the lung and gastrointestinal tract. For some it may be the first manifestation of malignancy (Biller et al. 1982; Kooiker et al. 1976; Bryan et al. 1969). Most commonly, however, the clinical manifestations of NBTE occur in the setting of known disseminated carcinoma.

Along with disseminated intravascular coagulation (DIC), NBTE constitutes the most frequent cause of symptomatic brain infarction in cancer patients, regardless of the concomitant occurrence of atherosclerotic risk factors (Graus et al. 1985; Rogers et al. 1981). Infarction in NBTE results from embolic arterial occlusion by fibrin/platelet material originating from sterile, small (usually less than 5 mm) vegetations on the surface of the mitral and/or aortic valves (Deppisch et al. 1976). The pathogenesis of these vegetations is poorly understood but various factors acting either singly or in combination may be responsible. These include cardiac valvular deformation or degeneration (MacDonald et al. 1957), the mucin by-product of adenocarcinomas (Min et al. 1980), and a hypercoagulable state that is relatively common in cancer patients (Rickles et al. 1983).

The common clinical presentation is that of a patient with disseminated adenocarcinoma of the lung who develops an acute focal neurological deficit which may or may not be accompanied by a diffuse encephalopathy. Emboli are seldom restricted to the brain and may involve the heart, viscera, and extremities (Graus et al. 1985). Cardiac murmurs are often absent due to the small size of the vegetations and subsequent relative lack of intracardiac hemodynamic disturbance (Biller et al. 1982). Echocardiography is typically unrevealing for the same reasons.

Measurable coagulation parameters in NBTE are seldom useful for diagnosis as there are no characteristic abnormalities (Graus et al. 1985; Biller et al. 1982). DIC may coexist with NBTE. However, full laboratory support for DIC will often be lacking.

Although heparin has been used, there is currently no satisfactory treatment to prevent the embolic consequences of NBTE.

Prosthetic Valves

Mechanical Prostheses

Generally speaking, mechanical valves carry a higher risk of thromboembolism than bioprostheses. The risk is lowered substantially with anticoagulation and is about 2 events per 100 patient years for aortic and 4 events per 100 patient years for mitral prostheses (Edmunds 1981; Murphy et al. 1979). These rates are similar to those of bioprosthetic valves without anticoagulation (Edmunds 1981; Cohn et al. 1978).

The greater thromboembolic risk of mechanical valves is related to the inherent thrombogenic potential of the materials used as well as the mechanical disturbance of laminar flow. Plasma beta-thromboglobulin and platelet factor 4, both products of the platelet release reaction, are elevated in patients with mechanical valves indicating increased platelet activation (Pumphrey et al. 1981; Dudczak et al. 1980). Platelet survival is also shortened and has been correlated with an increased incidence of thromboembolic events (Weily et al. 1974). Flow velocity studies have demonstrated turbulent flow which contributes to stasis of blood in and around mechanical valves thereby enhancing thrombogenicity (Barnhorst et al. 1975). The newer mechanical valves have diminished the effects of some if not all of these factors.

Bioprostheses

These are usually of porcine or bovine origin. Early thrombosis has been noted in the left atrium or around the sewing ring of the bioprosthestic mitral valves before lining by neointima has occurred.

Bioprostheses alone are less likely to cause thrombus formation as a concurrent relationship has been found with a large left atrial size, atrial fibrillation, and low-output state. Late thrombus has been noted in the cusp sinuses instead of the valve ring in patients who eventually develop mitral stenosis as a result of fibrosis and calcification (Thiene et al. 1980). Electron micrographs of degenerated valves have revealed denuded areas of endothelium with exposed basement membrane and subendothelial fibers as well as deposition of platelet-fibrin material which may also enhance embolic potential (Riddle et al. 1981).

Multiple factors have decreased the thromboembolic risk of prosthetic valves over the years: innovations in valve design, the use of bioprostheses, improvement of surgical technique, better patient selection and postoperative management, and particularly the use of anticoagulants in therapeutic doses. Atrial fibrillation is the single most important associated condition leading to thromboembolism especially in those patients who are not anticoagulated (Geha et al. 1982; Jamieson et al. 1981). Other potential risk factors include large atrial size, left atrial thrombus, prior history of emboli, congestive heart failure, and the first few postoperative months.

Disorders of Cardiac Walls

Myocardial Infarction

Stroke occurs in 2%–3% of patients after acute myocardial infarction (MI) (Komrad et al. 1984; Thompson et al. 1978). About 85% will occur within the 1st month (Komrad et al. 1984; Bean et al. 1938). Sometimes an underlying "silent" MI will be found in the course of investigation of an acute stroke. The majority of these patients fail to have any symptoms or signs of myocardial ischemia or infarction (Chin et al. 1977). When stroke complicates MI, mortality is significantly increased, with a 1-year mortality rate of about 70% (Komrad et al. 1984; Chin 1982).

Patients with a prior history of stroke and atrial arrhythmia are at increased risk for stroke after MI. Large transmural anterior or anterolateral wall infarction associated with low cardiac output also carries an increased stroke risk (Komrad et al. 1984; Thompson et al. 1978).

Thrombus formation is associated with apical dyskinesis which can be readily detected by two-dimensional (2-D) echocardiography. Indium-111 platelet scintigraphy can complement 2-D echocardiography by detecting mural thrombi that are small and actively incorporating platelets but that have been missed by 2-D echocardiography because of technical limitations (Ezekowitz et al. 1982). Forty-six percent of infarcts with apical dyskinesis develop overlying mural thrombus (Asinger et al. 1981) (Fig. 4.3). Mural thrombi formed within the first 2 weeks following infarction usually gradually decrease in size or completely resolve within months regardless of anticoagulant use (McEntee et al. 1981). Pedunculated, mobile thrombi that project into the left ventricular lumen may further predispose to embolism (Meltzer et al. 1984).

Left ventricular aneurysm formation may follow MI. Many aneurysms contain thrombus for months or even years whether or not oral anticoagulation is used. The long-term risk of embolism from ventricular aneurysm appears low (5%) but is greatest within the first few weeks after the MI (Reeder et al. 1981; Simpson et al. 1980). The reasons for the low incidence of late embolism from left ventricular aneurysms are probably related to the firm adherence of thrombus to the aneurysmal wall, the relatively small area of thrombus exposed to blood flow, and the loss of projectile force from the underlying damaged myocardium (Cabin et al. 1980).

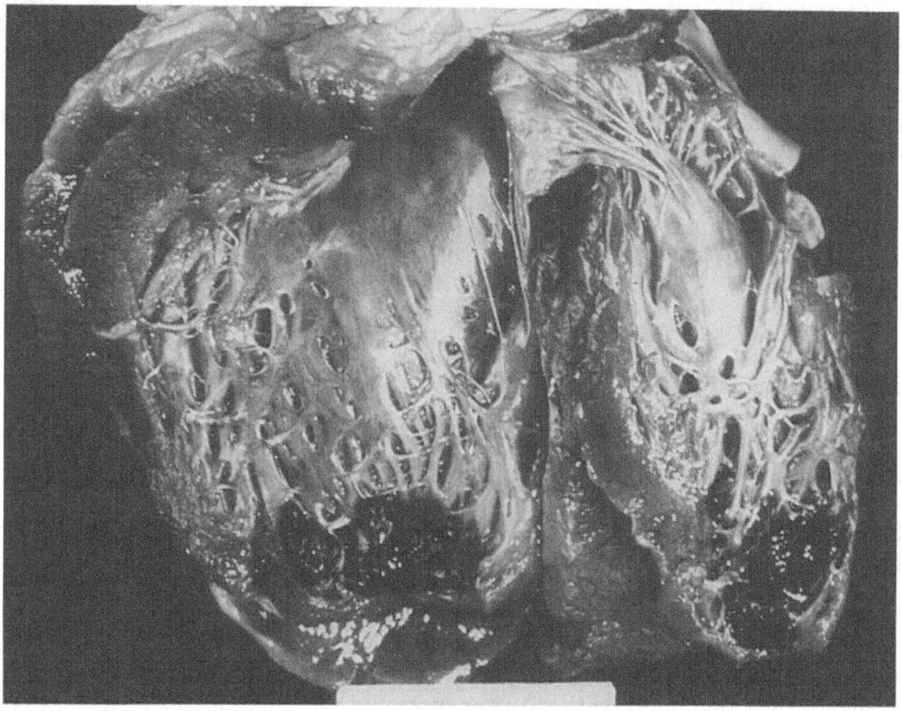

Fig. 4.3. Postmyocardial infarction apical mural thrombus. (Courtesy of Dr. H. Okazaki)

Cardiomyopathy

Brain embolism occurs in approximately 15% of patients with cardiomyopathy (Gottdiener et al. 1983; Fuster et al. 1981). Dilated and restrictive types have higher rates while the hypertrophic (idiopathic hypertrophic subaortic stenosis) type has a lower rate (Furlan et al. 1984; Fuster et al. 1981; Becker et al. 1953). Dilated and restrictive cardiomyopathies share certain characteristics which may predispose to embolism. These include increased left ventricular end-diastolic pressure, higher incidence of congestive heart failure, and increased incidence of mural thrombi. Atrial fibrillation is also more common in dilated cardiomyopathy than in the other two functional types.

Thrombogenicity can be enhanced by alteration of the left ventricular endocardium or wall motion as a result of infarction from coronary artery embolism. Intraluminal encroachment of the coronary arteries by amyloidosis or endomyocardial fibrosis can produce the same results (Rice et al. 1981).

Increased platelet activation has recently been reported in hypertrophic cardiomyopathy and may be a contributing factor in thromboembolic events (Longo et al. 1984).

Mural thrombi have been detected in up to 53% of autopsy cases of dilated cardiomyopathy (Roberts et al. 1974). However, embolism is not always correlated with the presence of thrombi on noninvasive studies (Gottdiener et al. 1983). Mural thrombi occur most frequently within the trabeculae carneae of the cardiac apex.

Paradoxical Emboli

Paradoxical emboli may be more common than previously believed. Most were not suspected during life and were found only at autopsy. A series of recent publications have increased awareness of this entity (Jones et al. 1983; Cheng 1976; Meister et al. 1972), and less invasive modalities have made diagnosis easier.

Paradoxical emboli are formed in the venous system and because of anomalous shunting of blood from the venous to the arterial side cause arterial embolism. The most frequent shunt occurs in the heart due to a patent foramen ovale or an atrial septal defect. Other cardiac structural anomalies have been less frequently implicated. Pulmonary arteriovenous fistulas as can occur with hereditary hemorrhagic telangiectasia may also serve as conduits for paradoxical emboli (Roman et al. 1978; Sisel et al. 1970).

A presumptive diagnosis can be made on the basis of (a) evidence of venous thrombosis (e.g., legs, pelvic plexus) or of pulmonary embolism, (b) right to left shunt, and (c) clinical evidence of systemic arterial embolism. Fifty percent of patients with pulmonary emboli may have no clinical evidence of deep venous thrombosis (Rosenow et al. 1981) and pulmonary embolism may occur with minimal or no symptoms. Therefore, paradoxical embolism must always be considered in any patient for whom there is no explanation for peripheral arterial embolism. It is not uncommon for emboli to travel to the coronary arteries, viscera, or limbs as well as brain in such patients. Predisposing factors included obesity, prolonged bed rest, anovulatory drugs, and malignancy (Jones et al. 1983).

Unsuspected patent foramen ovale is a common condition. A probe-patent foramen ovale was found in 35% of cases in a consecutive autopsy series (Thompson et al. 1930). While this anatomical variant alone is unlikely to result in shunting of blood, any condition that results in increased right atrial pressure can produce shunting (e.g., acute pulmonary embolism). Physiologically a valsalva maneuver will have the same effect.

Our ability to detect intracardiac shunting of blood has become much easier and safer with contrast echocardiography (Detrano et al. 1985; Higgins et al. 1984; Valdes-Cruz et al. 1976) (Fig. 4.4). Similar information can be obtained from indicator-dilution curves obtained after injecting Cardiogreen into the inferior vena cava or right heart and sampling from a systemic artery (Banas et al. 1971).

Cardiac Myxoma

Primary cardiac tumors are quite rare. Fifty percent are myxomas and 75% of these occur in the left atrium. The typical appearance of a cardiac myxoma is that of a pedunculated mass arising from the interatrial septum adjacent to the fossa ovalis. The tumor is gelatinous and friable and its histological appearance is rather benign. If it is large enough, left atrial outflow obstruction may result.

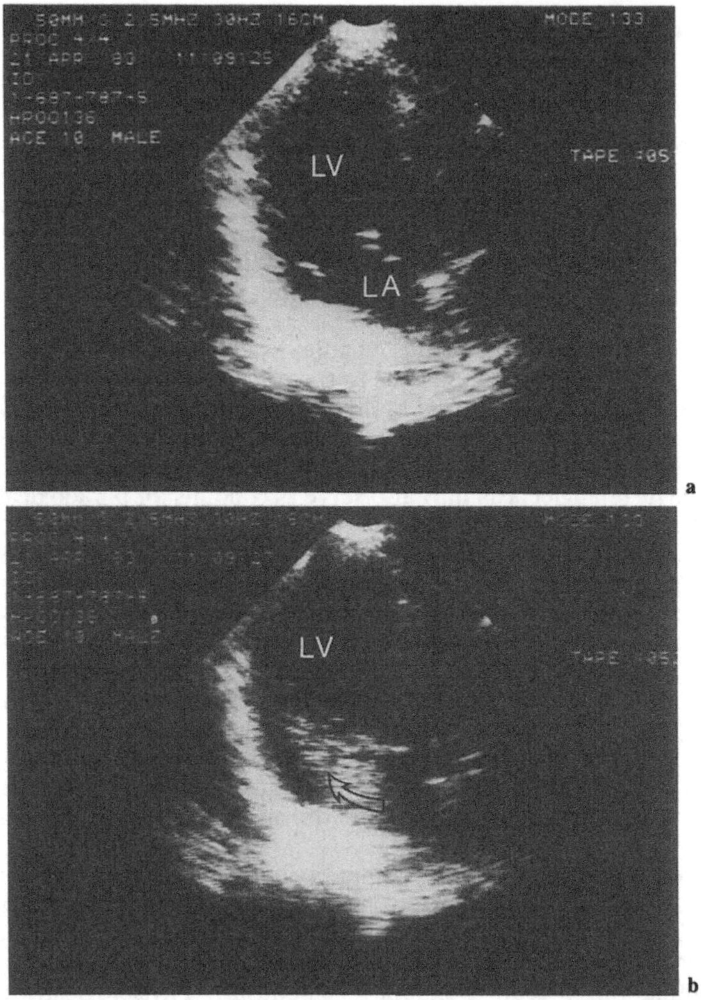

Fig. 4.4. a Apical two-chamber view in a patient with an atrial septal defect before arrival of contrast agent. **b** Same view after contrast agent has passed from the right to the left atrium. *LA*, left atrium; *LV*, left ventricle. (Detrano et al. 1985)

Systemic embolism occurs in 40% of cases and about half of these lodge in the brain (Sandok et al. 1980; Silverman et al. 1962). Emboli are of two types: platelet-fibrin and tumor fragments. The relative frequency with which each occurs is unknown but the latter has received more attention due to its potential invasive nature (Frank et al. 1979; Desousa et al. 1978; Price et al. 1970). Tumor emboli can invade cerebral vasculature giving rise to aneurysms, subarachnoid hemorrhage, intraparenchymal hemorrhage, or intraparenchymal metastatic deposits. Atrial fibrillation does not typically occur in these patients; hence its potential contribution to intraatrial thrombosis and embolism is negligible.

Patients most commonly present with symptoms secondary to cardiac outflow obstruction or constitutional symptoms (Sandok et al. 1980). Not infrequently, however, cerebral emboli may be the initial manifestation.

While 2-D echocardiography is the noninvasive diagnostic modality of choice in the diagnosis of cardiac myxoma, magnetic resonance imaging holds much promise (Go et al. 1985; Pflugfelder et al. 1984) (Fig. 4.5).

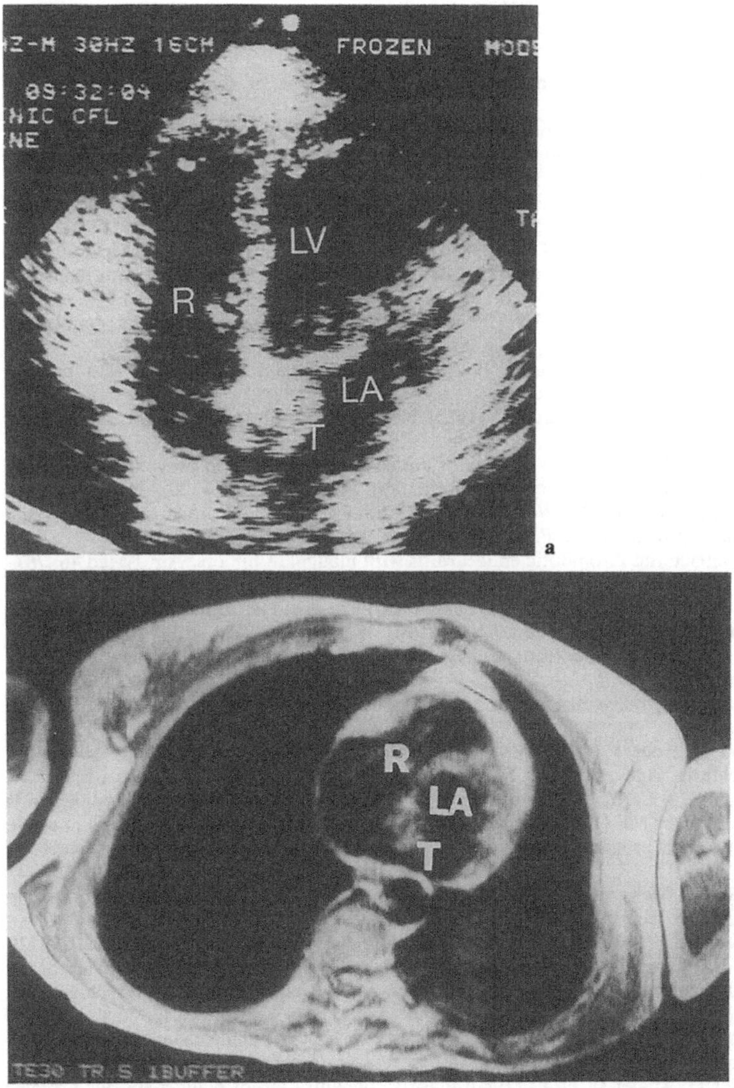

a

b

Fig. 4.5. Left atrial myxoma. **a** 2-D echocardiogram; **b** Spin-echo gated cardiac magnetic resonance image. *T*, tumor; *LA*, left atrium; *LV*, left ventricle; *R*, right heart chambers. (Courtesy of Dr. R. T. Go)

Other Cardioembolic Sources of Stroke

The more recently recognized cardioembolic sources of stroke, mitral valve prolapse, and mitral annulus calcification will be discussed in a separate chapter.

References

Abernathy WS, Willis PW (1973) Thromboembolic complications of rheumatic heart disease. Cardiovasc Clin 5: 131–175

Asinger RW, Mikell FL, Elsperger J, Hodges M (1981) Incidence of left ventricular thrombosis after acute transmural myocardial infarction: serial evaluation by two-dimensional echocardiography. N Engl J Med 305: 297–302

Banas JS, Meister SG, Gazzaniga AB, O'Connor NE, Haynes FW, Dalen JE (1971) A simple technique for detecting small defects of the atrial septum. Am J. Cardiol 28: 467–471

Barnhorst DA, Oxman HE, Connolly DC, Pluth JR, Danielson GK, Wallace RB, McGoon DW (1975) Long-term follow-up of isolated replacement of the aortic or mitral valve with the Starr-Edwards prosthesis. Am J Cardiol 35: 228–233

Bean WB (1938) Infarction of the heart. III. Clinical course and morphological findings. Ann Intern Med 12: 71–94

Becker BJP, Chatgidakis CB, van Lingen B (1953) Cardiovascular collagenosis with parietal endocardial thrombosis. Circulation 7: 345

Biller J, Challa VR, Toole JF, Howard VJ (1982) Nonbacterial thrombotic endocarditis. Arch Neurol 39: 95–98

Bjerkelung CJ, Orning OM (1969) The efficacy of anticoagulant therapy in preventing embolism related to D.C. electrical conversion of atrial fibrillation. Am J Cardiol 23: 208–216

Brand FN, Abbott RD, Kannel WB, Wolf PA (1985) Characteristics and prognosis of lone atrial fibrillation: 30-year follow-up in the Framingham study. JAMA 254(24): 3449–3453

Bryan CS (1969) Nonbacterial thrombotic endocarditis with malignant tumors. Am J Med 46: 787–793

Cabin HS, Roberts WC (1980) Left ventricular aneurysm, intra-aneurysmal thrombus and systemic embolus in coronary heart disease. Chest 77: 586–590

Cheng TO (1976) Paradoxical embolism: a diagnostic challenge and its detection during life. Circulation 53(3): 565–568

Chin PL (1982) Relationship between acute stroke and myocardial infarction in the elderly. IM 3(7): 45–52

Chin PL, Kaminski J, Rout J (1977) Myocardial infarction: coincident with cerebrovascular accidents in the elderly. Age and Aging 6: 29–37

Cohn LH, Collins JJ (1978) Cardiac valve replacement: tissue or prosthetic? Primary Cardiol, April

Come PC, Isaacs RE, Riley MF (1982) Diagnostic accuracy of M-mode echocardiography in active infective endocarditis and prognostic implications of ultrasound-detectable vegetations. Am Heart J 103: 839–847

Coulshed N, Epstein EJ, McKendrick CS, Galloway RW, Walker E (1970) Systemic embolism in mitral valve disease. Br Heart J 32: 26–34

Deppisch LM, Fayemi AO (1976) Nonbacterial thrombotic endocarditis. Am Heart J 92: 723–729

De Sousa AL, Muller J, Campbell RL, Batnitzky S, Rankin L (1978) Atrial myxoma: a review of the neurological complications, metastases, and recurrences. J Neurol Neurosurg Psychiatry 41: 1119–1124

Detrano R, Salcedo EE, Yiannikas J, Moodie DS (1985) Contrast two-dimensional echocardiography in the diagnosis of adult congenital heart disease. Cleve Clin Q 52: 229–238

Dudczak R, Niessner H, Thaler E, et al. (1980) Plasma concentration of platelet-specific proteins and fibrinopeptide A in patients with artificial heart valves. Haemostasis 10: 186–194

Edmunds LH (1981) Thromboembolic complications of current cardiac valvular prostheses. Ann Thorac Surg 34(1): 96–106

Ezekowitz MD, Wilson DA, Smith EO, Burow RD, Harrison LH, Parker DE, Elkins LRC, Peyton M, Taylor FB (1982) Comparison of indium-111 platelet scintigraphy and two-dimensional echocardiography in the diagnosis of left ventricular thrombi. N Engl J Med 306: 1509–1513

Fairfax AJ, Lambert CD (1976) Neurological aspects of sinoatrial heart blocks. J Neurol Neurosurg Psychiatry 39: 576–580

Fairfax AJ, Lambert CD, Leatham A (1976a) Systemic embolism in chronic sinoatrial disorders. N Engl J Med 295: 190–192

Frank RA, Shalen PR, Harvey DG, Berg L, Ferguson TB, Schwartz HG (1979) Atrial myxoma with intellectual decline and cerebral growths on CT scan. Ann Neurol 5: 396–400

Furlan AJ, Craciun AR, Raju NR, Hart N (1984) Cerebrovascular complications associated with idiopathic hypertrophic subaortic stenosis. Stroke 15(2): 282–284

Fuster V, Gersh BJ, Giuliani ER, Tajik AJ, Brandenburg RO, Frye RL (1981) The natural history of idiopathic dilated cardiomyopathy. Am J Cardiol 47: 525–531

Geha AS, Hammond GL, Laks H, Stansel HC, Glenn WWL (1982) Factors affecting performance and thromboembolism after porcine xenograft cardiac valve replacement. J Thorac Cardiovasc Surg 83: 377–384

Go RT, O'Donnell JK, Underwood DA, Feiglan DH, Salcedo EE, Pantoja M, MacIntyre WS, Meaney TF (1985) Comparison of gated cardiac MRI and 2D echocardiography of intracardiac neoplasms. AJR 145: 21–25

Gottdiener JS, Gay JA, Van Voorhees L, DiBianco R, Fletcher RD (1983) Frequency and embolic potential of left ventricular thrombus in dilated cardiomyopathy: Assessment by 2-dimensional echocardiography. Am J Cardiol 52: 1281–1285

Graus F, Rogers LR, Posner JB (1985) Cerebrovascular complications in patients with cancer. Medicine 64(1): 16–35

Harrison MJG, Marshall J (1984) Atrial fibrillation, TIAs and completed strokes. Stroke 15(3) 441–442

Hart RG, Sherman DG, Miller VT, Easton JD (1983) Diagnosis and management of ischemic stroke, part II. Selected controversies. Curr Probl Cardiol 8: 53–59

Hart RG, Coull BM, Hart D (1983a) Early recurrent embolism associated with nonvalvular atrial fibrillation: a retrospective study. Stroke 14(5): 688–693

Higgins JR, Strunk BL, Schiller NB (1984) Diagnosis of paradoxical embolism with contrast echocardiography. Am Heart J 107(2): 375–377

Jamieson WRE, Janusz MT, Miyagishima RT, Munro AI, Tutassura H, Gerein AN, Burr LH, Allen P (1981) Embolic complications of porcine heterograft cardiac valves. J Thorac Cardiovasc Surg 81: 626–631

Jones HR Jr, Caplan LR, Come PC, Swinton NW, Breslin DJ (1983) Cerebral emboli of paradoxical origin. Ann Neurol 13: 314–319

Jones HR Jr, Siekert RG, Geraci JE (1969) Neurologic manifestations of bacterial endocarditis. Ann Intern Med 71(1): 21–28

Kannel WB, Abbott RD, Savage DD, McNamara PM (1982) Epidemiologic features of chronic atrial fibrillation: the Framingham study. NEJM 306: 1018–1022

Kelley RE, Berger JR, Alter M, Kovacs AG (1984) Cerebral ischemia and atrial fibrillation: prospective study. Neurology 34: 1285–1291

Komrad MS, Coffey KS, McKinnis R, Massey EW, Califf RM (1984) Myocardial infarction and stroke. Neurology 34: 1403–1409

Kosiker JC, Maclean JM, Sumi SJ (1976) Cerebral embolism, marantic endocarditis and cancer. Arch Neurol 33: 260–264

Longo G, Cecchi F, Grossi A, Matucci M, Rafanelli D, Vannucchi AM, Casprini P, Vannini S, Morfini M, Dolara A (1984) Coagulation and platelet function in hypertrophic cardiomyopathy. Thromb Haemostas (Stuttgart) 51(2): 299

MacDonald RA, Robbins SL (1957) The significance of nonbacterial thrombotic endocarditis. An autopsy and clinical study of 78 cases. Ann Intern Med 46: 255–273

Martin RP, Meltzer RS, Chin BL, Stinson EB, Rakowski H, Popp RL (1980) Clinical utility of two-dimensional echocardiography in infective endocarditis. Am J Cardiol 46: 379–385

McEntee CW, Van Reet RE, Winters WL, Nelson JG, Waggoner AD, Miller RR, Quinones MA (1981) Incidence and natural history of mural thrombi in acute myocardial infarction by two-dimensional echocardiography. Circulation 64 (suppl IV): 93

Meister SG, Grossman W, Dexter L, Dalen JE (1972) Paradoxical embolism. Diagnosis during life. Am J Med 53: 292–298

Meltzer RS, Visser CA, Kan G, et al. (1984) Two-dimensional echocardiographic appearance of left ventricular thrombi with systemic emboli after myocardial infarction. Am J Cardiol 53: 1511–1513

Min KW, Gyorkey F, Satto C (1980) Mucin producing adenocarcinomas and nonbacterial thrombotic endocarditis: pathogenic role of tumor mucin. Cancer 45: 2374–2382

Mohr JP, Caplan LR, Melski JW, Goldstein RJ, Duncan GW, Kistler JP, Pessin MS, Bleich HL (1978) The Harvard Cooperative Stroke Registry: a prospective registry. Neurology 28: 754–762

Molinari GF, Amith L, Goldstein MN, Satran R (1973) Pathogenesis of cerebral myocotic aneurysms. Neurology 23: 325–332

Murphy ES, Kloster FE (1979) Late results of valve replacement surgery. II. Complications of prosthetic heart valves. Mod Concep Cardiovas Dis XLVIII (11): 59–66

Pflugfelder PW, Wisenberg G, Boughner DR (1985) Detection of atrial myxoma by magnetic resonance imaging. Am J Cardiol 55: 242–243

Price DL, Harris JL, New PFJ, Cantu RC (1970) Cardiac myxoma. A clinicopathologic and angiographic study. Arch Neurol 23: 558–567

Pruitt AA, Rubin RH, Karchmer AW, Duncan GW (1978) Neurologic complications of bacterial endocarditis. Medicine 57(4): 329–343

Pumphrey CW, Dawes J (1981) Elevation of plasma B-thromboglobulin in patients with prosthetic cardiac valves. Thromb Res 22: 147–155

Reeder GS, Lengyel M, Tajik AJ, Seward JB, Smith HC, Danielson GK (1981) Mural thrombus in left ventricular aneurysm. Incidence, role of angiography, and relation between anticoagulation and embolization. Mayo Clin Proc 56: 77–81

Rice GPA, Ebers GC, Newland F, Wysocki GP (1981) Recurrent cerebral embolism in cardiac amyloidosis. Neurology 31: 904–906

Rickles FR, Edwards RL, Barb C, Cronlund M (1982) Abnormalities of blood coagulation in patients with cancer. Cancer 51: 301–307

Riddle JM, Magilligan DJ Jr, Stein PD (1981) Surface morphology of degenerated porcine bioprosthetic valves four to seven years following implantation. J Thorac Cardiovasc Surg 81: 279–287

Roach MR, Drake CG (1965) Ruptured cerebral aneurysms caused by microorganisms. N Engl J Med 273: 240–244

Roberts WC, Ferrans VJ (1974) Pathological aspects of certain cardiomyopathies. Circulation Res 34/35 (suppl II): 128–144

Rogers LR, Chernik N, Posner JB (1981) Central nervous system vascular complications occurring in patients with cancer: changes within the past decade. Neurology 31(2): 44

Roman G, Fisher M, Perl DP, Poser CM (1978) Neurological manifestations of hereditary hemorrhagic telangiectasia (Rendu-Osler-Weber disease): report of 2 cases and review of the literature. Ann Neurol 4: 130–144

Rosenow EC III, Osmundson PJ, Brown ML (1981) Pulmonary embolism. Mayo Clin Proc 56: 161–178

Rubinstein JJ, Schulman CL, Yurchak PM, DeSanctis RW (1972) Clinical spectrum of the sick sinus syndrome. Circulation 46: 5–13

Samarasinghe HHR, Senanayake N (1973) Permanent neurologic deficits complicating sinoatrial block. Br Heart J 35: 503–506

Sandok BA, von Estorff I, Giuliani E (1980) CNS embolism due to atrial myxoma. Clinical features and diagnosis. Arch Neurol 37: 485–488

Shrestha NK, Moreno FL, Narciso FV, Torres L, Calleja HB (1983) Two-dimensional echocardiographic diagnosis of left atrial thrombus in rheumatic heart disease: a clinico-pathologic study. Circulation 67(2): 341–347

Silverman J, Olwin JS, Graethinger JS (1962) Cardiac myxomas with systemic embolization: review of the literature and report of a case. Circulation 26: 99–103

Simpson MT, Oberman A, Kouchoukos NT, Rogers WJ (1980) Prevalence of mural thrombi and systemic embolization with left ventricular aneurysm: effect of anticoagulation therapy. Chest 77: 463–469

Sisel RJ, Parker BM, Bahl OP (1970) Cerebral symptoms in pulmonary arteriovenous fistula: a result of paradoxical emboli (?). Circulation XLI: 123–128

Stafford WJ, Petch J, Radford DJ (1985) Vegetations in infective endocarditis: clinical relevance and diagnosis by cross-sectional echocardiography. Br Heart J 53: 310–313

Thiene G, Bortolotti U, Panizzon G, Miland A, Gallucci V (1980) Pathological substrates of thrombus formation after heart valve replacement with the Hancock bioprosthesis. J Thorac Cardiovasc Surg 80: 414–423

Thompson PL, Robinson JS (1978) Stroke after acute myocardial infarction: relation to infarct size. Br Med J 2: 457–459

Thompson T, Evans W (1930) Paradoxical embolism. Q J Med 23: 135–150

Turner JRB, Towers JRH (1965) Complications of cardioversion. Lancet 2: 612–614
Valdés-Cruz LM, Pieroni DR, Roland JMA, Varghese PJ (1976) Echocardiographic detection of intracardiac right-to-left shunts following peripheral vein injections. Circulation 54(4): 558–562
Wan SH, Lee GS, Toh CS (1972) The sick sinus syndrome. Br Heart J 34: 942–952
Weily HS, Steele PP, Davies H, Pappas G, Genton E (1974) Platelet survival in patients with substitute heart valves. N Engl J Med 290: 534–537
Wolf PA, Kannel WB, McGee DL, et al. (1983) Duration of atrial fibrillation and imminence of stroke: the Framingham study. Stroke 14(5): 664–667
Wolf PA, Dawber TR, Thomas HE, et al. (1978) Epidemiologic assessment of chronic atrial fibrillation and risk of stroke: the Framingham study. Neurology 28: 973–977

Chapter 5

Cerebral Ischemia with Mitral Valve Prolapse and Mitral Annulus Calcification

S. Lauzier and H. J. M. Barnett

Mitral Valve Prolapse

Historical Review

For more than a century, the mid-systolic click and late systolic murmur were thought to be innocent and extracardiac in origin. In 1913, Gallaverdin felt that a mid-systolic click was produced by pericardial adhesions causing traction on the myocardium during systole. The recognition of a valvular origin for the mid-systolic clicks and late systolic murmurs was first postulated by Reid in 1961 and confirmed by Barlow in 1963. They demonstrated phonocardiographic and angiographic evidence substantiating the association between these abnormal sounds and the ballooning or prolapsing of the mitral valve.

The multiple designations applied to the condition over the years underline the confusion and also the disagreement concerning the etiology and pathogenesis of this syndrome: floppy mitral valve, myxomatous degeneration of the mitral valve, ballooning mitral valve, redundant cusp syndrome, systolic click-murmur syndrome, Barlow syndrome, and finally mitral valve prolapse, which is today's most common nomenclature.

Prevalence and Distribution in the Population

Mitral valve prolapse (MVP) remains the most frequently diagnosed valvular cardiac abnormality. The prevalence figures vary widely, depending on the definition provided, whether by auscultation, echocardiography, or necropsy, and on the population selected, be it an unselected group or a clearly defined subgroup.

The prevalence of mitral valve prolapse ranges from 5% to more than 15% in the normal adult population. There is a slight preponderance of females, with a sex ratio prevalence of 6.5 females for 5 males (Jeresaty 1979). It is generally estimated that the prevalence of MVP in an otherwise healthy young female population varies from 6% to 17% (Procacci et al. 1976; Markiewicz et al. 1976) and in otherwise healthy young males from 4% to 7% (Sbarbaro et al. 1979; Hickey et al. 1980). MVP appears to occur in all races and all Caucasian groups. Its prevalence occurs at least as frequently in randomly selected populations of blacks (Savage et al. 1982)

With the renewed interest in MVP, we are now confronted with a multitude of epidemiologic studies, most of them biased by nonrandom subgroup selection (Table 5.1). However, in a large prospective survey of 4967 randomly selected cases, the Framingham Study (Savage et al. 1983) has identified an echocardiographic prevalence of MVP of 5% in the general population, 7% in the young population, and 3% in the elderly population. This study demonstrated a decline in the occurrence of MVP in older females: 17% in those in the 20s, 12.2% in the 40s, 7.5% in the 50s, and 1.4% in the 80s. A similar decline was not observed among the male population. The figure obtained ranged between 2% and 4% from the 2nd to 8th decades. The Framingham Study concluded that MVP was present in a significantly higher proportion of young females than among older females or males. This decreased prevalence in older patients was attributed to a tendency of the prolapsed mitral leaflets to become fibrotic, scarred, and less mobile after prolonged exposure to abnormal stress and, therefore, leading to a reduced degree of valvular prolapse in older people.

Table 5.1. Prevalence of mitral valve prolapse

	Population	Age	Phono	Echo (M-mode)	Necropsy
Framingham (1983)	4967 unselected general population	57		5%	
Markiewicz (1976)	100 healthy young women	17–35	17%	21%	
Procacci (1976)	1169 healthy young women		6.3%		
Rizzon (1973)	1009 female students	14–18	0.33%		
Lachman (1975)	12 500 South African School Children		1.4%		
Brown (1975)	520 women	17–40		6%	
	180 men	17–30		0.5%	
Chandraratna (1979)	100 newborn baby girls		3%	7%	
Sbabaro (1979)	100 male students	26	0%	4%	
Davies (1978)	1984 consecutive routine autopsies	50			0.6%
		70			6.3%
Lucas (1982)	1376 routine autopsies				7.4%
Barnett (1980)	60 controls	33		6.8%	
	141 controls	63		7.1%	

Three major necropsy studies carried out by Pomerance (1967), Hill et al. (1974), and Davies et al. (1978) concluded that the frequency of MVP in autopsy specimens increases progressively with age, reaching a plateau of 5.5% from the 7th through the 9th decades. In the Davies et al. study (1978), the prevalence of MVP was 0.6% for patients under 50 and 6.3% for patients over 70 years. This conflicts with the community surveys and clinical experience; according to this postmortem study, the less florid valvular changes seen in younger patients (isolated nonejection systolic click without murmur) may not be readily recognizable at autopsy.

Pathology

The anatomic substratum of the mitral leaflet prolapse is extremely variable. The amount of valvular involvement varies from a single posterior leaflet scallop to the entire valve, including its supporting chordae tendinae and the annulus itself. Prolapse is limited to the posterior leaflet in roughly 65% of patients and affects both leaflets in 25% of cases (Davies et al. 1978).

The prolapsed mitral valve is characterized by a significant thickening of the spongiosa layer which extends and replaces part of the fibrosa, resulting in loss of fibrous tissue. As a consequence of this loss of integrity, the leaflets become stretched and elongated. The basic pathologic process is a collagen disruption with primary infiltration by myxomatous material. In the central spongiosa and in the fibrosa encroached upon, there is a fragmentation of collagen bundles with disruption of the fibers associated with a proliferation of myxomatous tissue, rich in acid mucopolysaccharide. The chordae tendinae and the annulus may have deposits of the myxomatous material leading to chordal elongation and secondary rupture as well as dilatation of the mitral annulus (Cheitlin and Byrd 1984).

Davies et al. (1978) observed in their impressive series of 2000 floppy mitral valves obtained at autopsy or from surgical material a twofold increase in cross-linked procollagen and single-chain collagen. This accumulation of procollagen suggested a block in the synthesis of collagen at the level of the enzyme procollagen peptidase. The main issue of that observation, still strongly debated, is whether this represents a collagen *dissolution* as a result of chronic leaflet wear and tear or whether there is an initiating structural fault or collagen *dysgenesis*. In summary, a collagen abnormality of unknown etiology involving the pars fibrosa and the chordae tendinae appears to be the basic pathologic process responsible for the ballooning, billowing, and prolapsing mitral valve.

Several secondary changes related to abnormal mitral valve leaflet motion have been described (Lucas and Edwards 1982; Devereux and Brown 1983). One of these changes consists of a fibrosis and secondary thickening of the endocardial surfaces of the mitral leaflets. Presumably this is due to repeated trauma from the enlarged leaflets striking forcefully against each other and against the atrial and ventricular walls, resulting in a rigid and opaque valvular aspect. The chordae tendinae may undergo similar changes, becoming either elongated and attenuated and therefore prone to rupture or thickened and fibrotic. Also left ventricular friction lesions parallel to contiguous chordae have been observed resulting from friction between the chordae and the left ventricular wall. These fibrous patches sometimes result in entrapment of the chordae and might provide a nidus for the thrombus formation. Marked dilatation of the mitral annulus occurs, especially in patients having significant mitral regurgitation due to mitral prolapse.

Patients with mitral valve prolapse often demonstrate an associated prolapse of other cardiac valves. The tricuspid valve is the most frequently involved, sustaining some degree of prolapse in 25%–70% of patients with MVP (Lucas and Edwards 1982; Pomerance 1969; Morganroth et al. 1981; Davies et al. 1978). The aortic valve is variably affected in 3%–20% of the cases (Lucas and Edwards 1982; Morganroth et al. 1981; Beton et al. 1983; Davies et al. 1978).

Clinical Picture

Mitral valve prolapse is a common but variable syndrome occurring from early childhood to advanced years. However, clinical recognition is most common in the 3rd through 5th decades and two-thirds of the subjects are female. The sex distribution appears to be more equal in middle age and older life. Frequently patients complain of vague but occasionally disabling symptoms of angina or nonanginal chest pain, palpitations, syncope, dyspnea, and a high level of anxiety.

According to the Framingham survey, the cardiovascular symptoms are not more frequent in patients with MVP than among apparently healthy individuals, with the exception of complaints of palpitation, which are significantly more common in MVP patients (Savage et al. 1983).

The majority of patients with chest pain related to MVP experience an atypical nonischemic chest discomfort of musculoskeletal origin. This chest discomfort is often reproduced by pressure on or movement of the chest wall and it includes atypical features such as the length of time it lasts or unusual precipitating factors (Cheitlin and Byrd 1984). However, in a minority of patients, the discomfort is characteristic of angina, accounting for the unsettled problem of the relationship between MVP and coronary artery disease. MVP has been described as a direct result of coronary artery disease, i.e., left ventricular dysfunction induced by coronary insufficiency leads to a poor support of the mitral apparatus, so-called papillary muscle dysfunction. Steelman et al. (1971) and Crawford (1977), in their respective series, described the development of a typical nonejection click-late systolic murmur after the occurrence of symptomatic ischemic heart disease or myocardial infarction. However, the development of myocardial infarction in young patients with MVP and normal coronary arteriogram favors the fact that myocardial ischemia may be induced by MVP (Chesler et al. 1976; Imaizumi et al. 1978). Natarajan et. al (1975) observed the production of myocardial lactate during atrial pacing in 30% of 23 patients with MVP and chest pain. Several mechanisms have been suggested to explain this secondary myocardial ischemia: (1) small thrombus formation in mitral leaflet prolapse with secondary coronary emboli, (2) thrombus formation on a small plaque of the coronary artery with subsequent thrombolysis, (3) coronary artery spasm (Chesler et al. 1976; Buda et al. 1978), (4) increased myocardial tension associated with traction on the papillary muscles and on the left ventricular wall due to the prolapsing valve (Devereux et al. 1976; Le Winter et al. 1974), and (5) sympathetic overactivity and increased catecholamine levels and/or altered sensitivity to these amines (Abinader and Shahar 1982). But despite many reports of coexisting coronary artery disease and MVP, the prevalence of such an association remains unknown. The high prevalence in the population of coronary artery disease as well as mitral valve prolapse suggests that, many times, they are coincidental findings. The Framingham group confirmed that the prevalence of overt ischemic heart disease is nearly identical in subjects with MVP as compared with those without MVP.

Approximately half of the subjects with MVP complain of palpitations (Gooch et al. 1972). In general, there is a lack of correlation between symptoms and recorded arrhythmias (Winkle et al. 1975). All types of arrhythmias have been observed in mitral valve prolapse patients including atrial and ventricular ectopic beats and tachyarrhythmias, accelerated atrioventricular conduction, sinoatrial arrhythmias, and atrioventricular blocks of varying degree. The most frequent arrhythmia is ventricular premature contraction detected in roughly one-third of routine ECGs (Jeresaty 1973; Fontana et al. 1970; Sloman et al. 1972). However, supraventricular tachycardia represents the most common sustained arrhythmia in asymptomatic young patients (Devereux et al. 1976). Atrial fibrillation will be seen at all ages but occurs principally in the elderly or in the presence of long-standing mitral regurgitation associated with left atrial enlargement (Beton et al. 1983). Life-threatening arrhythmias probably are rare in MVP patients but more data on this subject will be needed to clarify their true prevalence. Up to 1977, 25 cases of sudden death had been reported and a further 21 patients who had developed ventricular fibrillation were successfully resuscitated.

Several theories have been proposed to explain the occurrence of arrhythmias in MVP: (1) myocardial ischemia induced by increased tension on the papillary muscle due to the prolapsing valve resulting in blood perfusion impairment of the subendocardium and myocardium (Pocock and Barlow 1971; Criley et al. 1973), (2) increased adrenergic tone (Pasternac et al. 1982), (3) prolongation of QT interval as the basis for ventricular arrhythmias (Paddu et al. 1983), (4) mechanical tension by the prolapsing mural leaflet on the left atrial wall (Leclerque et al. 1980), (5) stretched mitral valve acting as a site of ectopic impulse initiation with secondary propagation to the left atrium (Wit et al. 1973), (6) reentry mechanism: in Josephson's series (1978), 50% of patients with MVP and supraventricular tachycardia had intraatrial bypass tracts responsible for reentry rhythms, and (7) mitral insufficiency complicated by atrial and ventricular dilatation (Shah et al. 1982).

Despite the common occurrence of arrhythmias in MVP patients, the Framingham group showed that there was no significant difference in the prevalence of dysrhythmia in subjects under 40 years of age with MVP and in controls. However, in people over 40 years of age, there was a significant excess of dysrhythmia in patients with MVP (73%) compared with those without MVP (46%). It is postulated that the progression of the prolapse in older subjects (increased mitral regurgitation and/or histologic degeneration) might be reflected by a propensity to develop dysrhythmia (Savage et al. 1983).

The occurrence of significant cardiovascular symptoms and the frequent coexistence of marked anxiety and panic attacks in patients with MVP and trivial mitral regurgitation have suggested a disorder of autonomic cardiac regulation. Boudoulas et al. (1980) and Pasternac et al. (1982) have observed an excessive catecholamine excretion associated with an increased alpha and beta adrenergic tone in patients with prolapsing mitral leaflets. Subsequently Gaffney et al. (1979, 1980) reproduced the spontaneous symptoms of chest pain, palpitations, and anxiety in these patients after the infusion of isoproterenol or phenylephrine. Parasympathetic abnormalities have also been described by Coghlan et al. (1979), who reported an increased resting vagal tone and decreased parasympathetic responsiveness in subjects with MVP. The analogy of mitral valve prolapse with older clinical syndromes named differently under Da Costa syndrome, soldier's heart syndrome, effort syndrome, and neurocirculatory asthenia point to this dual autonomic and psychiatric involvement in the pathogenesis of the clinical constellation of MVP syndrome.

Clinical and Radiologic Findings

The elongation of mitral valvular leaflets, chordae tendinae, and mitral annulus allow the mitral valve to prolapse or balloon into the left atrium as ejection of blood during systole shrinks the left ventricular dimension below a critical level. The systolic click is generated during the ventricular systole when the mitral leaflet is suddenly checked in its normal anterior movement. It usually coincides with maximal prolapse of the leaflets and has been ascribed to a tautness of the elongated chordae tendinae (chordal snap) (Reid 1961) or to the leaflets themselves (Criley et al. 1966). The click occurs after the opening of the aortic valve and is therefore nonejection in timing. There may be multiple clicks resulting from the asynchronous prolapse of either the leaflets or the individual scallop of the posterior leaflet or to asynchronous chordal tautening (Wigle et al. 1976).

If there is sufficient slippage so that a portion of the mitral valve fails to coapt against the rest of the leaflet, a mitral regurgitant orifice is formed, generating mitral insuffiiciency with a systolic murmur. As the left ventricle continues to empty, the prolapsing mitral leaflet may further extend into the left atrium, increasing the mitral regurgitation, which results in a progressively louder systolic murmur that ends with the aortic component of the second sound (crescendo in quality). The systolic click occurs when the left ventricle reaches a volume specific for each individual patient (click volume) at which point the prolapsing portion of the mitral valve suddenly slips. Therefore the click is always triggered at the same left ventricular systolic volume and this remains constant despite differing left ventricular end-diastolic volume and rate of left ventricular emptying. Any maneuver that decreases the left ventricular end-diastolic volume (inspiration, standing position, Valsalva maneuver, amylnitrite, or isoproterenol infusion) or increases the left ventricular contractility (increased heart rate induced by atrial or ventricular pacing) causes click and murmur to occur earlier in systole. In other words, when left ventricular volume decreases, the chordae are relatively longer and permit earlier and greater prolapse to occur. Maneuvers that increase the left ventricular end-diastolic volume or decrease the velocity of the left ventricular contraction (squatting, supine or prone position, isometric handgrip, administration of phenylephrine or propranolol) move the click toward the second sound and delay onset of the murmur.

Echocardiography is much more sensitive than the routine physical examination in detecting evidence of MVP. The prevalence of cardiac signs in patients with echocardiographic prolapse was 8%–13% with systolic click, 3%–11% with systolic murmur, and 0%–2% with systolic click and murmur, according to the Framingham survey (Savage et al. 1983). A higher prevalence of up to 17% of ausculatory prolapse has been reported in clinical series (Darsee et al. 1979; Devereux et al. 1982; Savage et al. 1982; Markiewicz et al. 1976), probably imputable to selection bias in the population analyzed.

The usual criteria used for the diagnosis of MVP on M-mode echocardiogram is the presence of an abnormal posterior movement of the coapted anterior and/ or posterior leaflets of 2 mm or more from the C-D line during systole (the line connecting the closure point with the point of opening of the leaflets in diastole). There are two basic types of echocardiographic prolapse described: a midsystolic "buckling" and a pansystolic "hammocking" of the valvular leaflets (Shah and

Gramiak 1970; Kerber et al. 1971; Dillon et al. 1971; Popp et al. 1974; De Maria et al. 1974). Because M-mode echocardiogram strikes only a portion of the mitral valve, prolapse of the posteromedial and/or anterolateral scallop of the posterior leaflet may be missed. The echocardiographic features of chordal rupture complicating MVP are holosystolic prolapse with a coarse irregular diastolic fluttering of the leaflets. Two-dimensional (2-D) echocardiogram, which visualizes more of the mitral leaflets, is more accurate in identifying prolapse. The presence of any bulging toward the left atrium above the mitral annular ring confirms the diagnosis (Sahn et al. 1977; Gilbert et al. 1976; Morganroth et al. 1981). However, it must be stressed that the accuracy of echocardiogram in the diagnosis of MVP has never been fully validated.

Electrocardiographic abnormalities have been described in up to two-thirds of patients with MVP. The most characteristic change is nonspecific ST segment change and T-wave inversion in leads II, III, AVF and V5, V6, suggesting inferolateral myocardial ischemia. These findings are sometimes accompanied by tall, peaked T-waves in leads V2, V3. Prolongation of the Q-T interval has also been noted and is important in view of a presumed association with ventricular arrhythmias and sudden death. Accordingly, Winkle et al. (1975) have remarked on a higher incidence of episodic arrhythmia in these patients (72%) compared with 22.6% in patients showing a lesser degree of QT prolongation. The Framingham group did not notice more common ECG abnormalities of MVP patients compared with the controls (Savage et al. 1983).

Treadmill exercise testing induces ischemic ST segment depression in a high proportion of patients with MVP and without angiographically demonstrated coronary artery disease. The incidence of false-positive test results varies from 10% to 60% in prolapse patients with chest pain and normal coronary arteriogram (Sloman et al. 1972; Engel et al. 1979). Exercise testing has also demonstrated arrhythmias in as many as 75% of tested patients (Gooch et al. 1972). Ventricular arrhythmias (ventricular bigeminy, multifocal ventricular ectopic beats, and ventricular tachycardia) are especially provoked, appearing at the termination of exercise during deceleration of heart rate. Holter monitoring is more sensitive than treadmill testing in eliciting arrhythmia.

Ranganathan et al. (1970, 1973) have defined certain angiographic correlations of clinical findings in MVP patients. Thus patients with a nonejection click and late systolic murmur usually demonstrate isolated prolapse of the posterior leaflet with a mild to moderate mitral insufficiency. However, a pansystolic murmur usually corresponds to a combined posterior and anterior leaflet prolapse with severe mitral regurgitation. Ruptured chordae tendinae are commonly found in this last cetagory.

Various segmental abnormalities of left ventricular contraction have been described in up to 82% of ventriculograms in MVP patients (Scampardonis et al. 1973). The most frequently encountered abnormal pattern is a vigorous contraction ring of the basal inferior wall which may be associated with an anterolateral wall asynergy or bulging (Grossman et al. 1968; Gooch et al. 1972; Ranganathan et al. 1973). Despite the high prevalence of abnormal contraction patterns, the function of the left ventricle is not usually impaired (Crawford and O'Rourke 1984). However, intracardial pressures and cardiac output may become progressively abnormal as mitral regurgitation becomes more severe. These abnormalities of segmental contraction raise the long-standing conflict of whether a primary valvular involvement or a primary segmental cardiomyopathy forms the basis for the mitral leaflet prolapse syndrome. The hypothesis of a cardiac myopathy was raised a few years ago, when several authors reported histologic changes in the myocardium of patients with MVP, i.e., endocardial and interstitial fibrosis and degenerative mitochondria (Mason et al. 1978). The subsequent observation of the same histologic findings in patients with severe mitral regurgitation of different etiologies has weakened this hypothesis. Several factors favor a primary leaflet abnormality: the presence of specific histopathologic valvular changes, its association with different connective tissue disorders, the normal left ventricular function in the majority of subjects, and particularly the disappearance of the segmental contraction abnormalities after mitral valve replacement (Cobbs and King 1977; King et al. 1982). At present, the prevailing opinion supports the concept of a primary problem of the mitral valve and attributes the abnormal ventricular wall motion to the unusual stress exerted on the papillary muscles and on the supporting ventricular wall by the sudden tensing of the mitral leaflet.

Natural History and Complications

The MVP syndrome has always been considered a benign condition, with the vast majority of patients dying of unrelated cause at a normal expected age. However, the true risk of complications remains unknown, most of the studies reporting on the natural history being retrospective and involving selected subgroups. In summary, these studies conclude that 60%–80% of patients with MVP remain unchanged for a follow-up period varying between 10 and 24 years (Belardi et al. 1976; Allen et al. 1974; Mills et al. 1977; Koch and Hancock 1976; Appelblatt et al. 1975). Even in highly selected groups, the risk of major complications is roughly 13.5% for that period, representing an approximated risk of 1%–2%/year. According to several necropsy studies, MVP-related death varies from 4% (Lucas and Edwards 1982) to 17% (Davies et al. 1978), the main causes of death being bacterial endocarditis and mitral regurgitation from chordal rupture. Little relation is found between symptoms, physical signs, and complications, except that patients having severe mitral regurgitation and infective endocarditis tend to have holosystolic prolapse.

Infective endocarditis has been observed in patients who had only a nonejection click as well as in patients with pansystolic murmur. The risk for individual patients with MVP to develop infective endocarditis is extremely small and, until 1975, there were only 22 cases of infective endocarditis superimposed on MVP described in the literature. Its incidence among MVP patients has been variously reported, ranging from 0% (Koch and Hancock 1976) to 8% (Allen et al. 1974). Some authors suggest that antibiotic prophylaxis should be recommended in all patients with MVP undergoing procedures involving a risk of sepsis, whether or not a click and/or murmur is present, while others think that it is unnecessary to order prophylaxis in subjects who have MVP detected only by echocardiography.

Approximately 8% of MVP patients exhibit at some point severe mitral regurgitation leading to congestive heart failure and necessitating valve surgery (Belardi et al. 1976; Hill et al. 1974). The mitral regurgitation may occur suddenly by spontaneous rupture of the attenuated chordae tendinae (Goodman et al. 1974). Neither signs of infection or acute stress are recognizable in most of these patients. The spontaneous rupture is usually attributed to the marked degenerative changes localized at the site of primary chordal attachments. Patients may undergo a gradually progressive mitral regurgitation without readily identifiable cause. Unsuspected rupture of chordae tendinae is found in some of these patients, while in others the cause of advancing mitral insufficiency is a progressive prolapse of the mitral leaflets (McKay and Yacoub 1973; Hill et al. 1974). Leaflet or chordal rupture in the course of infective endocarditis must be kept in mind in cases of acute mitral regurgitation. Mitral valve replacement remains the treatment of choice. However, a number of reports have stressed a high incidence of valve dehiscence in patients treated surgically, presumably because of myxomatous change in the mitral annulus (Read and Thal 1966; McKay and Yacoub 1973).

The rarity of sudden death even in symptomatic MVP patients is underscored by its low incidence varying between 0% and 2% (Belardi et al. 1976; Allen et al. 1974; Mills et al. 1977; Appleblatt et al. 1975; Barlow and Pocock 1979). Included in that category is death explained neither by clinical nor pathologic evidence but in the presence of some degree of floppy mitral valve and without superimposed ruptured chordae or bacterial endocarditis. Ventricular tachyarrhythmias are the presumed mechanism of death in these patients. Review of the published cases has led to the identification of a group of MVP patients who are at risk of sudden death (Jeresaty 1976; Chesler et al. 1983; Bharati et al. 1983; Cheitlin and Byrd 1984): young to middle aged women with a clear-cut familial syndrome and who present late systolic or pansystolic murmur and marked prolapsing mitral leaflets usually involving both leaflets and associated with a mild to moderate mitral insufficiency. ECG in these patients usually discloses ST-T segment depression in the inferolateral leads and occasionally QT interval prolongation. Dysrhythmias (particularly multiple ventricular arrhythmias) are frequently identified in their Holter monitoring (Campbell et al. 1876; Koch and Hancock 1976). Lucas and Edwards (1982) in their necropsy material of 14 sudden deaths observed the presence of fibrin deposits at the mitral valve-left atrial junction without evidence of embolization to the coronary arteries in 21% of the cases and 69% showed an associated tricuspid valve prolapse.

Etiology and Pathogenesis (Table 5.2)

Mitral valve prolapse has been associated with several distinct clinical entities, suggesting that this syndrome is etiologically heterogeneous. Individuals with the systolic click-murmur syndrome but without any evidence of these underlying diseases are said to have the idiopathic form of mitral valve prolapse. A familial occurrence of this idiopathic form has been demonstrated in many family studies of MVP, the first-degree relative being affected in a uniformly high proportion of MVP patients (Sheele et al. 1976; Devereux et al. 1982). Indeed 30% of MVP subjects have at least one first-degree relative affected, according to the Framingham survey (Savage et al. 1983). Characteristic anthropometric traits and histologic features shared by many MVP patients provide strong evidence favoring a genetic etiology for this disease i.e., (1) an inherited pattern consistent with an autosomal dominant inheritance (Devereux and Brown 1983; Devereux et al. 1981; Scheele et al. 1976); (2) a distinct body habitus characterized by low body weight, long arm span, long gracilis fingers, and low blood pressure (Savage et al. 1983); (3) distinctive skeletal abnormalities including pectus excavatum, scoliosis, loss of kyphosis of the thoracic spine, and high-arched palate (Bon Tempo et al. 1975; Udeshi et al. 1979); (4) an increased frequency of arch patterns on the fingers of MVP patients (Swartz et al. 1976); and (5) possible HLA association especially with HLA-BW35 and HLA-A3 (Braun et al. 1977).

Table 5.2. Etiologic classification of MVP

Primary leaflet abnormality
Idiopathic: familial, nonfamilial
Connective tissue disorder: Marfan's syndrome, Ehlers-Danlos syndrome, osteogenesis imperfecta, pseudoxanthoma elasticum, relapsing polychondritis, von Willebrand syndrome
Secondary prolapse
Coronary artery disease
Rheumatic valve disease
Congenital cardiomyopathies: Duchenne muscular dystrophy, Berger muscular dystrophy, myotonic dystrophy
Myocardial diseases: congestive cardiomyopathy, myocarditis, left ventricular aneurysm
Collagen disorders: systemic lupus erythematosus, polyarteritis nodosa
Chromosomic aberrations: Turner syndrome, Klinefelter syndrome
Trauma
Mitral valve surgery
Left atrial myxoma
Functional prolapse
Hypertrophic cardiomyopathy
Secundum atrial septal defect
Decreased blood volume
Hypercontractile state: hyperthyroidism

Several genetic hypotheses have been suggested over the past 2 decades to explain this varied and variable clinical syndrome. The most attractive theory attributes the MVP syndrome to a basic connective tissue disorder affecting both the skeleton and the mitral valve, i.e., a forme fruste of Marfan's syndrome (Read et al. 1965). Supporting this conclusion of an underlying connective tissue abnormality of the fibrous support of the cardiac valves is the finding of concomitant tricuspid valve prolapse and aortic valve prolapse on one-third to one-half of MVP patients (Werner et al. 1978; Mardelli et al. 1981). A second hypothesis proposes an embryonal insult either by environmental agents or drugs between the 35th and 42nd day of fetal development (Davies 1963). This period of fetal life is concerned with differentiation of the mitral valve into its final form and the chondrification and ossification of the vertebral column and thoracic cage. An inborn error of metabolism involving collagen synthesis was subsequently described by Hammer et al. in 1979 following the discovery of an incompletely characterized collagen (absence of types III and AB collagen) in a few subjects with MVP. Finally a hereditary disorder of centrally mediated autonomic and adrenergic function for which MVP would represent a genetic marker has been suggested (Wooley 1983).

If MVP appears to be inherited in a autosomal dominant mode, its expression is affected by several factors: (1) sex: males generally have a lower incidence of MVP (Devereux et al. 1982). (2) age: a high incidence of 6% in neonates (Chandraratna et al. 1979) owing to the predominant role of the right ventricle in fetal circulation with an associated left ventricular underdevelopment drops sharply to a 1% prevalence in childhood and adolescence. A second decline is observed in elderly women, presumably attributed to a valvular thickening, thus lessening the valvular leaflet's motility and prolapse (Savage et al. 1983). (3) Cardiac geometry: as previously described, the left ventricular size and shape may either enhance or reduce MVP expression.

Therefore the idiopathic form of MVP remains etiologically obscure and as best summarized by Devereux (1983): "MVP is genetically heterogeneous with great clinical phenotypic variation, but there is still no evidence whether this reflects difference in etiology of MVP or alternatively whether there is a wide variability in expression of a single gene depending on interaction with environmental or other genetic factors."

Mitral valve prolapse is also an integral feature of several distinct connective tissue diseases including Marfan syndrome, Ehlers-Danlos I, II, IV, osteogenesis imperfecta, etc. There are no qualitative or quantitative differences between the MVP of Marfan syndrome and idiopathic MVP.

Secondary MVP may be induced by any disease that produces dysfunction of the mitral apparatus, either at the valvular level (leaflets, annulus, chordae tendinae cordis) or at the ventricular level (papillary muscles, left ventricular wall). Thus any cardiomyopathy, ischemic, degenerative, or inflammatory, which produces segmental contraction abnormalities might trigger prolapse of the mitral leaflets. Functional prolapse is usually caused by systemic diseases which through variation in heart rate or blood volume alter the left ventricular volume or contractility.

Neurologic Complications

Since 1974 when stroke and mitral valve prolapse were first associated (Barnett), various other neurologic complications have been reported in patients suffering from this abnormality. Syncope represents the most frequent of these manifestations but less common syndromes including stroke and transient global amnesia have also been documented. While most of these complications can be attributed to cardiovascular mechanisms, some remain unexplained.

Syncope

Approximately one-third of patients with MVP complain of lightheadedness, dizziness, and syncope (Litman and Friedman 1980). However, true syncope happens much less frequently than do other symptoms usually ascribed to near-syncopal episodes. In his series of 589 symptomatic patients with MVP and documented arrhythmias, Swartz et al. (1977) observed that 11.6% reported lightheadedness but only 4% sustained syncope.

Syncopal episodes usually occur in clusters over a few weeks or months; their numbers are small, the majority of patients having sustained one or two. They are observed mainly in women, onsetting in the latter part of the 3rd decade. In most cases, patients are unaware of warning abnormal cardiac beats. Neither is syncope precipitated by postural change or the usual triggering stimuli which suggest vasovagal attack (Horenstein et al. 1979).

In the MVP syndrome, syncope is attributed to hemodynamically significant arrhythmias resulting in transient fall of systemic arterial blood pressure and cerebral blood flow. Paroxysmal ventricular fibrillation/tachycardia, supraventricular tachyarrhythmia, and complete atrioventricular block represent reported arrhythmias resulting in syncope. The most clear-cut instance of tachyarrhythmias causing syncope is those episodes of self-limited ventricular fibrillation. Wigle et al. (1976) reported seven cases of MVP associated with well-documented bouts of ventricular fibrillation and syncope. Supraventricular tachycardia is often accompanied by near-syncopal symptoms but rarely by true syncope. However, supraventricular arrhythmias have been postulated as a mechanism of syncope in the MVP syndrome: the frequent demonstration of a concealed atrioventricular bypass tract in those patients might result in the rapid transmission of an atrial tachyarrhythmia leading to ventricular fibrillation through preexcitation and reentry mechanisms (Josephson et al. 1978). Finally Leightman et al. (1975) described three family members with MVP and sinus bradycardia/arrest experiencing recurrent bouts of syncope. These authors suggested that excessive vagal tone was responsible for both bradycardia and sinus arrest. Accordingly two patients were treated with permanent demand pacemakers followed by a complete resolution of their symptoms.

The usual treatment advocated for ventricular and supraventricular tacharrhythmia in MVP syndrome is propanolol, in accordance with the increased plasma cathecholamines and adrenergic tone demonstrated in these subjects (Pocock and Barlow 1970). Sometimes the addition of digitalis may be necessary for the treatment of supraventricular tachycardia as well as diphenylhydantoin for ventricular arrhythmias. There is a case report of MVP and refractory ventricular tachyarrhythmia which disclosed a complete abolition of the arrhythmia following mitral valve replacement (Ross et al. 1978). Severe bradyarrhythmia and sinus arrest must be treated with demand pacemaker implantation (De Silva and Shubrooks 1977; Leightman et al. 1975).

Repetitive syncopal attacks are sometimes misdiagnosed as epilepsy. Six patients with a similar picture and normal electroencephalogram sustained a complete remission following the discontinuation of anticonvulsant and the institution of antiarrhythmic treatment (Litman and Friedman 1980).

Seizure

Seizure represents an uncommon neurologic disorder associated with the MVP syndrome. The vast majority of these attacks are characterized by a focal and abrupt onset (Horenstein et al. 1979). They are invariably mild, of short duration, and restricted to a short period of usually less than 24 h. Generally a history of prior convulsions cannot be elicited in these patients. Localized abnormalities are occasionally observed on the electroencephalogram. Several mechanisms have been postulated to explain the paroxysmal occurrence of these focal seizures: (1) seizures may have resulted from an acute regional ischemia following embolization, i.e., occurring in the course of a cardioembolic stroke. The presence of a long-standing residual deficit in assocation with the appearance of an infarction on the CT scan corroborates that hypothesis in several patients (Horenstein et al. 1979; Barnett 1982). (2) Activation of a chronic, silent epileptogenic focus might have been triggered by an acute hemodynamic alteration induced by dysrythmia (Horenstein et al. 1979). (3) Spontaneous discharge of an independent epileptogenic focus unrelated to the cardiac function. Litman and Friedman (1980) reported two subjects with MVP and independent seizure disorder with characteristic epileptic abnormalities on their EEG.

Finally as a result of persisting complete atrioventricular block with prolonged secondary cerebral hypoxia, some patients may experience syncope complicated by generalized convulsions (Medina and Dreifus 1983). It usually occurs when the cerebral anoxia persists for more than 10–15 s. Woodley et al. (1977) reported a young man 24 years old with MVP and a history of epilepsy since the age of 8. His seizures were initially manifested by blackout spells and then by generalized tonic-clonic convulsions. They were refractory to anticonvulsant regimens and the EEG never showed any abnormality. Prolonged Holter monitoring revealed multiple episodes of complete AV block lasting up to 23 s. The patient's symptoms were totally corrected by implantation of a demand pacemaker.

Cerebral Ischemic Events

Over the past decade, numerous reports have recognized an association between prolapsing mitral valve and cerebral ischemic events. The first instance of this phenomenon was described by Barlow and Bosman in 1966, but its significance was unnoticed by these authors. A young woman 23 years old experienced a transient left upper limb weakness and was told that her heart was abnormal. No detail of any neurologic examination was reported and the possible relationship to the MVP was not considered.

The first suggestion of a possible relationship between MVP and ischemia in the cerebral circulation came in 1974 when Barnett reported four patients who had suffered cerebral ischemic events. He subsequently enlarged his number to 12 patients (Barnett et al 1976) and to 14 in 1977 (Kostuk et al. 1977). All these patients were young, ranging between 10 and 48 years old, and none of them presented the usual predisposing factors for atherosclerotic vascular diseases. The only abnormality found was prolapsing mitral valve on angiocardiogram performed in every patient. There was a complete absence of coronary disease or intracranial/extracranial atherosclerotic arterial disease. Barnett postulated that an embolic process originating from the abnormal mitral valve was responsible for the recurrent ischemic attack. The focal nature of the neurologic deficit, the involvement of both hemispheres at different times in three patients coupled with the six angiographic pictures of occluded intracranial arteries, all favored the embolic explanation.

Finally, Barnett et al. published in 1980 a case-control series strongly supporting a causal relationship between prolapsing mitral valve and cerebral/ retinal ischemic events in the young population group. They reported on 60 patients 45 years of age or younger admitted following transient ischemic attacks or minor nonprogressing stroke and studied on a protocol looking for all possible pathogenetic mechanisms. All were submitted to M-mode echocardiographic studies. There were an equal number of age- and sex-matched controls who did not sustain any neurologic or cardiac symptoms. Further data were obtained by submitting to the same protocol 141 patients who had entered into a platelet drug trial for cerebral ischemic events and were over 45 years of age. One hundred and forty-one controls without significant history of cardiac or neurologic complaints were matched to this older age group. Twenty-four of the 60 young patients (40%) evidenced mitral valve prolapse compared with only 5 of the 60 controls (6.8%). Of these 24 young patients with MVP and cerebral ischemic events, 6 presented other potential cause for stroke: birth control pill, hemiplegic migraine, prosthetic heart valve, systemic lupus erythematosus. Excluding these 6 cases, 18 of 60 patients (30%) did not show any recognizable cause for their stroke except MVP, meaning 4.5 times the control value. In the older age group, no significant differences were found in the incidence of MVP between the 141 patients (mean age, 64) with TIA or minor stroke (8/141 or 5.7%) and the 141 controls (mean age, 63) (10/141 or 7.1%).

Review of published cases of stroke patients who demonstrated an isolated prolapsing mitral valve permitted identification of some typical clinical features common to most of them (Table 5.3). Regarding the sex, a preponderance of females is present but not impressive. Indeed there is a disproportionately large number of males with cerebral ischemic events associated with MVP compared with patients found to have uncomplicated MVP, which is many times more common in women. Two series revealed a higher incidence of TIA/stroke in male patients with MVP (Kostuk et al. 1977; Watson 1979) which, according to Watson, might reflect some difference in basic clotting mechanisms between the sexes. MVP is significantly more common in patients under 45 with cerebral

Table 5.3. Clinical picture of cerebral ischemic events in MVP patients

	Kostuk (1977)	Watson (1979)	Hanson (1980)	Sandok (1982)	Jones (1982)	Kouvaras (1985)
Number of patients with MVP and cerebral ischemic events	14	11	24	40	9	16
M:F ratio	7:7	7:4	6:18	15:25	4:5	7:9
Age (x̄)	37	51	43	48	48	38
Neurologic presenting picture	14	–	20	–	–	–
Previous cardiac symptoms	10	1	12	–	–	14
Cardiac signs	11	3	13	37	–	16
Single attack	4	6	18	–	8	3
Multiple attacks	10	5	4	–	1	3
TIA	4	8	5	5	2	13
Stroke	10	3	17	35	7	3
Amaurosis fugax only	–	4	1	2	1	–
More than one hemisphere	3	0	3	3	0	–
Convulsions	0	0	2	0	0	0
Severity: no deficit	4	–	8	–	3	13
Residual deficit	10	3	16	–	6	3
Vascular territory: carotid	9	9	15	40	7	–
Vertebrobasilar	3	2	8	0	2	–
Angiogram: normal	8	7	13	–	4	13
Embolic occlusion	6	3	4	2	2	3
Holter: arrhythmias	9	2	5	–	–	0
Atrial fibrillation	3	–	–	5	–	0
Follow-up (years)	1–4	1	3	5	2	2

ischemic events but patients in and beyond the 6th decade must also be considered for this diagnosis. However, the high prevalence of primary carotid atherosclerosis in elderly stroke patients makes questionable a pathogenetic relation between MVP and cerebral ischemia in that age group. Two cases of childhood hemiplegic syndrome were described in association with MVP (Rice et al. 1980, 1981), mainly in the familial form of MVP.

The majority of patients going on to stroke have been unaware of the existence of prolapsing mitral valve. However, a totally negative cardiac history is uncommon and inquiry at the time of the neurologic illness often reveals the recognition of vague symptoms of nonspecific chest discomfort and palpitations. Characteristically no temporal relationship can be elicited between these two types of symptomatology. About one-third to one-half of patients report bouts of chest pain and periodic awareness of palpitations and few complain of lightheadedness or syncope. The auscultatory findings vary considerably in the reported series and depend, of course, on the determination with which they were sought and if the physician had appealed to the different maneuvers used to accentuate these findings. Nevertheless the majority of patients present an isolated mid or/and late systolic murmur while a smaller proportion have intermittent midsystolic click or a combination of nonejection click/murmur. Only one series (Jackson et al. 1984) report an exceptionally high prevalence of normal cardiac examination where 75% of their patients did not demonstrate the characteristic findings of a click or a murmur. Holter ECG monitoring has been done erratically in several of the published series for varying periods. Between 50% and 75% of the subjects submitted to this procedure had no significant abnormalities. However, in the acute stroke period, Holter monitoring cannot predict if the dysrhythmia is the cause of stroke or a secondary manifestation of stroke. Two series (Kostuk et al. 1977; Nishimura et al. 1985) described a high occurrence of atrial fibrillation among MVP patients experiencing cerebral ischemia. The impressive incidence of 60% in Nishimura's series led this author to conclude that MVP in the presence of normal sinus rhythm represented a low risk for cerebral ischemic events.

Ischemic events vary from mild and transient to moderate or severe. The major clinical features in 7 large series totaling 130 patients are summarized in Table 5.3. Of this number, 30% experienced transient ischemic attack (TIA) alone and stroke occurred in 89 of the 130 (68.5%). Approximately 20% of the patients sustained recurrent episodes which were generally separated by many months or several years, but in some the intervals were shorter. The more frequent episodes were typical of the abrupt onset of TIA with complete early resolution. The single event or those separated by several months or years tended to be associated with more prolonged and occasionally persistent disability. A significant neurologic deficit after the initial ischemic event occurred in 30% of the patients, but as a rule the majority eventually recovered almost completely. Only one series (Jackson et al. 1984) has looked at the recurrence rate of cerebral ischemic events. After a mean follow-up period of 8 years from the time of the first ischemic event, only one of 8 patients (12.5%) who presented with a TIA had a stroke. Also only one patient (4%) had a TIA before the first stroke, suggesting that subjects with MVP and cerebral ischemia appear less likely to have TIA before stroke than other patients with atherosclerotic carotid disease. Seven of the 24 patients with initial stroke had recurrent stroke after a mean interval of 3.5 years, a stroke recurrence rate of

6.8%/patient per year. They concluded that the prognosis after the diagnosis of MVP-associated ischemia was good with respect to recurrent ischemic events.

The cerebral hemispheres are the most common site of clinical signs and symptoms but as expected with an embolic source for ischemic events, a smaller proportion (1:5) have posterior circulation disturbances. In 8.5% of cases, the events have included more than one hemisphere or a hemisphere plus the brain stem in succeeding episodes. The embolic lesion appears clinically to affect mainly medium-sized or small arteries. The recognized occlusions on cerebral angiogram most often involve the main trunk or cortical branches of the middle or posterior cerebral arteries. Very rarely, patients may sustain an occlusion large enough to produce a proximal massive occlusion of the internal carotid artery complicated by cerebral edema and obtundation (Barnett 1982; Watson 1979).

Rice et al. (1980, 1981) reported two families with an autosomal dominant pattern of inheritance of mitral valve prolapse in which several younger subjects have developed cerebral or retinal ischemic events. In the most impressive family, 8 members of three generations involving 27 individuals were found to have MVP and 4 of these have been affected by 8 episodes of cerebral ischemia or infarction in the first 4 decades of life. The ischemic episodes were widely dispersed in time, occurring several years apart. The presence of such premature and multiple stroke in these eight patients and the absence of such a phenomenon in the other 19 strongly suggests a direct relationship between stroke and MVP. Also two examples of childhood hemiplegic syndrome associated with MVP were found among these two families, supporting a possible association between prolapse and childhood stroke. Neither family displayed the usual features characteristic of Marfan's syndrome.

Several retinal ischemic complications have been recognized in association with prolapsing mitral valve in the absence of complicating infective endocarditis. The retinal lesions have consisted of amaurosis fugax, central retinal artery and retinal arteriolar branch occlusions with persistent defects of retinal or optic nerve origin, an atypical form of Eale's disease, and central retinal vein thrombosis (Caltrider et al. 1980; Wilson et al. 1977; Kimball and Hedges 1977; Woldoff et al. 1975; Gonder et al. 1983; Baker et al. 1981). The repeated episodes of transient visual obscuration and the permanent monocular defects are usually attributed to fibrin and platelet microemboli originating from thrombus deposition on mitral leaflet. Atypical Eale's disease has also been described in association with MVP (Caltrider et al. 1980). In these atypical cases, there are recurrent small embolic arteriolar occlusions leading to areas of ischemia and secondary retinal neovascularization. The extensive process of neovascularization eventually causes a severe impairment of vision. The cause of central retinal vein obstruction in young adults is not well understood and routine medical and laboratory evaluation usually fails to reveal an obvious cause. However, in Gonder's series (1983) of 15 cases under 50 years of age, 7 showed mitral leaflet prolapse on echocardiogram and 4 of these 7 cases also had abnormalities of platelet function. Several pathogenic mechanisms have been postulated to explain the occurrence of central retinal vein thrombosis in the presence of MVP: (1) Primary central retinal artery occlusion evoking retinal ischemia and edema with secondary pressure and occlusion of the central retinal vein (Woldoff et al. 1975) and (2) platelet hyperactivity induced by MVP, culminating in venous obstruction induced by platelet aggregation at the level of the lamina cribrosa (Gonder et al. 1983). Therefore MVP remains a potential cause of unexplained retinal occlusive disease in young patients. However, in the age group at highest risk for stroke, the discovery of MVP should not routinely exclude evaluation for other sources of embolic stroke and should not be considered as the only explanation for retinal ischemia (Baker et al. 1981).

The most likely cause of the link between MVP and cerebral ischemia is a noninfective thromboembolism originating from the abnormal mitral valve. Pomerance (1969), in her series of 35 postmortem cases of myxomatous valves, described a noninflammatory fibrinous endocarditis which she attributed to changes in the underlying fibrous layer. Indeed the transformation of the normally rigid valve into loose myxomatous tissue allows stretching of the leaflet by the normal intraventricular pressures: this stretching might result in loss of endothelial continuity and rupture of subendothelial connective tissue fibers. These changes on the surface of the leaflet might initiate platelet adherence and aggregation with formation of a platelet-fibrin thrombus which could later become detached. In their observation, Pomerance and Davies (1977) felt that this fibrinous endocarditis was an improbable source for emboli of sufficient size to occlude the lumen of a major cerebral artery. Subsequent lesions of larger size have been described (Kostuk et al. 1977; Hanson et al. 1980), especially in the angle between the posterior leaflet of the mitral valve and the left atrial wall (Fig. 5.1). The formation of a thrombus adherent at the cul-de-sac created

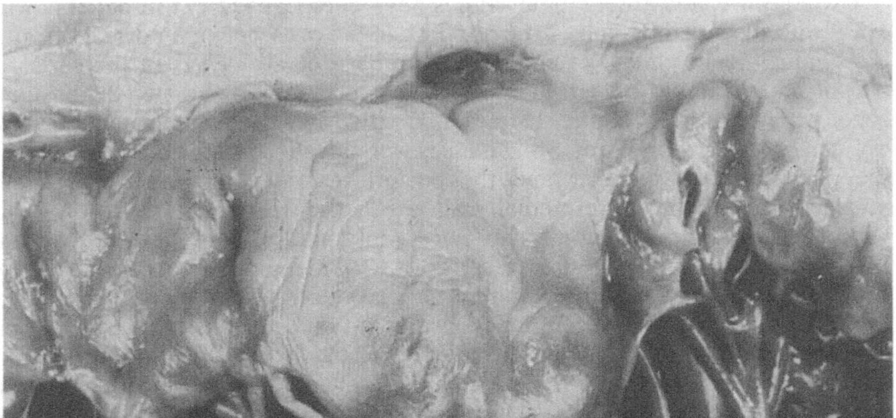

Fig. 5.1. Postmortem specimen indicates myxomatous valve degeneration, change in chordae tendinae, and small area of premortem thrombotic material attached to roughened area at valve insertion (Silver 1974).

between the ballooning posterior leaflet and the atrial wall is usually attributed to a localized jet of mitral regurgitation (Falicov 1977). During late systole, a localized jet of mitral regurgitation can be demonstrated on angiocardiogram. Subsequently (diastole) the regurgitant material is observed to swirl briefly into the left atrium and then to collect into a posterior-inferior cul-de-sac, remaining stagnant there until the end of diastole. Thrombus may form and subsequently embolize even in the absence of atrial fibrillation. A third site for thrombus formation was described in the ventricular fibrinous endocardial changes induced by friction between the chordae and the left ventricular wall (McKay and Yacoub 1973).

The very focal nature of the clinical presentation and the angiographic findings are highly suggestive of emboli. The usual picture is that of an occlusion of an intracranial artery with an abrupt cut-off of the artery with no proximal irregularities and without significant atheroma visualized in the cervical or intracranial portion of the larger arteries. In several instances, repeat angiograms revealed the disappearance of the obstructive lesion (Woldoff et al. 1975; Allcock 1967); either the thrombus had broken up and dissipated or the lesion had become recanalized. These "disappearing lesions" are strongly supportive of embolic obstructions. The descriptions and observations on retinal arteriolar lesions are also compatible with embolization. Several authors (Watson 1979; Caltrider et al. 1980; Barnett 1982; Donaldson et al. 1981) have produced photographic evidence of material compatible with platelet-fibrin emboli passing through retinal arterioles in patients afflicted with amaurosis fugax; no other explanation was found on detailed investigation to explain these events besides the MVP.

Two major echocardiographic studies have been carried out in patients with MVP who sustained embolic stroke or TIA in the presence of a normal cerebral angiogram (Nichol and Kertesz 1979; Rothbard et al. 1979). In the series of Nichol and Kertesz, left atrial masses were present on the two-dimensional echocardiogram in 8 of the 15 patients with MVP and associated ischemic events. These possibly thrombotic masses were localized in the angle formed by the posterior mitral leaflet and the posterior atrial wall and were usually attached behind the postermedial scallop. Of the 30 patients with MVP but without neurologic symptoms, no intraatrial masses were detected on the echocardiogram. In the Rothbard series of 62 patients with echocardiographic prolapsing mitral valve, three experienced embolic stroke and one of them was found to have small localized echodensities on anterior/posterior MV leaflets consistent with thrombi. Another case report (Saffro and Talano 1979), of a woman 26 years old with left hemisphere TIA, demonstrated on the M-mode echocardiogram a posterior leaflet prolapse in association with excessive echoes, suggesting thrombus on the atrial side of the leaflet. There is only one surgical confirmation of an echocardiographic pattern of thrombus formation, reported by Donaldson et al. (1981). This 36-year-old man, after a transient blindness of his left eye, demonstrated on 2-DE the presence of a slightly mobile mass on the posterior wall of the atrium in addition to echoes suggestive of thrombus near the posterior leaflet of the mitral valve. The presence of an atrial thrombus in the area of attachment of the valve was subsequently demonstrated at the time of the mitral valve surgery. Actually 2-D echocardiogram cannot differentiate between thrombus formation, artifact due to redundant myxomatous tissue folding up, and normal variants. Several authors (Boughner and Barnett 1985;

Hart and Easton 1982; Barletta et al. 1985) have recommended to await further data concerning the ultimate role of 2-D echocardiography in view of the actual variations in technical expertise.

Four postmortems have been conducted in patients known to have a mitral valve prolapse and afflicted with fatal cerebral embolism (Cook et al. 1978; Geyer and Franzini 1979; Bramlet et al. 1982; Schnee and Bucal 1983). The first postmortem (1978) performed on a patient with myotonic dystrophy and mitral valve prolapse who had sustained a severe hemiplegia 2 weeks prior to death demonstrated a myxomatous degeneration of the mitral valve and an occlusion of the main trunk of the middle cerebral artery. However, no ulcerative lesion or thrombus was detected on the valve. The second case died at 21 years old following the sudden onset of a left hemiplegia. The findings at postmortem indicated a myxomatous degeneration of the posterior leaflet with superimposed friable, granular yellow thrombus made of fibrin and platelets. Fibrin emboli were also demonstrated in the coronary arteries, in the intrarenal arteries, and in the small intracerebral arteries of the right frontal lobe. The third necropsy case revealed a lung carcinoma complicated by nonbacterial thrombotic endocarditis overlying prolapsing mitral valve leaflets. Multiple sites of systemic embolization were observed in renal, splenic, and middle cerebral arteries. The last patient experienced a sudden massive cerebral infarction complicating MVP in association with atrial fibrillation. The postmortem showed a floppy mitral valve and intracardiac thrombus embedded in the muscular trabeculae at the base of the mitral valve.

There is an equal frequency of systemic embolization complicating MVP as compared with retinal or cerebral embolism. Several reports of embolism to the heart, the bowel, and the kidneys have been published. However, the majority of systemic emboli usually involving small size arteries and arterioles are asymptomatic by contrast with retinal and cerebral emboli, which are symptomatic.

Abnormalities of platelet activity in patients with MVP and thromboembolism have been demonstrated by several authors (Walsh et al. 1980, 1981; Steele et al. 1979; Scharf 1982; Fisher et al. 1983). The observation of platelet hyperactivity in patients with MVP whether or not they had suffered from cerebral ischemic events was corroborated by the following abnormalities: (1) shortened platelet survival time (Steele et al. 1979), (2) platelet coagulant hyperactivity and increased proportion of circulating platelet aggregates (Walsh et al. 1980, 1981), and (3) elevation of beta-thromboglobulin and platelet factor 4 (Scharf et al. 1982; Fisher et al. 1983), which are platelet-specific proteins stored within the alpha-granules and released into the surrounding medium during platelet aggregation. These abnormalities are consistent with the view that platelet interaction with the valvular and endocardial pathology of mitral valve prolapse might give rise to in vivo platelet activation, resulting in intravascular thromboembolism. However, the same abnormal platelet pattern is found in other cardiac diseases (rheumatic mitral stenosis, prosthetic heart valves, coronary atherosclerosis) which are associated with an increased incidence of thromboembolism (Cheitlin 1979). Therefore in that group of diseases, patients prone to thromboembolism cannot be readily differentiated by these platelet abnormalities. Moreover, the demonstration of platelet hyperactivity in MVP patients with cerebral ischemia as well as in other cerebrovascular patients without MVP suggests that platelet activation might reflect secondary effects of ischemia or extensive intravascular thrombosis. In summary, these studies remain inconclusive because platelet stimulation may result either from varied valvular dysfunction or may represent secondary effects of cerebral infarction. The observation of an increase of beta-thromboglobulin and PF 4 in patients with focal migraine at the time of their attacks supports equally the possibility that activation of platelets in vivo could be related to transient spasm of cerebral vasculature (Scharf et al. 1981).

Subacute bacterial endocarditis occurs at an increased frequency in association with MVP, and in this setting stroke may occur. With the declining frequency of rheumatic heart disease, MVP may become an increasingly important cause of subacute bacterial endocarditis (Horowitz and Smith 1977; Gregoratus and Karliner 1979). However, septic embolization represents a very rare complication of prolapsing mitral valve. In a recent report (Nishimura et al. 1985) of 237 patients with an asymptomatic or minimally symptomatic MVP, 3 went on to develop bacterial endocarditis complicated by cerebral embolization in only 1 case. Each patient responded promptly to the antibiotic therapy. In consequence, infective endocarditis should be sought whenever there are retinal or cerebral ischemic events of the type described here.

Tachyarrhythmias occur in a high proportion of patients with MVP and may be invoked to explain diffuse cerebral symptoms such as dizziness and syncope but not to explain focal neurologic deficits. (Barnett 1983; De Bono and Warlow 1981). It has also been noted that the timing of these ischemic events has been poorly related to the occurrence of arrhythmias (Winkle et al. 1975). These latter may contribute to thrombogenesis by favoring stagnation and enhancing thrombosis in the left atrium when there is an ulcerative lesion and a change in rhythm (Falicov 1977; Fairfax et al. 1976). The occurrence of paroxysmal atrial fibrillation with MVP, however, cannot be denied as a contributory cause, being a well-known precursor to embolic episodes in patients both with and without valvular heart disease. It is quite possible that an arrhythmia could dislodge a small embolus from the abnormal valve with consequent cerebral or retinal embolization.

Several echocardiographic changes have been analyzed in an attempt to isolate a subgroup of patients with MVP at a higher risk of developing cerebral or retinal ischemic events. According to Barletta et al. (1985) and Jackson et al. (1984), no relation was found between the extent of mitral leaflet prolapse and the risk of embolic stroke. However, a relation between the number of valves involved and the potential of embolization has been demonstrated. Barletta et al. showed echocardiographic evidence of a higher incidence of combined aortic (62%) and tricuspid prolapse (31%) in MVP patients with stroke than in control MVP patients without stroke (aortic prolapse 34%; tricuspid prolapse, 24%). Conclusive demonstration of valvular thickness as a clinical predictor for embolization has not been done yet (Barletta et al. 1985; Nishimura et al. 1985). A higher incidence of cardiac complications and body habitus consistent with Marfan's syndrome has been observed in that group with excessive leaflet thickening (Devereux et al. 1976; Perloff 1982; Chandraratna et al. 1984). Barletta equally reported a higher occurrence of valve thickness in subjects with MVP and cerebral ischemic events (64%) as compared with the control group (46%). The significance and the specifity/sensitivity of this echocardiographic pattern remain unclear and the vigorous application of Chandraratna's criteria for valve thickness measurements has not been done (Chandraratna et al. 1984).

The same dilemma is faced in the case of the echocardiographic picture of an ulcerative lesion with attached thrombotic material on prolapsing leaflets (Barletta et al. 1985). Actually the resolution of 2-D echocardiography is not good enough to permit the differential diagnosis between thrombi adherent to the valve surface, localized myxomatous degeneration, and some normal variants. In fact, some localized enlargement of mitral valve echoes is often seen in healthy people.

The assessment of the importance of MVP as a cause of stroke remains to be satisfactorily determined. The skepticism about the role of MVP in producing stroke has been largely based on the infrequency with which subjects known to have MVP proceed to stroke. MVP is an important cause of cerebral infarction in young patients with otherwise unexplained ischemia (Table 5.4). Looking at the series published over the past few years (Barnett et al. 1980; Bensaid et al. 1980; Fieschi et al. 1983; Kouvaras and Bacoulas 1985), approximately one-third of stroke in young populations is due to MVP. On average, ischemic events occurred 15 years before those attributed to atherothrombotic stroke. However, cerebral ischemia rarely occurs in unselected young adults with MVP (Table 5.5). A considerable discrepancy exists between the rather frequent occurrence

Table 5.4. Prevalence of MVP in neurologic population

	Unselected stroke			Unexplained stroke[a]			
	Total No. of patients with stroke	Mean age	MVP	Total No. of patients with stroke	Mean age	MVP	Duration of follow-up (years)
Knopman and Anderson (1980)	100	70	1 (1%)				–
Bensaid and Cuisinier (1980)				20 116	<40 >40	4 (20%) 6 (5.2%)	2
Barnett (1980)	60 141	33.9 64.7	24 (40%) 8 (5.8%)				
Jones (1982)				43	45	9 (21%)	5
Fieschi (1983)				14 106	<45 >45	3 (21.5%) 3 (2.9%)	
De Bono and Warlow (1981)	117	57.9	13 (11%)				
Kouvaras and Bacoulas (1985)	66	38	23 (34.8%)				2

[a] Unexplained stroke: absence of risk factors, embolic cardiac diseases, arrhythmia, cerebrovascular atherosclerosis

Table 5.5. Prevalence of stroke in general population with MVP

	Total number of cases with MVP	Mean age	Unselected stroke in MVP patients	Unexplained stroke in MVP patients	Duration of Follow-up (years)
Bensaid and Cuisinier (1980)	72	46		10 (14%)	2
Bisset (1980)	119	9.9	1 (0.8%)		6.9
Jones (1982)	760	48	1 (0.13%)		5
Sandok and Giuliani (1982)	1138	48.4	40 (3.5%)	26 (2.9%)	5

of MVP in young stroke patients and the rarity of stroke in young MVP populations in clinical series (Boughner and Barnett 1985; Wolf et al. 1983; Hart and Easton 1982; Hart et al. 1985). The incidence of stroke in young patients under the age of 40 is low, being estimated at 3/100 000 per year. Assuming that one-third of stroke in young adults is attributed to MVP and that roughly 6% of the young population exhibit MVP, the incidence of MVP-related stroke in young patients is very low, calculated at 1/6000 per year (0.02%). Clearly no prophylactic treatment to prevent stroke is warranted in asymptomatic patients with prolapsing mitral leaflets. In summary the relative risk of stroke in young MVP patients remains high, mitral valve prolapse being one of the commonest factors causing strokes and TIA in patients under 40 years of age. However, the absolute risk of stroke in young populations with MVP is very low. An accurate estimation of these risks remains unknown and would be more likely to emerge from population-based studies rather than case studies of individual patients or groups of patients.

Such an association has not been demonstrated in older stroke patients in whom atherothrombotic mechanisms predominate. Sandok and Giuliani (1982), in Rochester, have showed that the incidence of MVP-associated cerebral ischemia does not vary with patient age, being 1/100 000 per year. Therefore, knowing that the incidence of stroke in the older adult population is approximately 80/100 000 per year, 1.25% of all strokes in older people is MVP related. Even if we assume a similar incidence of MVP-related stroke for all age groups, the observed incidence of MVP-related stroke is only 1%/year for all groups.

Certain principles should be followed in the investigation and treatment of MVP patients afflicted with cerebral or retinal ischemic events. A careful physical examination of the heart must be performed as well as 24- to 48-h cardiac monitoring necessary to determine the presence or absence of associated rhythm disorders. A careful search must be made to exclude other known causes of cerebral ischemia before involving prolapsing mitral valve. The treatable complications such as bacterial endocarditis must be excluded. Possible collagen disorders, polycythemia, sickle cell disease, other hematologic disorders involving coagulation abnormalities, and drugs such as the contraceptive pill liable to alter coagulation should all be investigated. Cerebral angiography is usually required to rule out premature atheroma, fibromuscular dysplasia, and spontaneous carotid or vertebral dissection.

Once it is determined that there is no detectable cause for the ischemic events other than MVP, a trial on platelet antiaggregants appears to be the first line of defense against further attacks. Pending the results of the British study on the appropriate prophylactic dosage of aspirin, 1200 mg aspirin daily is recommended on an empirical basis. Should infarction occur despite this therapy, a period of anticoagulant treatment is recommended again on an empirical basis. Anticoagulation is suggested for 3 months, keeping in mind that ischemic events in these patients tend to be separated by months or even years and the possibility exists that eroded lesions on the valves will heal spontaneously. Beta-blockers should be administered if cardiac arrhythmias appear to be contributing to symptomatology, as should standard drugs for the management of atrial fibrillation. Known risk factors for thromboembolism should be treated or avoided: hypertension, increased hematocrit, cigarette smoking, and the use of the birth control pill.

Transient Global Amnesia

Transient global amnesia (TGA) is a clinical syndrome characterized by the sudden onset of retrograde amnesia, inability to recall newly acquired information, and confusion with regard to the current situation; consciousness is preserved and personal identity is retained. Typical attacks last a few hours and amnesia for the period is the only residual deficit (Fisher and Adams 1964; Shuping et al. 1980; Logan and Sherman 1983). This syndrome occurs principally in individuals of middle age or beyond and single attacks are the rule. Although the etiology of TGA is uncertain, a localized epileptic discharge arising in the temporal lobe or an episode of ischemia involving the limbic system of the temporal lobe represent the two main theories. Several features argue against an epileptogenic origin: the age at onset, the infrequency of recurrent attacks, the absence of concomitant manifestations of epilepsy, and the usually normal EEG. Data from several series support the theory that TGA is produced by a thromboembolic mechanism (Shuping et al. 1980; Mathew and Meyer 1974; Fogelholm et al. 1975; Jensen and de Fine Olivarius 1981). Several cardiac and other embolic sources have been identified in patients experiencing TGA: MVP, mitral annulus calcification, prosthetic heart valves, and akinetic cardiac segments. TGA may also occur as a complication of cerebral angiography (Wales and Nov 1981; Cochran et al. 1982; Pexman and Coates 1983) and angiocardiogram (Shuttlework and Wise 1973), likely by emboli from atheromatous debris or catheter clot. Other etiologic conditions that have been reported in association with TGA include tumor, overdosage of diazepam, cardiac dysrhythmia resulting from digitalis intoxication, and migraine (Greenlec et al. 1975; Leak and Zimmerman 1975; Gilbert and Benson 1972; Crowell et al. 1984).

A study carried out by Jackson et al. in 1984 strongly supports an association between TGA and prolapsing mitral valve. Indeed MVP was present in 24.5% of the 53 patients with TGA, which was significantly higher than the 7.5% prevalence in the age and sex-matched control group. The mean age for TGA patients both with and without MVP was 66.1 years. Recurrent episodes of TGA were more common in patients with MVP (46%) than in those without MVP (17.5%). Subsequent neurologic events other than amnesia were experienced by five of these patients including generalized convulsions, syncope, mild hemispheric stroke, and hemispheric transient ischemic attack. Shuping et al. (1980) described a patient with MVP and multiple recurrences of TGA who achieved a complete remission following mitral valve replacement. In 12 consecutive cases of TGA reported by Crowell et al. (1984), echocardiography demonstrated MVP in 2 of the 6 patients submitted to this testing.

Therefore cardiac evaluation is recommended for all patients with TGA. In order to reduce the risk of recurrent episodes of TGA, the empirical usage of platelet antiaggregation therapy is recommended for patients with the combination of TGA and MVP. The possibility must be entertained of also giving platelet antiaggregants to patients with TGA but without MVP.

Cerebral Aneurysm

Jackson (1983) recently described five patients with MVP and intracranial aneurysms. Three of them had symptomatic rupture of aneurysms, while in the other two asymptomatic aneurysms were found during investigation of cerebral ischemic events subsequently considered secondary to MVP. The well-known association of MVP with hereditary connective tissue disorders including Marfan's syndrome, Ehlers-Danlos syndrome, and pseudoxanthoma elasticum and the high prevalence of intracranial aneurysm in each of these disorders suggest that the occurrence of cerebral aneurysm in MVP syndrome could be related to a mesodermal disturbance involving collagen and elastic tissue of the cerebral arteries. Indeed a similar collagen abnormality has been identified in patients with ruptured cerebral aneurysm and in type IV Ehlers-Danlos syndrome. Type III collagen deficiency has been reported in 11 of 17 ruptured cerebral aneurysm patients (Neil-Dwyer et al. 1983). Jaffe et al. (1981) demonstrated a decreased type III collagen on skin biopsy and MVP on echocardiography in eight family members of a patient with type IV Ehlers-Danlos syndrome. The same abnormality has been observed in patients with von Willebrand syndrome, which is also associated with prolapsing mitral valve and intracranial aneurysm (Andrews 1984; Pickering et al. 1981).

The frequent occurrence of MVP and cerebral aneurysm in the general population raises the possibility that they are associated by chance alone. Jackson suggested that a prospective, controlled study of cerebral aneurysms and mitral valve prolapse be undertaken to confirm this association and to elucidate the nature of any underlying connective tissue defect.

Migraine

Several studies have reported an association between migraine headache and MVP syndrome (Litman and Friedman 1978; Gamberini et al. 1984; Amat et al. 1982; Spence et al. 1984). In a retrospective study of 230 MVP patients, 28% had symptoms characteristic of migraine including throbbing, pulsating headache, teichopsia, visual scotoma, and repetitive neurologic deficit (Litman and Friedman 1978). There was a marked preponderance of Caucasian females and the majority had the onset of migraine during the (2nd and 3rd decades of life). Some authors have speculated that increased platelet aggregability might represent a common pathophysiologic mechanism of the two syndromes, as it relates both to emboli from an abnormal mitral valve and to strokes, which have been reported to occur at an increased rate in people who suffer from migraines.

However, the high prevalence of migraine headache among women in the general population, estimated at 20%, makes questionable any association between MVP and vascular headache. Most of these previous studies were retrospective and did not apply definite criteria for identification of migraine patients. Only a large population study completely randomized can ultimately confirm or deny this putative association between the two conditions.

Mitral Annulus Calcification

The increased use of echocardiography has focussed new attention on the subject of mitral annulus calcification (MAC) otherwise described as submitral (annular) calcification (Hirchfield et al. 1975; Gabor et al. 1976; D'Cruz et al. 1977). It has been established without equivocation that there is a relationship between this entity and ischemic stroke. It remains for much investigation to be done, and better techniques of cardiac and blood-vessel imaging to emerge, before the prevalence of MAC as a primary cause of cerebral and retinal ischemia can be recounted with accuracy.

Prevalence

The lesion is sufficiently common that it has been described as the most frequent pathologic background for systolic murmurs in elderly subjects (Pomerance 1968). McKeown (1975) detected this lesion in 27% of 100 elderly (nonagenarian) subjects examined at postmortem. At the time of the 16th biennial Framingham population examination, when the mean age of the original cohort generation was 70 years and the mean age of the offspring group was 44 years, all subjects were submitted to M-mode echocardiography (Savage et al. 1983). Of the total of 5694 subjects 2.8% had "evidence of posterior submitral calcification," 95% coming from the 40% of the study over 59 years of age. Women were more than twice as likely (3.8%) to have the findings as were men (1.7%) although the average age of men with the lesion was 73 years and of women 77 years.

Associated Risk Factors

In addition to age and female sex some reports claim that hypertension, possibly diabetes mellitus, and preexisting mitral valve prolapse are associated with increased prevalence of MAC (Kirk and Russell 1969; Fulkerson et al 1979). Nair et al. (1983), in an early report on 62 patients with MAC, found no increase of hypertension or diabetes mellitus; a later report by the same investigators involving 107 patients with age- and sex-matched controls detected a significant increase in diabetes mellitus and systemic hypertension, as well as increased prevalence of cardiomegaly by chest X-ray and of left atrial and left ventricular enlargement by echocardiography (Nair et al. 1984b). At Framingham there was a higher incidence of MAC among hypertensive males and among obese females (Savage 1983).

Cardiac Dysrythmias

The lesion of MAC is in close proximity to the atrioventricular node and the bundle of His. Thus it is not surprising that its cardiac complications include conduction system disease. In one review of patients requiring pacemaker implantation for heart block, 10% had MAC; conversely 51% of 80 patients with MAC had "evidence of significant atrioventricular or intraventricular block" (Fulkerson 1979). Atrial fibrillation, either paroxysmal or persistent, is common as it is in all conditions which give rise to a chronic increase of the left atrial pressure (Fulkerson 1979; Mellino et al. 1982). Sinus node dysfunction has been noted: it occurred in 9 of 80 patients described by Fulkerson et al. (1979) and 3 of 53 patients described by another group had sick sinus syndrome (Mellino et al. 1983). Focal cerebral ischemia is a very uncommon sequel to heart block (Reed et al. 1973) but is a common complication of atrial fibrillation and sick sinus syndrome (Barnett 1983—Neurologic Clinics).

Valvular Dysfunction

Mitral regurgitation, at times requiring valve replacement, and made more probable by preexisting myxomatous degeneration of the valve, is a recognized complication (Fulkerson 1979; Tajik et al. 1972). Left ventricular and left atrial enlargement are related to the degree of stenosis and regurgitation (Kirk and Russell 1969; Grossman et al. 1983). Bacterial endocarditis is known to occur superimposed upon this lesion (Burnside and DeSanctis 1972; Watanakunakuru 1973). Aortic stenosis as well as idiopathic hypertrophic subaortic stenosis and coronary artery disease with myocardial ischemia have all been described in association with MAC (Nair 1984a,b; Tajik et al. 1972, 1974).

Thromboembolism—Clinical Evidence

Thromboembolism complicates the condition. One report of 80 patients with MAC (Fulkerson 1979) described four instances of confirmed emboli: thrombus was removed surgically from the brachial, femoral, and popliteal arteries in three patients, and the embolic material was visualized as a calcific retinal embolus in the fourth. In the same series there were said to have been 11 patients with suggestive evidence of lesser embolic events, "usually causing transient ischemic attacks." Unfortunately no more detail was reported.

Clinical suspicion that MAC might be a cause of cerebral and retinal ischemia was stimulated particularly because of the report by de Bono and Warlow (1979). In a consecutive series of 151 patients (aged 64–78) afflicted with retinal or cerebral ischemic events by M-mode echocardiography, 8 of the 151 and none of the control group, matched for age and sex, had MAC. Emboli in the retinal arterioles, compatible in appearance with calcium, were observed in four of the eight. The totally negative findings in the control group of individuals are unexpected in view of the prevalence of MAC in population studies.

A major problem which clinicians face whenever a patient with retinal and cerebral ischemia is found to have MAC is to determine whether or not the MAC is the cause of the symptoms. Patients are at an age when other types of heart disease and when aortic and particularly carotid artery disease are very common. In de Bono and Warlow's series, only two of the patients had angiographic studies performed and this investigation was not available in the one patient said to have bilateral carotid bruits. A series of patients with ischemia were studied by Irino (Barnett 1983) with both arteriography and

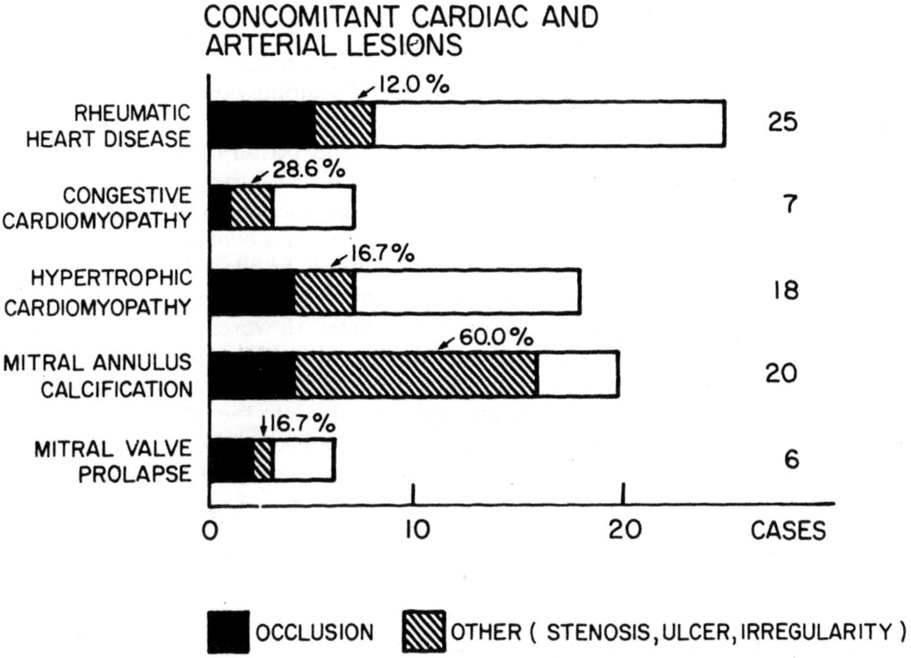

Fig. 5.2. A study of 76 patients with a variety of cardiac lesions in association with cerebral ischemic events. Cerebral angiography indicated the highest percentage of concomitant potentially thromboembolic lesions in patients with mitral annulus calcification (Irino 1983).

cardiac imaging. Figure 5.2 depicts the number of times, in a variety of lesions detected by echocardiography, that there was difficulty in determining which lesion was the causative mechanism in producing the ischemia. Sixty percent of 20 patients with MAC had recognizable stenotic ulceration or irregular change in the ipsilateral internal carotid artery; 20% had a carotid occlusion; and only 20% had a normal appropriate carotid artery.

A study involving 350 patients with ischemic stroke, in whom two-dimensional (2-D) echocardiography was carried out, detected MAC in 29 (8.3%) of the subjects, but in only 12 (3.4%) age- and sex-matched controls (Nishide et al. 1983). A similar study by 2-D echocardiography divided 105 patients with ischemic stroke into those without cardiac symptoms or signs (N=48) and those with evidence of heart abnormality (N=57). MAC was present in 3 (6.3%) of the former but in 11 (19.3%) of the latter groups respectively (Thal et al. 1982).

In elderly patients under investigation for cerebral ischemia, there exists at the present time no easy way to implicate the MAC as the sole possible causative factor. If the patient has atrial enlargement, atrial fibrillation, sick sinus syndrome, and possibly also associated aortic stenosis, a definitive relationship is probably stronger than with MAC alone. However, the possibility of an artery lesion will often remain as a possible cause because of the prevalence of arteriosclerosis with advancing years.

Thromboembolism—Pathologic Evidence

Pathologic studies, some correlated with the clinical histories of patients with MAC, have determined that there are a variety of complications of the condition which could lead to circulatory or embolic disorders affecting the brain and retina. The calcification has a predilection for the posterior segment of the annulus; massive calcification with complete closure of the ring is relatively infrequent at postmortem (Korn 1962). Thus a lesion severe enough to produce mitral insufficiency is frequent but mitral valve stenosis is considered rare (Geill 1951, 1950). In an early postmortem study 14 patients fulfilled the requirements of massive MAC, producing deformity of the atrium, without evidence of healed rheumatic disease or endocarditis (Korn et al. 1962). All were women of average age 75 (range 52-88). Calcific masses extended from the rigid ring by as much as 3.5 cm into the adjacent myocardium. Masses of calcific material were observed projecting superiorly toward the atrium and centrally into the ventricular cavity. In this particular group of 14 postmortem subjects, all were known to have been afflicted with mitral systolic murmurs and three with mitral diastolic murmurs. Aortic systolic murmurs had been heard in 6 of the 14, and aortic calcific material in irregular nodular masses with free cusp edges was observed in 5 of the 6. Coronary artery disease was evident in all 14 patients, slight in 10, moderate in 4, and occlusive in none. However, evidence of generalized arteriosclerosis was noted, severe in eight, moderate in two. The cardiac rhythm disorders in this group of 14 patients were impressive: nine had atrial fibrillation, one had complete heart block, and one a "bizarre" supraventricular tachycardia. Four of the 14 had massive (1) or bilateral (3) cerebral infarcts with evidence of embolic obstructions of the middle, posterior cerebral, and carotid arteries. Three of the four with cerebral embolic events had been known to be afflicted with atrial fibrillation; the fourth had complete heart block.

Two reports concern observations of calcific emboli to brain or retina. One is a clinical report by Fulkerson et al. (1979) concerning 80 patients, of mean age 73 and with a female to male ratio of 2.5:1, 5 of whom experienced arterial episodes: 4 had peripheral arterial embolectomy and 1 had recognizable calcific retinal emboli. In the other, multiple calcific emboli caused obstructive lesions of the coronary artery and in the anterior and posterior cerebral circulation; the lesions were examined at a postmortem conducted on a 53-year-old patient (Ridolfi et al. 1976).

Several types of material may produce the embolization in MAC. First of all there is no doubt that the calcified ring is prone to caseation (Fig. 5.3). In a study of 258 hearts with MAC, of which twice as many come from women as from men, Pomerance (1970) detected ulceration and extrusion of the calcium through the overlapping cusp in 12 hearts; 11 were from females and 1 from a male. Thrombi were attached to these ulcerated valves in 4 of the 12 (Fig. 5.4). Additional emboligenic lesions identified by Pomerance in this careful study included one instance of an acute hemorrhagic valvulitis and three instances of bacterial endocarditis. The latter, in one patient, had led to what was described as an emboligenic origin of a fatal bacterial meningitis. All of these lesions reflect potentially thromboembolic lesions and it is evident that the emboli may consist of calcific material, thrombus, or fragments of endocardial proliferative lesions accompanying infection.

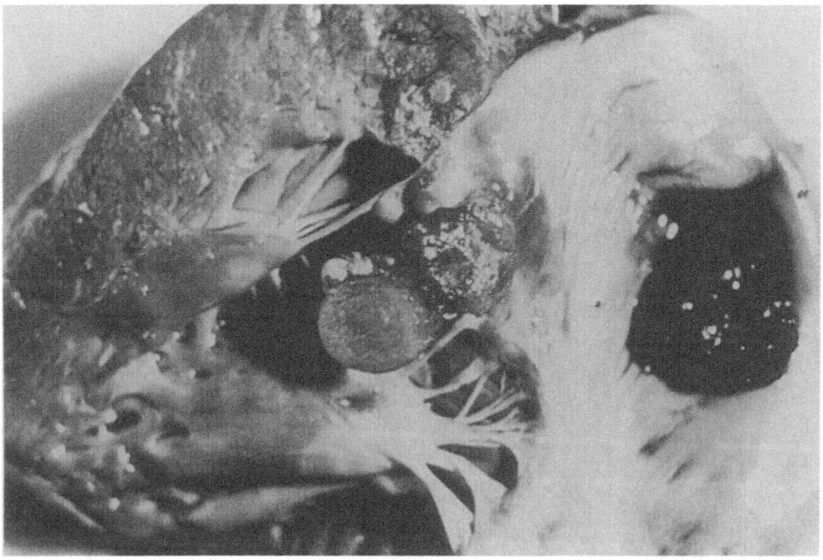

Fig. 5.3. Large thrombus attached to mitral annulus calcification—an incidental postmortem finding in an elderly patient (Pomerance 1970).

Prognosis for Patients with Mitral Annulus Calcification

One retrospective review of a series (N=63) of patients with MAC has been published by Furlan et al. (1984). Curiously the series was equally representative of men (32) as of women (31) and the average age at diagnosis was slightly younger than in most reported series (mean age 65, range 47–78). Four of the patients had presented with amaurosis fugax and two with hemispheric TIA. Coronary arteriosclerosis and hypertension were universally found, three had left atrial enlargement, five had congestive heart failure, and only one had atrial fibrillation at the time of diagnosis. In follow-up, averaging 3.4 years, 3 strokes (all fatal) occurred in the group of 63 patients, but 2 were related to intracerebral hemorrhage and one was caused by a pontine infarction. There were two TIAs in this follow-up; both were in the territory of arteries previously submitted to carotid endarterectomy but without persistent lesions of consequence visualized in repeat angiograms. These authors concluded, with justification, that the finding of MAC is to be regarded most particularly as a marker for the presence of generalized arteriosclerosis disease. Nevertheless pathologic observations make it very certain that MAC does cause cerebral ischemia. How often it is the main cause remains unknown and how to be sure of the relationship to the stroke in an individual patient remains difficult to establish.

Management of Patients with Embolism Related to Mitral Annulus Calcification

Treatment for patients who have evidence of retinal and cerebral ischemia in association with MAC is empirical. Firstly, the rhythm disorders of atrial

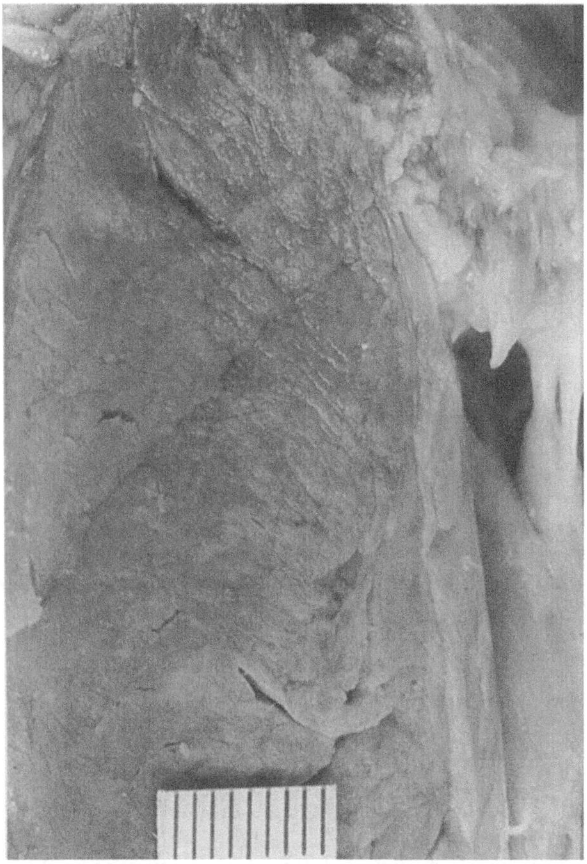

Fig. 5.4. A caseating mitral annulus calcific lesion in an elderly patient. These lesions are potentially capable of producing emboli containing this calcific material (Silver 1980).

fibrillation, heart block, and sinoatrial node dysfunction must receive appropriate therapy. A stenosing or regurgitant valve may require surgical replacement. Hypertension, which may be aggravating or even causative of the degenerative valvular process, demands diligent treatment. Antithrombotic agents have been dismissed by one group (de Bono and Warlow 1979) as not rational because of the fact that some of the embolic material is composed of fragments of calcium. However, thrombi have been seen on the valves attached to the ulcerating process and have been identified in surgical embolectomies; hence the empirical use of antithrombotics is a reasonable therapeutic strategy in selected patients (Traill et al. 1979). Should the patient have evidence of a recent major arterial embolus, the possibility of a large thrombus attached to the valve (as in Fig. 5.4) justifies a short 6- to 10-week) period on warfarin followed by long-term aspirin prophylaxis. If there is no clinical or echocardiographic evidence of a large thrombus in the heart, nor any evidence of major peripheral thromboembolism, the empirical utilization of aspirin as initial and continuing therapy is recommended.

References

Abinader EG, Shahar J (1982) Exercise testing in mitral valve prolapse before and after beta blockade. Br Heart J 48: 130–133

Allcock J (1967) Occlusion of middle cerebral artery: serial angiography as a guide to conservative therapy. J Neurosurg 27: 353–363

Allen H, Harris A, Leatham A (1974) Significance and prognosis of an isolated late systolic murmur: a 9- to 22-year follow up. Br Heart J 36: 525–532

Amat G, Loisy C, Jean Louis P, Centonze V, Pelage S (1982) Migraine and the mitral valve prolapse syndrome. In: Critchley M, Friedman AP, Gorini S, Sicuteri F (eds) Headache. Advances in neurology, vol 33, Raven, New York, pp 27–29

Andrews RJ (1984) Collagen in cerebral aneurysms, mitral valve prolapse and von Willebrand syndrome. Stroke 15: 917–918

Appelblatt NH, Willis PW, Lenhart JA Shulman JI, Walton JA Jr (1975) Ten to forty year follow-up of 69 patients with systolic click with or without apical late systolic murmur. Am J Cardiol 35: 119

Baker RS, Tibbs PA, Millett AJ (1981) Carotid-retinal embolism with coexistent mitral valve prolapse. Neurology 31: 1192–1193

Barletta CA, Gagliardi R, Benvenuti L, Fantini F (1985) Cerebral ischemic attacks as a complication of aortic and mitral valve prolapse. Stroke 16(2): 219–223

Barlow JB, Bosman CK (1966) Aneurysmal protrusion of posterior leaflet of the mitral valve. An auscultatory-electrocardiographic syndrome. Am Heart J 71: 166–178

Barlow JB, Pocock WA (1979) Mitral valve prolapse, the specific following mitral leaflet syndrome or an insignificant non-ejection systolic click. Am Heart J 97: 277–285

Barlow JB, Pocock WA, Marchand P, Denny M (1963) The significance of late systolic murmurs. Am Heart J 66: 443–452

Barnett HJM (1974) Transient cerebral ischemia: pathogenesis, prognosis and management. Ann R Coll Phys Surg Can 7: 153–173

Barnett HJM (1982) Embolism in mitral valve prolapse. Ann Rev Med 33: 489–507

Barnett HJM (1983) Heart in ischemic stroke—a changing emphasis. Neurol Clinics 1: 291–315

Barnett HJM, Boughner DR, Taylor DW, Cooper PE, Kostuk WJ, Nichol PM (1980) Further evidence relating mitral valve prolapse to cerebral ischemic events. N Engl J Med 302: 139–144

Barnett HJM, Jones MW, Boughner DR, Kostuk WJ (1976) Cerebral ischemic events associated with prolapsing mitral valve. Arch Neurol 33: 777–782

Belardi J, Lardani H, Manubens S, Sheldon WC, Moreyra A (1976) Idiopathic prolapse of the mitral valve. A follow-up study in 137 patients studied by angiography. Am J Cardiol 37: 120

Bensaid J, Cuisinier Y, Renaudin D, Vallat JM (1980) Accidents vasculaires cerebraux ischemiques: role etiologique du prolapsus valvulaire mitral-10 observations. Nouv Press Med 9: 1716

Beton DC, Brear SG, Edwards JD, Leonard JC (1983) Mitral valve prolapse: an assessment of clinical features, associated conditions and prognosis. Q J Med, New Series 52 (206): 150–164

Bisset GS, Schwartz DC, Meyer RA, James FW, Kaplan S (1980) Clinical spectrum and long- term follow-up of isolated mitral valve prolapse in 119 children. Circulation 62: 423–429

Bharati S, Bauernfeind R, Miller LB, Strasberg B, Lev M (1983) Sudden death in three teenagers. Conduction system studies. J Am Cardiol 1: 879–886

Bon Tempo CP, Ronan JA Jr, de Leon AC Jr, Twigg HL (1975) Radiographic appearance of the thorax in systolic click—late systolic murmur syndrome. Am J Cardiol 36: 27–31

Boudoulas H, Reynolds JC, Mazzaferri E, Wooley CF (1980) Metabolic studies in mitral valve prolapse syndrome: a neuroendocrine—cardiovascular process. Circulation 61: 1200–1205

Boughner D, Barnett HJM (1985) The enigma of the risk of stroke in mitral valve prolapse. Stroke 16: 175–177

Bramlet DA, Dicker EL, Floyd (1982) Nonbacterial thrombotic endocarditis as a cause of stroke in mitral valve prolapse. South Med J 75: 1133–1135

Braun WE, Ronan J, Schacter B, Gardin J, Isner J, Grececk J (1977) HLA antigens in mitral valve prolapse. Transplant Proc 9: 1862–1871

Brown OR, Kloster FE, Demots H (1975) Incidence of mitral valve prolapse in the asymptomatic normal. Circulation 52 [Suppl II]: 651–662

Buda AJ, Levene DL, Myers MG, Chisholm AW, Shane SJ (1978) Coronary artery spasm and mitral valve prolapse. Am Heart J 95: 457–462

Burnside JW, de Sanctis RW (1972) Bacterial endocarditis on calcification of the mitral annulus fibrosis. Ann Intern Med 76: 615

Caltrider ND, Irvine AR, Kline HJ, Rosenblatt A (1980) Retinal emboli in patients with mitral valve prolapse. Am J Ophtalmol 90(4): 534–539
Campbell RWF, Godman MG, Fiddler GI, Marquis RM, Julian DG (1976). Ventricular arrhythmias in syndrome of balloon deformity of mitral valve: definition of a possible high risk group. Br Heart J 38: 1053–1057
Caplan LR, Weiner H, Weintraub RM, Austen WG (1976) "Migrainous" neurologic dysfunction in patients with prosthetic cardiac valves. Headache 16: 218–221
Chandraratna PAN, Nimalasuruja A, Kawanishi D, Duncan P, Rosin B, Rahimtoola SH (1984) Identification of the increased frequency of cardiovascular abnormalities associated with mitral valve prolapse by two-dimensional echocardiography. Am J Cardiol 54: 1283–1287
Chandraratna PAN, Vlahovich G, Kong Y, Wilson D (1979) Incidence of mitral valve prolapse in one hundred clinically stable newborn baby girls: an echocardiographic study. Am Heart J 98: 312–314
Cheitlin MD (1979) Thromboembolic studies in the patient with the prolapsed mitral valve. Has Salome dropped another veil? Circulation 60(1): 46–47
Cheitlin MD, Byrd RC (1984) Prolapsed mitral valve: the commonest valve disease? Curr Probl Cardiol 8(10): 3–53
Chesler E, King RA, Edwards JE (1983) The myxomatous mitral valve and sudden death. Circulation 67: 632–639
Chesler E, Matisonn RE, Lakier JB, Pocock WA, Obel IWP, Barlow JB (1976) Acute myocardial infarction with normal coronary arteries: a possible manifestation of the billowing mitral leaflet syndrome. Circulation 54: 203–209
Cochran JW, Morrell F, Huckman MS, Cochran EJ (1982) Transient global amnesia after cerebral angiography: report of seven cases. Arch Neurol 39: 593–594
Cobbs BW Jr, King SB (1977) III: Ventricular buckling: a factor in the abnormal ventriculogram and peculiar hemodynamics associated with mitral valve prolapse. Am Heart J 93 (6): 741–758
Coghlan HC, Phares P, Cowley M, Copely D, James TN (1979) Dysautonomia in valve prolapse. Am J Med 67: 236–244
Cook AW, Bird TD, Spence AM, Pagon RA, Wallace FJ (1978) Myotonic dystrophy, mitral valve prolapse and stroke. Letter to the editor. Lancet 1: 335
Crawford MH (1977) Mitral valve prolapse due to coronary artery disease. Am J Med 62: 447–451
Crawford MH, O'Rourke RA (1984) Mitral valve prolapse: a cardiomyopathic state? Prog Cardiov Dis 27 (2): 133–139
Criley JM, Lewis KB, Humphries JO, Ross RS (1966) Prolapse of the mitral valve: clinical and cineangiographic findings. Br Heart J 28: 488–496
Criley JM, Zeilenga DW, Mosgin MT (1973). Mitral dysfunction: a possible cause of arrhythmias in the prolapsing mitral leaflet syndrome. Trans Am Clin Climatol Assoc 85: 44–53
Crowell GF, Stump DA, Biller J, McHenry LC, Toole JF (1984). The transient global amnesia-migraine connection. Arch Neurol 41: 75–79
D'Andrea G, Toldo M, Cortelazzos, Ferro Milane F (1982) Platelet activity in migraine. Headache 22: 207–212
Darsee JR, Mickolich JR, Nicoloff NB, Lesser LE (1979) Prevalence of mitral valve prolapse in presumably healthy young men. Circulation 59: 619–622
Davies J (1963) Human development anatomy. Ronald, New York. pp 81, 276, 278
Davies MJ, Moore BP, Braimbridge MV (1978) The floppy mitral valve: study of incidence, pathology and complications in surgical, necropsy, and forensic material. Br Heart J 40: 468–481
D'Cruz IA, Cohen HC, Prabhu R, Bisla V, Click G (1977) Clinical manifestations of mitral annulus calcification with emphasis on its echocardiographic features. Am Heart J 94: 367–377
De Bono DP, Warlow CP (1979) Mitral annulus calcification and cerebral or retinal ischemia. Lancet II: 383
De Bono DP, Warlow CP (1981) Potential sources of emboli in patients with presumed transient cerebral or retinal ischemia. Lancet I: 343–346
De Maria AN, King JF, Bogren HG, Lies JE, Mason DT (1974). The variable spectrum of echocardiographic manifestations of the mitral valve prolapse syndrome. Circulation 50: 33–41
De Silva RA, Shubrooks SJ (1977) Mitral valve prolapse with atrioventricular and sinoatrial node abnormalities of long duration. Am Heart J 93: 772–775
Devereux RB, Brown WT (1983) Genetics of mitral valve prolapse. Prog Med Genetics 5: 139–161
Devereux RB, Brown WT, Kramer-Fox R, Sachs I (1981) Inheritance of mitral valve prolapse: autosomal dominant with reduced expression in children and adult males. (Abstr) Clin Res 29: 412A
Devereux RB, Brown WT, Kramer-Fox R, Sachs I (1982) Inheritance of mitral valve prolapse: effects of age and sex on gene transmission. Ann Intern Med 97: 826–832

Devereux RB, Kramer-Fox R, Brown WT, Hartman N, Kligfield P, Lutas EM (1982) Is there a clinically distinct mitral valve prolapse syndrome? Clin Res 30: 480a
Devereux RB, Perloff JK, Reichek N, Josephson ME, Sachs I, Litwin SD (1976) Mitral valve prolapse. Circulation 54: 3–14
Dillon JC, Haine CL, Chang S, Feigenbaum H (1971) Use of echocardiography in patients with prolapsed mitral valve. Circulation 43: 503–507
Donaldson RM, Emanual RW, Earl CJ (1981) The role of two-dimensional echocardiography in the detection of potentially embolic intracardiac masses in patients with cerebral ischemia. J Neurol Neurosurg Psych 44: 803–809
Engel PJ, Alpert BL, Hickman JR Jr (1979) The nature and prevalence of the abnormal exercise electrocardiogram in mitral valve prolapse. Am Heart J 98: 716–724
Fairfax AJ, Lambert CD, Leatham A (1976) Systemic embolism in chronic sinoatrial disorder. N Engl J Med 295: 190–192
Falicov RE (1977) Strokes: a compilation of mitral-leaflet prolapse? Letter to the editor. Lancet I: 335
Falicov RE (1977) Strokes: a complication of mitral leaflet prolapse? Letter to the editor. Lancet 2: 923
Fieschi C, Francia A, Allori L, Argentino L, Bernardi S, Bertazzoni G (1983) Mitral valve prolapse as a risk factor for TIA. Eur Neurol 22: 233–239
Fisher CM, Adams RD (1964) Transient global amnesia syndrome. Acta Neurol Scand 40 (Suppl 9): 7–82
Fisher M, Weiner B, Ockene IS, Forsberg A, Duffy CP, Levine PH (1983) Platelet activation and mitral valve prolapse. Neurology 33: 384–386
Fogelholm R, Kivalo E, Bergstrom L (1975) The transient global amnesia syndrome—an analysis of 35 cases. Eur Neurol 13: 72–84
Fontana ME, Pence HL, Leighton RF, Wooley CL (1970) The varying clinical spectrum of the systolic click—late systolic murmur syndrome. Circulation 41: 807–816
Fulkerson PK, Beaver BM, Auseon JC, Graver HL (1979) Calcification of the mitral annulus — etiology, clinical associations, complications and therapy. Am J Med 66: 967–977
Furlan AJ, Craciun AR, Salcedo EE, Mellino M (1984) Risk of stroke in patients with mitral annulus calcification. Stroke 15: 801–803
Gabor GE, Mohr BC, Goel PC, Cohen B (1976) Echocardiographic and clinical spectrum of mitral annular calcification. Am J Cardiol 38: 836–842
Gaffney FA, Karlsson ES, Campbell W, Schutte JE, Nixon JV, Willerson JT, Blomquist CG (1979) Autonomic dysfunction in women with mitral valve prolapse syndrome. Circulation 59: 894–901
Gaffney FA, Bastian BC, Taylor WF, Schutte JE, Graham RM, Pettinger WA, Blomquist CG (1980) Adregenic control mechanisms in the mitral valve prolapse syndrome (Abstr.) Circulation 62 [Suppl III]: 206
Gallavardin L (1913) Pseudo-dedoublement du deuxieme bruit du coeur: simulant le dedoublement mitral par bruit extracardiaque telesystolique surajoute. Lyon Medicale 121: 409
Gamberini G, D'Alessandro R, Labriola E, Poggi V, Manzoni GC, Carpeggiana P, Sacquegna T (1984) Further evidence on the association of mitral valve prolapse and migraine. Headache 24: 39–40
Geill T (1950) Calcification of left annulus fibrosus (230 cases). Acta Med Scandivania 138 [Suppl 239]: 153–156
Geill T (1951) Calcification of left annulus fibrosus. J Gerontol 6: 327–333
Geyer SJ, Franzini DA (1979) Myxomatous degeneration of the mitral valve complicated by nonbacterial thrombotic endocarditis with systemic embolization. Am J Clin Path 72: 489–492
Gilbert BW, Schatz RA, Von Ramm OT, Behar VS, Kisslo JA (1976) Mitral valve prolapse: Two-dimensional echocardiographic and angiographic correlation. Circulation 54: 716–723
Gilbert JJ, Benson DF (1972) Transient global amnesia. Report of two cases with definite etiologies. J Nerv Mental Dis 154: 461–464
Gonder JR, Magargal LE, Walsh PN, Rao K, Denenberg BE (1983) Central retinal vein obstruction associated with mitral valve prolapse. Can J Ophthalmol 18 (5): 220–222
Gooch AS, Vicencio F, Maranhao V, Goldberg H (1972) Arrhythmias and left ventricular asynergy in the prolapsing mitral leaflet syndrome. Am J Cariol 29: 611–620
Goodman D, Kimbiris D, Linhart JW (1974) Chordae tendinae rupture complicating the systolic click—late systolic murmur syndrome. Am J Cardiol 33: 681–684
Greenlee JE, Crampton RS, Miller JQ (1975) Transient global amnesia associated with cardiac arrhythmia and digitalis intoxication. Stroke 6: 513–516
Gregoratus G, Karliner JS (1979) Infective endocarditis. Diagnosis and management. Med Clin North Am 63: 173–199

Grossman H, Fleming RJ, Engle MA, Levin AH, Ehlers KH (1968) Angiocardiography in the apical systolic click syndrome. Radiology 91: 898–904
Grossman RJ, Abbasi AS, DeCristofaro D, Ungar I (1983) Mitral regurgitation in patients with calcified mitral annulus. Circulation 68: 241
Hammer D, Leier EV, Baba N, Vasko JS, Wooley CF, Pinnell SR (1979) Altered collagen composition in a prolapsing mitral valve with ruptured chordae tendinae. Am J Med 67: 863–866
Hanson MR, Conomy JP, Hodgman JR (1980) Brain events associated with mitral valve prolapse. Stroke 11 (5): 499–506
Hart RG, Easton JD (1982) Mitral valve prolapse and cerebral infarction. Stroke 13 (4): 429–430
Hart RG, Sherman DG, Wolf PA, Kannel WB (1985) Mitral valve prolapse and embolic stroke. Letter to the editor. Stroke 16 (2): 334
Hickley AJ, Wilcken DEL (1980) Prevalence of mitral valve prolapse in an Australian population. Lancet 1: 1366
Hill DG, Davies MJ, Braimbridge MV (1974) The natural history and surgical management of the redundant cusp syndrome (floppy mitral valve). J Thorac Cardiovas Surg 67: 519–525
Hirschfeld DS, Emilson BB (1975) Echocardiogram in calcified mitral annulus. Am J Cardiol 36: 354–356
Horenstein S, Taylor D, Williams G, Wiens R (1979) Syncope, seizure and stroke in the mitral valve prolapse syndrome. Neurology 29: 537 (abstr)
Horowitz MS, Smith LG (1977) Vegetative bacterial endocarditis in the prolapsing mitral valve. Arch Intern Med 137: 788–790
Imaizumi T, Chandraratna PAN, Whayne TF Jr, Schechter E, Bhatia SK (1978) Transmural myocardial infarction: with the prolapsing mitral leaflet syndrome and normal coronary arteries. Arch Intern Med 138: 1354–1355
Jackson AC (1983) Association of mitral valve prolapse and intracranial aneurysms. South Med J 76: 712–713
Jackson AC, Boughner DR, Barnett HJM (1984) Mitral valve prolapse and cerebral ischemic events in young patients. Neurology 34: 784–787
Jackson AC, Boughner DR, Bolton CF, Hopkins M, Barnett HJM (1985) Transient global amnesia associated with mitral valve prolapse. Neurology 35 [Suppl I]: 215 (Abstract)
Jaffe AS, Geltman EM, Rodey GE, Uitto J (1981) Mitral valve prolapse: a consistent manifestation of type IV Ehlers-Danlos syndrome. Circulation 64: 121–125
Jenson TS, de Fine Olivarius (1981) Transient global amnesia—its clinical and pathophysiological basis and prognosis. Acta Neurol Scand 63: 220–230
Jeresaty RM (1976) Sudden death in the mitral valve prolapse—click syndrome. Am J Cardiol 37: 317–318
Jeresaty RM (1973) Mitral valve prolapse—click syndrome. Prog Cardiovasc Dis 15: 623–652
Jeresaty RM (1979) Mitral valve prolapse. Raven, New York
Jones HR, Naggar CZ, Selijan MP, Downing ZZ (1982) Mitral valve prolapse and cerebral ischemic events. A comparison between a neurology population with stroke and a cardiology population with mitral valve prolapse observed for five years. Stroke 13 (4): 451–453
Josephson ME, Horowitz LN, Kastor JA (1978) Paroxysmal supraventricular tachycardia in patients with mitral valve prolapse. Circulation 57: 111–115
Kerber RE, Isaeff DM, Hancock EW (1971) Echocardiographic patterns in patients with syndrome of systolic click and late systolic murmur. N Engl J Med 284: 691–693
Kimball RW, Hedges TR (1977) Amaurosis fugax caused by prolapsed mitral valve leaflet in the midsystolic click—late systolic murmur syndrome. Am J Ophtalmol 83: 469–470
King BD, Clark MA, Baba N, Hilman JW, Wooley CF (1982) "Myxomatous" mitral valve: collagen dissolution as the primary defect. Circulation 66 (2): 288–296
Kirk RS, Russell JGB (1969) Subvalvular calcification of mitral valve. Br Heart J 31: 684–692
Knopman D, Anderson DC, Greenland P, Mikell F, Asinger R, Good D (1980) Mitral valve prolapse and cerebral ischemic events in the elderly. Letter to the editor. N Engl J Med 303: 641
Koch LH, Hancock EW (1976) Ten-year follow-up of forty patients with midsystolic click/late systolic murmur syndrome. Am J Cardiol 37: 149
Korn D, De Sanctis RW, Sell S (1962) Massive calcification of the mitral annulus. A clinicopathological study of fourteen cases. New Engl J Med 267: 900–909
Kostuk WJ, Boughner DR, Barnett HJM, Silver MD (1977) Strokes: a complication of mitral-leaflet prolapse? Lancet 2: 313–316
Kouvaras G, Bacoulas G (1985) Association of mitral leaflet prolapse with cerebral ischemic events in the young and early middle-aged patient. J Med, New Series 55 (219): 387–392

Lachman AS, Bramwell-Jones DM, Lakier JB, Pocock WA, Barlow JB (1975) Infective endocarditis in the billowing mitral syndrome. Br Heart J 37: 326–330
Leak RP, Zimmerman RA (1975) Transient global amnesia due to dominant hemisphere tumor. Arch Neurol 34: 317–318
Leclerqu JF, Malergue MC, Milosevic D, et al. (1980) Troubles due rythme ventriculaire et prolapsus mitral. Arch Mal Coeur 73: 276–287
Leightman D, Nelson R, Gobel F, Alexander CS, Cohn J (1975) Bradyarrhythmia in familial mitral valve prolapse syndrome: a potential mechanism of sudden death. Circulation 52 [Suppl 2]: 92
Le Winter MM, Hoffman JR, Shell WE, Karliner JS, O'Rourke RA (1974) Phenylephrine-induced atypical chest pain in patients with prolapsing mitral valve leaflets. Am J Cardiol 34: 12–18
Litman GI, Friedman HM (1978) Migraine and the mitral valve prolapse syndrome. Am Heart J 96: 610–614
Litman GI, Friedman HM (1980) Neurological manifestations of mitral valve prolapse. Update III: the heart. In: Hurst JW (ed) McGraw Hill, New York, pp 53–58
Logan W, Scherman DG (1983) Transient global amnesia. Stroke 14: 1005–1007
Lucas RV, Edwards JE (1982) The floppy mitral valve. Curr Probl Cardiol 7 (4): 5–48
Mardelli TJ, Morganroth J, Chen CC, Naito M, Vergel J (1981) Tricuspid valve prolapse diagnosed by cross-sectional echocardiography. Chest 79: 201–205
Markiewicz W, Stoner J, London E, Hunt SA, Popp RL (1976) Mitral valve prolapse in one hundred presumably healthy young females. Circulation 53: 464–473
Mason JW, Koch FH, Billingham ME, Winkle RA (1978) Cardiac biopsy evidence for a cardiomyopathy associated with symptomatic mitral valve prolapse. Am J Cardiol 42: 557–562
Mathew NT, Meyer JS (1974) Pathogenesis and natural history of transient global amnesia. Stroke 5: 303–311
McKay R, Yacoub MH (1973) Clinical and pathological findings in patients with "floppy" valves treated surgically. Circulation 48 [Suppl III]: 63–72
McKeoun EF (1975) De senectu: the FE Williams Lecture. J Roy Coll Phys (London) 10: 79
Medina RP, Dreifus LS (1983) Syncope. Current Probl Cardio 6 (8): 8–50
Mellino M, Salcedo EE (1983) Mitral annulus calcification: clinical implications. Cleveland Clin Q 50: 6–10
Mellino M, Salcedo EE, Lever HM, Vasudevan G, Kramer JR (1982) Echographic-quantified severity of mitral annulus calcification: prognostic correlation to related hemodynamic, valvular, rhythm, and conduction abnormalities. Am Heart J 103: 222–225
Mills P, Rose J, Hollingsworth J, Amara I, Craige E (1977) Long-term prognosis of mitral valve prolapse. N Engl J Med 297: 13–18
Morganroth J, Mardelli TJ, Naito M, Chen CC (1981) Apical cross-sectional echocardiography: standard for the diagnosis of idiopathic mitral valve prolapse syndrome. Chest 79: 23–28
Nair CK, Aronow WS, Sketch MH, Mohiuddin SM, Pagano T, Esterbrooks DJ, Hee TT (1983) Clinical and echocardiographic characteristics of patients with mitral annular calcification. Comparison with age- and sex-matched control subjects. Am J Cardiol 51: 992–995
Nair CK, Aronow WS, Stokke K, Mohiuddin SM, Thomson W, Sketch MH (1984) Cardiac conduction defects in patients older than 60 years with aortic stenosis with and without mitral anular calcium. Am J Cardiol 53: 169–172
Nair CK, Sudhakaran C, Aronow WS, Thomson W, Woodruff MP, Sketch MH (1984). Clinical characteristics of patients younger than 60 years with mitral anular calcium. Comparison with age- and sex-matched control subjects. Am J Cardiol 54: 1286–1287
Natarajan G, Nakhjavam FK, Kahn D, Yazdanfar S, Sahibzada W, Khawaja F, Goldberg H (1975) Myocardial metabolic studies in prolapsing mitral leaflet syndrome. Circulation 52: 1105–1110
Nichol P, Kertesz A (1979) Two-dimensional echocardiographic (2DE) detection of left atrial thrombus in patients with mitral valve prolapse and strokes. Circulation 59/60 [Suppl II]: 18
Neil-Dwyer G, Bartlett JR, Nicholls AC, Narcisi P, Pope FM (1983) Collagen deficiency and ruptured cerebral aneurysms: a clinical and biochemical study. J Neurosurg 59: 16–20
Nishide M, Tadayoshi I, Gotoh M, Naka M, Tsuji K (1983) Cardiac abnormalities in ischemic cerebrovascular disease studied by two-dimensional echocardiography. Stroke 14: 541–561
Nishimura RA, McGoon MD, Shub C, Miller FA, Ilstrup DM, Tajik AJ (1985) Echocardiographically documented mitral valve prolapse. Long-term follow-up of 237 patients. N Engl J Med 313(21): 1305–1309
Oakley CM (1985) Mitral valve prolapse: Q J Med, New Series 56 (219): 317–320
Paternac A, Tubau JF, Puddu PE, Krol RB, deChamplain J (1982) Increased plasma catecholamine levels in patients with symptomatic mitral valve prolapse. Am J Med 73: 783–789
Perloff JK (1982) Evolving concepts of mitral valve prolapse. N Engl J Med 307: 369–370

Pexman JHW, Coates RK (1983) Amnesia after femorocerebral angiography. Am J Neuroradiol 4: 979–983
Pickering NJ, Brody JI, Barrett MJ (1981) Von Willebrand syndrome and mitral valve prolapse: linked mesenchymal dysplasias. N Engl J Med 305: 131–134
Pocock WA, Barlow JB (1970) Post exercise arrhythmias in the billowing posterior mitral leaflet syndrome. Am Heart J 80: 740–745
Pocock WA, Barlow JB (1971) Etiology and electrocardiographic features of the billowing posterior mitral leaflet syndrome. Am J Med 51: 731–739
Pomerance A (1967) Ageing changes in human heart valves. Br Heart J 29: 222–231
Pomerance A (1969) Ballooning deformity (mucoid degeneration) of atrioventricular valves. Br Heart J 31: 343–351
Pomerance A (1970) Pathological and clinical study of calcification of the mitral valve ring. J Clin Path 23: 354–361
Pomerance A, Davies MJ (1977) Strokes: a complication of mitral leaflet prolapse. Letter to the editor. Lancet 2: 1186
Popp RL, Brown OR, Silverman JF, Harrison DC (1974) Echocardiographic abnormalities in the mitral valve prolapse syndrome. Circulation 44: 428–433
Procacci PM, Savran SV, Schreiter SL, Bryson AL (1976) Prevalence of clinical mitral valve prolapse in 1169 young women. N Eng J Med 294: 1086–1088
Puddu PE, Pasternac A, Tubau JF, Krol R, Farley L, de Champlain J (1983) QT interval prolongation and increased plasma catecholamine levels in patients with mitral valve prolapse. Am Heart J 105: 422–428
Ranganathan N, Lam JHC, Wigle ED, Silver MD (1970) Morphology of the human mitral valve: II. The valve leaflets. Circulation 41: 459–467
Ranganatham N, Robinson T, Silver MD, Patt NL, Wilson JK (1973) Angiographic clinical correlation in mitral click syndrome. Circulation 48 (4): 206 (Abstr.)
Ranganathan N, Silver MD, Robinson T, Kostuk WJ, Felderhof CH, Patt NL, Wilson JK, Wigle ED (1973) Angiographic-morphological correlation in patients with severe mitral regurgitation due to prolapse of the posterior mitral valve leaflet. Circulation 48: 514–518
Read RC, Thal AP (1966) Surgical experience with symptomatic myxomatous valvular transformation (the floppy valve syndrome). Surgery 59: 173–182
Read RC, Thal AP, Wendt VE (1965) Symptomatic valvular myxomatous transformation: a possible forme frustre of the Marfan syndrome. Circulation 32: 897–910
Reed RL, Siekert RG, Merideth J (1973) Rarity of transient focal cerebral ischemia in cardiac dysrhythmia. JAMA 223: 893
Reid JVO (1961) Mid-systolic clicks. S Afr Med J 35: 353–355
Rice GPA, Boughner DR, Stiller C, Ebers GC (1980). Familial stroke syndrome associated with mitral valve prolapse. Ann Neurol 7: 130–134
Rice GPA, Ebers GC, Bondar RL, Boughner DR (1981) Mitral valve prolapse: a cause of stroke in children? Develop Med Child Neurol 23: 352–356
Rizzon P, Biasco G, Brindicci G, Mauro F (1973) Familial syndrome of midsystolic click and late systolic murmur. Br. Heart J 35: 245–259
Ross A, DeWeese JA, Yu PN (1978) Refractory ventricular arrythmias in a patient with mitral valve prolapse: successful control with mitral valve replacement. J. Electrocardiol 11(3): 289–295
Rothbard RL, Nanda NC, Fleck G, Heinle RA (1979) Mitral valve prolapse and stroke: detection of potential emboli by real-time two-dimensional echocardiography. Circulation 59/60 [Suppl II]: 99
Saffro R, Talano JV (1979) Transient ischemic attack association with mitral systolic clicks. Arch Intern Med 139: 693–694
Sahn DJ, Wood J, Allen HD, Peoples W, Goldberg SJ (1977) Echocardiographic spectrum of mitral valve motion in children with and without mitral valve prolapse: the nature of false positive diagnosis. Am J Cardiol 39: 422–431
Sandok BA, Giuliani ER (1982) Cerebral ischemic events in patients with mitral valve prolapse. Stroke 13 (4): 448–450
Savage DD, Devereux RB, Donahue R, et al. (1982) Mitral valve prolapse in blacks. J Natl Med Assoc 74: 895–900
Savage DD, Devereux RB, Garrison RJ, Castelli WP, Anderson SJ, Levy D, Thomas HE, Kannel WB, Feinleib M (1983) Mitral valve prolapse in the general population. 2 Clinical features. The Framingham Study. Am Heart J 106: 577–581
Savage DD, Garrison RJ, Castelli WP, McNamara PM, Anderson SJ, Kannel WB, Feinleib M (1983): Prevalence of submitral (anular) calcium and its correlates in general population-based sample (The Framingham Study) Am J Cardiol 51: 1375–1378

Savage DD, Garrison RJ, Devereux RB, Castelli WP, Anderson SJ, Levy D, McNamara PM, Stokes J, Kannel WB, Feinleib M (1983) Mitral valve prolapse in the general population. 1. Epidemiologic features. The Framingham Study. Am Heart J 106: 571–576
Savage D, Levy D, Garrison R, Castelli WP, Kligfield P, Devereux RB, Anderson SJ, Kannel WB, Feinleib M (1983) Mitral valve prolapse in the general population. 3. Dysrythmias: The Framingham Study. Am Heart J 106: 582–586
Sbarbaro JA, Mehlman DJ, Wu L, Brooks HL (1979) A prospective study of mitral valvular prolapse in young men. Chest 75: 555–559
Scampardonis G, Yang SS, Maranhao V, Goldberg H, Gooch AS (1973) Left ventricular abnormalities in prolapsed mitral leaflet syndrome. Circulation 48: 287–297
Scharf RE, Hennerici M, Bluschke V, Lueck J, Kladetzky RG (1982) Cerebral ischemia in young patients: is it associated with mitral valve prolapse and abnormal platelet activity in vivo? Stroke 13 (4): 454–458
Scharf RE, Hennerici M, Schneider W (1981) In vivo platelet release reaction in patients with "classic" migraine. International Vascular Symposium, London 1981. Abstract 200, Macmillan, London
Scheele W, Allen HN, Kraus R, Rubin TG (1976) Familial prevalence and genetic transmission of mitral valve prolapse syndrome. Circulation 54 [Suppl III]: 3
Schnee MA, Bucal AA (1983) Fatal embolism in mitral valve prolapse. Chest 83 (2): 285–287
Shah PM, Gramiak R (1970) Echocardiographic recognition of mitral valve prolapse. Circulation 42 (3): 45 (Abstr.)
Shah AA, Quinones MA, Waggoner AD, et al. (1982) Pulsed Doppler echocardiographic detection of mitral regurgitation in mitral valve prolapse: correlation with cardiac arrhythmias. Cathet Cardiovasc Diagn 8: 437–444
Shuping JR, Rollinson RD, Toole JF (1980) Transient global amnesia. Ann Neurol 7: 281–285
Shuttleworth EC, Wise GR (1973) Transient global amensia due to arterial embolism. Arch Neurol 29: 340–342
Silver M (1974) Rheumatic carditis: acute and chronic atrioventricular valve disease. In: Edwards J, Lev M, Abel M (eds) The heart. William and Wilkins, Baltimore, pp 87–109
Silver M (1980) Cardiovascular pathology. Churchill Livingstone, New York
Sloman G, Wong M, Walker J (1972) Arrhythmias on exercise in patients with abnormalities of the posterior leaflet of the mitral valve. Am Heart J 83: 312–317
Spence JD, Wong DG, Melendez LJ, Nichol PM, Brown JD (1984) Increased prevalence of mitral valve prolapse in patients with migraine. Can Med Assoc J 131: 1457–1461
Steele P, Weily H, Rainwater J, Vogel R (1979) Platelet survival time and thromboembolism in patients with mitral valve prolapse. Circulation 60 (1): 43–45
Steelman RB, White RS, Hill JC, Nagle JP, Cheitlin MD (1971) Midsystolic clicks in arteriosclerotic heart disease: a new facet in the clinical syndrome of papillary muscle dysfunction. Circulation 44: 503–515
Swartz MH, Herman MV, Teichholz LE (1976) Dermatoglyphic patterns in patients with mitral valve prolapse: a clue to pathogenesis. Am J Cardiol 38: 588–593
Swartz MH, Teichholz LE, Donosco E (1977) Mitral valve prolapse: a review of associated arrhythmias. Am J Med 62: 377–389
Tajik AJ, Giuliani ER, Frye RL, Davis GD (1972) Mitral valve and/or annulus calcification associated with idiopathic hypertrophic sub-aortic stenosis (IHSS). Circulation 45, 46 [Suppl]: 228
Tajik AJ, Giuliani ER, Weidman WH, Brandenburg RO, McGoon DC (1974) Idiopathic hypertrophic subaortic stenosis—long-term surgical follow-up. Am J Cardiol 34: 815–822
Thal, H, et al. (1982) Abstract. Am Coll of Chest Phys
Traill TA, Fortuin NJ (1979) Mitral annulus calcification and cerebral ischemia. Lancet II: 860
Udeshi MS, Shah A, Fisher VJ, Dolgin M (1979) Incidence of mitral valve prolapse in subjects with throracic skeletal abnormalities. Am Heart J 97: 303–311
Wales LR, Nov AA (1981) Transient global amnesia: complicaton of cerebral angiography. Am J Neuroradiol 2: 275–277
Walsh PN, Kansu TA, Corbett JJ, Savino PJ, Goldburgh W, Schatz NJ (1980) Platelets, thromboembolism and mitral valve prolapse. Circulation 62 [Suppl 3]: 276
Walsh PN, Phil D, Kansu TA, Corbett JJ, Savino PJ, Goldburgh WP, Schatz NJ (1981) Platelets, thromboembolism and mitral valve prolapse. Circulation 63 (3): 552–559
Watanakunakorn C (1973) *Staphylococcus aureus* endocarditis on the calcified mitral annulus fibrosus. Am J Med Sci 266: 219–223
Watson RT (1979) TIA, stroke and mitral valve prolapse. Neurology 29: 886–889
Weksler BB, Gillick M, Pink J (1977) Effects of propanolol on platelet function. Blood 49: 185–196

Werner JA, Schiller NB, Prasquier R (1978) Occurrence and significance of echocardiographically demonstrated tricuspid valve prolapse. Am Heart J 96: 180–186
Wigle ED, Rakowski H, Ranganathan N, Silver MD (1976) Mitral valve prolapse. Am Rev Med 27: 165–180
Wilson LA, Keeling PWN, Malcolm AD, RossRussell RW, Webb-PePloe MM (1977) Visual complications of mitral leaflet prolapse. Br Med J 2: 86–88
Winkle RA, Lopes MG, Fitzgerald JW, Goodman DJ, Schroeder JS, Harrison DC (1975) Arrhythmias in patients with mitral valve prolapse. Circulation 52: 73–81
Wit AL, Fenoglio JJJr, Wagner BM, Bassett AL (1973) Electrophysiological properties of cardiac muscle in the anterior mitral valve leaflet and the adjacent atrium in the dog: possible implications for the genesis of atrial dysrhythmias. Circ Res 32: 731–745
Woldoff HS, Gerber M, Desser KB, Benchimol A (1975) Retinal vascular lesions in two patients with prolapsed mitral valve leaflets. Am J Ophthalmol 79: 382–385
Wolf PA, Savage DD, Kannel WB, Castelli WP (1983) Mital valve prolapse and risk of stroke. Stroke 14 (6): 1010–1011
Woodley D, Chambers W, Starke H, Dzindzio B, Forker AD (1977) Intermittent complete atrioventricular block masquerading as epilepsy in the mitral valve prolapse syndrome. Chest 72 (3): 369–372
Wooley CF (1983) The mitral valve prolapse syndrome. Hosp Prac 18: 163–174

Chapter 6

Infarct of Unclear Cause

J. P. Mohr

Historical Overview

Despite a liberal resort to CT scanning and angiography, clinicians have been disappointed in their hopes that a definite diagnosis as to stroke mechanism requires merely the application of sensitive laboratory procedures. Considerable progress has been made with parenchymatous hemorrhage, diagnosed easily in its early stages by CT scan, but less success has been encountered with infarction. In the latter diagnosis, complex problems abound nowadays trying to assess the role of risk factors, the size of vessel deemed involved, the source of alleged embolic particles, whether the occluding lesion is still in situ or already gone, and what the image on CT scan or angiogram represents.

Earlier studies made heavy use of risk factors in the diagnosis of ischemic stroke subtype (Aring and Merritt 1935; Hyland 1933; Mohr et al. 1978). Advanced age, hypertension, diabetes mellitus, and absence of cardiac valvular disease or atrial arrhythmias were factors favoring a diagnosis of thrombosis; the young with valvular heart disease and atrial arrhythmia usually implied embolism.

Then more detailed studies of the distribution of atherosclerotic lesions suggested most of the primary lesions, at least those in the carotid system, were extracranial, while most of the intracranial lesions were embolic in nature (Samuel 1956; Castaigne et al. 1965, 1970; Fisher et al. 1965; Torvik and Jorgensen 1967). These observations made a clinical diagnosis of embolism a reasonable bet when faced with a case of ischemic stroke associated with a single intracranial arterial occlusion.

When angiography became common practice, it was soon clear that large artery atheromatous lesions were uncommon, even in the elderly, where atherosclerosis was often assumed to be the cause of stroke. Instead, the frequent finding was intracranial disease involving one or more branches far beyond the usual sites found affected by atherosclerotic plaques in studies of autopsy material. These branch occlusions corresponded to embolic occlusions found at autopsies and were soon recognized as embolic in nature on angiography as well (Ring 1966; Davis et al. 1969). After this point was well established, another problem in diagnosis was posed by the frequent normal angiogram in the territory clinically involved in a case of recent stroke. Once a few studies indicated that an initial occlusion could disappear between two angiographic studies a mere few days apart (Delal et al. 1965; Rodriquez et al. 1979), the unstable nature of embolic material was demonstrated in life just as it had been years before in autopsy studies. In rare instances, the moving embolus could be tracked through the arterial tree (Liebeskind et al. 1971). These findings opened the way to a diagnosis of embolic ischemic stroke in the presence of a normal angiogram.

The radiographic diagnosis of embolism based on demonstrated or inferred intracranial arterial trunk or branch occlusions has been found much easier than the often low yield search for a source of the embolus. Ample documentation supports the casual acceptance of a causal association between cerebral embolism and cardiac disease of many kinds (Gazengel 1966), especially atrial fibrillation (Wolf et al. 1978), sinoatrial disorder (Fairfax et al. 1976), recent myocardial infarction (especially anteroseptal), marantic (Neufield et al. 1960) or subacute bacterial endocarditis (Harrison and Hampton 1967), cardiac tumors (Joynt et al. 1965; Yufe et al. 1976), and artificial valves. However, in all too many cases have the stroke, the angiographic finding, or a CT scan indicated highly circumscribed surface infarction, but no source is apparent (Adams and Graham 1957). Search for occult cardiac disease, by means of prolonged monitoring (Åbdon et al. 1982), blood cultures (Harrison and Hampton 1967), echocardiology (Starling et al. 1983), and the like may yield a few potential sources but not as often as they prove normal or diagnostically unhelpful.

Lacking evidence of obvious cardioembolic sources, it became easy to seek a source of embolism in the walls of the aortic arch and the extracranial vessels (Wood and Correll 1966; Imparato et al. 1979). Embolism has been diagnosed frequently in recent years in association with extracranial disease, and documented in a few instances with the acute appearance of ulceration (David et al. 1963; Zatz et al. 1965), and even after considerable delay in instances of carotid occlusion (Barnett et al. 1978; Finklestein et al. 1980). This interest has become so acute that the original correlation of carotid occlusive diseases with cerebral infarction from perfusion failure was deemphasized and almost forgotten (Pessin et al. 1979). With these general correlations established, the question arose how severe a stroke could occur from how trivial an extracranial source. Calcific plaques have only rarely been described as producing large embolic strokes (David et al. 1963; Zatz et al. 1966), but the conviction of an association with embolic stroke led to smaller and smaller suspicious lesions being found at surgery (Edwards et al. 1979). Once such sources were put forward, the meaning of the term "embolism" had to be expanded to include these noncardiac sources.

One final complicating point was the demonstration that embolic material could vary considerably in size. Fibrin-platelet complexes and those also laden with bacteria vary considerably, some so huge that they have obstructed the stem of the middle cerebral (Friedlich et al. 1967) while others have been too small to cause symptoms. Although the smaller particle might be considered less dangerous, experience with noncompressible objects such as shotgun pellets (Kase et al. 1981) has shown that particles as small as a few millimeters are large enough to cause major stroke.

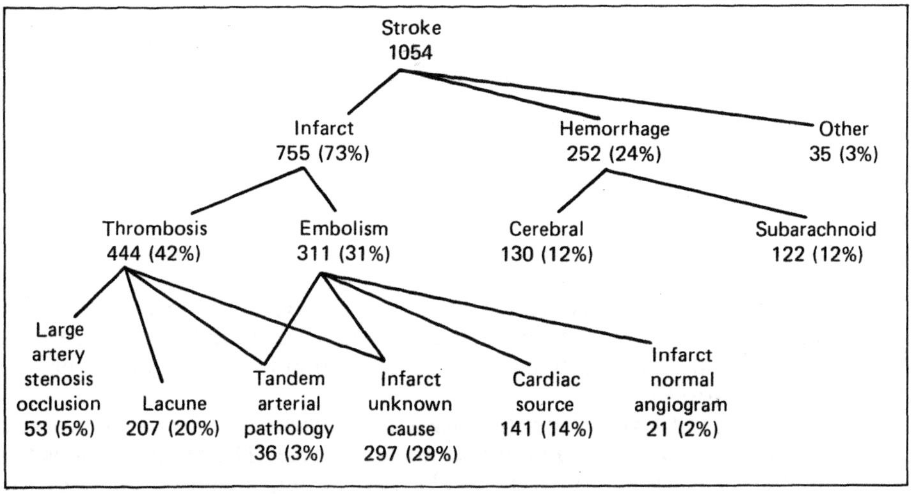

Fig. 6.1. National Institute of Neurological, Communicative Disorders and Stroke, stroke data bank 1983–1985.

These many factors have confounded what was once a less cluttered series of terms defining stroke of various causes. Nowadays, the plethora of tests has created as many important exceptions as it has confirmed earlier rules. The traditional terms used to classify strokes have had to be supplemented by new ones designed to accommodate the clinically unclear subtypes of stroke. The ongoing full phase of the National Stroke Data Bank project has been attempting to address these problems in diagnosis categories (Kunitz et al. 1984).

In the work done in the Data Bank project over the past few years, little difference has been observed in the incidence of the broad diagnostic categories of infarction versus hemorrhage compared with those determined by previous studies (Mohr et al. 1985). However, the incidence of the traditional diagnostic categories of large artery thrombosis and cardiac embolism have proved disappointingly low, even in prospective population-based studies (Gross et al. 1984). Most frustrating has been the high incidence of infarct of undetermined cause (Fig. 6.1). This high incidence has not resulted from inadequate efforts to pursue the diagnosis: the frequency of this diagnosis has been the highest in those centers where CT scanning and angiogram studies are used extensively. This point was especially noticeable during the pilot phase of the Stroke Data Bank project when the participating center with the greatest effort at CT scanning and angiogram had the highest incidence of ischemic stroke of undetermined mechanism.

Difficulties Establishing the Cause of Infarction

Despite efforts to arrive at a diagnosis, the cause of the infarction in a discouragingly large number of cases remains undetermined. The most frequent explanations are the failure to perform the appropriate tests, the improper timing of otherwise appropriate tests, and normal findings or findings subject to ambiguity in interpretation on appropriate tests performed at the appropriate time.

Failure To Perform the Appropriate Tests

Advanced age, coexisting severe disease with a poor prognosis, patient or physician unwillingness to undergo special tests, and casual confidence in a diagnosis based on clinical grounds are the most common of the many reasons for deferring a workup.

Advanced age and severe coexisting disease as reasons for inadequate workup of a diagnosis of stroke should no longer be acceptable. The main reason is the large number of minimally invasive studies which help diagnose many of the major types of stroke. For example, an extracranial hemodynamic internal carotid stenosis that might lead to an endarterectomy can be diagnosed in many instances by an easily performed modern range-gated duplex Doppler study. Lacunar infarction can be pursued by CT scan alone. More dramatic illnesses such as subacute bacterial endocarditis (Pruitt et al. 1978) and marantic endocarditis (Kookier et al. 1976) may begin as a minor focal deficit, suggesting embolism of unclear source, and be uncovered by the simple expedient of a blood culture. In subacute bacterial and marantic endocarditis, the rate of reembolization is high and the size of the particle and the seriousness of the stroke it produces are unpredictable and not merely a function of the first attack.

The frequent unwillingness of the patient and the physician to engage in a workup for stroke subtype is often a function of the stroke severity and perception of prognosis. Few patients or physicians prove resistant to CT scanning, especially if angiography or surgery are deferred in all but the less severely affected, or in those younger patients whose CT scan is negative or shows such a focus that no determination can be made as to the mechanism of the infarct.

At one time almost taken for granted, the confidence in the diagnosis of stroke subtype on clinical grounds alone has been heavily eroded in recent years. Only a handful of syndromes have survived studies with CT scanning and emerged intact with clinicopathologic correlations or as reliable predictors of stroke etiology. Causes other than stroke have been so often reported with most of the classical focal brain syndromes in recent years that the point need not be labored. Among the many syndromes casually attributed to ischemia, only the Wallenberg syndrome has yet to be reported from hematoma. Lacunar syndromes, in particular, seem to have been accepted on clinical grounds for many years, but no longer (Poirier and Derouesne 1985). The characteristic features of all of the lacunar syndromes have been their relative purity and their failure to involve higher cerebral functions such as language, praxis, behavior controlled by the nondominant hemisphere, memory, and vision. Efforts to expand the diagnosis into new formulae have shaken the earlier purity of the syndromes, but have both opened up new opportunties for research and confounded the appealing simplicity of the initial syndromes (Fisher 1982).

Computed tomography scanning is positive for only half of the most common form of lacune, pure motor stroke. Positive CT scans in the capsule and adjacent corona radiata have been reported on occasion for ataxic-hemiparesis, dysarthria-clumsy hand syndrome, and hemiballism. Thus far, CT scan abnormalities have not been associated with cases of pure sensory stroke (presumed from thalamic infarction), as the lesions have been so small they have required autopsy studies for their demonstration. Whether pure sensory stroke from low densities in the centrum semiovale are lacunar has not been corroborated neuropathologically, although surface infarction has been demonstrated. Nuclear magnetic resonance (NMR) scanning holds out the promise of providing important information in this area in the future. Because the vascular lesion lies in vessels some 200–400 μm in diameter, it is perhaps no surprise the angiogram is normal. In at least one autopsied case, the vessel feeding the lacune was widely patent, suggesting microembolus. The probability the CT will be positive is roughly a function of the severity of the deficit. The larger deep infarcts, some of which have been called "super lacunes" or "giant lacunes," may be seen by CT scan as a focal, deep site of infarction without involvement of the cerebral surface. A problem arises in the interpretation of these deep lesions, since an embolus may arrest itself initially in the stem of the middle cerebral artery, causing a large swath of infarction scattered through the lenticulostriate territories. When accompanied by a cerebral surface low density, such large deep infarcts are easily reclassified as examples of embolism, nonthrombotic infarction, or infarction of other cause.

Because some of the cases of pure motor stroke have been associated with middle cerebral artery stenosis, the mere presence of such a syndrome cannot be used to predict the status of the major artery in question. Angiography has been required to settle the matter, and remains our policy in cases where the CT scan shows a large area of low density, one spanning several sections, and one whose base extends down to the affected basal ganglia. Such a large infarct is not easily accounted for by primary disease in the penetrating artery itself, justifying angiography to seek stenosis of the middle cerebral stem. The prognosis for later hemisperhal symptoms in cases with stem stenosis presenting as a lacunar infarct is unknown.

Improper Timing of Tests

The second common cause for failure to determine the cause of an infarct is improper timing of the appropriate laboratory studies. The usual problems arise from CT scans done too early and angiograms done too late.

Angiograms for embolism over 48 h after the ictus have a yield as low as 15% for evidence of the responsible occlusion (Delal et al. 1965; Mohr et al. 1978), even in those whose angiogram was initially positive. CT scans performed once only within a few hours of the onset of an ischemic stroke have a similarly low yield (Tatemichi et al. 1985).

Test Results Without Conclusive Findings

As many as 40% of the cases of ischemic stroke of undetermined cause fall into the third category, in which no conclusive findings are reached despite appropriate laboratory studies performed at the proper time (Gross et al. 1984). This last group of cases poses special problems for research in stroke diagnosis.

Computed tomography scanning may be positive and still leave the etiology of the infarction unclear. This point is especially so in the larger infarcts that include the territories supplied by the stem of a major cerebral artery, since occlusion of the stem may be embolic or thrombotic, and the differentiation cannot be accomplished by CT scanning alone (Araki 1978). CT scans performed no matter how often may remain negative in some cases of small lacunar infarction when the lesion is below the limits of resolution of the CT scan technique (Mohr 1983). CT scanning of the brain stem may often be negative when NMR is positive (Kistler et al. 1984).

Angiography contains many findings that continue to pose diagnostic problems, including such seemingly straightforward findings as occlusion and stenosis (Corston et al. 1984; Irino et al. 1977). Although branch occlusion in the absence of other occlusive disease elsewhere has long been accepted as a feature of embolism (Bladwin 1964; Davis et al. 1969; Ring 1966), isolated branch occlusions may occur in arteritis (Ferris 1973). In the case of occlusions of the middle cerebral artery stem, atheromatous disease is now well established as a cause, especially in blacks (Caplan et al. 1983), while intracranial arterial dissection, still a rarity, is always a possibility (Johnson et al. 1977). Stenosis would seem to be a fairly reliable sign of atherosclerosis in extracranial vessels, yet recanalizing intracranial embolus has been shown to mimic all the angiographic features of atherosclerosis (Irino et al. 1977), and stenosis has also been encountered with dissection and with arteritis (Ferris 1973). Only when the angiogram is repeated within days of the one demonstrating occlusion, and the initial occlusion is gone, can a diagnosis of embolism be made with confidence, but this aggressive a diagnostic effort is usually deemed excessive for patient management. At most, thrombosis appears to account for a mere 2% of ischemic events in the middle cerebral artery territory (Lhermitte et al. 1968), making a diagnosis of embolism, source unclear or not, an easy inference. Multisegmental stenoses are a feature of arteritis, whether the result of primary arterial disease (Leeds and Goldberg 1971) or disease secondary to meningeal infiltrates, but are also seen in the remission phase of so-called vasospasm from embolism, primary subarachnoid hemorrhage, and trauma.

For brain stem syndromes, basilar occlusion demonstrated by angiogram is usually considered the explanation for the stroke. Yet in many such cases the clinical syndrome fits the criteria for lacune (Caplan 1979, 1980; Fisher and Caplan 1971). For some, the infarction is in the field of supply of a vessel which may be thrombosed incidental to a mural atheroma of the basilar artery which is too small to produce flow alteration in the basilar itself (Fisher 1977). Basilar stenosis may also give rise to stroke by means of local embolism (Castaigne et al. 1973). Thus far, no useful criteria have been developed to differentiate these various forms of ischemia which produce brainstem syndromes (Ausman et al. 1985).

Differential Diagnosis

All the unusual forms of ischemic stroke could be enumerated in this section. A brief review of those entities often considered in differential diagnosis is worthwhile, if only to show how infrequently any of them apply. Once the more unusual ones have been considered, the unhappy clinician is faced with the probability that the most common explanation is embolism, even though current efforts at identifying the source are frustratingly inadequate.

Migraine

In the autopsy material that is available, infarctions affecting the distal internal carotid (Oppenheim 1890), the stem (Sinclair 1953), branch (Polyak 1957), or multiple branches (Guest and Wolf 1964) of a major cerebral artery have been reported. Although many of the cases had only a migrainous history and no obvious cause for arterial occlusion to support a migrainous mechanism, in a few the onset occurred during a typical attack of migraine. It is suspected this cause of infarction is rare (Marshall 1982), and more than one stroke in the same patient attributed to migraine seems even more rare. If so, it may be fortunate for the puzzled clinician faced with therapeutic decisions, since no useful means have yet been developed to settle the role of migraine in the genesis of cerebral infarction.

Rejected in this discussion is the notion that headache after a stroke is a sign that the cause is migraine. Such headaches occur often after strokes (Fisher 1965) and are widely recognized to occur with a variety of mechanisms, including such common entities as embolism, although they are especially common in arterial dissection.

Migraine seems unlikely as an explanation for any but a handful of the cases of infarct of unclear cause.

Arteritis

Intracranial arteritis as a cause of stroke is a condition that plagues physicians constantly, not because of its rarity but because the diagnosis is made only with difficulty under the best of conditions, cannot be ruled out by any set of tests singly or in combination, and does not reliably respond to any form of therapy.

Temporal arteritis, although not rare (Hauser et al. 1971), is not often a cause of stroke and some studies even suggest there is no increased incidence of stroke in this population (Huston et al. 1978). Although there are usually associated systemic signs of temporal arteritis, a few instances have been reported with stroke as the first manifestation (Howard et al. 1984). The small number of cases reported suggest a relative predominance of vertebrobasilar location of the infarcts.

Granulomatous arteritis confined to the central nervous system has proved to be a very difficult condition to diagnose. With fewer than 50 cases in the literature and an inconstant clinical picture, it is likely to be the rarity, not the rule, to reach the diagnosis on clinical grounds. The predicted accompaniments of spinal fluid signs of inflammation, elevated sedimentation rate, and fever may be absent. The smaller leptomeningeal arteries are the vessels most commonly affected. Although a widespread involvement might be expected, some cases have been limited to a single vessel or group of vessels (Shuangshoti 1979). Episodes of focal deficit may occur over days to months. In some cases the angiogram has been normal. Response to steroids is inconstant. In short, this condition may defy all efforts at diagnosis including meningeal biopsy.

Considering their rarity, neither form of arteritis is a candidate to explain the large number of infarcts of unclear cause.

Binswanger Disease

This poorly understood entity has come into prominence in recent years mainly because of diagnostic difficulties posed by CT scan findings of low densities scattered along the cerebral convexity and its subjacent white matter. Although Binswanger did not actually document an example of the disorder that bears his name, the eponym has been used because his description corresponded to these high convexity and centrum semiovale lesions (Binswanger 1894). Some authors have suggested the findings may occur in as many as 4% of CT scans performed on elderly patients (Goto et al. 1981).

Efforts have been made to define a characteristic clinical and radiographic picture (Caplan and Schoene 1978; Hurwitz et al. 1984). The most common elements are hypertension, repeated acute or subacute neurologic deficits, especially asymmetric bilateral weakness and pseudobulbar palsy, periods in which the clinical deficits stabilized or even improve, and a CT scan picture which includes hydrocephalus.

Even accepting the notion of a Binswanger disease per se, none of the radiologic, clinical, or epidemiologic features have proved unique. The CT picture of high convexity and centrum semiovale lesions has also been documented in anoxic-ischemic encephalopathy (DeReuck and Schaumberg 1972) and in "distal field infarction" from internal carotid artery occlusion (Mohr 1979); after whole brain irradiation (DeReuck and van der Eecken 1975); in adrenoleukodystrophy (Inoue et al. 1983); and even in a wide variety of metabolic diseases such as the aminoacidurias, Alexander's disease, Canavan's disease, and Reye's syndrome (Kendall 1982; Heinz et al. 1979; Ludwig et al. 1983). The infarcts, even to the extent of a lacunar state, have been speculated to be an accompaniment of the hydrocephalus and not a separate entity (Fisher 1982). Similar clinical syndromes may occur in a variety of settings.

Binswanger disease, if a separate entity, is not likely to prove a common explanation for the many examples of infarct of unclear cause.

Embolism of Undetermined Source

This group probably accounts for the majority of these cases. The clinician is either unlucky in his efforts at diagnosis or the source of the particle sufficiently large to cause the stroke is too small to be detected by image technology, does not produce clinically evident emboli elsewhere, or has actually disappeared before it can be discovered.

Unusual sources of particle release which can block one or more arterial branches on the cerebral surface include: mitral valve prolapse (Barnett et al. 1976), cardiac myxoma (Yufe et al. 1976), marantic embolus (Kookier et al. 1976; Neufield et al. 1966), mucin and emulsified fat from breast metastasis (Deck and Lee 1978), endocaritis due to candida (Glew 1979), arterial wall fragments after resuscitation (Gulkin and Asbury 1967), spontaneous dissection of the internal carotid artery from fibromuscular hyperplasia (Ringel et al. 1977), traumatic internal carotid dissection (Stringer and Kelly 1980), calcific material from the ipsilateral internal carotid (Chiari 1905), internal carotid occlusion from various causes (Barnett et al. 1978), and giant fusiform MCA aneurysm (Auld and Shafey 1976). Those whose particle(s) has/have been large enough to occlude the middle cerebral artery stem itself include: mitral valve prolapse (Bluschke et al. 1982), marantic embolus (Kookier et al. 1976), a "paradoxical" embolus from a leg vein source (Friedlich et al. 1967; Gleysteen and Silver 1970), fibrin-platelet complexes from a nonobstructing internal carotid artery plaque (David et al. 1963), shotgun pellet (Kase et al. 1982), traumatic dissection of the internal carotid artery (Duman and Syephans 1963; Hollin et al. 1966), and internal carotid occlusion of various causes (Pessin et al. 1979). No useful advice can be given to ensure such causes will be uncovered in a given case; a prompt and thorough workup is the mainstay for making any of these diagnoses. In some cases, the clinical syndrome from embolism has been so short lived a diagnosis of transient ischemic attack has been made (Beal et al. 1981; Perrone et al. 1979).

Later diagnosis of the original cause is an uncommon event. However, it has become clear that several systemic illnesses which cause embolism may present as stroke before other elements of the illness have developed. Subacute bacterial endocarditis may present as stroke alone, the systemic disease appearing as late as the autopsy (Kookier et al. 1976). Paradoxical embolism can occur with no evidence of the primary source despite detailed investigation. And the course of a nonhemodynamic, modest-appearing carotid lesion remains so poorly understood that no coherent policy has yet been devised for its proper management.

Frustrating though it might be, the cause of embolism is often not demonstrated despite a focal cerebral infarction sufficient to produce considerable clinical disability.

Characteristics of Infarcts of Unclear Cause

Having discussed the many pitfalls and disappointments in attempting to arrive at an etiologic diagnosis, what then are the features of the strokes currently classified, by default, in the category of infarct of unclear cause?

Clinical Features

The essential clinical features of such infarcts are all negative: the absence of those items which carry the distinctive stamp of a syndrome or mechanism of ischemia. The cases categorized as infarcts of unclear cause show none of the risk factors commonly associated with large artery thrombosis, such as a bruit in the extracranial vessels or over the eye, or ipsilateral TIA affecting eye or brain in the days or weeks prior to the stroke. Likewise, they have none of the risk factors for cardiogenic embolism, such as atrial fibrillation, atrial tachycardia, subacute bacterial endocarditis, anterior wall myocardial infarction, myocardial infarction within the past 6 weeks, and patent foramen ovale. Infarct of unclear cause also excludes elements typical of lacunar infarction as reflected in the standard syndromes of pure motor stroke, pure sensory stroke, sensorimotor stroke, ataxic hemiparesis, all of which admittedly have been due to causes other than lacune but which have had a high correlation with small, deep infarcts.

On the positive side, the diagnosis of infarcts of unclear cause is used for those cases whose deficit entails at least a combined system disturbance, such as sensorimotor stroke with accompanying disturbance in eye movements, coordination, vision, praxis, language, memory, or brain stem function. This reservation has been used to set aside trivial disturbances in cerebral function to emphasize the point that the diagnosis often applies to infarcts of truly huge size (Fig. 6.2).

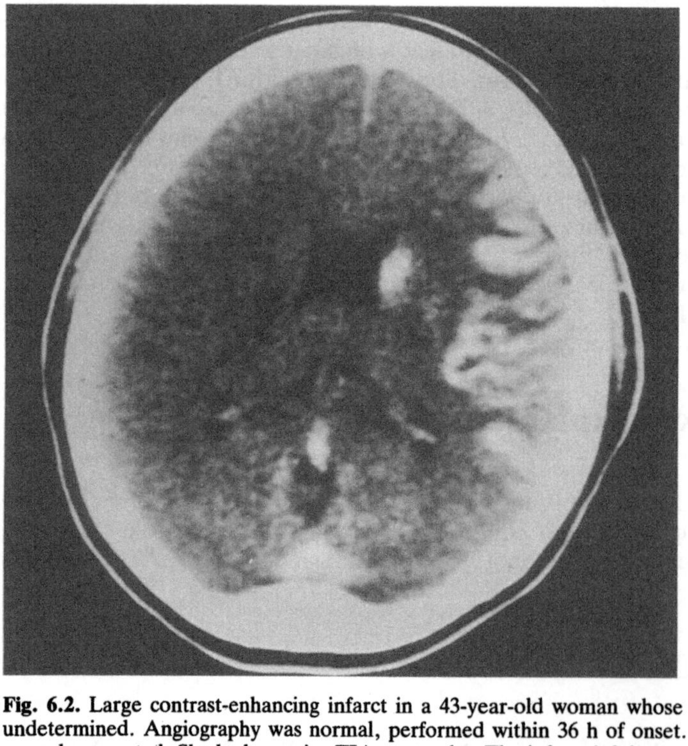

Fig. 6.2. Large contrast-enhancing infarct in a 43-year-old woman whose cause of infarction was undetermined. Angiography was normal, performed within 36 h of onset. No cardiac risk factors were documented. She had no prior TIAs or stroke. The infarct left her permanently aphasic, with right hemiplegia.

Laboratory Features

The following survey indicates that the findings on commonly used studies document an abnormality without clarifying its source or mechanism.

Computed tomographic scanning performed within 7 days may be normal, or may show a large zone of low density or contrast (not ring) enhancement affecting regions larger than that accounted for by infarction of a single branch territory.

The CT scan has been interpreted using the criteria developed from study of autopsy material. When the cause is thrombus, the usual occlusion persists, preventing reperfusion of the infarcted region, resulting in pale, anemic, or bland infarction. When hemorrhagic infarction occurs, the concentration of red cells is enough to make a high-density appearance consistent with blood on CT scan, whether concentrated as a single mass—which is indistinguishable from a hematoma—or with a variegated appearance thought to reflect hemorrhagic foci ranging from a few scattered petechiae through a more confluent collection of such foci. Because hemorrhagic infarction has long been a consequence of embolization, its occurrence is commonly accepted as a sign of embolism, even if the source is unclear. At times, the arterial occlusion may be apparent on CT scan (Gacs et al. 1983), a point which still does not settle the mechanism of the occlusion.

Angiography may be normal, or when occlusion is found it affects a major cerebral artery stem or the top of the basilar. Because these latter foci of occlusion can be from thrombotic or embolic cause (Castaigne et al. 1970, 1973; Lhermitte et al. 1968), their demonstration does not settle the mechanism; only if the extreme effort of repeat angiography is undertaken and the occlusion is gone can a diagnosis of embolism be made. Many instances will be found of single branch occlusion, sufficient to satisfy a diagnosis of embolism on radiographic grounds; yet the source eludes discovery despite extensive laboratory investigation (Fig. 6.3).

Stroke Severity

It would be comforting if most of these cases fell among those with milder deficits, perhaps accounting for the negative laboratory studies by virtue of the relative insensitivity of such tests to smaller lesions. Yet the scanty data on the subject indicates they are not: they are roughly as severe as ischemic strokes for which a cause is found (Mohr 1984) and the 30-day survival is as bad as any form of ischemic stroke.

Risk of Recurrence

All this effort at diagnosis is made because of the difficulty arriving at the risk of recurrence. The recurrence rate of stroke of unclear cause may not be trivial. It

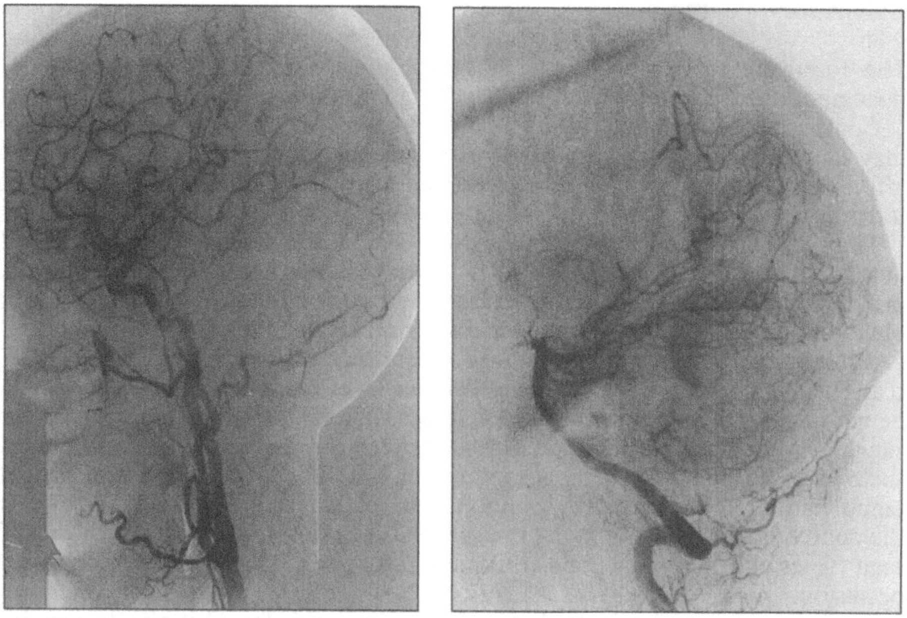

a b

Fig. 6.3a,b Branch occlusion of the ascending parietal artery seen on middle cerebral angiography done within 48 h of onset of infarction in a 62-year-old woman with no risk factors for stroke and no prior TIAs or stroke. Full workup for cardiac source was negative.

approaches that encountered in embolism associated with an obvious cardiac source. The recurrence rate more closely approximates this subtype of ischemic stroke than any other.

Management Options

To the extent that the findings indicate that many examples of infarct of unclear cause are from cardiac embolism which eludes efforts at source detection, the treatment might well be the same as when a source is apparent. The mere demonstration of an arterial branch occlusion and the known poor functional outlook for many examples of intracranial embolism prompt many physicians to undertake anticoagulant therapy when the angiographic data are in support of embolus, whether or not a "source" for the embolus can be found. Others advise prophylactic endarterectomy under the assumption that a tiny plaque may be the source of the embolus. If no branch occlusion is found, many would opt for antiplatelet therapy.

Lacking proof of the cause of the stroke, classifying such cases this way may prove useful in eventually determining if this group differs in some way from those in which the mechanism of stroke is better defined. At present, little is known of the risk for recurrence and proper therapy for strokes of unclear cause. At the least, the findings thus far justify feelings of frustration, but not those of complacency, when the clinician faces yet another example of the disorder.

References

Abdon NJ, Zettervall O, Carlson J, Berglund S, Sterner G, Tejler L, Turesson I (1982) Is occult atrial disorder a frequent cause of non-hemorrhagic stroke? Long-term ECG in 86 patients. Stroke 13: 832–837

Adams JH, Graham DI (1967) Twelve cases of fatal cerebral infarction due to arterial occlusion in the absence of atheromatous stenosis or embolism. J Neurol Surg Psychiatr 30: 479–488

Adams HP, Gross CE (1981) Embolism distal to stenosis of the middle cerebral artery. Stroke 12: 228–229

Adams RD, Fisher CM (1961) Pathology of cerebral arterial occlusion. In: Fields WS (ed) Houston symposium on pathogenesis and treatment of cerebrovascular disease. Charles C Thomas, Springfield, Ill

Araki G (1978) Small infarctions of the basal ganglia with special reference to transient ischemic attacks. Rec Adv Gerontol 469: 161

Aring CD, Merritt HH (1935) Differential diagnosis between cerebral hemorrhage and cerebral thrombosis. Arch Intern Med 56: 435

Auld AW, Shafey S (1976) Transient ischemic attacks not produced by extracranial vascular disease: a plea for early and complete angiographic evaluation. South Med J 69: 722

Ausman JI, Shrontz CE, Pearce JE, Diaz FG, Crecelius JL (1985) Vertebrobasilar insufficiency. Arch Neurol 42: 803–808

Barnett HJM, Jones MW, Boughner DR, Kostuk WJ (1976) Cerebral ischemic events associated with prolapsing mitral valve. Arch Neurol (Chic) 33: 777–782

Barnett HJM, Peerless SJ, Kaufmann JCE (1978) "Stump" of internal carotid artery—a source for further cerebral embolic ischemia. Stroke 9: 448–456

Beal MF, Williams RS, Richardson EP, Fisher CM (1981) Cerebral embolism as a cause of transient ischemic attacks and cerebral infarction. Neurology (Ny) 31: 860–865

Binswanger O (1894) Die Abgrenzung der allgemeinen progressiven Paralyse. Klin Wochenschr 31: 1103

Blackwood W, Bratty P, Mair WGP (1963) In: Jakob H (ed) Observations on occlusive vascular disease of the brain, vol 3. Thieme, Stuttgart, p 146

Bladin PF (1964) A radiologic and pathologic study of embolism of the internal carotid-middle cerebral arterial axis. Radiology 82: 615–625

Bluschke V, Hennerici M, Scharf RE, et al. (1982) Mitralklappenprolaps-Syndrom und Thrombozytenaktivität bei jungen Patienten mit zerebralen Ischämien. Deuts Med Wochenschr 107: 410

Bounds JV, Sandok BA, Barnhorst DA (1976) Fatal cerebral embolism following aorto-coronary bypass graft surgery. Stroke 7: 611–614

Caplan LR (1979) Occlusion of the vertebral or basilar artery. Follow up analysis of some patients with benign outcome. Stroke 10: 277–282

Caplan LR (1980) "Top of the basilar" syndrome. Neurology 30: 72–79

Caplan LR, Schoene WC (1978) Clinical features of subcortical arteriosclerotic encephalopathy (Binswanger's disease) (1978) Neurology 28: 1206–1215

Caplan LR, Hier DB, D'Cruz I (1983) Cerebral embolism in the Michael Reese Stroke Registry, Stroke 14: 530–536

Castaigne P, Lhermitte F, Gautier JC (1965) Role des lesions arterielles dans les accidents ischemiques cerebraux de l'atherosclerose. Rev Neurol (Paris) 113: 1

Castaigne P, Lhermitte F, Gautier J-C, Escourolle R, Derouesne C (1970) Internal carotid artery occlusion: a study of 61 instances in 50 patients with post-mortem data. Brain 93: 231–258

Castaigne P, Lhermitte F, Gautier JC, Escourolle R, Derouesne C, Der Agopian P, Popa C (1973) Arterial occlusions in the vertebro-basilar system—a study of forty-four patients with post-mortem data. Brain 96: 133–154

Castaigne P, Lhermitte F, Buge A, Escourolle R, Hauw JJ, Lyon-Caen O (1981) Paramedian thalamic and midbrain infarcts: clinical and neuropathological study. Ann Neurol 10: 127–148

Chiari H (1905) Ueber das Verhalten des Teilungswinkels der Carotis communis bei der Endarteritis chronic deformans. Verh Dtsch Ges Path 9: 326
Cohen MM, Hemalatha CP, D'Addario RT, Goldman HW (1980) Embolism from a fusiform middle cerebral artery aneurysm. Stroke 11: 158–161
Corston RN, Kendall BE, Marshall J (1984) Prognosis in middle cerebral artery stenosis. Stroke 15: 237–241
David NJ, Gordon KK, Friedberg SJ, Dillon M (1963) Fatal atheromatous cerebral embolism associated with bright plaques in the retinal arterioles. Neurology 13: 708–713
Davis DO, Rumbaugh CL, Gilson JM (1969) Angiographic diagnosis of small-vessel cerebral emboli. Acta Radiol (Stockh) 9: 264–271
Deck JHN, Lee MA (1978) Mucin embolism to cerebral arteritis: a fatal complication of carcinoma of the breast. J Canad Sci Neurol 5: 327
Delal PM, Shah PM, Aiyar RR (1965) Arteriographic study of cerebral embolism. Lancet 2: 358–361
DeReuck J, Schaumberg HH (1972) Periventricular atherosclerotic leukoencephalopathy. Neurology 22: 1094–1097
DeReuck J, van der Eecken H (1975) The anatomy of late radiation encephalopathy. Eur Neurol 13: 481–494
Derouesne C, Mas JL, Bolgert AF, Castaigne P (1984) Pure sensory stroke caused by a small cortical infarct in the middle cerebral artery territory. Stroke 15: 660–662
Dratz HM, Woodhall B (1947) Traumatic dissecting aneurysm of left internal carotid, anterior cerebral and middle cerebral arteries. J Neuropath Exp Neurol 6: 286
Duman S, Stephans KW (1963) Post-traumatic middle cerebral artery occlusion. Neurology 13: 613–616
Edwards JH, Kricheff II, Riles T, Imparato A (1979) Angiographically undetected ulceration of the carotid bifurcation as a cause of embolic stroke. Radiology 132: 369–373
Fairfax AJ, Lambert CD, Leatham A (1976) Systemic embolism in chronic sinoatrial disorder. N Engl J Med 295: 190–192
Ferris H, Levine HL (1973) Cerebral arteritis: classification. Radiology 109: 327–341
Finklestein S, Kleinman GM, Cuneo R, Baringer JR (1980) Delayed stroke following carotid occlusion. Neurology 30: 84–88
Fisher CM (1965) Headache in cerebrovascular disease. In: Vinken PJ, Buyn GW (eds) Handbook of clinical neurology, vol 5. North Holland, Amsterdam
Fisher CM (1977) Bilateral occlusion of basilar artery branches. J Neurol Neurosurg Psychiatr 40: 1182
Fisher CM (1982) Lacunar strokes and infarcts: a review. Neurology 32: 871–876
Fisher CM, Adams RD (1951) Observations on brain embolism with special reference to the mechanism of hemorrhagic infarction. J Neuropathol Exp Neurol 10: 92–94
Fisher CM, Caplan LR (1971) Basilar artery branch occlusion: a cause of pontine infarction. Neurology (Minneapolis) 21: 900–905
Fisher CM, Karnes WE (1965) Local embolism. J Neuropathol Exp Neurol 24: 174
Fisher CM, Pearlman A (1967) The non-sudden onset of cerebral embolism. Neurology (Minneapolis) 17: 1025–1032
Fisher CM, Gore I, Okabe N, White PD (1965) Atherosclerosis of the carotid and vertebral arteries—extracranial and intracranial. J Neuropath Exp Neurol 24: 455–476
Frielich AL, Castleman B, Mohr JP (168) Case records of the Massachusetts General Hospital. N Eng J Med 278: 1109–1118
Gacs G, Fox AJ, Barnett HJM, Vinuela F (1983) CT visualization of intracranial arterial thromboembolism. Stroke 14: 756–762
Gazengel JGL (1966) Etude de 276 emboles cerebrales d'origine cardiaque. These Faculte de Medecine de Paris. Editions AGEMP, Paris, p 123
Gleysteen JJ, Silver D (1970) Paradoxical arterial embolism: collective review. Am Surg 36: 47–54
Glew RH (1979) Case records of the Massachusetts General Hospital. New Engl J Med 301: 34–42
Goto K, Ishii N, Fukasawa H (1981) Diffuse white-matter disease in the geriatric population. Radiology 141: 687–695
Gross CR, Kase CS, Mohr JP, Cunningham SC (1984) Stroke in south Alabama: incidence and diagnostic features. Stroke 15: 249–255
Guest IA, Woolf AL (1964) Fatal infarction of brain in migraine. Br Med J 1: 225–226
Gulkin TA, Asbury AK (1967) Fragment of great-vessel wall causing cerebral embolism. N Engl J Med 277: 751–752
Harrison MJG, Marshall J (1977) Evidence of silent cerebral embolism in patients with amaurosis fugax. J Neurol Neurosurg Psychiatr 40: 651

Harrison MJG, Hampton JR (1977) Neurologic presentation of bacterial endocarditis. Br Med J 2: 148
Hauser WA, Ferguson RH, Holley KE, Kurland LT (1971) Temporal arteritis in Rochester, Minnesota, 1951 to 1967. Mayo Clin Proc 46: 597–602
Heinz ER, Drayer BP, Haenggeli CA, et al. (1979) Computed tomography in white-matter disease. Radiology 130: 371–378
Hinton RC, Kistler JP, Fallon JT, Friedlich AS, Fisher CM (1977) Influence of etiology of atrial fibrillation on incidence of systemic embolism. Am J Cardiol 40: 509–513
Hinton RC, Mohr JP, Ackerman RA, Adair LB, Fisher CM (1979) Symptomatic middle cerebral artery stem stenosis. Ann Neurol 5: 152–157
Hollin SA, Sukoff MH, Silverstein A, Gross SW (1966) Post-traumatic middle cerebral artery occlusion. J Neurosurg 25: 526
Howard GF, Ho SU, Kim KS, Wallach J (1984) Bilateral carotid occlusion resulting from temporal arteritis. Ann Neurol 15: 204–207
Hulqvist GT (1942) Ueber Thrombose und Embolie der Arteria carotis und herbei vorkommende Gehirnveränderungen. Eine pathologish-anatomische Studie. Fischer, Stockholm
Hurwitz BJ, Heyman A, Drayer B, Utley C (1984) Cerebral white matter hypodensity in computed tomographical scans: an indication of Binswanger's disease? (1984) Ann Neurol 16: 155
Huston KA, Hunder GG, Lie JT, Kennedy RH, Elveback LR (1978) Temporal arteritis: 25-year epidemiologic, clinical, and pathologic study. Ann Intern Med 88: 162–167
Hyland HH (1933) Thrombosis of intracranial arteries. Arch Neurol Psychiatr 30: 342
Imparato AM, Riles TS, Gorstein F (1979) The carotid bifurcation plaque: pathologic findings associated with cerebral ischemia. Stroke 10: 238–245
Inoue Y, Fukuda T, Takashima F, et al. (1983) Adrenoleukodystrophy: new CT findings. Am J Neuroradiol 4: 951
Irino T, Tandea M, Minami T (1977) Angiographic manefestations in postrecanalized cerebral infarction. Neurology 27: 471–475
Johnson AC, Graves VB, Pfaff JP Jr (1977) Dissecting aneurysm of intracranial arteries. Surg Neurol 7: 49–52
Joynt RJ, Zimmerman G, Khalifett R (1965) Cerebral emboli from cardiac tumors. Arch Neurol 12: 84–91
Kase CS, White L, Vinson L, Eichelberger P (1981) Shotgun pellet embolus to the middle cerebral artery. Neurology 31: 458–461
Kendall B (1982) Cranial CT scans in metabolic diseases involving the CNS of children. Resident Staff Physician 28 (2): 33
Kistler JP, Buonanno FS, Dewitt LD (1984) Vertebral basilar posterior cerebral territory stroke—delineation by proton nuclear magnetic resonance imaging. Stroke 15: 417–426
Kooiker JC, MacLean JM, Sumi SM (1976) Cerebral embolism, marantic endocarditis, and cancer. Arch Neurol 33: 260–264
Krayenbuehl HA, Yasargil MG (1984) Cerebral angiography, 2nd edn. Butterworths, London
Kunitz S, Gross CR, Heyman A, Kase CS, Mohr JP, Price TR, Wolf PA (1984) The pilot stroke data bank: definition, design, data. Stroke 15: 740–746
Leeds NE, Goldberg HI (1971) Angiographic manifestations in cerebral inflammatory disease. Radiology 98: 595–604
Lhermitte F, Gautier JC, Derouesne C, Guiraud B (1968) Ischemic accidents in the middle cerebral artery territory (a study of the causes in 122 cases). Arch Neurol 19: 248–256
Lhermitte F, Gautier JC, Derouesne C (1970) Nature of occlusions of the middle cerebral artery. Neurology (Minneapolis) 20: 82–88
Liebeskind A, Chinichian A, Schechter MM (1971) The moving embolus seen during serial cerebral angiography. Stroke 2: 440–443
Little JR, Shawhan B, Weinstein M (1980) Pseudo-tandem stenosis of the internal carotid artery. Neurosurg 7: 574–577
Ludwig B, Kishikawa T, Wemde S, et al. (1983) Cranial computed tomography in disorders of complex carbohydrate metabolism and related storage diseases. Am J Neuroradiol 4: 431
Marshall J (1982) The cause and prognosis of strokes in people under 50 years. J Neurol Sci 53: 473–488
Mohr JP (1979) Neurologic complications of cardiac valvular disease and cardiac surgery. In: Vinken PJ, Bruyn GW (eds) Handbook of clinical neurology, vol. 34, medical conditions. North Holland, Amsterdam
Mohr JP (1983) Lacunar infarctions. In: Barnett HJM (ed) Neurological clinics of North America. Philadelphia, Saunders

Mohr JP, Caplan LR, Melski JW, Duncan GW, Goldstein RJ, Kistler JP, Pessin MS, Bleich HL (1978) The Harvard cooperative stroke registry: a prospective registry of cases hospitalized with stroke. Neurology 28: 754–762

Nelson RF, Pullicino P, Kendall BE, Marshall J (1980) Computed tomography on patients presenting with lacunar syndromes. Stroke: 11: 256–261

Neufield HN, Cadman NL, Miller AW, Edwards JE (1960) Embolism from marantic endocarditis as a manifestation of occult carcinoma. Proc Mayo Clin 35: 292

Oppenheim H (1980) Casuistischer Beitrag zur Prognose der Hemikranie. Charite-Annalen 15: 298

Perrone P, Candelise L, Scotti G, DeGrandi C, Scalfa G (1979) CT evaluation in patients with transient ischemic attack. Correlation between clinical and angiographic findings. Eur Neurol 18: 217–221

Pessin MS, Hinton RC, Davis KR, Duncan GW, Mohr JP (1979) Mechanisms of acute carotid stroke: a clinicoangiographic study. Ann Neurol 6: 245–252

Polyak S (1957) The vertebrate visual system. University of Chicago Press, Chicago

Pruitt AA, Rubin RH, Karchanev AW, Duncan GW (1978) Neurologic complications of bacterial endocarditis. Medicine 57: 329

Rascol A, Clanet M, Manelfe C (1982) Pure motor hemiplegia: CT study of 30 cases. Stroke 13: 11–17

Ring BA (1966) Diagnosis of embolic occlusions of smaller branches of the intracerebral arteries. Am J Roentgenol Radium Ther Nucl Med 97: 575–582

Ringel SP, Harrison SH, Norenberg MD, Austen JH (1977) Fibromuscular dysplasia: multiple "spontaneous" dissecting aneurysms of the major cervical arteries. Ann Neurol 1: 301–304

Samuel KC (1956) Atheroclerosis and occlusion of the internal carotid artery. J Path Bact 71: 391

Santamaria J, Graus F, Rubio F (1983) Cerebral infarction of the basal ganglia due to embolism from the heart. Stroke 14: 911–914

Shuangshoti S (1979) Localized granulomatous (giant cell) angiitis of brain with eosinophil infiltration and saccular aneurysm. J Med Assoc Thai 62: 281

Sinclair W (1953) Dissecting aneurysm of the middle cerebral artery associated with migraine syndrome. Am J Pathol 29: 1083

Starling MR, Crawford MH, Sorenson SG, Grover FL (1983) Comparative value of invasive and noninvasive techniques for identifying left ventricular mural thrombi. Am Heart J 106: 1143–1149

Stringer WL, Kelly DL (1980) Traumatic dissection of the extracranial internal carotid artery. Neurosurg 6: 123

Torvik A, Jorgensen L (1966) Thrombotic and embolic occlusions of the carotid arteries in an autopsy material. Part 2. Cerebral lesions and clinical course. J Neurol Sci 3: 410

Waddington M, Ring BA (1968) Syndromes of occlusion of middle cerebral artery branches, angiographic and clinical correlation. Brain 91: 685–696

Whisnant JP (1982) Multiple particles injected may all go to the same cerebral artery branch. Stroke 13: 720

Wolf PA, Dawber TR, Thomas HE, Kannel WB (1978) Epidemiologic assessment of chronic atrial fibrillation and risk of stroke: the Framingham Study. Neurology (Minneapolis) 28: 973–977

Wood EH, Correll JW (1969) Atheromatous ulceration in major neck vessels as a cause of cerebral ebolism. Acta Radiol [Diag] 9: 520–536

Yufe R, Karpati G, Carpenter S (1976) Cardiac myxoma: a diagnostic challenge for the neurologist. Neurology 26: 1060–1065

Zatz LM, Iannone AM, Eckman PB, Hecker SP (1965) Observations concerning intracerebral vascular occlusion. Neurology 15: 389–401

Chapter 7

Prevention and Treatment of Cardioembolic Stroke

R. G. Hart

Introduction

About 15% (11%–23%) of all ischemic strokes are caused by cardiogenic embolism (Mohr et al. 1978; Wolf et al. 1983; Caplan et al. 1983; Herman et al. 1982; Chambers et al. 1983). Since many potential cardiogenic sources of emboli are identifiable prior to stroke, prevention would seem possible. However, two major problems limit preventive efforts. First, only a fraction of patients with cardiac disorders predisposing to embolism experience embolic stroke (Table 7.1). Unless subgroups of patients at particularly high risk for stroke can be identified, many patients with potentially emboligenic heart disease will need to be treated to prevent stroke that is destined to occur in only a small minority. Second, currently available prophylactic treatments, both medical and surgical, either carry a substantial risk or are of unproven benefit. So despite burgeoning clinical data suggesting that one in six ischemic strokes is due to cardiogenic embolism, effective preventive measures have been largely lacking.

The concept of emboli migrating within the arterial circulation to occlude distal vessels has been present for over 100 years, since its description by Virchow. However, adequate studies of treatment of patients with cardioembolic stroke are few. The difficulty in establishing cardiogenic embolism as the cause of brain ischemia in individual patients has been a major problem in clinical research studies and in everyday patient management. As a consequence, treatment recommendations often remain empiric and must be viewed with skepticism.

The presence of a potential cardiac source of emboli in a patient with cerebral ischemia does not a priori establish cardiogenic embolism as the cause. Many patients with ischemic stroke have both a potential cardiac source of emboli and risk factors for cerebrovascular disease. Clinical differentiation is imperfect and is commonly based on analysis of several clinical features (Table 7.2). Correlation of these clinical features with autopsy findings is not available. Even autopsy results can be equivocal. There is currently no clinical "gold standard" for diagnosing cardioembolic stroke (Ramirez-Lassepas et al. 1984). Ancillary studies can be supportive. CT evidence of hemorrhagic infarct, angiographic

Table 7.1. Sources of cardioembolic stroke[a]

Source	Fraction of all embolic stroke	Estimated stroke risk
Nonrheumatic atrial fibrillation	45%	5%/year
Ischemic heart disease		
Acute myocardial infarct	15%	3% within 4 weeks
Ventricular aneurysm[b]	10%	5% prevalence
Rheumatic heart disease	10%	20% prevalence
Prosthetic cardiac valves	10%	1%–4%/year
Other, less common sources	10%	
Mitral valve prolapse		0.02%/year
Mitral annulus calcification		–
Nonbacterial thrombotic endocarditis		30% prevalence
Calcific aortic stenosis		–
Cardiac myxoma		35% prevalence
Nonischemic dilated cardiomyopathy		20% prevalence
Bacterial (infective) endocarditis		20% native valve 50% prosthetic valve

[a] Estimates from data summarized by the Cerebral Embolism Task Force (1986); see text for specific references

[b] Includes left ventricular dyskinesis remote from acute myocardial infarct

findings of "vanishing occlusions" and of absence of atherosclerosis, and imaging of cardiac thrombi with sonographic or radiographic techniques can be helpful (Cerebral Embolism Task Force 1986). A constellation of clinical evidence is required, as no single feature is sufficiently predictive (Table 7.2).

Clinically, the brain is involved in about 70% of emboli from the heart. The prevalence of embolic stroke (Table 7.1) may be much lower than that of occult systemic emboli. Systemic emboli are usually unrecognized during life but are frequent in autopsy studies (Hinton et al. 1977; Easton and Sherman 1980).

Depending upon the cardiac source, emboli can be composed predominantly of platelets (nonbacterial thrombotic endocarditis); laminated, red, fibrin-rich thrombi (ventricular aneurysm); calcific material (aortic stenosis); or tumor (atrial myxoma). Thus, antithrombotic therapy that is effective for one cardioembolic source cannot be assumed to be effective in another.

Table 7.2. Predictive value of clinical features for cardioembolic stroke[a]

	Likelihood of embolism	
	Present	Absent
Potential cardiac source	56%	1%
Prior TIA	5%	21%
Maximal deficit at onset	20%	7%
Onset while awake	19%	10%
Hemorrhagic infarct on CT	50%	15%

[a] Figures derived from Caplan et al. (1983) and Hakim et al. (1983) in which the diagnosis of cardioembolic stroke was based on a constellation of clinical data including the above variables, without independent postmortem confirmation. Predictive value of combinations of features are not derivable. The above estimates are based on the assumption that 15% of ischemic strokes are due to cardiogenic embolism (i.e., pretest likelihood of 15%)

While clinical concepts of cardiogenic embolism remain rudimentary, knowledge about cardioembolic disorders is increasing rapidly. Because each specific source of cardioembolic stroke has a unique natural history, prevention and treatment will be considered separately for each type of cardiac disorder. The risk, optimal intensity, and timing of initiation of anticoagulation following acute embolic stroke will then be considered.

Atrial Fibrillation

Patients with nonrheumatic atrial fibrillation have about five times the risk of ischemic stroke compared with age-matched patients without this dysrhythmia (Wolf et al. 1978; Hinton et al. 1977; Aberg 1968). The fraction of these strokes that are due to cardiogenic embolism versus coexistent cerebrovascular disease is uncertain. Clinical estimates of the fraction that are embolic vary from 19% to 71% (Hart et al. 1983a; Britton et al. 1985; Mohr et al. 1978). Autopsy studies suggest that 50%–71% are due to cardiogenic embolism (Jorgensen and Torvik 1966; Britton et al. 1985). From epidemiologic data, it is estimated that a maximum of 78% of ischemic strokes in patients with nonrheumatic atrial fibrillation can be due to embolism (Wolf et al. 1978). It is therefore likely that one-half to two-thirds of ischemic strokes associated with nonrheumatic atrial fibrillation are on the basis of cardiogenic embolism. Nonrheumatic atrial fibrillation is associated with increased risk of stroke, but not transient ischemic attack (TIA) (Harrison and Marshall 1984; Bogousslavsky et al 1986).

Nonrheumatic atrial fibrillation encompasses a wide range of heart disease. It can be questioned whether the dysrhythmia itself is responsible for cardioembolic stroke or whether the dysrhythmia is only a marker of underlying cardiac disease which is the actual source of emboli. Clinical data are conflicting. Several studies of patients with "lone" atrial fibrillation, unassociated with other clinical evidence of cardiac disease, have reported a low risk of embolism, while others have reported a substantial risk of embolism in these patients (Table 7.3). The

Table 7.3. "Lone" atrial fibrillation and ischemic stroke[a]

	Study type	*N*	Stroke prevalence	Stroke incidence
Sherman et al. (1984)	Consecutive clinical	15	20%	–
Kannel et al. (1982)	Epidemiologic	5	20%	2%/year
Close et al. (1979)[b]	Consecutive clinical	75	1%	0.2%/year
Hinton et al. (1977)	Autopsy	14	21%	–
Evans and Swan (1954)[b]	Anecdotal	20	0%	–
Hanson and Rutledge (1949)[b]	Consecutive clinical	10	0%	0%/year
Brand et al. (1985)	Epidemiologic	32	28%	2.6%/year

[a] "Lone" atrial fibrillation means no other clinical, ECG, or radiographic evidence of heart disease "Lone" AF usually comprises 4%–10% of all AF patients and occurs predominantly in men with a mean age of 54

[b] These studies included only constant (nonparoxysmal) "lone" AF. Takahashi et al. (1981) studied paroxysmal "lone AF" only, and reported one brain and one renal embolus in two of 23 patients (8%) with a mean estimated follow-up of 24 months

embolism risk in patients with thyrotoxic atrial fibrillation, which is usually not associated with structural heart disease, averages 12% and argues that the dysrhythmia itself is at least partly the culprit (Bar-Sela et al. 1981; Staffurth et al. 1977; Yuen et al. 1979; Hurley et al. 1981).

It is probable that within the diverse spectrum of nonrheumatic atrial fibrillation there are those subgroups with higher and lower risks of ischemic stroke. Identification of such subgroups would have clear implications for prevention of embolism. In one study, atrial fibrillation associated with congestive heart failure carried a 60% further increased risk of stroke compared with similar patients without congestive failure (Wolf et al. 1978). The risk of embolism appears to be greatest in the months immediately following the onset of the dysrhythmia; the stroke risk may be three times higher during the 1st year of atrial fibrillation (Wolf et al. 1983; Hart et al. 1983b). The relative risk of embolism from constant versus intermittent atrial fibrillation is uncertain. Reversion of atrial fibrillation into sinus rhythm has been postulated to be a risk factor for embolism, as resumption of atrial contraction might dislodge stasis-induced thrombi. Support for this hypothesis is found in studies of thyrotoxic atrial fibrillation (Bar Sela et al. 1981; Staffurth et al. 1977) and of embolism following iatrogenic cardioversion (Bjerklund and Orning 1969). However, most patients with stroke and associated nonrheumatic atrial fibrillation have chronic, sustained atrial fibrillation (Hart et al. 1983a; Bharucha et al. 1981; Sherman et al. 1984). The influence of left atrial size on embolic potential has not been systematically studied.

Prevention of stroke in patients with nonrheumatic atrial fibrillation is an important clinical issue since this dysrhythmia affects 2%–5% of people over age 64 (Morris and Hurst 1980), and 35% of these patients will experience ischemic stroke (Kannel et al. 1982; Fisher 1979; Sherman et al. 1984; Godtfredsen 1983). Conventional practice is to withhold antithrombotic therapy until there is evidence of embolism. The high likelihood of stroke as the initial manifestation of embolism makes this approach unsatisfactory; death or severe disability occurs in more than half of initial strokes associated with atrial fibrillation (Fisher 1979; Sherman et al. 1984; Hart et al. 1983a). Prophylactic anticoagulation has been advocated, extrapolating from its apparent efficacy in reducing embolism in patients with rheumatic heart disease and prosthetic cardiac valves (Fisher 1971; Easton and Sherman 1980). While it is a reasonable hypothesis that anticoagulation may lower the risk of stroke, the dangers of chronic anticoagulation in these relatively elderly patients are considerable. The risk of brain hemorrhage may reach 1%/year, and major systemic bleeding may occur in an additional 2%/year (Whisnant et al. 1978; Sixty-plus Reinfarction Research Group 1982; Forfar 1982; Loeliger 1984; Wintzen et al. 1984). The optimal intensity of oral anticoagulation to prevent embolism in patients with nonrheumatic atrial fibrillation is not known. Less intensive anticoagulation than conventionally deemed therapeutic has been effective in preventing venous thrombosis and has been associated with fewer hemorrhagic complications (Hull et al. 1982).

The role of platelet antiaggregating agents in stroke prophylaxis in patients with nonrheumatic atrial fibrillation is also unknown. Based on their efficacy in stroke prevention following transient ischemic attacks (Canadian Cooperative Study Group 1980; Bousser et al. 1983) and following prosthetic cardiac valve implantation (Cheseboro et al. 1983; Nunez et al. 1984; Gallo et al. 1984), antiplatelet agents have been suggested for use in patients with atrial fibrillation. Platelet antiaggregating agents are inexpensive, easy to administer, and relatively free of life-threatening adverse reactions—facts which contribute to their widespread use despite unproven clinical benefit. There are no data regarding their use in nonrheumatic atrial fibrillation, and consequently the optimal type of agent and dose are purely speculative (Hirsh 1985).

In short, although the presence of atrial fibrillation identifies patients at increased risk of ischemic (mostly cardioembolic) stroke, there are currently no data about how to protect them. In the 10% or less of atrial fibrillation patients with longstanding "lone" atrial fibrillation, anticoagulation prophylaxis does not appear to be warranted (Table 7.3). In thyrotoxic atrial fibrillation, especially if paroxysmal, short-term anticoagulation seems prudent. For the remaining majority, the optimal preventive course is unclear.

In atrial fibrillation patients who have already experienced an initial stroke, prevention of a second stroke has not been systematically studied. The risk of recurrent stroke is 10%–20% within 1 year (Sage and VanUitert 1984; Wolf et al. 1983; Hart et al. 1983a; Fisher 1969; Sherman et al. 1984; Darling 1967). If cardioembolism is the likely cause of stroke, chronic anticoagulation is recommended for suitable candidates (Easton and Sherman 1980; Fisher 1979).

Acute Myocardial Infarction

Stroke occurs within 1 month of acute myocardial infarction (MI) in about 3% of patients (Table 7.4) (Cerebral Embolism Task Force 1986). The majority of these strokes are due to embolism from left ventricular thrombi, while a minority are attributable to embolism from atrial thrombi, to hypotension, or to other mechanisms (Komrad et al. 1984; Johannessen et al. 1984; Weinrich et al. 1984). Patients with transmural, anterior MI, especially if complicated by echocardiographic evidence of ventricular thrombus, appear to be at especially high risk (Table 7.5).

Table 7.4. Acute MI, stroke risk, and anticoagulation

	N	Stroke risk	
		Nonanticoagulated	Anticoagulated
Veterans study	999	3.8%	0.8%
MRC study	1427	2.5%	1.1%
Bronx Hospital	1136	2.3%	1.7%
Aggregate	3562	2.9%	1.2%
Hemorrhage in anticoagulated patients (n=2348)			
Minor bleed	7%		
Major bleed	1.5%		
CNS bleed	0.05%		
Fatal bleed	0%		

[a] Results of three randomized studies: Veterans Cooperative Studies (1973), Medical Research Council (1969) and Drapkin and Mersky (1973), as modified from the report of the Cerebral Embolism Task Force (1986)

Table 7.5. Acute MI, mural thrombi, and embolism[a]

	Follow-up period	Nonanticoagulated *N*	Nonanticoagulated Embolism	Anticoagulated *N*	Anticoagulated Embolism
Weinreich et al. (1984)	4 months	18	7	25	0
Keating et al. (1983)	3 months	7	6	10	0
Friedman et al. (1982)	?1 month	2	1	9	1
Aggregate	4 months	27	14 (52%)	44	1 (2%)

[a] Retrospective studies of consecutive patients; selection for anticoagulation was nonrandomly done. Mural thrombi were detected by echocardiography; includes brain and systemic emboli

A 3% stroke prevalence is not high, but acute MI is a common disorder and thousands of strokes occur yearly in this setting. Since many of these strokes occur during hospitalization for treatment of acute MI, there is the potential for their prevention. Three controlled clinical trials have shown that stroke risk is reduced in patients with acute MI who are anticoagulated (Table 7.4). However, major hemorrhagic complications occurred in 1.5% of anticoagulated patients. Because of the relatively low prevalence of stroke in unselected patients with acute MI and potential hemorrhagic complications, anticoagulation is not routinely administered at most institutions.

Subgroups of acute MI patients with ventricular dyskinesis and ventricular thrombi have a higher stroke risk and may benefit from anticoagulation. Three recent nonrandomized studies reported that stroke risk was substantially increased in patients with acute MI complicated by mural thrombi who were not anticoagulated (Table 7.5). The potential efficacy of platelet antiaggregating agents or low-dose, subcutaneous heparin in this setting has not been studied systematically (Ezkowitz et al. 1984).

Pending further data, the proper use of antithrombotic therapy to minimize embolic stroke after acute MI is uncertain. The risk of stroke following inferior MI or nontransmural MI appears to be quite low, unless atrial fibrillation is present or prior infarcts have contributed to dyskinesis. At present it is uncertain if patients with acute anterior MI should routinely undergo early echocardiography to define a subset with mural thrombi who have a substantial risk of imminent stroke. The issue requires further study before general recommendations can be made. Ventricular dykinesis, mural thrombi, and stroke often occur very early, within days of MI, so that echocardigraphy and/or anticoagulation may need to be carried out shortly after admission to be maximally effective (Asinger et al. 1981; Komrad et al. 1984; Meizlish et al. 1984). Determination of the optimal type and intensity of antithrombotic prophylaxis in high-risk subsets of acute MI patients awaits further study.

While most ischemic strokes in the weeks following acute MI are cardioembolic, other mechanisms should be considered if the stroke occurs in a setting of profound hypotension, following iatrogenic instrumentation, or without ventricular dyskinesis on echocardiography. If the stroke is deemed cardioembolic, anticoagulation is recommended to prevent recurrent embolism. The efficacy and the duration of antithrombotic therapy has not been studied. If echocardiography repeated 3–6 months after acute MI demonstrates improvement or resolution of dyskinesis, further anticoagulation may not be needed. Persistent left ventricular dyskinesis remote from acute MI may well have a different embolic potential.

Persistent Ventricular Aneurysm

Thrombi associated with persistent ventricular dyskinesis in healed MI can embolize to cause stroke (Haugland et al. 1981; Cabin and Roberts 1980; Reeder et al. 1981; Simpson et al. 1980; Meltzer et al. 1984). Surgical, pathologic, and echocardiographic studies all agree that about half of left ventricular aneurysms have overlying mural thrombi (Cabin and Roberts 1980; Reeder et al. 1981; Simpson et al. 1980; Hochman et al. 1984). However, the rate of embolism associated with mural thrombi remote from MI appears to be low. Although the incidence cannot be estimated from the literature, only about 5% of such patients appear to experience stroke in studies with months to years of observation (Haugland et al. 1981; Cabin and Roberts 1980; Reeder et al. 1981; Simpson et al. 1980; Meltzer et al. 1984). Preliminary studies suggest that the embolic potential may be related to the shape of mural thrombus and the type of wall motion abnormality (Cabin and Roberts 1980; Haugland 1981; Gottdiener et al. 1983; Kinney 1985). Thrombi that project into the lumen, especially if mobile, appear to be especially prone to embolization (Meltzer et al. 1984; Haugland et al. 1981).

At present, when ventricular aneurysm with or without mural thrombus is discovered remote from acute MI and in the absence of embolism, anticoagulation is usually not recommended because of the presumed low embolic potential. Platelet antiaggregating agents have been shown to interrupt platelet deposition in ventricular thrombi (Stratton and Ritchie 1984) but the implications of this observation concerning embolic potential are uncertain.

When a patient with TIA or stroke is found to have ventricular dyskinesis remote from acute MI, the relationship of the cardiac abnormality to cerebral ischemia may not necessarily be cause to effect. Patients with cerebrovascular disease often suffer from coexistent ischemic heart disease. Because of the relatively low embolic potential of ventricular dyskinesis, other mechanisms of stroke should be considered before attributing ischemia to cardiogenic embolism. If the typical clinical features of embolic stroke are present (Table 7.2), and a protruding thrombus overlies the dyskinetic segment, the likelihood of cardioembolic stroke is high. The absence of overlying ventricular thrombus does not exclude cardioembolic stroke. Echocardiography following stroke will not detect thrombi that have already embolized to the brain (Arvan et al. 1985). Further, small thrombi beyond the resolution of echocardiography may yet be large enough to embolize and cause stroke. The clinical situation is seldom straightforward, and the likelihood of embolism must be weighed in the absence of quantitative guidelines.

Rheumatic Heart Disease

About 20% of patients with rheumatic mitral stenosis clinically experience embolism, with an estimated incidence of about 3%/year (Szekely 1964; Deverall et al. 1968; Coulshed et al. 1979; Fukuda and Nakamura 1984; Fleming and Bailey 1971; Neilson et al. 1978). Embolism occurs with all degrees of mitral stenosis and may be the presenting symptom (Wood 1956; Hart and Miller 1983). The presence of atrial fibrillation in patients with mitral stenosis increases the risk of embolism by three to seven times over those with mitral stenosis alone (Coulshed et al. 1970; Fleming and Bailey 1971; Szekely 1964). Other clinical features, such as patient age, left atrial size, valve calcification, and degree of stenosis, are less reliably correlated with embolism risk independent of atrial fibrillation (Levine 1981).

It is widely accepted that anticoagulation will reduce the occurrence of embolism (Owren 1963; Szekely 1964; Fleming and Bailey 1971; Adams et al. 1974). The efficacy of platelet antiaggregation agents in embolism prevention in this setting has not been convincingly established (Steele et al. 1980). It is recommended that all patients with rheumatic mitral stenosis and atrial fibrillation, chronic or paroxysmal, receive anticoagulants (Levine 1981; Easton and Sherman 1980). The risk-to-benefit of anticoagulants and other antithrombotic therapy in patients with rheumatic heart disease without atrial fibrillation is controversial (Levine 1981).

Recurrent embolism follows initial embolus in 30%–65% of patients with rheumatic heart disease, occurring at a rate of almost 10% annually (Darling et al. 1967; Fleming and Bailey 1971; Daly et al. 1951; Szekely 1964; Carter 1965). The weeks and months following the initial embolus are particularly high risk periods (Daly et al. 1951; Szekely 1964; Santamaria et al. 1982; Darling et al. 1967). Retrospective, but convincing, data indicate that the risk of recurrent embolism is reduced by more than two-thirds in anticoagulated patients (Adams et al. 1974; Szekely 1964; Fleming and Bailey 1971; Owren 1963). The efficacy of platelet antiaggregation agents in this setting has not been established.

Prosthetic Cardiac Valves

Embolism is a feared complication of prosthetic cardiac valve implantation. The continuing introduction of new valves, the modifications of existing models, and the wide variety of antithrombotic regimes have led to a large, complex and confusing literature concerning embolism prevention (McGoon 1984).

There is general consensus about some issues. In adults, mechanical heart valves (e.g., Starr-Edwards, Bjork-Shiley, St. Jude Medical) require permanent anticoagulation, although the optimal intensity of anticoagulation has not been determined. Prosthetic mitral valves have shown a consistently greater risk of embolism compared with similar model aortic valves, perhaps due to the higher prevalence of atrial fibrillation associated with prosthetic mitral valves. In anticoagulated patients with mechanical valves, the embolism risk is 4% yearly for mitral valves and 2% yearly for aortic valves (Edmunds 1982; Burkhardt et al. 1984; Rahimtoola 1983). Addition of platelet antiaggregating agents may further reduce this rate (Cheseboro et al. 1983; Dale et al. 1977).

Bioprosthetic valves (e.g., Hancock, Carpentier-Edwards, Ionescu-Shiley) have a lower embolic potential than mechanical valves. In nonanticoagulated patients with aortic bioprotheses and in anticoagulated patients with mitral bioprotheses, the embolism risk is 1%–2% yearly and is even lower in the absence of coexistent atrial fibrillation (Nunez et al. 1984; Gallo et al. 1984;

Williams et al. 1980; Jamieson et al. 1984). Anticoagulation is usually recommended for both bioprosthetic aortic and mitral valves during the first 3 months after insertion. A single report showed a low embolism risk in patients treated only with aspirin in the postoperative period (Nunez et al. 1984). In the absence of atrial fibrillation, many patients with bioprosthetic mitral valves may not require long-term anticoagulation (Jamieson et al. 1984; Nunez et al. 1984; Gonzalez-Lavin et al. 1984). Recent studies have reported low rates of embolism in patients with bioprosthetic mitral valves with atrial fibrillation who were treated with platelet antiaggregation agents (Nunez et al. 1984; Gonzalez-Lavin et al. 1984; Silverton et al. 1984). Others have reported a high risk of embolism without anticoagulation in this setting (Gallo et al. 1984; Geha et al. 1982), and further data are needed to define the correct course (Table 7.6).

Table 7.6. Bioprosthetic mitral valves, atrial fibrillation, and embolism

	Valve type[a]	*N*	Dose	Embolism risk
I. Anticoagulation				
Geha et al. (1982)	Porcine	61	–	0%/3 years
Gallo et al. (1984)	Porcine	27	–	1.3%/year
Hertzer et al. (1982)	Porcine	147	–	2.3%/year
Nunez et al. (1982)	Porcine	151	–	2.3%/year
II. Platelet antiaggregants				
Geha et al. (1982)	Porcine	16	ASA+DYP	12%/year
Gallo et al. (1984)	Porcine	16	?	2.8%/year
Nunez et al. (1984)	Porcine	135	ASA 1 g/day	1.3%/year
Nunez et al. (1984)	Porcine	219	ASA 0.5 g/day	0.3%/year
III. No antithrombotic therapy[b]				
Gonzalez-Lavin et al. (1984)	Bovine	209	–	0.2%/year
Gallo et al. (1984)	Porcine	90	–	2.7%/year

Abbreviations: ASA, aspirin; DYP, dipyridimole
[a] Porcine xenobioprostheses are Hancock and Carpentier-Edwards; bovine pericardial bioprostheses are Ionescu-Shiley
[b] Some patients may have received platelet antiaggregation agents

Children may require less intensive antithrombotic therapy than adults with similar valve models and similar risk factors, although this tenuous hypothesis is based on retrospective comparison between clinical studies (Pass et al. 1984; Schaff et al. 1984; Weinstein et al. 1981). Management of pregnant patients with prosthetic valves who require anticoagulation is a difficult dilemma with no satisfactory solution; bioprosthetic valves are recommended for women who wish to bear children (Salazar et al. 1984; Larrea et al. 1984).

Treatment of Less Common Sources of Cardioembolic Stroke

The risk of stroke in unselected young patients with *mitral valve prolapse* is estimated to be about 1/5000 per year (Hart and Easton 1982), and no antithrombotic therapy is usually recommended for asymptomatic people. In patients with cerebral ischemia attributed to mitral valve prolapse, recurrent ischemic events are common, although usually TIAs (Jackson et al. 1984). Based on isolated observations of platelet-fibrin emboli in mitral valve prolapse patients with cerebral ischemia, platelet antiaggregation agents have been recommended as initial treatment (Barnett et al. 1980; Barnett 1982).

Mitral annulus calcification in stroke patients is more often a marker of atherosclerotic cardio- and cerebrovascular disease than a primary embolic source (Fulkerson et al. 1979; Savage et al. 1983; Furlan et al. 1984; Nestico et al. 1984), although it has been clinically and pathologically linked to cerebral and retinal ischemia (DeBono and Warlow 1979; Korn et al. 1962; Ridolfi and Hutchins 1976; Nishide et al. 1983). The natural history and treatment of the embolic complications of this disorder have not been established (Furlan et al. 1984).

Nonbacterial thrombotic endocarditis (NBTE) is complicated by cardioembolic stroke in 35% of patients (Cerebral Embolism Task Force 1986; Biller et al. 1982; Rosen and Armstrong 1973; Graus et al. 1985; Rogers et al. 1982). While NBTE is found in about 1% of consecutive autopsies from academic hospitals, it is usually unsuspected during life (Biller et al. 1982; Barron et al. 1960; Deppisch et al. 1976).

The diagnosis of NBTE-associated embolism should be considered when multiple brain and/or systemic emboli occur in patients with malignancy or wasting illness, especially if coagulation abnormalities or thrombophlebitis coexists. Prevention and treatment have not been systematically studied; at least five patients have experienced recurrent embolism during intravenous heparin therapy (Kearsley and Tattersall 1982; Graus et al. 1985).

While *calcific aortic stenosis* only rarely serves as a source of cardioembolic stroke (Dry and Willis 1939; Kumpe and Bean 1948; Rotman et al. 1971; Kapila and Hart 1986), calcific retinal emboli have been associated with this disorder (Brockmeier et al. 1981; Jabbari et al. 1980; Holley et al. 1963; Penner and Font 1969). Prospective studies of the embolic risk and treatment have not been undertaken. Platelet antiaggregation agents have been employed based on the observation of platelet-fibrin deposits on disrupted valvular endothelium in surgical specimens (Stein et al. 1977).

From 27% to 55% of patients with left *atrial myxoma* have associated emboli, which are usually composed of tumor fragments (Sandok et al. 1980; Marvaste et al. 1984; Larrieu et al. 1982). Treatment is surgical and, although thrombi are visible on the friable surface of surgical specimens, there appears to be little role for antithrombotic therapy (Sandok et al. 1980; Barnett 1983).

Brain embolism is conceded to be frequent in patients with nonischemic *dilated cardiomyopathies* of all types. The prevalence of embolic stroke is difficult to estimate, but is in the order of 20% (Fuster et al. 1981; Gottdiener et al. 1983; Segal et al. 1965; Segal et al. 1978; Demakis et al. 1974). There is a consensus that anticoagulation is indicated for all patients with dilated cardiomyopathy, with or without echocardiographically defined ventricular thrombus (Segal et al. 1978; Fuster et al. 1981) (Gottdiener et al. 1983; Johnson and Palacios 1982). Atrial fibrillation associated with dilated cardiomyopathy is associated with a particularly high risk of embolism (Segal et al. 1978).

Embolic stroke occurs in about 20% of patients with *native valve endocarditis* (Pruitt et al. 1978; O'Brien and Geiser 1984; Carpenter et al. 1983; Pelletier et al. 1977; Le Cam et al. 1984). Experimental evidence and anecdotal clinical observations caution that anticoagulation can result in secondary brain hemorrhage (Pruitt et al. 1978; Kanis 1974; Foote et al. 1978; Lieberman et al. 1978). Anticoagulation is not recommended for most patients with native valve endocarditis (Carpenter et al. 1983; O'Brien and Geiser 1984). Patients with valvular vegetations detected echocardiographically may have a higher risk of embolism (O'Brien and Geiser 1984; Stafford et al. 1985).

Prosthetic valve endocarditis is associated with a higher rate of embolism, approaching 50% in nonanticoagulated patients (Wilson et al. 1978; Garvey et al. 1979). Anticoagulation appears to reduce this risk, but increases the risk of brain hemorrhage in patients with mechanical prosthetic valve endocarditis (Wilson et al. 1978; Carpenter et al. 1983; Karchmer et al. 1978). Hence the use of anticoagulants in mechanical prosthetic valve endocarditis is controversial, with many clinicians favoring cautious, careful continuation of anticoagulation in these patients. The embolic risk of nonanticoagulated patients with bioprosthetic valve endocarditis cannot be determined from the handful of available case reports (Carpenter et al. 1983; Nagata et al. 1984), but appears to be lower than with mechanical valves.

Management of endocarditis patients who develop stroke is likewise controversial, as brain hemorrhage has sometimes resulted when anticoagulation was initiated or continued in this setting (Pruitt et al. 1978; Lieberman et al. 1978). Discontinuing or postponing anticoagulation for at least 48–72 h followed by CT scan to exclude hemorrhagic infarct before initiation of anticoagulation has been recommended (Wilson et al. 1982; Cerebral Embolism Task Force 1986).

Risk and Intensity of Chronic Anticoagulation Therapy

Chronic anticoagulation with warfarin is associated with important risks of major hemorrhagic complications. The magnitude of these risks is critical when considering prophylactic anticoagulation to prevent embolism. The risk of major hemorrhagic complications in conventionally anticoagulated patients with prosthetic cardiac valves is estimated to be 2%/year (Edmunds 1982; Rahimtoola 1983). In patients who are anticoagulated following myocardial infarction, major hemorrhage occurs in 2%–4%/year (Sixty-Plus Re-infarction Research Group 1982; EPSIM Research Group 1982). In large numbers of patients anticoagulated for mixed indications, the risk of major hemorrhage is 4%–6%/year (Forfar 1982; Errichette et al. 1984).

Hemorrhagic complications of chronic anticoagulation are directly related to the degree of anticoagulation, assessed by any of several laboratory monitoring tests (Kelton and Hirsh 1980; Hull et al. 1982; Coon and Willis 1974; Husted and Andreassen 1976; Moschos et al. 1964). Other factors variably correlated with hemorrhagic complications include age, uncontrolled hypertension, concomitant aspirin use, multiple concomitant medications, alcoholism, and recent surgery (Kelton and Hirsh 1980; Coon and Willis 1974; Davis and Sczupak 1979; Husted and Andreassen 1976). Patient cooperation, the experience of the physician in prescribing anticoagulants, and the adequacy of laboratory monitoring are further factors postulated to relate to the risk of hemorrhage (Husted and Andreassen 1976; Loeliger et al. 1984; Forfar 1982).

Intracerebral hemorrhage is the most feared and least treatable complication of chronic anticoagulation. The risk of intracerebral hemorrhage is increased about eight times in these patients (Whisnant et al. 1978; Sixty-Plus Re-infarction Research Group 1982; Wintzen et al. 1984; Ericksson and Link 1983). The risk of intracerebral hemorrhage approaches 1%/year in conventionally anticoagulated patients (Sixty-Plus Re-infarction Research Group 1982; Trent and Andersson 1980; Olsson 1980; Ericksson and Link 1983). The occurrence of intracerebral hemorrhage is not entirely predictable. While advanced age and excessive anticoagulation appear to be overrepresented in patients who experience this complication, many such patients are not hypertensive and are not excessively anticoagulated at the time of hemorrhage (Kasē et al. 1984; Whisnant et al. 1978; Sixty-Plus Re-infarction Research Group 1982).

Less intensive anticoagulation has been explored in several clinical settings in an attempt to minimize hemorrhagic complications (Hull et al. 1982; Loelinger 1979; Loelinger et al. 1983). The optimal therapeutic range of anticoagulant therapy for prevention of cardioembolic stroke is uncertain for most clinical situations. The conventional level of oral anticoagulation in North America has usually been considered to be reached when the prothrombin time (one-stage, rabbit-brain thromboplastin) is prolonged by 1.5–2.5 times control values. This therapeutic range is largely based on recommendations for prevention of venous thrombosis generated almost 40 years ago. North American patients have generally received more intensive anticoagulation than patients in western Europe due to different sensitivities of thromboplastins (Loelinger 1979; Loelinger et al. 1983). Consequently, clinical studies from western Europe have usually reported fewer bleeding complications than those from North American, although methodologic differences preclude direct comparison. In particular, thromboplastins used in North American laboratories are less sensitive to the effects of anticoagulants compared with European thromboplastins (Hirsh et al. 1986).

An important step in resolving the confusion caused by this difference in thromboplastin sensitivities is the use of international standards for reference thromboplastins to generate a common value, the international normalized ratio (INR) (van den Besslaar et al. 1984). The INR value allows accurate comparison of intensity of oral anticoagulation not only between local laboratories using different commercial thromboplastins, but also between laboratories from different parts of the world.

Analysis using INRs reveals that North American patients generally receive more intensive anticoagulation than European patients, explaining the more frequent hemorrhages. Hence, reporting of anticoagulation monitoring using the INR should be mandatory in the medical literature, otherwise results cannot be compared except with laboratories using the same type, brand, and even batch of thromboplastin.

Critical analysis of results of earlier trials using the INR (Hirsh et al. 1986; Moschos et al. 1964) and of more recent studies of different intensities of oral anticoagulation leads to important revisions in the optimal therapeutic range of oral anticoagulation applicable to most North American patients (Table 7.7) (Hull et al. 1982). Previously recommended levels of anticoagulation are needlessly high in most situations, resulting in unnecessary and often serious

Table 7.7. Recommended intensity of oral anticoagulation

Clinical state	Standardized human brain (INR)	Equivalent rabbit brain ratio[a]
Prophylaxis—venous thromboembolism	2.0–3.0	1.2–1.5
Treatment of deep vein thrombosis or pulmonary embolism	2.0–3.0	1.2–1.5
Prevention of embolism in atrial fibrillation, valvular heart disease, tissue heart valves, or acute MI	2.0–3.0	1.2–1.5
Mechanical prosthetic heart valves, recurrent systemic embolism	3.0–4.5	1.5–2.0

[a] As most North American laboratories use rabbit-brain thromboplastins, these approximate the conventional prothrombin time (Hirsh et al. 1986)

hemorrhage. Clinical antithrombotic effect appears to be adequate at lower intensities and the risk of hemorrhage is reduced by two-thirds (Hirsh and Levine 1986).

Timing of Anticoagulation After Acute Nonseptic Embolic Stroke

Embolic infarcts are often hemorrhagic at postmortem (Fisher and Adams 1951). Hemorrhagic infarcts may vary from minimal petechiae, beyond the resolution of CT, to dense areas of confluent purpura resembling hematoma (Fig. 7.1). Hemorrhagic transformation of embolic infarcts can be delayed for hours after stroke onset, even in nonanticoagulated patients, and can be unassociated with clinical worsening (Fig. 2) (Cerebral Embolism Study Group 1984).

The dilemma of the timing of initiation of anticoagulation in patients with cardioembolic stroke balances the risk of recurrent embolism against that of secondary brain hemorrhage. Recurrent embolism to the brain follows within 14 days of initial stroke in about 12% of patients who are not anticoagulated (Table 7.8). The recurrent rate appears to be similar for most major cardiac sources of embolism and is spread fairly evenly over the first 2 weeks with about 1%/day risk (Cerebral Embolism Study Group 1983; Cerebral Embolism Study Group 1984). Clinical data from several restrospective studies and one prospective study suggest that immediate anticoagulation with heparin lessens the risk of early recurrent brain embolism (Cerebral Embolism Study Group 1984; Cerebral Embolism Study Group 1983).

The risk of secondary brain hemorrhage in cardioembolic stroke patients who are immediately anticoagulated ranges from 0% to 14% (Cerebral Embolism Study Group 1984; Martin and Biller 1984; Calendre et al. 1984). Retrospective analysis of patients who have experienced secondary brain hemorrhage in this setting suggests that patients with large infarcts are at particular risk and that spontaneous hemorrhagic transformation may be delayed for 24–48 h after stroke onset (Cerebral Embolism Study Group 1984; Lodder 1984).

Table 7.8. Risk of early recurrent brain embolism

	No. of studies	Stroke risk[a] Mean (range)
Nonrheumatic atrial fibrillation	4	11% (2%–20%)
Rheumatic heart disease	6	12% (2%–19%)
Acute myocardial infarct	1	14% –
Mixed cardiac sources	9	12% (5%–22%)

[a] Recurrent embolism to brain only during the 14 days following initial stroke. Data from mostly retrospective studies summarized by the Cerebral Embolism Task Force (1986)

High-quality CT is probably a better test than CSF examination for detection of minimal hemorrhagic infarct. Ruff and Dougherty (1981) reported five patients with hemorrhagic infarct on CT with normal CSF. Further, a few red blood cells (RBCs) are often present in the CSF in nonhemorrhagic infarcts due to "traumatic taps." In an autopsy series, Lee et al. (1975) reported that 26% (7/27) of hemorrhagic infarcts had more than 50 RBCs/mm in the CSF, but that 17% (3/18) of *non*hemorrhagic infarcts also had more than 50 RBCs/mm^3. Thus, the positive predictive value (true positive rate) of more than 50 RBCs/mm^3 for hemorrhagic infarct (assuming that 10% all infarcts are hemorrhagic infarcts) is only 15%. Higher CSF RBC counts (more than 500/mm^3) appear to have greater specificity for hemorrhagic infarct, but the timing of appearance of RBCs in the CSF and comparison with CT has not been studied. If high-quality CT is not available or motion artifact precludes adequate study, CSF examination for detection of hemorrhagic infarct should be done prior to anticoagulation. Anticoagulation following lumbar puncture should be delayed for at least 4–6 h to minimize spinal hematoma (Ruff and Dougherty 1981; Ramirez-Lassepas and Quinones 1984; Walsh et al. 1984).

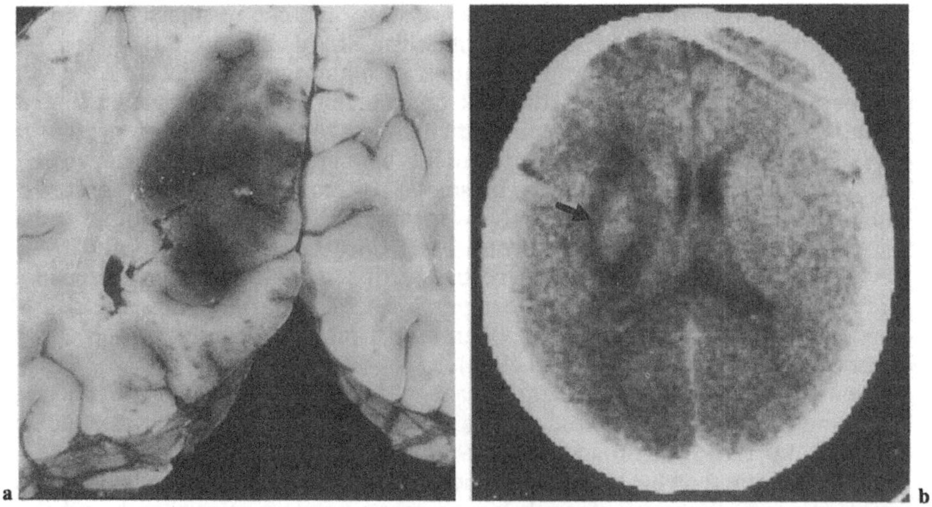

Fig. 7.1a,b. Hemorrhagic infarction. **a** Gross specimen showing multifocal petechial extravasations. **b** CT appearance of hemorrhagic infarction, showing mottled increased density (*arrow*) within a larger area of hypodense, pale infarction and relatively minimal mass effect.

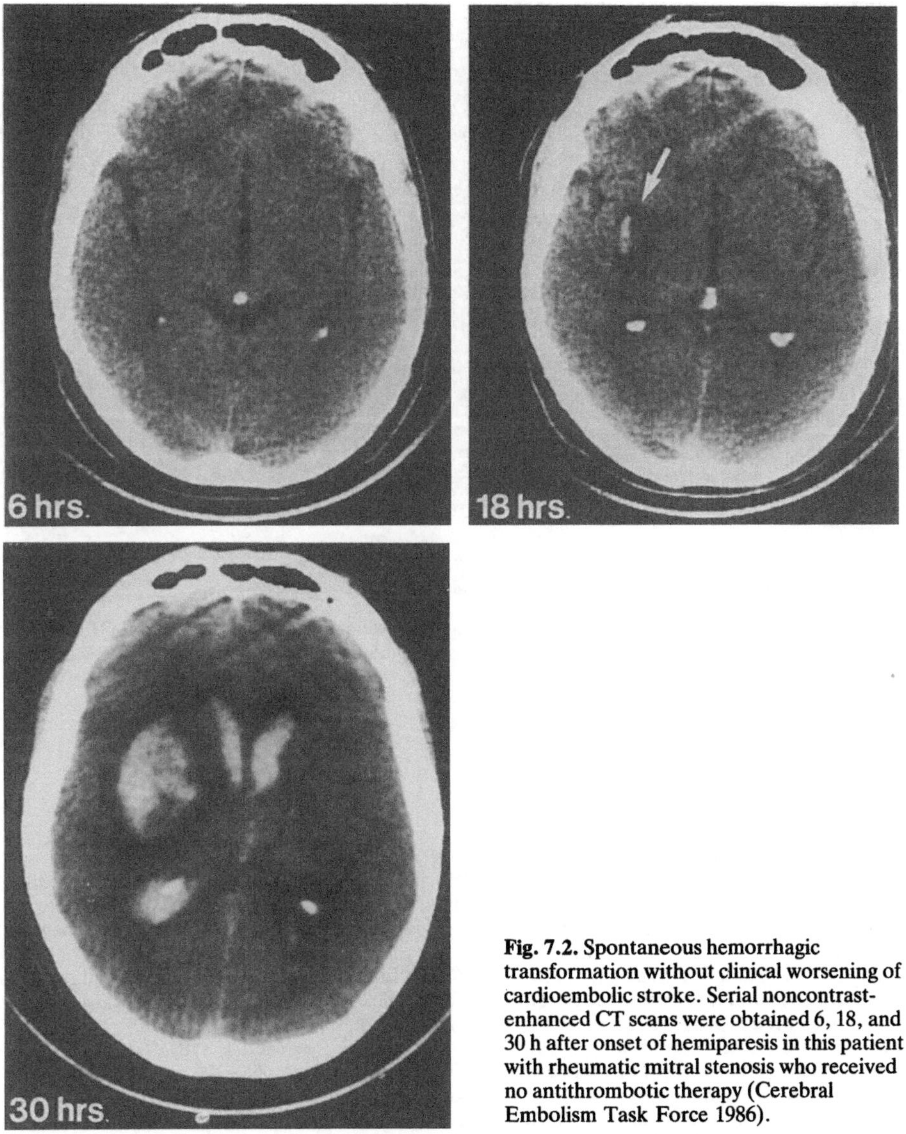

Fig. 7.2. Spontaneous hemorrhagic transformation without clinical worsening of cardioembolic stroke. Serial noncontrast-enhanced CT scans were obtained 6, 18, and 30 h after onset of hemiparesis in this patient with rheumatic mitral stenosis who received no antithrombotic therapy (Cerebral Embolism Task Force 1986).

Given the available data, the proper management of acute nonseptic embolic stroke is uncertain. While iatrogenic brain hemorrhage may not be entirely avoidable, immediate anticoagulation with heparin of small to moderate-sized cardioembolic strokes may be of overall benefit if CT performed 24–48 h after stroke is nonhemorrhagic. Blood pressure should be carefully monitored and bolus injections of heparin empirically avoided. Patients with large embolic infarcts appear to be at special risk for delayed hemorrhagic transformation; postponing anticoagulation for at least 7 days is probably judicious despite the risk of recurrent embolism.

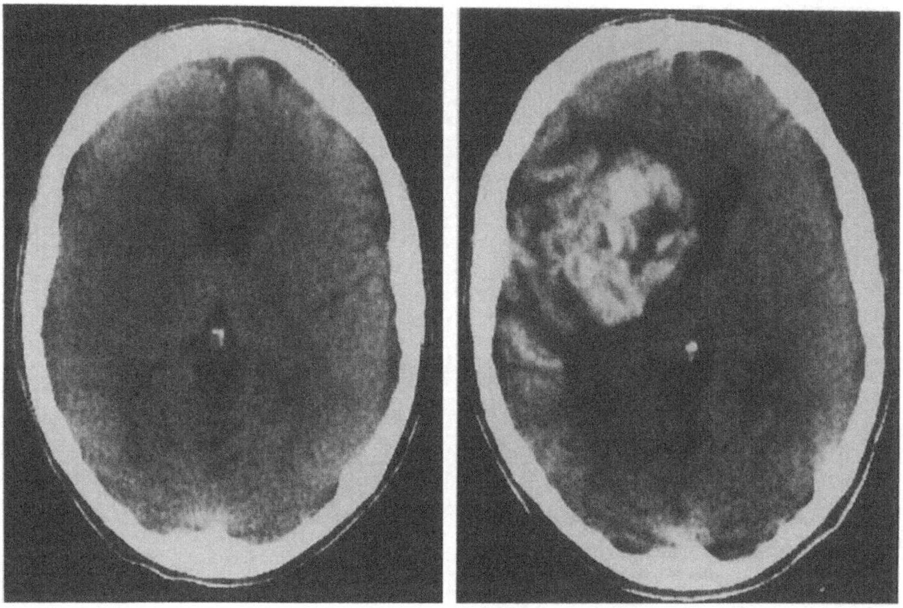

a b

Fig. 7.3. Anticoagulation-related brain hemorrhage following embolic stroke. **a** Initial CT done 12 h after stroke shows no hemorrhage. **b** Following anticoagulation, the patient abruptly worsened, and repeat CT showed massive brain hemorrhage.

References

Aberg H (1968) Atrial fibrillation. Acta Med Scand 185: 373–379

Adams GF, Merrett JD, Hutchinson WM, Polock AM (1974) Cerebral embolism and mitral stenosis: survival with and without anticoagulants. J Neurol Neurosurg Psych 37: 378–383

Arvan S (1985) Persistent intracardiac thrombi and systemic embolization despite anticoagulant therapy. Am Heart J 109: 178–180

Asinger RW, Mikell FL, Elsperger J, Hodges M (1981) Incidence of left-ventricular thrombosis after acute transmural myocardial infarction: serial evaluation by two-dimensional echocardiography. N Engl J Med 305: 297–302

Barnett HJM (1982) Embolism in mitral valve prolapse. Ann Rev Med 33: 489–507

Barnett HJM (1983) Heart in ischemic stroke. Neurologic Clinics 1: 292–316

Barnett HJM, Boughner DR, Taylor DW, Cooper PE, Kostuk WJ, Nichol PM (1980) Further evidence relating mitral valve prolapse to cerebral ischemic events. N Engl J Med 302: 139–144

Barron KD, Siqueira E, Hivano A (1960) Cerebral embolism caused by nonbacterial thrombotic endocarditis. Neurology 10: 391–397

Bar-Sela S, Ehrenfeld M, Elialiam M (1981) Arterial embolism in thyrotoxicosis with atrial fibrillation. Arch Int Med 141: 1191–1192

Bharucha NE, Wolf PA, Kannel WB, McNamara PM (1981) Epidemiological study of cerebral embolism: The Framingham Study. Ann Neurol 10: 105

Biller J, Challa VR, Toole JF, Howard VJ (1982) Nonbacterial thrombotic endocarditis. Arch Neurol 39: 95–98

Bjerkland CJ, Orning OM (1969) The efficacy of anticoagulant therapy in preventing embolism related to DC electrical conversion of atrial fibrillation. Am J Cardiol 23: 208–213

Block PC, DeSanctis RW, Weinberg AN, Austen WG (1979) Prosthetic valve endocarditis. J Thoracic Cardiovasc Surg 60: 540–546

Bogousslavsky J, Hachinski VC, Boughner DR, Fox AJ, Vinuela F, Barnett HJM (1986) Cardiac

and arterial lesions in carotid transient ischemic attacks. Arch Neurol 43: 223–228
Bousser MG, Eschwege E, Haguenau M, Lefaucconnier JM, Thibultn N, Touboul D, Touboul PJ (1983) "AICLA" Controlled trial of aspirin and dypridamole in secondary prevention of atherothrombotic-cerebral ischemia. Stroke 14: 5–13
Brand FN, Abbott RD, Kannel WB, Wolf PA (1985) Characteristics and prognosis of lone atrial fibrillation. JAMA 254: 3449–3453
Britton M, Gustafson C (1985) Nonrheumatic atrial fibrillation as a risk factor for stroke. Stroke 16: 182–188
Brockmeier LB, Adolph RJ, Gustin BW, Holmes JC, Sacks JG (1981) Calcium emboli to the retinal artery in calcific aortic stenosis. Am Heart J 101: 32–37
Burckhardt D, Hoffman A, Vogt S, Pfisterer M, Hasse J, Grädel E (1984) Clinical evaluation of the St. Jude Medical heart valve prothesis. J Thorac Cardiovasc Surg 88: 432–438
Cabin HS, Roberts WC (1980) Left ventricular aneurysm, intra-aneurysmal thrombus and systemic embolus in coronary heart disease. Chest 77: 586–590
Calendre L, Ortego JF, Bermejo F, Portera A (1984) Anticoagulation and hemorrhagic infarction in cerebral embolism secondary to rheumatic heart disease. Arch Neurol 41: 1152–1154
Canadian Cooperative Study Group (1978) A randomized trial of aspirin and sulfinpyrazone in threatened stroke. N Engl J Med 299: 53–59
Caplan LR, Hier D, D'Cruz I (1983) Cerebral embolism in the Michael Reese Stroke Registry. Stroke 14: 530–537
Carpenter JL, McAllister CK, US Army Collaborative Group (1983) Anticoagulation in prosthetic valve endocarditis. South Med J 76: 1372–75
Carter AB (1965) Prognosis of cerebral embolism. Lancet 2: 514–519
Cerebral Embolism Study Group (1983) immediate anticoagulation of embolic stroke: a randomized trial. Stroke 14: 668–676
Cerebral Embolism Study Group (1984) Immediate anticoagulation embolic stroke: brain hemorrhage and management options. Stroke 15: 779–789
Cerebral Embolism Task Force (1986) Cardiogenic brain embolism. Arch Neurol 43: 71–84
Chambers BR, Donnan GA, Bladen PF (1983) An analysis of the first 700 consecutive admissions to the Austin Hospital Stroke Unit. Aust NZ J Med 13: 57–64
Chesebro JH, Fuster V, Elveback LR, McGoon DC, Pluth JR, Puga FJ, Wallace RB, Danielson GK, Orszulak TA, Piehler JM, Schaff HV (1983) Trial of combined warfarin plus dipyridamole or aspirin therapy in prosthetic heart valve replacement: danger of aspirin compared with dipyridamole. Am J Cardiol 51: 1537–1541
Close JB, Evans DW, Bailey SW, (1979) Persistent lone atrial fibrillation—its prognosis after clinical diagnosis. J Royal Coll Gen Prac 29: 547–549
Coon WW, Willis PW (1974) Hemorrhagic complications of anticoagulant therapy. Arch Intern Med 133: 386–392
Coulshed N, Epstein EJ, McKendrick CS, Galloway RW (1970) Systemic embolism in mitral valve disease. Br Heart J 32: 26–34
Dale J, Myhre E, Stortstein O, Stormorken H, Efskind L (1977) Prevention of arterial thromboembolism with acetylsalicyclic acid: a controlled clinical study in patients with aortic ball valves. Am Heart J 94: 101–111
Daly R, Kattingly TW, Holt CL, et al. (1951) Systemic arterial embolism in rheumatic heart disease. Am Heart J 42: 556–581
Darling RC, Austin WC, Linton RR (1964) Arterial embolism. Surg Gynecol Obstet 124: 106–114
Davis FB, Sczupak CA (1979) Outpatient oral anticoagulation. Guidelines for longterm management. Postgrad Med 66: 100–109
DeBono DP, Warlow CP (1979) Mitral-annulus calcification and cerebral or retinal ischemia. Lancet 2: 383–385
Demakis JG, Proskey A, Rahimtoola SH, Jamil M, Sutton GC, Rosen KM, Gunnar RM, Tobin JR (1974) The natural course of alcoholic cardiomyopathy. Ann Int Med 80: 293–297
Deppisch LM, Fayemi AO (1976) Nonbacterial thrombotic endocarditis. Am Heart J 92: 723–729
Deverall PB, Olley PM, Smith DR, Watson DA, Whitaker W (1968) Incidence of embolism before and after mitral valvulotomy. Thorax 23: 530–540
Drapkin A, Mersky C (1972) Anticoagulant therapy after acute myocardial infarction: relation of therapeutic benefit to patient's age, sex and severity of infarction. JAMA 222: 541–549
Dry TJ, Willius FA (1939) Calcareous disease of the aortic valve: a study of 228 cases. Am Heart J 17: 138–145
Easton JD, Sherman DG (1980) Management of cerebral embolism of cardiac origin. Stroke 11: 433–442

Edmunds LH (1982) Thromboembolic complications of current cardiac valvular prosthesis. Ann Thorac Surg 34: 96–106
EPSIM Research Group (1982) A controlled comparison of aspirin and oral anticoagulants in prevention of death after myocardial infarction. N Engl J Med 307: 701–708
Eriksson SE, Link H (1983) Evaluation of anticoagulants in patients with cerebral infarction with slight to moderate neurological deficit. Acta Neurol Scand 68: 96–106
Errichetti AM, Holden A, Ansell J (1984) Management of oral anticoagulant therapy. Arch Int Med 14: 1966–1968
Evans W, Swann P (1954) Lone auricular fibrillation. Br Heart J 16: 189–194
Ezekowitz MD, Kellerman DJ, Smith EO, Streitz TM (1984) Detection of active left ventricular thrombosis during acute myocardial infarction using indium-111 platelet scintigraphy. Chest 86: 35–39
Fisher CM (1972) Treatment of chronic atrial fibrillation. Lancet 1: 1284
Fisher CM (1979) Reducing risks of cerebral embolism. Geriatrics 34: 59–66
Fisher CM, Adams RD (1951) Observations on brain embolism with special reference to the mechanism of hemorrhagic infarction. J Neurol Exp Neuropath 10: 92–93
Fleming HA, Bailey SM (1971) Mitral valve disease, systemic embolism and anticoagulants. Postgrad Med J 47: 599–604
Foote RA, Reagan TJ, Sandok BA (1978) Effects of anticoagulants in an animal model of septic cerebral embolization. Stroke 9: 573–79
Forfar JC (1982) Prediction of hemorrhage during long-term oral coumarin anticoagulation by excessive prothrombin ration. Am Heart J 103: 445–447
Friedman MJ, Carlson K, Marcus FI, et al. (1982) Clinical correlations in patients with acute myocardial infarction and left ventricular thrombus detected by two-dimensional echocardiography. Am J Med 72: 894–898
Fukuda Y, Nakamura K (1984) The incidence of thromboembolism and hemocoagulative background in patients with rheumatic heart disease. Jpn Circ J 48: 59–66
Fulkerson PK, Beaver BM, Auseon JC, Graber HL (1979) Calcification of the mitral annulus: etiology, clinical associations, complications and therapy. Am J Med 66: 967– 975
Furlan AJ, Cracuin AR, Salcedo E, Mellino M (1984) Risk of stroke in patients with mitral annular calcification. Stroke 15: 801–803
Fuster V, Gersh BJ, Guiliani ER, et al. (1981) The natural history of idiopathic dilated cardiomyopathy. Am J Cardiol 47: 525–531
Gallo I, Ruiz B, Duran CG (1984) Isolated mitral valve replacement with the Hancock Porcine Bioprosthesis in rheumatic heart disease: analysis of 213 operative survivors followed up 4.5–8.5 years. Am J Card 53: 178–181
Garvey GJ, Neu HC (1979) Infective endocarditis: an evolving disease. Medicine 57: 105–26
Geha AS, Hammond GL, Laks H, Stansel HC, Glenn WWL (1982) Factors affecting performance and thromboembolism after porcine xenograft cardiac valve replacement. J Thorac Cardiovasc Surg 83: 377–384
Godtfredson J (1982) Atrial fibrillation; course and prognosis—a follow-up study of 1212 cases. In: Kulbertus HE, Olsson SB, Schlepper M. atrial fibrillation. AB Hassle, Molndal, Sweden
Gonzalez-Laven L, Tandon AP, Chi S, Blair TC, McFadden PU, Lewis B, Daughters G, Ionescu M (1984) The risk of thromboembolism and hemorrhage following mitral valve replacement. J Thorac Cardiovasc Surg 87: 340–351
Goodnight SH (1980) Editorial: antiplatelet therapy for mitral stenosis? Circulation 62: 466–468
Gottdiener JS, Gay JA, VanVoorhees L, DiBianco R, Fletcher RD (1983) Frequency and embolic potential of left ventricular thrombus in dilated cardiomyopathy: 2-D echocardiography. Am J Card 52: 1281–1285
Graus F, Rogers JB (1985) Cerebrovascular complications in patients with cancer. Medicine 64: 16– 35
Hakim AM, Ryder-Cooke A, Melanson D (1983) Sequential computerized tomographic appearance of strokes. Stroke 14: 893–897
Hanson HH, Rutledge DI (1949) Auricular fibrillation in normal hearts. N Engl J Med 240: 947–954
Harrison MJG, Marshall J (1984) Atrial fibrillation, TIAs and completed strokes. Stroke 15: 441–442
Hart RG, Easton JD (1982) Mitral valve prolapse and cerebral infarction. Stroke 13: 429–430
Hart RG, Easton JD, Sherman DG (1983b) Duration of nonvalvular atrial fibrillation and stroke. Stroke 14: 827
Hart RG, Coull BM, Hart D (1983a) Early recurrent embolism associated with nonvalvular atrial fibrillation. Stroke 14: 688–693
Hart RG, Miller VT (1983b) Cerebral infarction in young adults: a practical approach. Stroke 14: 110–114

Haugland JM, Asinger RW, Mikell FL, Elsperger KJ, Hodges M (1981) Embolic potential of left ventricular thrombus detected by two-dimensional echocardiography. Am J Cardiol 47: 471

Herman B, Leyten ACM, Luijk JH, Frenken CWGM, Op de Coul AAW, Schulte BPM (1982) Epidemiology of stroke in Tilburg, The Netherlands. Stroke 13: 629–634

Hetzer R, Topalidis, Borst HG (1982) Thromboembolism and anticoagulation after isolated mitral valve replacement with porcine heterografts. In: Cohn LH, Gallucci V (eds). Proceedings, second international symposium on cardiac bioprosthesis. Yorke Medical Books, New York

Hinton RC, Kistler JP, Fallon JT, Friedlich AL, Fisher CM (1977) Influence of etiology of atrial fibrillation on incidence of systemic embolism. Am J Cardiol 40: 509–513

Hirsh J (1985) The relationship between dose of aspirin, side-effects and antithrombotic effectiveness. Stroke 16: 1–4

Hirsh J, Deykin D, Poller L (1986) "Therapeutic range" for oral anticoagulant therapy. Chest 89 [Suppl]: 11–15

Hirsh J, Levine M (1986) Therapeutic range for the control of oral anticoagulant therapy. Arch Neurol 43: 1162–1164

Hochman JS, Platia EB, Bulkley BH (1984) Endocardial abnormalities in left ventricular aneurysms. Ann Int Med 100: 29–35

Holley KE, Bahn RC, McGoon DC, Manlein HT (1963) Spontaneous calcific embolization asociated with calcific aortic stenosis. Circulation 27: 197–205

Hull R, Hirsh J, Jay R, Carter C, England C, Gent M, Turpie AGG, McLoughlin D, Dodd P, Thomas M, Raskob G, Ockelford P (1982) Different intensities of oral anticoagulant therapy in treatment of proximal vein thrombosis. N Engl J Med 307: 1676–1680

Hurley DM, Hunter AN, Hewett MJ, Stockigt JR (1981) Atrial fibrillation and arterial embolism in hyperthyroidism. Aust NZ J Med 11: 391–393

Husted S, Andreassen F (1976) Problems encountered in long-term treatment with anticoagulants. Acta Med Scanda 200: 379–384

Jabbari B, Lawrence PJ, Houtt AD (1983) Aortic stenosis and calcific cerebral embolization. Med State Med J 33–38

Jackson AC, Boughner DR, Barnett HJM (1984) Mitral valve prolapse and cerebral ischemic events in young patients. Neurology 34: 784–787

Jamieson WRE, Pelletier LC Janusz MT, Chaitman BR, Tyers FO, Miyagishima RT (1984) Five year evaluation of the Carpentier-Edwards porcine bioprothesis. J Thorac Cardiovasc Surg 88: 324–333

Johannessen KA, Nordrehaug JE, Von der Lippe G (1984) Left ventricular thrombosis and cerebrovascular accident in acute myocardial infarction. Br Heart J 51: 553–556

Johnson RA, Palacios I (1982) Dilated cardiomyopathies of the adult. N Engl J Med 307: 1051–1058

Jorgensen L, Torvik A (1966) Ischemic cerebrovascular disease in an autopsy series. J Neurol Sci 3: 490–509

Kanis JA (1974) The use of anticoagulants in bacterial endocarditis. Postgraduate Med J 50: 312–313

Kannel WB, Abbott RD, Savage DD, McNamara PM (1982) Epidemiologic features of chronic atrial fibrillation: The Framingham Study. N Engl J Med 306–1018–1022

Kapila A, Hart RG (1986) Calcific cerebral emboli and aortic stenosis: detection by computed tomography. Stroke 17: 622–625

Karchmer AW, Dismukes WE, Buckley MJ, Austen WG (1978) Late prosthetic valve endocarditis. Am J Med 64: 199–206

Kase CS, Robinson KR, Stein RW, et al. (1984) Anticoagulant-related intracerebral hemorrhage. Neurology 34 [Suppl]: 201

Kearsley JH, Tattersall MHW (1982) Cerebral embolism in cancer patients. J Med 203: 279–291

Keating EC, Gross SA, Schlamowitz RA, Glassman J, Mazur JH, Pitt WA, Miller D (1983) Mural thrombi in myocardial infarctions. Am J Med 74: 989–995

Kelton JG, Hirsh J (1980) Bleeding associated with antithrombotic therapy. Sem Hemat 17: 259–291

Kinney EL (1965) The significance of left ventricular thrombi in patients with coronary heart disease. Am Heart J 109: 191–194

Komrad MS, Coffey CE, Coffey KS, McKinnis R, Massey EW, Califf RM (1984) Myocardial infarction and stroke. Neurology 34: 1403–1409

Korn D, DeSanctis RW, Sell S (1962) Massive calcification of the mitral annulus: a clinical pathological study of 14 cases. N Engl J Med 267: 900–909

Kumpe CW, Bean WB (1948) Aortic stenosis: a study of the clinical and pathologic aspects of 107 proved cases. Medicine 27: 139–153

Larrea JL, Nunez L, Reque JA, Aguado MG Matarros R, Minguez JA (1984) Pregnancy and mechanical valve prostheses: a high-risk situation for the mother and the fetus. Ann Thorac Surg 36: 459–465

Larrieu AJ, Jamieson WRE, Tyers GFO, Burr LH, Munro AI, Miyagishima RT, Gerein AN, Allen P (1982) Primary cardiac tumors. J Thorac Cardiovasic Surg 83: 339–348
LeCam B, Guivarch G, Boles JM, Garre M, Cartier F (1984) Neurologic complications in a group of 86 bacterial endocarditis. Europ Heart J 5 [Suppl C]: 97–100
Lee MC, Heaney LM, Jacobsen RL, Klassen AC (1975) CSF in cerebral hemorrhage and infarction. Stroke 6: 638–642
Levine HJ (1981) Which atrial fibrillation patients should receive anticoagulation? J Cardiovasc Med 6: 483–487
Lieberman A, Hass WK, Pinto R, Som WO, Kupermsith M, Bear G, Chase R (1978) Intracranial hemorrhage and infarction in anticoagulated patients with prosthetic heart valves. Stroke 9: 18–24
Lodder J (1984) CT-detected hemorrhagic infarction; relation with size of infarct, and presence of midline shift. Acta Neurol Scanda 70: 329–335
Loelinger EA (1979) The optimal therapeutic range in oral anticoagulation. Thromb Haemost 42: 1141–1152
Loeliger EA, Besselar AM, Broekmans AW (1983) Intensity of oral anticoagulation in patients monitored with various thromboplastins. N Engl J Med 308: 1228–1229
Loeliger EA, Van Dijk-Wierda CA, Van den Besselaar AM, et al. (1984) Anticoagulant control and risk of bleeding. In: Meade TW (ed) Anticoagulants and myocardial infarction: a reappraisal. Wiley, New York
Martin GJ, Biller J (1984) Non-septic cerebral emboli of cardiac origin. Arch Int Med 144: 1997–1999
Marvaste MA, Obeid AI, Potts JL (1984) Approach to the management of atrial myxoma with long-term follow-up. Ann Thorac Surg 38: 53–56
McGoon DC (1984) The risk of thromboembolism following valvular operations: how does one know? J Thorac Cardiovasc Surg 88: 782–786
Medical Research Council (1969) Assessment of short-term anticoagulant administration after cardiac infarction. Br Med J 1: 335–342
Meizlish JL, Berger HJ, Plankey M, Errico D, Levy W, Zaret BL (1984) Functional left ventricular aneurysm formation after acute anterior transmural myocardial infarction: incidence, natural history, and prognostic implications. N Engl J Med 311: 1001–1005
Meltzer RS, Visser CA, Kan G, Roelart J (1984) Two-dimensional echocardiographic appearance of left ventricular thrombi with systemic emboli after myocardial infarction. Am J Card 53: 1511–1513
Mohr JP, Caplan LR, Melski JW, et al. (1978) The Harvard Cooperative Stroke Registry: a prospective registry. Neurology 28: 745–762
Morris DC, Hurst JW (1980) Atrial fibrillation. Curr Probl Cardiol 5 (#1): 1–50
Moschos CB, Wong PCY, Sise HS (1964) Controlled study of the effective level of long-term anticoagulation. JAMA 190: 799–805
Nagata S, Park YD, Nagae Y, Beppu S, Kawazoe K, Fujita T, Sakakibara H, Nimura Y (1984) Echocardiographic features of bioprosthetic valve endocarditis. Br Heart J 51: 263–266
Neilson GH, Galea EG, Hossack KF (1979) Thromboembolic complications of mitral valve disease. Aust NZ J Med 8: 372–376
Nestico PF, Depace NL, Morganroth J, Kotler MN, Ross T (1984) Mitral annular calcification: clinical pathophysiology, and echocardiographic review. Am Heart J 107: 989–996
Nishide M, Irino T, Gotoh M, Naka M, Tsuji K (1983) Cardiac abnormalities in ischemic cerebrovascular disease studied by two-dimensional echocardiography. Stroke 14: 541–549
Nunez L, Aguado MG, Larrea JL, Celemin D, Oliver J (1984) Prevention of thromboembolism using aspirin after mitral valve replacement with porcine bioprosthesis. Ann Thoracic Surg 37: 84–87
Nunez L, Gill AM, Celemin D, Iglesias A, Larrea JL (1982) Aspirin or Coumadin as the drug of choice for valve replacement with porcine bioprosthesis. Ann Thorac Surg 33: 354–361
O'Brien JT, Geiser EA (1984) Infective endocarditis and echocardiography. Am Heart J 108: 386–394
Olsson JE (1980) Recent advances in the treatment of cerebrovascular disorders. Acta Neurol Scand [Suppl 78] 62: 77–95
Owren PA (1963) The results of anticoagulant therapy in Norway. Arch Int Med 111: 240–247
Pass HI, Sade RM, Crawford FA, Hohn AR (1984) Cardiac valve prostheses in children without anticoagulation. J Thorac Cardiovasc Surg 87: 832–835
Pelletier LL, Petersdorf RG (1977) Infective endocarditis: a review of 125 cases. Medicine 56:287–314

Penner R, Font RL (1969) Retinal embolism from calcified vegetations of aortic valve. Arch Opthalmol 81: 565–570
Pruitt AA, Rubin RH, Karchmer AW, Duncan GW (1978) Neurologic complications of bacterial endocarditis. Medicine 57: 329–343
Rahimtoola SH (1983) Valvular heart disease: a perspective. J Am Coll Card 1: 199–215
Ramirez-Lassepas M, Cipolle RJ, Bjork RJ, Weber JC, Stein SD (1984) Is there a neurologic profile for embolic stroke? Circulation Abstract of the 57th Scientific Sessions (Miami, November 12–15)
Ramirez-Lassepas M, Quinones MR (1984) Heparin therapy for stroke: hemorrhagic complications and risk factors for intracerebral hemorrhage. Neurology 34: 114–117
Reeder GS, Lengyel M, Tajik AJ, Smith HC, Danielson GK (1981) Mural thrombus in left ventricular aneurysm. Mayo Clinic Proc 56: 77–81
Ridolfi RL, Hutchins GM (1976) Spontaneous calcific emboli from calcific mitral annulus fibrosis. Arch Patho Lab Med 100: 117–120
Rogers L, Choes HB, Posner JB (1982) Cerebral embolization for nonbacterial thrombotic endocarditis. Neurology 32 [Suppl 2]: 156 (abstract)
Rosen P, Armstrong D (1973) Nonbacterial thrombotic endocarditis in patients with malignant neoplastic disease. Am J Med 54: 23–29
Rotman M, Morris JJ, Behar VS, Peter RH, Kong Y (1971) Aortic valvular disease: comparison of types and their medical and surgical management. Am J Med 51: 241–247
Ruff RL, Dougherty JL (1981) Evaluation of acute cerebral ischemia for anticoagulant therapy. Neurology 31: 736–740
Sage JI, Van Uitert RL (1983) Risk of recurrent stroke with atrial fibrillation: differences between rheumatic and arteriosclerotic heart disease. Stroke 14: 537–540
Salazar E, Zajarias A, Gutierrez N, Iturbe I (1984) The problem of cardiac valve prosthesis, anticoagulants, and pregnancy. Circulation 70 [Suppl I]: I–169–I–177
Sandok BA, von Estorff I, Giuliani ER (1980) CNS embolism due to atrial myxoma. Arch Neurol 37: 485–488
Savage DD, Garrison RJ, Castelli WP, McNamara PM, Anderson SJ, Kanell WB, Feinleib M (1983a) Prevalence of submitral calcium and its correlates in a general population-based sample: The Framingham Study. Am J Cardiol 51: 1375–1378
Schaff HV, Danielson GK, DiDonato RM, Pugh FJ, Mair DD, McGoon DC (1984) Late results after Starr-Edwards valve replacement in children. J Thorac Cardiovasc Surg 88: 583–589
Schwartzman RJ, Hill JB (1982) Neurologic complications of disseminated intravascular coagulation. Neurology 32: 791–797
Segal JP, Harvey P, Gurel T (1965) Diagnosis and treatment of primary myocardial disease. Circulation 27: 837–845
Segal JP, Stapleton JF, McClellan JR, Wallter BF, Harvey WP (1978) Curr Probl Cardiol 3 (#6): 1–45
Sherman DG, Goldman L, Whiting RB, Jurgensen K, Kaste M, Easton JD (1984) Thromboembolism in patients with atrial fibrillation. Arch Neurol 41: 708–710
Simpson MT, Oberman A, Kouchoukos NT, Rogers WJ (1980) Prevalence of mural thrombi and systemic embolization with left ventricular aneurysm. Chest 77: 463–469
Silverton NP, Abdulali SA, Yakirevich VS, et al. (1984) Embolism, thrombosis and anticoagulant hemorrhage in mitral valve disease. A prospective study of patients having valve replacement with the pericardial xenograft. Europ Heart J 5 [Suppl D]: 19–25
Sixty-plus Reinfarction Study Research Group (1982) Risks of longterm oral anticoagulant therapy in elderly patients after myocardial infarction. Lancet 1: 64–68
Stafford WJ, Petch J. Reford DJ (1985) Vegetations in infective endocarditis. Br Heart J 53: 310–313
Staffurth JS, Gibberd MC, Tang-Fui SN (1977) Arterial embolism in thyrotoxicosis with atrial fibrillation. Br Med J 2: 688–690
Steele P, Rainwater J (1980) Favorable effect of sulfinpyrazone on thromboembolism in patients with rheumatic heart disease. Circ 62: 462–465
Stein PD, Sabbah HN, Pitha JV (1977) Continuing process of calcific aortic stenosis. Am J Cardiol 39: 159–163
Stratton JR, Ritchie JL (1984) The effects of anti-thrombotic drugs in patients with left ventricular thrombi: assessment with indium-111 platelet imaging and two-dimensional echocardiography. Circulation 69: 561–569
Szekeley P (1964) Systemic embolism and anticoagulant prophylaxis in rheumatic heart disease. Br Med J 1: 209–212
Terent A, Andersson B (1980) The outcome of patients with TIA and stroke treated with anticoagulants. Acta Med Scand 208: 359–365

van den Besselaar AMHP, Granlnick HR, Lewis SM (1984) Thromboplastin calibration and oral anticoagulant control. Martinus Nijhoff (Boston)

Veterans Cooperative Study (1973) Anticoagulants in acute myocardial infarction: results of a cooperative trial. JAMA 225: 724–729

Walsh MN, Fisher GG, Anderson D, Mastri A (1984) Fatal intracranial extension of spinal hemorrhage after lumbar puncture. Arch Neurol 41: 987–989

Weinreich DJ, Burke JF, Pauletto FJ (1984) Left ventricular mural thrombi complicating acute myocardial infarction. Ann Int Med 100: 789–794

Weinstein GS, Mavroudis C, Ebert PA (1981) Preliminary experience with aspirin for anticoagulation in children with prosthetic cardiac valves. Ann Thorac Surg 33: 549–555

Whisnant JP, Cartlidge NEF, Elveback LR (1978) Carotid and vertebral-basilar transient ischemic attacks: effect of anticoagulants, hypertension and cardiac disorders on survival and stroke occurrence. Ann Neurol 3: 107–115

Williams, JB, Karp, RB, Kirlin JW, Kouchoukos, NT, Pacifico AD, Zorn GL, Blackstone EH, Brown RN, Piantadosi S, Bradley EL (1980) Considerations in selection and management of patients undergoing valve replacement with glutaraldehyde-fixed porcine bioprostheses. Ann Thorac Surg 30: 247–258

Wilson WR, Geraci JE, Danielson GK, Thompson RL, Sphtell JA, Washington JAII, Giuliani ER (1978) Anticoagulant therapy and central nervous system complications in patients with prosthetic valve endocarditis. Circulation 57: 1004–1007

Wilson WR, Guiliani ER, Danielson GK, Geraci JE (1982) Management of complications of infective endocarditis. Mayo Clin Proc 57: 162–170

Wintzen AR, de Jonge H, Loelinger EA, Bots GTA (1984) The risk of intracerebral hemorrhage during oral anticoagulant treatment: a population study. Ann Neurol 16: 553–558

Wolf PA, Dawber TR, Thomas HE, Kannel WB (1978) Epidemiologic assessment of chronic atrial fibrillation and risk of stroke: The Framingham Study. Neurology 28: 973–977

Wolf PA, Kannel W, McGee DL, Meeks SL, Bharucha NE, McNamara PM (1983) Duration of atrial fibrillation and imminence of stroke: The Framingham Study. Stroke 14: 664–667

Wood P (1956) Diseases of the heart and circulation. Lippincott, Philadelphia

Yuen RW, Gutteridge DH, Thompson PL, Robinson JS (1979) Embolism in thyrotoxic atrial fibrillation. Med J Aust 1: 630–631

Ziment I (1969) Nervous system complications of bacterial endocarditis. Am J Med 47: 593–607

Chapter 8

Cardioactive Drugs in Cerebrovascular Disease

J. R. Little and S. C. Jones

Introduction

During the past 10 years many new cardioactive drugs have been identified and some of them have been introduced into clinical practice. Many of these drugs have potential in the treatment of cerebrovascular diseases. Two groups of drugs, the Ca^{2+} entry blocking agents and the beta-receptor blocking agents, have attracted considerable attention and are being evaluated in a wide range of cerebrovascular disorders in both the clinical and experimental setting. The object of this chapter is to review current knowledge of these two groups of drugs in the treatment of cerebrovascular disease.

Calcium Entry Blocking Agents

The calcium ion (Ca^{2+}) is normally maintained at a 10 000 to 1 extracellular to intracellular gradient across the plasma membrane. Transport of Ca^{2+} out of the cell is mediated by two systems: (a) an adenosine triphosphate (ATP) and Mg^{2+}-dependent pump that is induced by Ca^{2+}-activated calmodulin (Penniston et al. 1980) and (b) a partially ATP-dependent Na^+–Ca^{2+} exchange pump that transports one Ca^{2+} out of the cell for three Na^+ into the cell (Blaustein 1974; Carafoli 1978). The influx of Ca^{2+} into cells is thought to be the result of: (a) depolarization-dependent entry activated by increased extracellular K^+ and intracellular Na^+ (Blaustein 1974; Blaustein et al. 1972); (b) a depolarization-independent steady state entry system (Dipoli 1979); and (c) changes in the membrane fluidity related to shifts in membrane phospholipid content (Hirata et al. 1979).

Mitochondria and sarcoplasmic reticulum (i.e., in smooth muscle cells) play an important role in intracellular Ca^{2+} homeostasis. Increased concentrations of cytosolic Ca^{2+} stimulate an energy-consuming uptake of Ca^{2+} into the mitochondria in exchange for protons (Lehninger 1974). The sarcoplasmic reticulum also actively pumps and binds Ca^{2+} in a process that requires Mg^{2+} and ATP and is accompanied by proton exchange (Madeira 1980).

Vascular smooth muscle contraction is initiated when cytosolic intracellular Ca^{2+} concentration rises to a critical level (Hartshorne and Mrwa 1982). The Ca^{2+} then links to calmodulin and activates it. The Ca^{2+}-calmodulin interacts with myosin light chain kinase which triggers the development of cross linkages between myosin and actin, leading to mechanical shortening. Vasodilatation can be produced by a variety of mechanisms which lower intracellular Ca^{2+}.

In most systemic arteries, smooth muscle contraction is initiated by the intracellular flux of Ca^{2+}. In contrast, cerebrovascular smooth muscle cells are more dependent upon extracellular Ca^{2+} than is other vascular smooth muscle (Allen et al. 1976; Allen 1977). Constriction of cerebral arteries appears to be initiated by the influx of extracellular Ca^{2+} into the smooth muscle cells.

Pharmacology

Ca^{2+} entry blockers are agents with the common ability to reduce transmembrane transport of extracellular Ca^{2+} and thereby produce selective blockade of the slow inward current. They constitute a heterogeneous family of compounds which have dissimilar structural, electrophysiological, and pharmacological properties (Henry 1980). The three basic groups of Ca^{2+} entry blockers and their prototypes include: phenylalkylamine (verapamil), dihydropyridine (nifedipine), and benzothiazepine (diltiazem). Other groups of agents will undoubtedly be identified in the future.

Of the three current groups of agents, those in the dihydropyridine group appear to hold the most promise in the treatment of cerebrovascular disorders. This potential is largely related to their aparent affinity and selective action upon cerebrovascular smooth muscle (Muller-Schweintzer and Neumann 1980). For this reason, most of the following discussion will concentrate on two drugs in the dihydropyridine group, nifedipine and nimodipine, which have been studied most extensively up to this time.

Nifedipine and nimodipine are dihydropyridine derivatives that bear no structural similarity to other known vasoactive drugs. They are readily absorbed when taken orally and are largely bound to plasma proteins. Both agents are lipid soluble and should cross the blood-brain barrier with little difficulty (Henry 1980).

Ca^{2+} entry blockers are generally thought to enhance cerebral blood flow, with the dihydropyridine derivatives having the most potent effect. Nifedipine and nimodipine have been shown to increase substantially cerebral blood flow in a variety of experimental animals including rats, cats, dogs, and baboons (Kazda and Towart 1982; Sandahl et al. 1978; Mohamed et al. 1985; Kazda et al. 1979; Harper et al. 1981). Information is currently limited regarding the effect of these drugs upon cerebral blood flow in man. Doses of these drugs high enough to reduce systemic arterial blood pressure, however, may reduce or eliminate any increases in cerebral blood flow.

Potential Uses of Ca^{2+} Entry Blockers

Brain Ischemia

The complete sequence of events leading to irreversible cell damage in ischemia has not been established. Recently, considerable interest has been directed toward the role of altered Ca^{2+} homeostasis in this process (Farber et al. 1981). Failure of membrane ionic pumps at critical levels of ischemia is thought to lead to elevated cystosolic free Ca^{2+}. Increased Ca^{2+} could paradoxically stimulate mitochondria, resulting in further ATP depletion, and activate endogenous phospholipases, resulting in degradation of mitochondrial, endoplasmic, and plasma membranes. If this hypothesis is correct, the altered Ca^{2+} metabolism would be an important, if not critical, factor in producing cell death. With increased cytosolic Ca^{2+}, vascular smooth muscle cells would also be stimulated to contract. This could result in arterial constriction and spasm and reduce further the perfusion of the ischemic zone (Raichle 1982).

Global Cerebral Ischemia. The results of some studies using Ca^{2+} entry blocking agents in treating acute global cerebral ischemia have been encouraging. Kazda et al (1979) produced complete brain ischemia in cats using a neck tourniquet technique. They found an initial postischemic phase of hyperemia followed by a secondary phase of cerebral blood flow reduction to less than 50% of normal. Pretreatment with nimodipine did not modify the immediate postischemic hyperemia but it eliminated the subsequent delayed reduction of cerebral blood flow. Mortality was reduced from 90% in the untreated group to 10% in those animals pretreated with nimodipine. The beneficial effect of nimodipine, and specifically the prevention of the delayed postischemic hypoperfusion, was thought to be the result of inhibition of transmembrane influx of extracellular Ca^{2+} in the face of K^+ leaking out of the intracellular space.

Steen et al. (1983) treated dogs exposed to 10 min of complete cerebral ischemia with nimodipine. Treatment before the induction of ischemia improved both the postischemic cerebral blood flow and the neurological outcome. Treatment after ischemia had similar effects on cerebral blood flow as pretreatment but there was no improvement in neurological outcome (Steen et al. 1984). In contrast to the studies by Kazda et al. (1979), the findings of the investigations by Steén et al. suggested that mechanisms other than those related to modification of circulation after ischemia play a major role in reducing ischemic damage.

Information about the biochemical effects of the Ca^{2+} entry blockers in global cerebral ischemia is limited. In a recent study, Hossman et al. (1983) attempted to correlate brain Ca^{2+} content with biochemical and electrophysiological recovery in cats following global ischemia. They found that ischemia and the subsequent recirculation of blood led to a substantial increase in total tissue Ca^{2+}. This increase in Ca^{2+}, however, did not appear to interfere with the early postischemic electrophysiological and biochemical recovery. Treatment with the Ca^{2+} entry blocker, flunarizine, did not reduce tissue Ca^{2+} or improve functional and metabolic recovery.

Focal Cerebral Ischemia. Harris et al. (1981) measured extracellular Ca^{2+} in the cortex of baboons undergoing middle cerebral artery (MCA) occlusion. They reported a decrease in extracellular Ca^{2+} after MCA occlusion which produced a cerebral blood flow reduction to the 5- to 10-ml g/min range. The decrease in the extracellular Ca^{2+} concentration followed an increase in the extracellular K^{+} concentration. They postulated that the decrease of extracellular Ca^{2+} was the result of an extracellular to intracellular shift of Ca^{2+}. These changes appeared to precede irreversible tissue injury.

Verapamil (Reedy et al. 1983; Roy et al. 1985) and nimodipine (Harris et al. 1982; G. Barnett et al. 1986) have been studied in models of acute focal cerebral ischemia. The results of these studies have been less encouraging than those with global cerebral ischemia. Reedy et al. (1983) treated cats undergoing MCA occlusion with an intracarotid infusion of verapamil. Regional cerebral blood flow, electroencephalographic findings, breakdown of the blood-brain barrier, and morphological changes were not modified by treatment. Roy et al. (1983), using a similar model, were also unable to show any beneficial effect by treating with verapamil.

Harris et al. (1982) treated baboons undergoing MCA occlusion with nimodipine. Basal cerebral blood flow and postocclusion cerebral blood flow were increased by the intracarotid infusion of nimodipine in animals with a large craniectomy over the ipsilateral cerebral hemisphere. Cerebral blood flow, however, was not improved in the closed skull preparation. The threshold levels of regional cerebral blood flow for the development of cortical edema and for disturbance of ion homeostasis were increased, which suggested that nimodipine might, in fact, have a deleterious effect upon cellular energy metabolism and increase the susceptibility of tissue to ischemic injury. Barnett et al. (G. Barnett et al. 1986), using cats and an open skull, were unable to demonstrate any beneficial effects of nimodipine upon cerebral blood flow after MCA occlusion in cats despite the continuous intracarotid infusion of nimodipine. In their study, electroencephalographic changes and infarct size were not favorably modified.

Data regarding the effects of Ca^{2+} entry blockers in treating focal cerebral ischemia in humans are too little at this time to draw any conclusions. Encouraging results have been reported by Gelmers (1984), who studied 60 patients with acute cerebral ischemia in a prospective, single-blind, randomized trial. Twenty-nine patients received nimodipine for a 28-day period and 31 patients were untreated. The results indicated a significant reduction in morbidity and mortality in the treated group. In another study, Gelmers (1982) showed an increase in regional cerebral blood flow in ischemic areas using the xenon-133 clearance technique after treatment with nimodipine. More extensive evaluation will be required, however, before a definitive statement about the role of Ca^{2+} entry blockers in treating acute focal cerebral ischemia in man can be made.

Cerebral Vasospasm

Cerebral vasospasm is a leading cause of morbidity and mortality in patients suffering a subarachnoid hemorrhage from a saccular aneurysm. The vasospasm usually develops 4–7 days after the hemorrhage (i.e., so-called "delayed" or "chronic" vasospasm) and often results in ischemic neurological deficit or death. Contraction of the cerebrovascular smooth muscle cells is thought to play an important, if not primary, role in this process. Consequently, attention has been directed toward the Ca^{2+} entry blockers as potential therapeutic agents. Experimental studies have shown that these agents generally inhibit cerebrovascular smooth muscle constriction and possibly prevent delayed vasospasm (Allen 1977; Allen and Banghart 1979; Allen and Bahr 1979; Cohen and Allen 1980; Tanaka et al. 1982; Svengaard et al. 1983). The dihydropyridines appear to have a more selective effect upon the cerebrovasculature than the other groups of Ca^{2+} entry blockers. Nimodipine, in particular, has been shown to have a greater affinity for cerebrovascular smooth muscle slow Ca^{2+} channels and a more potent vasodilatory effect than nifedipine.

In a multi-institution, prospective, double-blind, randomized, placebo-controlled trial, the effects of nimodipine treatment starting within 96 h of subarachnoid hemorrhage were evaluated (Allen et al. 1983). There were 116 patients in the study, including 56 receiving nimodipine and 60 receiving placebo. Analysis of results revealed a significant reduction of severe ischemic neurological deficits in the treated group. There were no side effects from the treatment. Further studies using larger doses of nimodipine as well as studies combining nimodipine and epsilon aminocaproic acid are currently being performed.

Migraine

Ca^{2+} entry blockers have been proposed as potential therapeutic agents in the prophylaxis of the migraine syndrome (Solomon et al. 1983; Kahan et al. 1983). Information available at this time does not allow a definitive statement but early reports have been favorable.

Verapamil is the Ca^{2+} entry blocking agent most frequently used in treating migraine. This is partly related to its early availability for clinical use. Undoubtedly more information will become available when other Ca^{2+}-blocking agents are used in this setting.

The mechanism of action of Ca^{2+} entry blockers in preventing migraine remains speculative. Most migraines are thought to include a prodromal phase of cerebrovascular vasoconstriction. If this vasoconstriction can be blocked by a Ca^{2+} entry blocking agent, it is possible that the secondary headache produced by vasodilation would not develop.

Beta-Receptor Blocking Agents

Radioligand-binding techniques have been used to identify beta-adrenergic receptors in various tissues including erythrocytes, heart, and brain. Although distributed throughout the brain, the highest density of beta-receptors is found in the cerebral cortex and corpus striatum (Alexander et al. 1975; Bylund and

Snyder 1976; Sporn and Molinoff 1976). The exact localization of beta-receptors on neurons and/or glial cells has not been determined. The presence of a high density of beta-receptors in regions with no adrenergic input, as well as the finding that there is no beta-adrenergic receptor change subsequent to kaniac acid-induced neuronal cell death (Zahniser et al. 1979), has prompted the suggestion of predominant glial rather than neuronal localization in the corpus striatum.

Both radioligand binding and beta-receptor-stimulated adenylate cyclase in purified preparations of brain and blood vessels have verified the presence of blood vessel beta-receptors (Palacious and Kuhar 1980; Nathanson and Glaser 1979). These receptors, however, constitute only a fraction of the total brain beta-receptor population and microvessels constitute less than 1% of whole brain homogenate and 1%–2% of the cortical gray matter (Petroutka et al. 1980; Lierse 1968). The beta-receptor density in the microvessel fraction is much less than in the whole brain homogenate (Minneman 1981). Culvenar and Jarrott (1981) have presented evidence that although the density of the beta-receptors in cortical microvessels is half that in gray matter membranes, the affinity for binding antagonists is six times greater. Both beta 1 and beta 2 receptors are thought to be present in the cerebral vasculature (Nathanson and Glaser 1979; Petroutka et al. 1980).

The extent to which the autonomic nervous system influences control of the cerebral circulation and blood flow has yet to be established despite the considerable investigative effort in this area. In general terms, stimulation of alpha-receptors increases cerebral vascular tonus and stimulation of beta-receptors decreases tonus. Extrinsic innervation arising from the superior cervical ganglia supplies the large arteries at the base of the brain, the epicerebral arteries, and some intraparenchymal arterioles. This network is vasoconstrictor in nature and acts through alpha receptors. An intrinsic system originating in the locus ceruleus has widespread influence upon intraparenchymal arteries (Dillier et al. 1978; Hoffer 1971). Activation of this system can produce vasodilatation mediated by the beta-receptors (Rosendorff et al. 1976).

The intrinsic adrenergic system has also been shown to affect neuronal discharge. Inhibition of firing of cerebellar, cortical, and hippocampal neurons results from stimulation of the locus ceruleus. Injection of a beta-blocking agent into the locus ceruleus blocks this inhibitory influence (Phillis and Kostopoulos 1977; Segal and Bloom 1974).

Pharmacology

Propranolol was the first beta-adrenergic antagonist to be used clinically. It is a highly potent, nonselective beta-adrenergic blocking agent with no intrinsic sympathomimetic activity. Most of the beta-adrenergic blocking agents, including propranolol, are derivatives of the beta-receptor agonist isoproterenol. Because of its widespread clinical use and the availability of information regarding its central nervous system actions, the remainder of this discussion will focus on propranolol.

Commercially available propranolol (i.e., Inderal) is a racemic mixture of the *d*-isomer and *l*-isomer. The beta-receptor blocking activity resides almost completely in the *l*-isomer.

Propranolol is readily absorbed when taken orally. Much of the administered drug, however, is metabolized by the liver during its first pass through the portal system and only one-third reaches the systemic circulation. Up to 90% of propranolol is bound to plasma proteins. Approximately 66% of propranolol in the blood crosses the blood-brain barrier in a single passage, an extraction rate similar to water (Olesson et al. 1978; Cruikshank et al. 1980).

The effects of propranolol upon the cerebral circulation have not been completely defined. Blocking of the cerebral vascular beta-receptors could potentially impair any decrease in arterial tonus that would result from beta stimulation. Micropipette studies of the pial arterial reactions in vivo reported by Wahl et al. (1974) failed to demonstrate a significant beta-adrenergic influence on vessel diameter. Over a wide range of concentrations, no change in arterial diameter was produced by propranolol.

Administration of propranolol to humans and experimental animals has been shown either to have no effect or to reduce slightly cerebral blood flow (Olesson et al. 1978; Laubie and Drouillat 1968; McKenzie et al. 1976; Nies et al. 1973). Oleson et al. (1978) studied the effects of intracarotid injections of propranolol upon cerebral blood flow in humans. No significant change in flow was seen and autoregulation remained intact. In those studies showing cerebral blood flow reduction with propranolol, the reduced flow was usually thought to be the result of a lowered rate of cerebral metabolism which propranolol has been shown to produce.

Potential Uses of Beta-Receptor Blocking Agents

Brain Ischemia

Propranolol has been found to have a protective effect in experimental myocardial ischemia (Maroka et al. 1971; Reimer et al. 1973). Protection of ischemic kidneys was subsequently demonstrated following treatment with propranolol (i.e., racemic *d,l*-propranolol) and its weak beta-blocking isomer, *d*-propranolol (Stowe et al. 1981).

A number of actions of propranolol and/or *d*-propranolol could potentially play a role in protecting ischemic brain. Pendleton et al. (1972) found a shift to the right of the hemoglobin-oxygen dissociation curve of erythrocytes with propranolol and *d*-propranolol. In their study, the weak beta-blocking *d*-isomer produced a greater shift than racemic *d,l*-propranolol. This action could increase the availability of oxygen to the ischemic tissue. Because the *d*-isomer was equally or more effective in shifting the curve than the racemic mixture, this action was not attributed to the beta-blocking properties of the *l*-isomer.

Racemic propranolol and *d*-propranolol appear to have "membrane stabilizing" effects. Langslet (1977) has shown both that racemic propranolol and *d*-propranolol inhibit osmotically induced erythrocyte lysis. This membrane-stabilizing effect was confirmed by Pendleton et al. (1972). As well, these agents have been shown to have local anesthetic effects which are comparable to those of lidocaine.

Weksler et al. (1977) demonstrated that propranolol inhibits platelet aggregation and serotonin release by adenosine diphosphate (ADP), epinephrine, collagen, and thrombin. The *d*-isomer, which has little beta-blocking activity, was equally effective in preventing platelet aggregation as the *l*-isomer. All platelet activities affected by propranolol were Ca^{2+} dependent, suggesting that the drug interferes with Ca^{2+} availability. Propranolol's membrane-stabilizing effects were previously theorized by Mills and Roberts (1967) to result in inhibition of catecholamine-induced platelet aggregation. As abnormal platelet function has been noted both in experimental ischemia and during acute cerebral ischemia in humans, propranolol's antiplatelet activity may be beneficial in preserving the microcirculation.

The role of Ca^{2+} as a mediator of cell death has been reviewed in the preceding section. Propranolol may interfere with Ca^{2+} influx into cells by reducing the population of receptor-operated channels and abolishing cyclic adenosine monophosphate (AMP)-dependent protein kinase mediated phosphorylation of slow inward current channels (Braunwald 1982; Lindemann 1982). Propranolol also reduces Ca^{2+}-dependent phospholipase A_2 activity in platelets and mouse lymphoma cells (van der Hoek and Feinstein 1978; Levine and Moskowitz 1979). The enzyme, phospholipase, promotes release of a number of free fatty acids, including arachidonic acid, and has been implicated in the disruption of organelle and plasma membrane structure and function. In addition, release of arachidonic acid increases production of potentially deleterious substances such as the prostaglandins F_2 and E_2, thromboxane A_2, and the leukotrienes.

In addition to propranolol's effect on precursor production of the prostaglandin cascade, it has also been shown to inhibit thromboxane A_2 production in human platelets through inhibition of thromboxane synthetase (Campbell et al. 1981; Johnson and Campbell 1980). Prostacyclin release from endothelial cells is not affected by propranolol (Callahan et al. 1980). In fact, the ability of media from cultured endothelial cells to inhibit platelet aggregation, presumably due to prostacyclin production, was greatly enhanced with propranolol.

Other experiments have suggested potential for enhancement of blood flow. Prostacyclin vasodilator response in rabbit-isolated hearts was significantly augmented by the addition of propranolol or sotolol (Gillespie et al. 1981). As *d*-propranolol possesses little beta adrenergic blocking properties and sotolol no membrane-stabilizing activity (Frishman 1979), the authors assumed that a non-beta-adrenergic effect was operative. Ca^{2+} antagonist activity was suggested as the mechanism by which propranolol inhibits contractions of isolated human basilar artery to locally applied prostaglandins (Boullin and Mohan 1977), and contractions of isolated dog coronary artery to exogenous Ca^{2+} (Sakanshi and Katsuhide 1981).

Preliminary reports suggest a potential role for propranolol and its *d*-isomer in the treatment of acute focal brain ischemia. Considerable investigative effort, however, will be needed to establish its role (if any). At this point there is no evidence to indicate a deleterious effect.

Little et al. (Little et al. 1982; Standefeder et al. 1986) studied the effects of propranolol and its isomer, *d*-propranolol, upon the evolution of cerebral infarction in cats undergoing MCA occlusion. Treatment with these agents reduced infarct size in lightly anesthetized cats undergoing 3 h of occlusion and unanesthetized cats undergoing 6 h of occlusion followed by 6 h of recirculation. Regional cerebral blood flow was not adversely affected by these agents.

Meyer et al. (1974, 1974) injected propranolol into the carotid artery of patients suffering a subacute ipsilateral cerebral ischemic event. They found that propranolol lowered cerebral oxygen consumption and glucose metabolism. They observed a concomitant reduction of hemispheric regional cerebral blood flow and attributed this partly to the reduced rate of metabolism.

Subarachnoid Hemorrhage

A preliminary report by Walter et al. (1982) suggests a potential role for propranolol in reducing neurological morbidity in subarachnoid hemorrhage. Treatment with propranolol was started within 48 h of subarachnoid hemorrhage. The mechanism of action was not defined but possibilities included a direct protective effect of propranolol upon ischemic brain and/or reduction in severity of cerebral vasospasm. The results of the study, however, have to be evaluated cautiously because of the lack of clear-cut statistical significance in the analysis of the data and the reports of Sundt et al. (1973) indicating a beneficial effect by treating subarachnoid hemorrhage patients with the beta-agonist, isoproterenol.

Migraine

During the past 10 years, propranolol has become one of the mainstays in the prophylactic treatment of the migraine syndrome. Other beta-blocking agents which also appear to provide benefit include nadolol, timolol maleate, atenolol, and metoprolol. Overall, the nonselective beta-blockers appear to be more effective in migraine prophylaxis than are the more cardiac-selective drugs.

The mechanism of action of propranolol and other beta blocking-agents in treating the migraine syndrome has not been established. There is no clear-cut evidence to support the hypothesis that benefit is directly related to beta-receptor blockade. The onset of a migraine headache appears to be associated with heightened sympathetic activity. The nonselective beta-blocking agents could produce a beneficial effect in part by decreasing sympathetic activity in the autonomic nervous system. In a recent report, Gengo et al. (1984) demonstrated periodic fluctuations in blood propranolol concentrations. In a patient with these fluctuations, migraine headaches recurred when propranolol concentrations were low. This variation of propranolol concentration might explain the inconsistent response in treating some patients.

Conclusions

Beta-blocking agents and Ca^{2+} entry blocking agents constitute two groups of cardioactive drugs which have become an integral part of the medical armamentarium during the past 10 years. These agents have also been found to have important effects upon the cerebral circulation and could play a role in the treatment of such cerebrovascular disorders as brain ischemia, cerebral vasospasm, and the migraine syndrome.

During the coming years, many new cardioactive drugs will be introduced. Some of these will have a direct effect upon the cerebral circulation and the potential to modify certain cerebrovascular disorders. The development of these drugs will provide an exciting challenge to those individuals committed to the investigation and treatment of cerebrovascular diseases.

References

Alexander RW, Davis JN, Lefkowitz RJ (1975) Direct identification and characterization of beta-adrenergic receptors in rat brain. Nature 258: 437–440

Allen GS (1977) Cerebral arterial spasm: a discussion of present and future research. Neurosurgery 1: 142–148

Allen GS, Bahr HL (1979) Cerebral arterial spasm. 10 Reversal of acute and chronic spasm in dogs with orally administered nifedipine. Neurosurgery 4: 43–47

Allen GS, Banghart SB (1979) Cerebral arterial spasm. In vitro effects of nifedipine on serotonin, phenylephrine, and potassium induced contractions of canine basilar and femoral arteries. Neurosurgery 4: 37–42

Allen GS, Gross CJ, Henderson LM, Chou SN (1976) Cerebral arterial spasm: part 4. In vitro effects of temperature, serotonin analogues, large nonphysiological concentration of serotonin, and extracellular calcium and magnesium or serotonin induced contractions of the canine basilar artery. J Neurosurg 44: 585–593

Allen GS, Ahn HS, Preziosi TJ, Battye R, Boone SC, Chou SN, Kelly DL, Weir BK, Crabbe RA, Lavile PJ, Rosenbloom SB, Dorsey FC, Ingram CR, Mellits DE, Bertsch LA, Boisvert DPJ, Hundley MB, Johnson RK, Strom JH, Transon CR (1983) Cerebral arterial spasm—a controlled trial of nimodipine in patients with subarachnoid hemorrhage. N Eng J Med 308: 619–624

Annual Meeting of the American Association of Neurological Surgeons, Washington: 60–61, 1983

Barnett GH, Bose B, Little JR, Jones SC, Friel HT (1986) Effects of nimodipine on acute focal cerebral ischemia. Stroke 17: 884–890

Blaustein MD (1974) The interrelationship between sodium and calcium fluxes across cell membranes. Rev Physiol Biochem Pharmacol 70: 33–82

Blaustein MP, Johnson EM, Needleman P (1972) Calcium dependent norepinephrine released from synaptic terminals. Proc Natl Acad Sci USA 69: 2237–2240

Boullin DJ, Mohan J (1977) Effects of (+) and (−) propranolol on the responses of the human isolated basilar artery to cerebrospinal fluid obtained from patients with subarachnoid hemorrhage and cerebral arterial spasm. Br J Clin Pharm 4: 27–31

Braunwald E (1982) Mechanism of action of calcium channel blocking agents. N Engl J Med 307: 1618–1627

Bylund DB, Snyder SH (1976) Beta-adrenergic receptor binding in membrane preparations from mammalian brain. Mol Pharm 12: 568–580

Callahan KS, Campbell WB, Johnson AR (1980) Antiplatelet activity of propranolol: interaction with PGI_2 and endothelial cells. Fed Proc 39: 392

Campbell WB, Johnson AR, Callahan KS, Graham R (1981) Antiplatelet activity of beta-adrenergic antagonists: inhibition of thromboxane synthesis and platelet aggregation in patients receiving long-term propranolol treatment. Lancet 2: 1382–1384

Carafoli E, Crompton M (1978) The regulation of intracellular calcium. Curr Top Memb Trans 10: 151–173

Cohen RJ, Allen GS (1980) Cerebral arterial spasm: the role of calcium in in vitro and in vivo analysis of treatment with nifedipine and nimodipine. In Wilkins RH (ed) Cerebral arterial spasm. Williams and Wilkins, Baltimore. pp. 527–532

Cruickshank M, Neil-Dwyer G, Cameron M, McAinsh J (1980) Beta-adrenoreceptor blocking agents and the blood-brain barrier. Clin Sci [Suppl] 6: S453–S455

Culvenor AJ, Jarrott B (1981) Comparison of beta-adrenoreceptors in bovine intracerebral microvessels and cerebral gray matter by (3H) dihydroalprenolol binding. Neuroscience 6: 1643–1648

Dillier N, Laslo J, Muller B, Koella WP, Olpe H-R (1978) Activation of an inhibitory noradrenergic

pathway projecting from the locus coeruleus to the angulate cortex of the rat. Brain Res 154: 61–68
DiPolo R (1979) Calcium influx in internally dialyzed giant squid axons. J Gen Physiol 73: 91–113
Farber JL, Chien KR, Mittnacht S (1981) The pathogenesis of irreversible cell injury in ischemia. Am J Pathol 102: 271–281
Frishman W (1979) Clinical pharmacology of the new beta-adrenergic blocking drugs. Part 1. Pharmacodynamics and pharmacokinetic properties. Am Heart J 97: 663–670
Gengo FM, Fagan SC, Kinkel W, McHugh WB (1984) Serum concentrations of propranolol and migraine prophylaxis. Arch Neurol 41: 1306–1307
Gelmers HJ (1982) Effect of nimodipine (Bay e 9736) on postischemic cerebrovascular reactivity, as revealed by measuring regional cerebral blood flow. Acta Neurochir 63: 283–290
Gelmers HJ (1984) The effects of nimodipine on the clinical course of patients with acute ischemic stroke. Acta Neurol Scand 69: 232–239
Gillespie MN, Atkinson JE, Turbeck JA, Diamond L (1981) Propranolol and sotolol augment the coronary vasodilatory action of prostacyclin (PGI_2) in rabbit isolated hearts. Eur J Pharm 75: 155–158
Harper AM, Craigen L, Kazda S (1981) Effect of the calcium antagonist, nimodipine, on cerebral blood flow and metabolism in the primate. J Cereb Blood Flow Metab 1: 349–356
Harris RJ, Branston NM, Symon L, Bayhan M, Watson M (1982) The effects of a calcium antagonist, nimodipine, upon physiological responses of the cerebral vasculature and its possible influence upon focal cerebral ischemia. Stroke 13: 759–766
Harris RJ, Symon L, Branston NM, Bayhan M (1981) Changes in extracellular calcium activity in cerebral ischemia. J Cereb Blood Flow Metab 1: 203–209
Hartshorne DJ, Mrwa V (1982) Regulation of smooth muscle actomyosin. Blood Vessels 19: 1–18
Henry PD (1980) Comparative pharmacology of calcium antagonists: nifedipine, verapamil and diltiazem. Am J Cardiol 46: 1047–1058
Hirata F, Steittmatter WJ Axebrod J (1979) Beta-adrenergic receptor increases phospholipid methylation membrane fluidity and beta-adrenergic receptor adenylate cyclase coupling. Proc Natl Acad Sci USA 76: 368–372
Hoffer BJ, Siggins GR, Bloom FE (1971): Studies on norepinephrine and related substances administered by microiontophoresis. Brain Res 25: 523–524
Hossmann KA, Paschen W, Csiba L (1983) Relationship between calcium accumulation and recovery of cat brain after prolonged cerebral ischemia. J Cereb Blood Flow Metab 3: 316–353
Johnson A, Campbell WB (1980) Antiplatelet activity or propranolol: inhibition of thromboxane synthetase. Fed Proc 39: 392
Kahan H, Weber S, Amor B, Guerin F, Degeorges M (1983) Nifedipine in the treatment of migraine in patients with Raynaud's phenomenon. N Engl J Med: 308: 1102–1103
Kazda S, Towart R (1982) Nimodipine: a new calcium antagonist drug with a preferential cerebrovascular action. Acta Neurochir 63: 259–265
Kazda S, Hoffmeister F, Garthoff B, Towart R (1979) Prevention of the postischemic impaired reperfusion of the brain by nimodipine (Bay e 9736) Acta Neurol Scand 60 [Suppl 72]: 302–303
Langslet A (1970) Membrane stabilization and cardiac effects of *d,l*-propranolol *d*-propranolol, and chlorpromazine. Eur J Pharmacol 13: 6–14
Laubie M, Drouillat M (1968) Effets hemodynamiques due propranolol chez le chien. Arch Int Pharmacodyn Ther 175: 470–481
Lehninger AL (1974) Role of phosphate and other proton-donating cations in respiration—coupled transport of calcium by mitochondria. Proc Natl Acad Sci USA 71: 1520–1524
Levine L, Moskowitz MA (1979) Alpha- and beta-adrenergic stimulation of arachidonic acid metabolism of cells in culture. Proc Nat Acad Sci USA 76: 6632–6636
Lierse W (1968) The capillary density of mammal's brain. In: *Oxygen transport in blood and tissues*. Lubbers DW, Luft VL, Thews G (eds) Theime, Stuttgart, pp 115–117
Lindemann JP, Bailey JC, Watanabe AM (1982) Potential biochemical mechanisms for regulation of the slow inward current: theoretical basis for drug action. Am Heart J 103: 746–756
Little JR, Latchaw JP, Slugg RM, Lesser RP, Stowe NP (1982) Treatment of acute focal cerebral ischemia with propranolol. Stroke 13: 302–307
Madeira VMC (1980) Proton movements across the membranes of sarcoplasmic reticulum during the uptake of calcium. Arch Biochem Biophys 200: 319–325
Maroka PR, Kjesus JK, Sobel BE, Watanabe I, Covell JW, Ross J, Braunwald E (1971) Factors influencing infarct size following experimental coronary artery occlusion. Circulation 43: 67–82
McKenzie ET, McCulloch J, Harper HM (1976) Influence of endogenous epinephrine on cerebral blood flow and metabolism. Am J Physiol 231: 489–494

Meyer JS, Okamoto S, Sari A, Koto A, Itoh Y, Ericsson AD (1974a) Effects of beta-adrenergic blockade on cerebral autoregulation and chemical vasomotor control in patients with stroke. Stroke 5: 167–179

Meyer JS, Okamoto S, Shimazu K, Koto A, Ohuchi T, Sari A, Ericsson AD (1974b) Cerebral metabolic changes during treatment of subacute cerebral infarction by alpha- and beta-adrenergic blockade with phenoxybenzamine and propranolol. Stroke 5: 180–195

Mills DCB, Roberts GCK (1967) Effects of adrenaline on human blood platelets. J Physiol 193–443–453

Minneman KP (1981) Adrenergic receptor molecules. In: Yamamura H, Enna SJ (eds) Neurotransmitter receptors, part 2. Biogenic amines. Chapman and Hall, New York, pp 188–268

Mohamed AA, Mendelow AD, Teasdale GM, Harper AM, McCulloch J (1985) Effect of the calcium antagonist nimodipine and local cerebral blood flow and metabolic coupling. J Cereb Blood Flow Metab 5: 26–33

Muller-Schweinitzer E, Neumann P (1983) In vitro effects of calcium antagonists PN 200–110, nifedipine and nimodipine on human and canine cerebral arteries. J Cereb Blood Flow Metab 3: 354–361

Nathanson JH, Glaser GH (1979) Identification of beta-adrenergic sensitive adenylate cyclase in intracranial blood vessels. Nature 278: 567–569

Nies AS, Evans GH, Shand DG (1973) Regional hemodynamic effects of beta-adrenergic blockade with propranolol in the unanesthetized primate. Am Heart J 85: 97–102

Olesson J, Hougard K, Hertz M (1978) Isoproterenol and propranolol ability to cross the blood-brain barrier and effects on the cerebral circulation in man. Stroke 9: 344–349

Palacios JM, Kuhar MJ (1980) Beta-adrenergic receptor localization by light microscopic autoradiography. Science 208: 1378–1380

Pendleton RG, Newman DJ, Sherman SS, Brann EG, Maya WE (1972) Effect of propranolol on the hemoglobin-oxygen dissociation curve. J Pharm Exp Ther 180: 647–656

Penniston JT, Graf E, Hano T (1980) Calmodulin regulation of the calcium pump of erythrocyte membranes. Ann NY Acad Sci 356: 245–257

Petroutka SJ, Moskowitz MH, Rheinhart JF, Snyder SH (1980) Neurotransmitter receptor binding in bovine cerebral microvessels. Science 208: 610–612

Phillis JW, Kostopoulos GK (1977) Activation of noradrenergic pathway from brainstem to rat cerebral cortex. Gen Pharmacol 8: 207–211

Raichle ME (1982) The pathophysiology of brain ischemia and infarction. Clin Neurosurg 29: 379–389

Reedy DP, Little JR, Capraro JA, Slugg RM, Lesser RP (1983) Effects of verapamil on acute focal cerebral ischemia. Neurosurgery 12: 272–276

Reimer KA, Rasmussen MM, Jennings B (1973) Reduction by propranolol of myocardial necrosis following temporary coronary occlusion in dogs. Circ Res 33: 353–363

Rosendorff C, Mitchell G, Scriven DRL, Shapiro C (1976) Evidence for a dual innervation affecting local blood flow in the hypothalamus of the conscious rabbit. Circ Res 38: 140–145

Roy MW, Dempsey RJ, Meyer KL, Donaldson DL, Tibbs PA, Young AB (1985) Effects of verapamil and diltiazem on acute strokes in cats. J. Neurosurg. 63: 629–636.

Sakanshi M, Katsuhide N (1981) Relaxation of isolated dog coronary artery induced by propranolol. Eur J Pharm 70: 83–85

Sandahl B, Anderson KE, Aronsen KF, Ulmsten V (1978) Effect of the calcium antagonist nifedipine on uterine blood flow in nontreated and oestradiol treated rats. Gynec Obstet Invest 9: 238–243

Segal M, Bloom FE (1974) Action of norepinephrine in the rat hypocampus II activation of the input pathway. Brain Res 72: 99–114

Solomon GD, Steel JG, Spaccavento LJ (1983) Verapamil prophylaxis of migraine. JAMA 250: 2500–2504

Sporn JR, Molinoff PB (1976) Beta-adrenergic receptors in rat brain. J Cyclic Nucleotide Res 2: 149–161

Standefer M, Little JR (1986) Improved neurological outcome in experimental focal cerebral ischemia treated with propranolol. Neurosurgery 18: 136–140

Steen PA, Newberg LA, Milde JH, Michefelder JD (1983) Nimodipine improves cerebral blood flow and neurologic recovery after complete cerebral ischemia in the dog. J Cereb Blood Flow Metab 3: 38–43

Steen PA, Newberg LA, Milde JH, Michenfelder JD (1984) Cerebral blood flow and neurologic outcome when nimodipine is given after complete cerebral ischemia in the dog. J Cereb Blood Flow Metab 4: 82–87

Stowe N, Magnussen M, Novick A, Palleschi J, Pechan W, Khairallah P, Gifford R, Straffon R (1981) Pharmacologic protection against prolonged ischemia during harvesting and preservation of canine kidneys. Transplant Proc 13: 699–701

Sundt TM, Onofrio BM, Merideth J (1973) Treatment of cerebral vasospasm from subarachnoid hemorrhage with isoproterenol and lidocaine hydrochloride. J Neurosurg 38: 557–560

Svengaard NA, Brisman J, Delgado T, Egund N, Owman C, Rodacki MA, Sahlin C, Salford LG (1983) Late cerebral arterial spasm: the cerebrovascular response to hypercapnia, induced hypertension and the effect of nimodipine on blood flow (auto) regulation in experimental subarachnoid hemorrhage in primates. Gen Pharmacol 14: 167–172

Tanaka K, Gotoh F, Muramatsu F, Fukuchi Y, Okayasu H, Suzuki N, Kobari M (1982) Effect of nimodipine, a calcium antagonist, on cerebral vasospasm after subarachnoid hemorrhage in cats. Arzneim Forsch 32: 1529–1534

Van der Hoek JY, Feinstein MB (1978) Local anesthetics, chlorpromazine and propranolol inhibit activation of phospholipase A_2 in human platelets. Mol Pharm 16: 171–180

Wahl M, Kuschinsky W, Bosse O, Neiss H (1974) Micropuncture evaluation of beta-receptors in pial arteries of cats. Pfluegers Arch 348: 293–303

Walter P, Neil-Dwyer G, Cruickshank JM (1982) Beneficial effects of adrenergic blockade in patients with subarachnoid hemorrhage. Br Med J 284: 1661–1664

Weksler BB, Gillick M, Pink J (1977) Effects of propranolol on platelet function. Blood 49: 185–196

Zahniser NR, Minneman KP, Molinoff PB (1979) Persistence of beta-adrenergic receptors in rat striatum following kaniac acid administration. Brain Res 178: 589–595

Section B

CARDIOVASCULAR NEUROBIOLOGY

Chapter 9

Role of the Central Nervous System in Cardiovascular Regulation

K. L. Barnes and C. M. Ferrario

Introduction

Although the participation of the central nervous system (CNS) in the regulation of cardiovascular function has been known for more than a century, the pervasive significance of neural mechanisms has only been recognized quite recently. In addition to the well-established role of the CNS in regulating the balance of sympathetic and parasympathetic outflow and controlling cardiovascular reflexes, it is now becoming clear that endocrine mechanisms are integrated with neural factors into a complex system of neuroendocrine control of cardiovascular regulation. These findings are being combined with pharmacological, molecular biological, and clinical areas of investigation into an emergent discipline of "cardiovascular neurobiology." This chapter focuses selectively upon evidence for the importance of medullary pathways in CNS cardiovascular regulation, particularly the afferent functions of the area postrema and nucleus tractus solitarii, the efferent mechanisms of the ventrolateral medulla, and the significance of these regions for neuroendocrine integration.

Cardiovascular Functions of the Autonomic Nervous System

It is well accepted that both central nervous system and peripheral components of the autonomic nervous system play important roles in the control of arterial blood pressure and heart rate by means of reciprocally balanced activities of sympathetic and parasympathetic innervation of blood vessels and the heart. However, evidence is also growing rapidly for the involvement of autonomic pathways in the control of vasoactive hormone release and the integration of cardiovascular functions with behavior (Ferrario 1985; Abboud 1982; Korner 1979).

The structures innervated by the peripheral autonomic nervous system are connected to the CNS by both afferent and efferent pathways, which provide functionally integrated neural control of the cardiovascular system (Hilton 1975). The cardiovascular afferent pathways transmit information to the CNS from arterial and cardiopulmonary baroreceptors and chemoreceptors through the IX and X cranial nerves. Sympathetic afferents from the heart and aorta enter the CNS via the spinal afferent pathways. These inputs are integrated within the CNS with somatic, visceral, and other sensory afferents which also contribute to cardiovascular regulation (Korner 1979). Efferent pathways include hypothalamic, medullary, and spinal centers with cardiovascular actions which regulate sympathetic and parasympathetic effector pathways. Autonomic control of vasomotor tone appears to be mediated predominantly by sympathetic efferents, in contrast to cardiac rate and output, which are regulated according to the balance between parasympathetic and sympathetic influences (Korner 1979). However, the sympathetic adrenergic vasoconstrictor mechanisms are modulated by neurogenic vasodilator mechanisms involving sympathetic cholinergic, histaminergic, dopaminergic, and beta-adrenergic pathways (Abboud 1982; Folkow 1982).

The autonomic nervous system also affects cardiovascular function through influences on electrolyte and fluid balance and hormonal mechanisms. CNS and peripheral autonomic pathways to the kidney influence sodium excretion (Edwards 1982) and renin release (Brosnihan 1984; Ganong 1982). Although some of the interactions between the autonomic nervous system and the release of pituitary vasopressin have been known for a long time (Share 1974), recent evidence has uncovered complex neurohormonal interactions which suggest new importance for this hormone in cardiovascular regulation (Ferrario 1985). The mechanisms by which the CNS can activate sympathetic outflow to increase adrenal medullary secretion of catecholamines (Lewis 1975) have now been shown by Brosnihan and Ferrario (1981) to include an action of angiotensin II (Ang II) mediated by the area postrema, a circumventricular organ in the IV ventricle.

Brain Stem Mechanisms of Cardiovascular Regulation

The concept of centers within the mammalian brain stem possessing counterbalancing pressor and depressor mechanisms dates back more than 100 years to the work of Dittmar (1870) and Owsjannikow (1871). Although Ranson and Billingsley (1916) mapped central autonomic function early in the present century, it was the investigations by Alexander (1945) and Bard (1960) that established the concept of a medullary "vasomotor center" which regulates arterial pressure, cardiac output, and the distribution of blood flow to different organs. It is now well accepted that the medullary vasomotor neurons operate in conjunction with more rostral structures to coordinate endocrine and autonomic neural outflow (Brooks 1979). In addition, the medullary center functions relatively autonomously to mediate visceral and somatic reflexes (Korner 1979).

In recent years two adjacent structures in the dorsal medulla have been shown by us and others to have important counterbalancing influences on cardiovascular regulation—the area postrema (AP) pressor and nucleus tractus solitarii (nTS) depressor mechanisms. Studies conducted in this laboratory (Ferrario 1979; Ferrario 1981) have shown in the dog that stimulation and ablation of these structures produce diametrically opposite cardiovascular effects; moreover, chronic removal of either structure produces lasting alterations in cardiovascular control mechanisms. The nTS has long been known to contain the first central synapse of the high-pressure baroreceptor afferents from the carotid sinus and aortic arch, and to receive the primary projections of chemoreceptor and respiratory afferents. Although it appears that most baroreceptor afferents are myelinated A fibers, nonmyelinated C fiber baroreceptors have also been identified in several species (Ferrario 1983). While the role of baroreceptor C fibers in tonic blood pressure regulation is somewhat controversial, they may become significant in hypertension, since their threshold appears to be higher than that of A fibers (Thoren 1980).

The recent development of new neuroanatomical methods for visualizing neuronal pathways within the brain utilizing axonal transport of horseradish peroxidase or lectins has now provided much more precise information about the trajectories and terminations of the baroreceptor afferents in a number of species. Kalia and Welles (1980) showed in the cat that the aortic nerve afferents terminate primarily in the dorsolateral and medial subnuclei of the nTS, and extend over 6 mm in the rostrocaudal dimension. They also identified a previously unknown heavy projection of aortic afferents to the area postrema, and confirmed that the aortic nerve in cat is purely afferent. Essentially the same findings were reported by Ciriello et al. (1981). A study in the rabbit (Wallach 1980) showed a sparse but similar projection of aortic afferents into the dorsal and medial nTS, although no labeling was seen in the AP. In the dog Chernicky et al. (1984) showed that the vagal afferents, which include the aortic baroreceptors, project heavily into the dorsal and medial nTS over a distance of 8 mm, and innervate the AP as well. In all species contralateral as well as ipsilateral projections were found.

Both Berger (1979) and Panneton and Loewy (1980) showed that the primary projections of the carotid sinus nerve in the cat were to the dorsal, dorsolateral, and commissural portions of the nTS, although the latter study also found projections into the AP. A subsequent investigation by Davies and Kalia (1981) also found carotid sinus afferents projecting to the ventrolateral medulla in the region of the nucleus ambiguus. Ciriello et al. (1981) reported carotid sinus afferent projections to ventrolateral external cuneate and the dorsolateral spinal trigeminal tract. In the dog Chernicky et al. (1983) found a pattern of carotid sinus nerve projections into the nTS and AP similar to that reported by Davies and Kalia (1981) in the cat. However, in contrast to the cat, where the afferents begin to distribute into the nTS as soon as they reach the solitary tract (Davies 1981), the carotid sinus afferents in the dog enter in the IX root 8–9 mm anterior to the obex, course dorsomedially to the solitary tract, and turn caudally. They remain in the tract, joined at 7 mm anterior by the vagal afferents, until about 5 mm anterior to the obex, before distributing into the adjacent structures. Thus the canine baroreceptor afferents are bundled together in the solitary tract for about 2 mm before beginning to send terminations into the nTS. This configuration has allowed Barnes et al. (1984) to interrupt the baroreceptor afferents with bilateral rostral solitary tract lesions, producing acute neurogenic hypertension in the dog. It appears that transection of the rostral solitary tracts in the dog produces a more complete and selective interruption of the baroreflex afferent pathway than can be accomplished with electrolytic destruction of the nTS itself, employed in previous studies in dog (Laubie 1979; Ferrario 1981), cat (Nathan 1977), and rat (Doba 1973).

In addition to receiving baroreceptor afferent projections, the area postrema differs strikingly from the adjacent nTS in its features as a circumventricular organ, with fenestrated capillaries which provide a leaky blood-brain barrier. Evidence for a chemosensory function of the AP dates back to 1950, when Borison and Brizzee (1951) found that it contained the receptive site for the emetic reflex. The possibility that the AP participates in cardiovascular regulation was uncovered by hypertension physiologists attempting to determine whether blood-borne Ang II acts within the CNS to facilitate sympathetic vasoconstrictor outflow (Ferrario 1972). In the late 1960s both Ferrario et al. (1970) and Joy and Lowe (1970), working independently, found that small doses of Ang II, which did not increase arterial pressure if given intravenously, elevated blood pressure by an action mediated within the brain stem when infused into the vertebral arteries of the dog. This central pressor effect of Ang II was localized to the AP because either ablation or local cooling of this structure abolished the rise in blood pressure (Ferrario 1972).

More recently, Barnes et al. (1979) showed that the pressor effects of intravertebral Ang II in the dog could be mimicked by electrical stimulation of the AP, which activated sympathetic vasoconstrictor pathways in much the same way as intravertebral Ang II (Barnes 1981; Barnes 1984b). Additional studies (Barnes 1984a) demonstrated that the AP pressor mechanism does not require an intact baroreceptor pathway, but appears to have an inhibitory influence upon the central baroreflex mechanism. Furthermore, persistence of the AP pressor response following midcollicular transection but elimination of pressor effects after destruction of AP neurons with kainic acid suggests that the AP pressor mechanism in the dog is mediated by a medullary pathway activated by neurons in the AP.

Because the studies just described were performed in anesthetized animals, experiments in conscious dogs were undertaken to determine whether the Ang II-sensitive AP is involved in the long-term regulation of blood pressure in both normal and hypertensive states. Chronic inactivation of the AP in normal animals produced modest hypotension accompanied by a significant decrease in the variability of arterial pressure, heart rate, and cardiac output (Ferrario 1979). These effects persisted during 6 weeks of observation, and were diametrically opposite to the hypertension and increased hemodynamic lability seen by Ferrario et al. (1981) in dogs after chronic destruction of the baroreceptor relay in the adjacent nTS. Furthermore, the pressor effects of Ang II given intravenously were markedly reduced following AP removal, suggesting a role for the AP in the cardiovascular effects of systemic Ang II (Ferrario 1979). Because the vasoconstrictor effects of norepinephrine were not reduced after AP lesions, the suppressed responsiveness to i.v. Ang II could not be explained by increased baroreceptor activity.

The logical extension of these studies was to determine whether the AP might contribute to the rise in blood pressure in dogs during the development of experimental renal hypertension associated with elevated blood levels of endogenous Ang II. One kidney, one clip renal hypertension has now been produced in dogs 2 weeks following either coagulation of the AP or sham AP lesion (Ferrario 1983). Most interestingly, the hypertension produced by constriction of the remaining renal artery was considerably attenuated in the AP-lesioned animals compared with the sham AP group, although plasma renin activity was elevated similarly in both groups of dogs. Therefore, elimination of the Ang II-sensitive AP in the dog may retard, or even permanently alter, the development of this form of renal hypertension. These findings suggest that the area postrema functions as a neuroendocrine transducer, sensing a hormonal signal transmitted from the kidney via the blood, resulting in altered cardiovascular function in both normal and pathological states (Ferrario 1972). Thus it appears that in the dog the AP pressor mechanism, normally counterbalanced by the baroreflex depressor functions in the adjacent nTS, provides an important component of the CNS control of the cardiovascular system.

Although these observations appear to hold true for a number of species including man, the same is not the case for the rat (Brody 1980). In the rat the CNS sites which mediate the central actions of Ang II appear to reside in the anterior third ventricle (AV3V region), and probably include the organum vasculosum of the lamina terminalis (OVLT) and subfornical organ (SFO). Destruction of these rostral third ventricular structures, but not of the AP, has been shown to prevent the development of renal hypertension in the rat (Brody 1980). On the other hand, rostral brain stem structures in the dog appear to mediate the pressor and dipsogenic actions of Ang II given into a lateral cerebral ventricle, because midcollicular transection (Gildenberg 1973) or electrolytic destruction of the anterior third ventricle (Marson 1984) abolish these effects. Hence it appears that in the dog, but not the rat, two different brain regions are responsible for the cardiovascular and endocrine actions of Ang II: the OVLT and/or SFO mediate the effects upon drinking, electrolytes, the release of vasopressin, and the AP mediates the cardiovascular actions of the blood-borne peptide.

Because neuroanatomical studies have shown that AP neurons are small and appear to have relatively short projections (Chernicky 1980), it is likely that they act on the medullary vasomotor neurons to produce their sympathoexcitatory effects rather than projecting directly to the spinal sympathetic preganglionic cells. Evidence from a number of species now suggests that the elusive "vasomotor center" may reside in the rostral ventrolateral medulla (RVLM). Both electrical and glutamate stimulation in rat (Ross 1983) and rabbit (Goodchild 1984) produce large increases in arterial pressure, while bilateral lesions or cooling reduce pressure to levels comparable to spinal transection (Reis 1984). Many neurons in this region have been shown to project directly to the intermediolateral cell column of the thoracic spinal cord, which contains the preganglionic sympathetic cell bodies (Amendt 1979). Using single neuron recording techniques, Brown and Guyenet (1984) in rat and Caverson et al. (1984) in cat have identified neurons in RVLM which both respond to cardiovascular input (blood pressure changes, cardiac cycle, baroreceptors) and project to the intermediolateral thoracic spinal cord. Reis and colleagues (1984) have now shown that in the rat the majority of neurons in the RVLM which project to the spinal cord contain PNMT, suggesting that the medullary vasomotor neurons may be adrenergic (C1 adrenergic cell group). They have also shown heavy PNMT-labeled fiber innervation of spinal intermediolateral neurons which project to the adrenal medulla. Anatomical demonstration of projections from the nTS to C1 neurons in the RVLM has now been given a functional relationship to the baroreflex pathway, because either electrolytic lesions or destruction of the neurons of the C1 region with the excitotoxin kainic acid abolishes the vasodepressor component of the baroreflex (Granata 1983).

On the other hand, not everyone agrees that the RVLM vasomotor neurons are necessarily adrenergic. Howe et al. (1983) have proposed that serotonergic neurons projecting to the spinal intermediolateral cell column have a vasomotor function, since destruction of these cells with the toxin 5,7-dihydroxytryptamine (5,7-DHT) lowered resting blood pressure and attenuated the pressor effects of stimulating the region. There is now considerable evidence which supports a prominent role for substance P in ventral medullary vasomotor neurons. Helke et al. (1982) showed that substance P immunoreactive neurons project to the intermediolateral cell column, where Charlton and Helke (1985) have found a high concentration of substance P binding sites, shown by Takano and Loewy (1985) to be associated with sympathetic preganglionic neurons. Loewy and Sawyer (1982) demonstrated that intraspinal administration of a substance P antagonist lowered resting blood pressure to spinal transection levels and blocked the pressor response produced by kainic acid applied to the surface of the RVLM. They also showed that the kainic acid pressor effects were not abolished by prior destruction of serotonergic neurons with 5,7-DHT. Recently Keeler and Helke (1985) have also shown that the pressor effects of bicuculline applied to the ventral medullary surface are blocked by intrathecal substance P antagonists, but not by pretreatment with a serotonin neurotoxin. Direct iontophoresis of substance P has also been shown to excite identified spinal sympathetic preganglionic neurons (Backman 1984; Gilbey 1983). An intriguing possibility for answering the question of whether the medullary vasomotor neurons are adrenergic or substance P-containing has been suggested recently by Lorenz et al. (1985), who report colocalization of these two substances in 50%–75% of ventrolateral medullary neurons which project to the thoracic spinal cord. However, it does seem clear that the noradrenergic A1 neurons of the ventral medulla are not candidates for the vasomotor neurons, because their destruction produces severe hypertension with massive increases in the plasma levels of epinephrine and vasopressin, while electrical or glutamate stimulation of these cells elicits a fall in blood pressure (West 1984). Thus the A1 noradrenergic neurons appear to exert a tonic inhibitory influence upon sympathetic vasomotor outflow and pituitary release of vasopressin.

Autonomic Interactions with Neuroendocrine Mechanisms

It is becoming increasingly evident that attempts to separate endocrine from neural factors in cardiovascular regulation may be forcing an artificial division upon an integrated neuroendocrine system with important effects upon cardiovascular function (Ferrario 1985). Hormones such as Ang II and vasopressin clearly exert important cardiovascular effects by means of actions within the CNS as well as directly upon vascular tissues. Adrenal steroids have been shown to act both presynaptically and postsynaptically to influence neurotransmitter uptake and release, and even alter the synthesis of neuronal proteins (McEwen 1979). The distinction between peripheral peptide hormones and brain neuropeptides has now become all but meaningless, since almost all of the classical peptide hormones have been localized within the brain (Iversen 1983). It appears that brain peptides exert their effects predominantly via mechanisms of neuromodulation rather than synaptic neurotransmission (Scharrer 1977), and that CNS peptidergic neurons may be quite similar to peripheral glandular hormone-producing cells. On the other hand, the brain monoamines are thought to function primarily by means of classical neurotransmission (Moore 1978, 1979).

Evidence for the importance of brain monoamines, especially the catecholamines, in CNS cardiovascular regulation has been accumulating for more than 20 years. Beginning with the work of Dahlstrom and Fuxe (1964, 1965), anatomical studies have localized noradrenergic, adrenergic, and serotonergic cell bodies in many regions of the brain stem with well-established cardiovascular importance. In the ventrolateral medulla these include the A1 and A5 noradrenergic, C1 adrenergic, and B1 and B3 serotonergic cell groups. Neurons in the A1 group provide the major noradrenergic innvervation of hypothalamus, including vasopressinergic cells in paraventricular and supraoptic nuclei (Sawchenko 1981). Cells in the A2 region of the dorsal medulla have also been shown to project to these structures. Whether the major source of noradrenergic innervation of the spinal cord intermediolateral cell column is A5 or A1 may differ between rat (Loewy 1979) and cat (Fleetwood-Walker 1981), but the adrenergic projections appear to originate in C1 (Ross 1981). Loewy and McKellar (1981) have also demonstrated projections of B1 and B3 serotonergic neurons to thoracic intermediolateral cells.

Physiological studies are providing functional cardiovascular relevance for these catecholaminergic pathways. Microinjection of norepinephrine or epinephrine into the nTS decreases blood pressure and heart rate (DeJong 1976), while injections of serotonin elicit dose-dependent increases in pressure (Coote 1981). Destruction of the A1 noradrenergic region in the rabbit produces marked hypertension and bradycardia (Blessing 1981), in contrast to the collapse of arterial pressure to spinal transection levels which follows inactivation of C1 neurons (Reis 1984). On the other hand, either electrolytic or neurochemical destruction of A2 cells in rat produced only increased lability of blood pressure without affecting the mean level (Reis 1979). With respect to participation of catecholamines in models of hypertension, Gordon et al. (1979) showed that widespread destruction of CNS noradrenergic neurons by intraventricular 6-hydroxydopamine prevented the development of one-kidney, one-clip renal hypertension in rats. The same treatment blocked deoxycorticosterone-salt and genetic hypertension in other studies (Reid 1975).

In considering the peptide hormones, the contribution of the peripheral renin-angiotensin system to the regulation of arterial pressure and the control of extracellular fluid volume is clearly established (Ferrario 1985). As discussed above, circulating Ang II has also been shown to act via circumventricular organs to activate sympathetic vasomotor outflow. Other CNS effects of this peptide include stimulation of thirst, natriuresis, and the release of pituitary hormones including vasopressin and ACTH (Reid 1983), probably mediated through the circumventricular structures of the anterior third ventricle (OVLT, SFO).

Evidence is also accumulating rapidly to support the formation of Ang II within the CNS by a brain renin-angiotensin system. The presence of immunoreactive Ang II in CSF (Finkielman 1972) and brain (Fischer-Ferraro 1971) was reported more than 10 years ago. In recent years some studies have indicated that the chemical composition of brain angiotensin may differ from the plasma form (Bumpus 1984). The presence of the precursor protein, angiotensinogen, in brain and CSF is also well established, but its source(s) remains unclear. Although Campbell et al. (1984) have demonstrated the presence of the messenger RNA for angiotensinogen in rat brain, it has not been determined whether the major portion of brain angiotensinogen is produced within the CNS or derived from the periphery. Itoh et al. (1980) showed that angiotensinogen from human CSF was immunologically different from the plasma material, providing additional support for the possibility of structural differences between the brain and peripheral forms of angiotensinogen. Renin-like activity which cannot be attributed to acid proteases such as cathepsin D has been demonstrated in brain tissue by Hirose et al. (1978) and Osman et al. (1979). A widespread distribution of renin-like immunoreactivity in rat brain has also been found by Slater (1981). Finally, specific, high-affinity Ang II binding sites suggestive of receptors have been localized by in vitro autoradiography in OVLT, SFO, nTS, AP, and the dorsal motor nucleus of the vagus (dmnX), regions which also contain cells and fibers immunoreactive for Ang II (Lind 1985), in both rat (Mendelsohn 1984) and dog (Speth 1985). These studies together suggest that Ang II may be produced within the CNS by means of a renin-angiotensin system distinct from that in the periphery. Furthermore, the centrally generated Ang II may act upon different brain structures, either alone or in association with blood-borne Ang II, to modulate the actions of CNS pathways upon blood pressure, thirst, electrolyte balance, and fluid volume. Recent studies by Diz et al. (1984) have revealed that very small amounts of Ang II (8–800 fmol) microinjected into the dmnX of the rat produce hypotension and bradycardia. In the dog, microinjection of Ang II into the AP and medial nTS evoked increases in blood pressure and heart rate (Averill, Diz, Barnes, and Ferrario, unpublished work). These observations provide a functional correlate for the Ang II binding sites found in these same areas.

Although the antidiuretic hormone vasopressin (AVP) was previously considered not to play a role in cardiovascular regulation under physiological conditions, recent evidence suggests that this may not be the case. A recent review by Doris (1984) summarizes the interactions between AVP and CNS mechanisms of cardiovascular regulation. AVP is clearly present both as a circulating peptide hormone and as a brain neuropeptide. Vasopressin appears to be produced by neuronal cell bodies in the hypothalamus, primarily within the paraventricular (PVN) and supraoptic (SON) nuclei (Scharrer 1954). Recent studies combining immunocytochemical identification of vasopressin neurons with retrograde tracer demonstration of their projections (Sawchenko 1983; Sofroniew 1983) have revealed that magnocellular neurosecretory cells in the PVN and SON provide vasopressinergic projections to the median eminence and the neurohypophysis capillary beds, where the peptide is released into the circulation. However, the more recently identified AVP-containing pathways within the brain appear to arise from smaller neurons, principally located in the paraventricular and suprachiasmatic nuclei (Sofroniew 1983). With respect to CNS cardiovascular regulation, vasopressinergic innervation of neurons in the nTS and dorsal motor nucleus of the vagus suggests that this peptide may play a role in modulating the baroreflex and vagal pathways. As described above for Ang II, a high density of specific binding sites for AVP has also been localized with the nTS (Biegon 1984).

It is well established that release of vasopressin from the pituitary can be altered by both osmotic and baroreceptor stimuli. Almost 30 years ago Jewell and Verney (1957) proposed that the osmotic effects are mediated centrally by osmoreceptive cells located in the hypothalamus. Recent studies by Sladek and colleagues employing a hypothalamo-neurohypophyseal explant in vitro support this localization, since hyperosmotic media increase secretion of AVP by the tissue (Sladek 1977), whereas lesions of the anterior third ventricle abolish AVP release from the explants (Sladek 1983). Stimulation of cardiopulmonary (atrial) or sinoaortic baroreceptors has been shown to inhibit vasopressin release, leading to diuresis (Share 1976).

It now appears that the reason that large amounts of AVP are required to elicit pressor effects in intact animals is the buffering effect of the baroreceptors. This possibility was uncovered by Rocha e Silva and Rosenberg (1969) in anesthetized dogs and by Cowley et al. (1974) in conscious baroreceptor denervated dogs, who found that baroreflex interruption led to specific enhancement of the pressor effects of AVP compared with other pressor agents. Recent work by Liard et al. (1981) in conscious dogs and Undesser et al. (1985) in conscious rabbits has now shown that intravertebral administration of AVP elicits reduced pressor effects with enhanced braycardia compared with the i.v. route, whereas chronic AP removal prevents the AVP-induced enhancement of the baroreflex-mediated inhibition of renal sympathetic nerve activity. In addition, projections of hypothalamic vasopressinergic neurons to the vicinity of the primary baroreflex synapse in the nTS, in combination with a high density of putative AVP receptors, provide the anatomical substrate for an interaction between endogenous brain AVP and the circulating peptide in the modulation of cardiovascular regulation at the level of the dorsomedial medulla. On the other hand, Barnes et al. (1984) have now shown that central baroreceptor deafferentation at the level of the rostral solitary tract in dogs produces an acute hypertension which is dependent upon increased release of pituitary vasopressin, since pressure reverts to the same level as sham-lesioned animals after i.v. administration of an antagonist of the vascular effects of AVP. The possibility of an interaction between AVP and Ang II at the level of the medulla has also been suggested by experiments from Michelini et al. (1984), demonstrating that the pressor effects of intravertebral Ang II mediated by the area postrema are abolished by prior administration of an antagonist of the vascular actions of vasopressin directly into the cisterna magna. It appears that the dorsomedial medulla may have an important integrative function, allowing circulating hormones to interact with both CNS cardiovascular pathways and peripheral baroreceptor and cardiopulmonary inputs to modulate the efferent CNS systems involved in cardiovascular regulation. Our concept of how this system may be organized is diagrammed in Fig 9.1. The dorsomedial medulla contains the counterbalanced AP Ang II-sensitive pressor and nTS baroreflex depressor mechanisms. Anatomical studies of the projections of these neuronal systems suggest that they may exert their effects upon sympathetic outflow via the vasomotor neurons of the rostral ventrolateral medulla (VLM), which may be adrenergic. It now appears that Ang II in very small amounts can produce

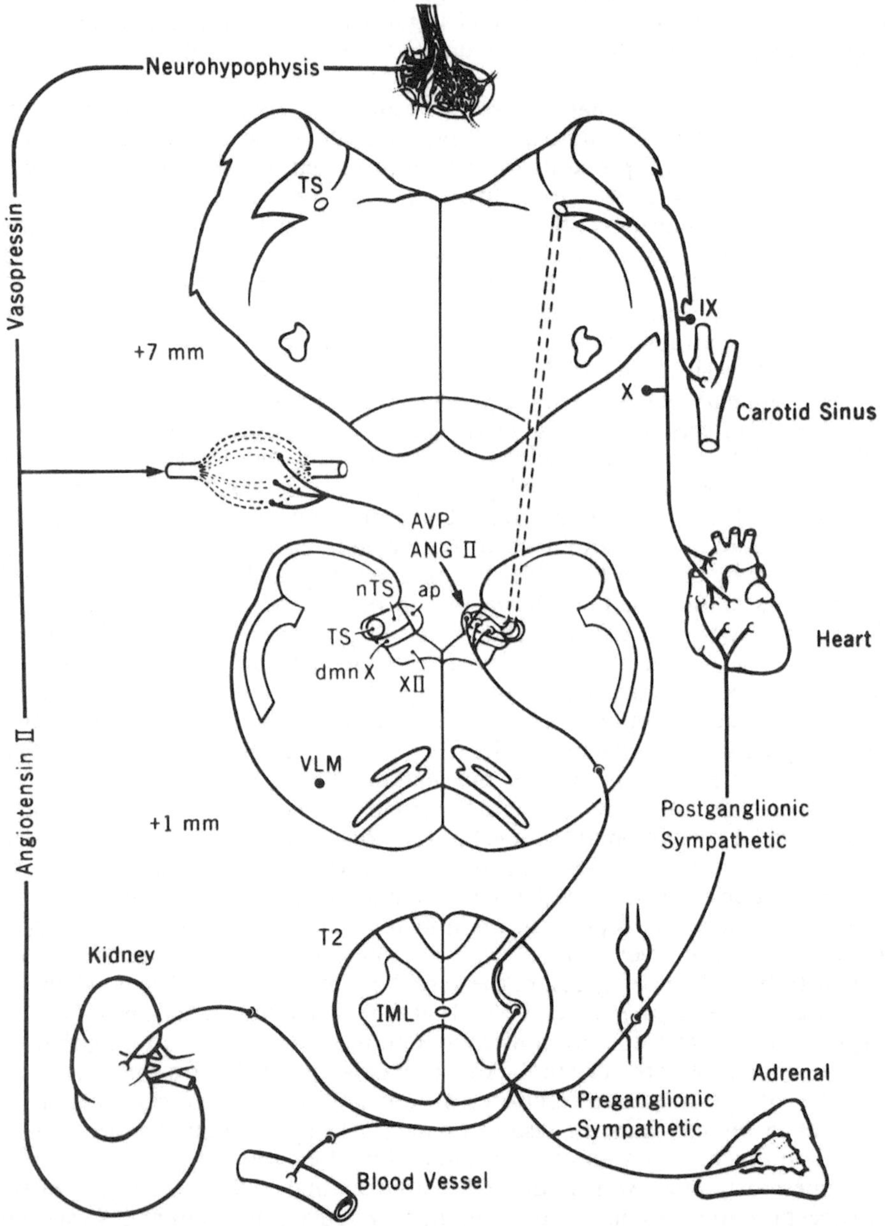

Fig. 9.1. Proposed schematic of the area postrema pressor pathway and its relationship to neurohormonal stimuli (*ANG II, AVP*) and the baroreceptor afferents, and to the effector pathways comprising the medullary vasomotor centers and the pre- and postganglionic sympathetic neural innervation. Medullary section levels are indicated by distance in millimeters anterior to the obex. *ap*, area postrema; *ANG II*, angiotensin II; *AVP*, arginine vasopressin; *dmnX*, dorsal motor nucleus of the vagus; *IML*, intermediolateral cell column; *nTS*, nucleus tractus solitarii; *TS*, tractus solitarius; *T2*, second thoracic spinal segment; *VLM*, ventrolateral medulla; *IX*, glossopharyngeal nerve; *X*, vagus nerve; *XII*, hypoglossal nucleus.

cardiovascular effects when injected into the dmnX, as well as when delivered to the circulation supplying the AP. Both Ang II and vasopressin have been shown immunocytochemically to be contained in medullary neural systems, thus exhibiting both hormonal and neuropeptide characteristics. Thus the dorsomedial medulla may be uniquely configured to integrate hormonal signals with neural inputs from peripheral cardiovascular receptors and rostral CNS structures to modulate CNS effector mechanisms regulating cardiovascular function.

References

Abboud FM (1982) The sympathetic system in hypertension. Hypertension 4 [Suppl II]: II-208–II-225

Alexander RS (1945) The effects of blood flow and anoxia on spinal cardiovascular centers. Am J Physiol 143: 698–708

Amendt J, Czachurski J, Dembowski K, Seller H (1979) Bulbospinal projections to the intermediolateral cell column: a neuroanatomical study. J Auton Nerv Syst 1: 103–117

Backman SB, Henry JL (1984) Effects of substance P and thyrotropin-releasing hormone on sympathetic preganglionic neurones in the upper thoracic intermediolateral nucleus of the cat. Can J Physiol Pharmacol 62: 248–251

Bard P (1960) Anatomical organization of the central nervous system in relation to control of the heart and blood vessels. Physiol Rev 40 [Suppl 4]: 3–26

Barnes KL, Averill DB, Ferrario DM (1984) Contribution of vasopressin to hypertension after solitary tract lesioning in the dog. J Hypertension 2 [Suppl 3]: 33–36

Barnes KL, Ferrario CM (1981) Anatomical and physiological characterization of the sympathofacilitative area postrema pathways in the dog. In: Buckley JP, Ferrario CM (eds) Central nervous system mechanisms in hypertension. Raven, New York, pp 25–36

Barnes KL, Ferrario CM (1984) Localization within the dog's brain stem of the area postrema pressor pathway. Hypertension 6: 482–488

Barnes KL, Ferrario CM, Chernicky CL, Brosnihan KB (1984) Participation of the area postrema in cardiovascular control in the dog. Fed Proc 43: 2959–2962

Barnes KL, Ferrario CM, Conomy JP (1979) Comparison of the hemodynamic changes produced by electrical stimulation of the area postrema and NTS in the dog. Circ Res 45: 136–143

Berger AJ (1979) Distribution of carotid sinus nerve afferent fibers to solitary tract nuclei of the cat using transganglionic transport of horseradish peroxidase. Neurosci Lett 14: 153–158

Biegon A, Terlou M, Voorhuis TD, deKloet ER (1984) Arginine-vasopressin binding sites in rat brain: a quantitative autoradiographic study. Neurosci Lett 44: 229–234

Blessing WW, West MJ, Chalmers J (1981) Hypertension, bradycardia and pulmonary edema in the conscious rabbit after brain stem lesions coinciding with the A1 group of catecholamine neurons. Circ Res 49: 949–958

Borison HL, Brizzee KR (1951) Morphology of emetic chemoreceptor trigger zone in cat medulla oblongata. Proc Soc Exp Biol Med 77: 38–42

Brody MJ, Johnson AK (1980) Role of the anteroventral third ventricle region in fluid and electrolyte balance, arterial pressure regulation and hypertension. In: Martini L, Ganong WF (eds) Frontiers in neuroendocrinology. Raven, New York, pp 249–292

Brooks C Mc, Koizumi K, Sato A (eds) (1979) Integrative functions of the autonomic nervous system. Elsevier, New York

Brosnihan KB, Ferrario CM (1982) Central mediation of adrenal catecholamine release by angiotensin II in normal and sodium depleted dog. Proc 64th annual meeting of the Endocrine Society, p 11

Brosnihan KB, Ferrario CM (1984) Central regulation of renin release. In: Guthrie GP Jr, Kotchen TA (eds) Hypertension and the brain. Futura, Mt. Kisco, NY, pp 83–112

Brown DL, Guyenet PG (1984) Cardiovascular neurons of brain stem with projections to spinal cord. Am J Physiol 247: R1009–R1016

Bumpus FM, Ferrario CM (1984) Extrarenal renin angiotensin system: comments on its occurrence and cardiovascular role. In: Villarreal H, Sambhi M (eds) Topics in pathophysiology of hypertension. Martinus Nijhoff, Boston, pp 407–416
Campbell DJ, Beuhnik J, Menard J, Corvol P (1984) Identity of angiotensinogen precursors of rat brain and liver. Nature 308: 206–208
Caverson MM, Ciriello J, Calaresu FR (1984) Chemoreceptor and baroreceptor inputs to ventrolateral medullary neurons. Am J Physiol 247: R872–R879
Charlton CG, Helke CJ (1985) Autoradiographic localization and characterization of spinal cord substance P binding sites: high densities in sensory, autonomic, phrenic, and Onuf's motor nuclei. J Neurosci 5: 1653–1661
Chernicky CL, Barnes KL, Conomy JP, Ferrario CM (1980) A morphological characterization of the canine area postrema. Neurosci Lett 20: 37–43
Chernicky CL, Barnes KL, Ferrario CM (1983) Brain stem distribution of the carotid sinus nerve in the dog. Neurosci Abstr 9: 1158
Chernicky CL, Barnes KL, Ferrario CM, Conomy JP (1984) Afferent projections of the cervical vagus and nodose ganglion in the dog. Brain Res Bull 13: 401–411
Ciriello J, Hrycyshyn AW, Calaresu FR (1981) Horseradish peroxidase study of brain stem projections of carotid sinus and aortic depressor nerves in the cat. J Auton Nerv Syst 4: 43–61
Coote JH, Macleod VN, Fleetwood-Walker S, Gilbey MP (1981) The response of individual sympathetic preganglionic neurones to microelectrophoretically applied endogenous monoamine. Brain Res 215: 135–145
Cowley AW Jr, Monos E, Guyton AC (1974) Interaction of vasopressin and the baroreceptor reflex system in the regulation of arterial blood pressure in the dog. Circ Res 34: 505–514
Dahlstrom A, Fuxe K (1964) Evidence for the existence of monoamine containing neurons in the central nervous system. I. Demonstration of monoamines in the cell bodies of brain stem neurons. Acta Physiol Scand 62 [Suppl 232]: 1–55
Dahlstrom A, Fuxe K (1965) Evidence for the existence of monoamine-containing neurons in the central nervous system. II. Experimentally induced changes in the intraneuronal amine levels of bulbospinal neuron system. Acta Physiol Scand 64 [Suppl 247]: 5–36
Davies R, Kalia M (1981) Carotid sinus nerve projections to the brain stem in the cat. Brain Res Bull 6: 531–544
DeJong W, Nijkamp FP (1976) Centrally induced hypotension and bradycardia after administration of α-methylnoradrenaline into the area of the nucleus tractus solitarii of the rat. Br J Pharmacol 58: 593–598
Dittmar C (1870) Ein neuer Beweis fur die Reizbarkeit der centripetalen Fasern des Ruckenmarks. Ber Sachs Ges (Akad) Wiss 22: 18–48
Diz DI, Barnes KL, Ferrario CM (1984) Hypotensive actions of angiotensin II microinjected into the dorsal motor nucleus of the vagus. J Hypertension 2 [Suppl 3]: 53–56
Doba N, Reis DJ (1973) Acute fulminating neurogenic hypertension produced by brainstem lesions in the rat. Circ Res 32: 584–593
Doris PA (1984) Central cardiovascular regulation and the role of vasopressin: a review. Clin Exp Hypertens—Theory and Practice A6: 2197–2217
Edwards CRW, Al-Dujaili EAS, Boscaro M, Gow I, Williams BC (1982) Peptidergic and monoaminergic regulation of aldosterone secretion. In: Mantero F, Biglieri EG, Edwards CRW (eds) Endocrinology of hypertension. Academic, London, pp 11–18
Ferrario CM (1983) Central nervous system mechanisms of blood pressure control in normotensive and hypertensive states. Chest 83S: 331S–335S
Ferrario CM, Barnes KL, Szilagyi JE, Brosnihan KB (1979) Physiological and pharmacological characterization of the area psotrema pressor pathways in the normal dog. Hypertension 1: 235–245
Ferrario CM, Barnes KL, Bohonek S (1981) Neurogenic hypertension produced by lesions of the nucleus tractus solitarii alone or with sinoaortic denervation in the dog. Hypertension 3 [Suppl II]: II–112–II–118
Ferrario CM, Dickinson CJ, McCubbin JW (1970) Central vasomotor stimulation by angiotensin. Clin Sci 39: 239–245
Ferrario CM, Gildenberg PL, McCubbin JW (1972) Cardiovascular effects of angiotensin mediated by the central nervous system. Circ Res 30: 257–262
Ferrario CM, Schiavone MT, Barnes KL, Brosnihan KB, Speth RC (1985) Role of central mechanisms in the development of endocrine hypertension. In: Edwards CRW, Carey RM (eds) Essential hypertension as an endocrine disease. Butterworths, London, pp 1–39
Ferrario CM, Takishita S (1981) Baroreceptor reflexes and hypertension. In: Kuchel O, Hamet P,

Cantin M (eds) Hypertension: physiopathology and treatment. McGraw-Hill, New York, pp 161–170
Finkelman S, Goldstein DJ, Fischer-Ferraro C, Diaz A, Nahmod VE (1972) In vitro production of angiotensin and renin release by isolated glomeruli. Medicina 32 [Suppl 1]: 37–39
Fischer-Ferraro C, Nahmod VE, Goldstein DJ, Finkielman S (1971) Angiotensin and renin in rat and dog brain. J Exp Med 133: 353–361
Fleetwood-Walker SM, Coote JH (1981) The contribution of brain stem catecholamine cell groups to the innervation of the sympathetic lateral cell column. Brain Res 205: 141–155
Folkow B (1962) Physiological aspects of primary hypertension. Physiol Rev 62:347–504
Ganong WF, Barbier C (1982) Neuroendocrine components in the regulation of renin secretion. In: Ganong WF, Martini L (eds) Frontiers in neuroendocrinology. Raven, New York, pp 231–262
Gilbey MP, McKenna K, Schramm L (1983) Effects of substance P on sympathetic preganglionic neurons. Neurosci Lett 41: 157–159
Gildenberg PL, Ferrario CM, McCubbin JW (1973) Two sites of cardiovascular action of angiotensin II in the brain of the dog. Clin Sci 44: 417–420
Goodchild AK, Moon EA, Dampney RAL, Howe PRC (1984) Evidence that adrenaline neurons in the rostral ventrolateral medulla have a vasopressor function. Neurosci Lett 45: 267–272
Gordon FJ, Brody MJ, Fink GD, Buggy J, Johnson AK (1979) Role of central catecholamines in the control of blood pressure and drinking behavior. Brain Res 178: 161–173
Granata AR, Ruggiero DA, Park DH, Joh TH, Reis DJ (1983) Lesions of epinephrine neurons in the rostral ventrolateral medulla abolish the vasodepressor components of baroreflex and cardiopulmonary reflex. Hypertension 5 [Suppl V]: V80–V84
Helke CJ, Neil JJ, Massari VJ, Loewy AD (1982) Substance P neurons project from the ventral medulla to the intermediolateral cell column and ventral horn in the rat. Brain Res 243: 147–152
Hilton SM (1975) Ways of viewing the central nervous system control of the circulation—old and new. Brain Res 87: 213–219
Hirose S, Yokosawa H, Inagami T (1978) Immunochemical identification of renin in rat brain and distinction from acid proteases. Nature 274: 392–393
Howe PRC, Kuhn DM, Minson JB, Stead BH, Chalmers JP (1983) Evidence for a bulbospinal serotonergic pressor pathway in the rat brain. Brain Res 270: 29–36
Ito T, Eggena P, Barrett JD, Katz D, Metter J, Sambhi MP (1980) Studies on angiotensinogen of plasma and cerebrospinal fluid in normal and hypertensive human subjects. Hypertension 2: 432–436
Iverson IL (1983) Nonopioid neuropeptides in mammalian CNS. Ann Rev Pharmacol Toxicol 23: 1–27
Jewell PA, Verney EB (1957) An experimental attempt to determine the site of the neurohypophysial osmoreceptors in the dog. Philos Trans R Soc London B240: 197–324
Joy MD, Lowe RD (1970) Evidence that the area postrema mediates the central cardiovascular response to angiotensin II. Nature 228: 1303–1304
Kalia M, Welles R (1980) Brain stem projections of the aortic nerve in the cat: a study using tetramethyl benzidine as the substrate for HRP. Brain Res 188: 23–32
Keeler JR, Helke CJ (1985) Spinal cord substance P mediates bicuculline-induced activation of cardiovascular responses from the ventral medulla. J Auton Nerv Syst 13: 19–34
Korner PI (1979) Central nervous control of autonomic cardiovascular function. In: Berne RM (ed) Handbook of physiology, section 2, vol 1, American Physiological Society, Bethesda, pp 691–739
Laubie M, Schmitt H (1979) Destruction of the nucleus tractus solitarii in the dog: comparison with sinoaortic denervation. Am J Physiol 236: H736–H743
Lewis GP (1975) Physiological mechanisms controlling secretory activity of adrenal medulla. In: Blaschko H, Sayers G, Smith AD (eds) Handbook of physiology, sect 7, vol VI. American Physiological Society, Washington, DC, pp 309–320
Liard JF, Dériaz O, Tschopp M, Schoun J (1981) Cardiovascular effects of vasopressin infused into the vertebral circulation of conscious dogs. Clin Sci 61: 345–347
Lind RW, Swanson LW, Ganten D (1985) Organization of angiotensin II immunoreactive cells and fibers in the rat central nervous system. Neuroendocrinology 40: 2–24
Loewy AD, Gregorie EM, McKellar S, Baker RP (1979) Electrophysiological evidence that the A5 catecholamine cell group is a vasomotor center. Brain Res 178: 196–200
Loewy AD, McKellar S (1981) Serotonergic projections from the ventral medulla to the intermediolateral cell column in the rat. Brain Res 211: 146–152
Loewy AD, Sawyer WB (1982) Substance P antagonist inhibits vasomotor responses elicited from ventral medulla in rat. Brain Res 245: 379–383
Lorenz RG, Saper CB, Wong DL, Ciaranello R, Loewy AD (1985) Co-localization of substance P

and PNMT-like immunoreactivity in neurons of ventrolateral medulla that project to the spinal cord: potential role in control of vasomotor tone. Neurosci Lett 55: 255–260

Marson O, Chernicky CL, Barnes KL, Averill DB, Ferrario CM (1984) What is the role of the AV3V region in the production of the neurogenic actions of angiotensin II in the dog? Clin Exp Hypertens A6: 1927–1932

McEwen BS, Davis PG, Parsons B, Pfaff DW (1979) The brain as a target for steroid hormone action. Ann Rev Neurosci 2: 65–112

Mendelsohn FAO, Quirion R, Saavedra JM, Aguilera G, Catt KJ (1984) Autoradiographic localization of angiotensin II receptors in rat brain. Proc Natl Acad Sci USA 81: 1575–1579

Michelini LC, Barnes KL, Ferrario CM (1983) Argnine vasopressin modulates the central action of angiotensin II in the dog. Hypertension 5 [Suppl V]: V94–V100

Moore RY, Bloom FE (1978) Central catecholamine neuron systems: anatomy and physiology of the dopamine systems. Ann Rev Neurosci 1: 129–169

Moore RY, Bloom FE (1979) Central catecholamine neuron systems: anatomy and physiology of the norepinephrine and epinephrine systems. Ann Rev Neurosci 2: 113–168

Nathan MA, Reis DJ (1977) Chronic labile hypertension produced by lesions of the nucleus tractus solitarii in the cat. Circ Res 40: 72–81

Osman MY, Smeby RR, Sen S (1979) Separation of dog brain renin-like activity from acid protease activity. Hypertension 1: 53–60

Owsjannikow P (1871) Die tonischen und reflectorischen centren der gefassnerven. Ber Sachs Ges (Akad) Wiss 23: 135–147

Panneton WM, Loewy AD (1980) Projections of the carotid sinus nerve to the nucleus of the solitary tract in the cat. Brain Res 191: 239–244

Ranson SW, Billingsley PR (1916) Vasomotor reactions from stimulation of the floor of the fourth ventricle. Studies in vasomotor reflex arcs III. Am J Physiol 41: 85–90

Reid IA (1983) Salt and water regulation. In: Krieger DT, Brownstein MJ, Martin JB (eds) Brain peptides. Wiley, New York, pp 333–348

Reid JL, Zivin JA, Kopin IJ (1975) Central and peripheral adrenergic mechanisms in the development of deoxycorticosterone-saline hypertension in rats. Circ Res 37: 569–579

Reis DJ, Joh TH, Nathan MA, Renaud B, Snyder DW, Talman W (1979) Nucleus tractus solitarii: catecholaminergic innervation in normal and abnormal control of arterial pressure. In: Meyer P, Schmitt H (eds) Nervous system and hypertension. Wiley, New York, pp 147–164

Reis DJ, Ross CA, Ruggiero DA, Granata AR, Joh TH (1984) Role of adrenaline neurons of ventrolateral medulla (the C1 group) in the tonic and phasic control of arterial pressure. Clin Exp Hypertens [A] 6: 221–241

Rocha e Silva M, Rosenberg M (1969) The release of vasopressin in response to haemorrhage and its role in the mechanism of blood pressure regulation. J Physiol (London) 202: 535–557

Ross CA, Armstrong DM, Ruggiero DA, Pickel VM, Joh TH, Reis DJ (1981) Adrenaline neurons in the rostral ventrolateral medulla innervate thoracic spinal cord: a combined immunocytochemical and retrograde transport demonstration. Neurosci Lett 25: 257–262

Ross C, Ruggiero DA, Joh TH, Park DH, Reis DJ (1983) Adrenaline synthesizing neurons in the rostral ventrolateral medulla: a possible role in tonic vasomotor control. Brain Res 273: 356–361

Sawchenko PE, Swanson LW (1981) Central noradrenergic pathways for the integration of hypothalamic neuroendocrine and autonomic responses. Science 214: 685–687

Sawchenko PE, Swanson LW (1982) Immunohistochemical identification of neurons in the paraventricular nucleus of the hypothalamus that project to the medulla or to the spinal cord in the rat. J Comp Neurol 205: 260–272

Scharrer B (1977) Peptides in neurobiology: historical introduction. In: Gainer H (ed) Peptides in neurobiology. Plenum, New York, pp 1–8

Scharrer E, Scharrer B (1954) Hormones produced by neurosecretary cells. Recent Prog Horm Res 10: 183–240

Share L (1974) Blood pressure, blood volume, and the release of vasopressin. In: Knobil E, Sawyer WH (eds) Handbook of physiology, Sect 7, Endocrinology, vol 4, The pituitary gland and its neuroendocrine control. American Physiological Society, Washington, DC, pp 243–255

Share L (1976) Role of cardiovascular receptors in the control of ADH release. Cardiology 61 [Suppl I]: 51–64

Sladek CD, Johnson AK (1983) Effect of anteroventral third ventricle lesions on vasopressin release by organ-cultured hypothalamo-neurohypophyseal explants. Neuroendocrinology 37: 78–84

Sladek CD, Knigge KM (1977) Osmotic control of vasopressin release by rat hypothalamo-neurohypophyseal explants in organ culture. Endocrinology 101: 1834–1838

Slater EE (1981) Brain renin: progress in research. In: Buckley JP, Ferrario CM (eds) Central nervous system mechanisms in hypertension. Raven, New York, pp 293–300
Sofroniew MV (1983) Morphology of vasopressin and oxytocin neurones and their central and vascular projections. In: Cross BA, Leng G (eds) The neurohypophysis: structure, function and control. Elsevier, London, pp 101–114 (Progress in brain research, vol. 60)
Speth RC, Wamsley JK, Gehlert DR, Chernicky CL, Barnes KL, Ferrario CM (1985) Angiotensin II receptor localization in the canine CNS. Brain Res 326: 137–143
Takano Y, Loewy AD (1985) Reduction of [^{3}H] substance P binding in the intermediolateral cell column after sympathectomy. Brain Res 333: 193–196
Thoren P (1980) Characteristics of aortic baroreceptors with non-medullated afferents in rabbits and rats. In: Sleight P (ed) Arterial baroreceptors and hypertension. Oxford University Press, Oxford, pp 17–22
Undesser KP, Hasser EM, Haywood JR, Johnson AK, Bishop VS (1985) Interactions of vasopressin with the area postrema in arterial baroreflex function in conscious rabbits. Circ Res 56: 410–417
Wallach JH, Loewy AD (1980) Projections of the aortic nerve to the nucleus tractus solitarius in the rabbit. Brain Res 188: 247–251
West MJ, Elliott J, Chalmers J (1984) The sympatho-adrenal system and vasopressin in cardovascular responses to A1 lesions. Clin Exp Hypertens [A] 6: 157–170

Chapter 10

Cardiac Dysfunction Following Stroke

J. W. Norris and V. C. Hachinski

> Every affection of the mind that is attended with either pain or pleasure, hope or fear, is the cause of an agitation whose influence extends to the heart.
>
> *William Harvey (1628)*

The powerful effects of the emotions on the heart have been acknowledged since ancient times, when it was known that people "died of fright." Since then, the brain has displaced the heart as the seat of the emotions (Smith and DeVitto 1984) but it continues to express itself through it. The pathways activated by emotions are probably those disinhibited by stroke. Current "lie detector" methods depend upon cardiovascular responses to psychogenic stress. Whether these physiological curiosities had pathological equivalents was not known until the early days of ECG, when abnormal cardiac electrical activity was found associated with brain tumors and subarachnoid hemorrhage (Aschenbrenner and Bodechtel 1938; Byer et al. 1947).

More recently there has been considerable interest and investigation into the brain-heart influence, and the emergent data indicate that this may have considerable clinical impact. Secondary cardiac dysfunction after ischemic and hemorrhagic stroke, especially following subarachnoid hemorrhage, probably contribute to early death and morbidity.

Pathways connecting brain and brain stem centers involved in cardiovascular regulation have been demonstrated, and both their stimulation and ablation affect cardiac function (Fig. 10.1). Experimental hemorrhagic and ischemic stroke can alter cardiac function directly by destruction of structures involved in cardiac regulation and indirectly by increasing intracranial pressure. Autonomic nervous system blockers prevent some of these effects.

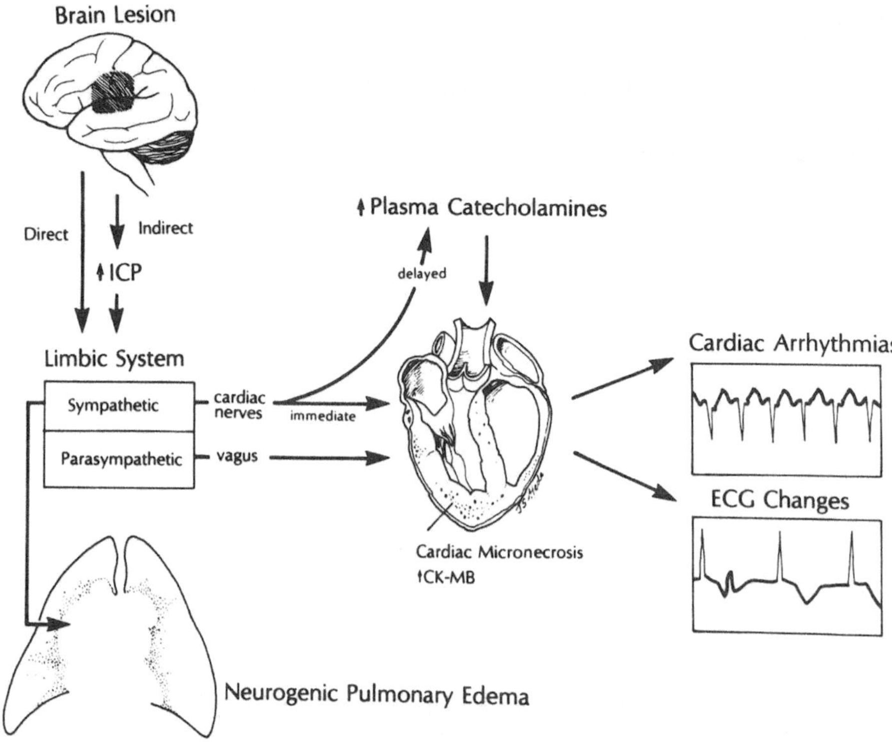

Fig. 10.1. Suggested pathways for the effect of cerebral lesions on the heart (Norris 1983).

Experimental Evidence

Cardiac Arrhythmias

Nauta (1964) described a frontocortical-brain stem pathway in the monkey coursing through the subthalamus, posterior hypothalamus, and fields of Forel. Blocking this pathway with a cryogenic probe prevented or delayed ventricular fibrillation after coronary artery occlusion in conscious stressed pigs (Skinner and Reed 1981). On the other hand, stimulation of the midbrain in dogs with induced coronary artery occlusion increased the chance of ventricular fibrillation tenfold (Satinsky et al. 1971).

Removal of central nervous system input to the heart by sectioning the sympathetic and vagus nerves protected cats against arrhythmias produced by coronary artery occlusion. Animals without neural input survived twice as long and had a significant decrease in the incidence of ventricular fibrillation (Gillis 1971).

Estanol et al. (1977) showed that almost all dogs with experimental subarachnoid hemorrhage developed cardiac dysrhythmias, but only those with intact cervical sympathetic nerves, spinal cord, or both had ventricular arrhythmias.

These stimulation and ablation experiments indicate an important role for the central nervous system in the initiation or facilitation of various cardiac arrhythmias, including lethal ventricular fibrillation.

Myocardial Damage

Electrostimulation of the orbital frontal cortex in the monkey (Hall et al. 1977) and the posterior hypothalamus (Melville et al. 1963) produced cardiac arrhythmias and myocardial lesions similar to those induced by the infusion of catecholamines (Chappel et al. 1959; Lepeschkin et al. 1960). Pigs subjected to restraint stress or sham amygdalectomies experience tachycardia, elevated blood catecholamine levels (especially noradrenaline), and widespread foci of myocardial necrosis (Johansson et al. 1982). Those with previous bilateral amygdalectomies experienced only mild elevations in heart rate, lower noradrenaline levels, and no myocardial necrosis or myocardial damage. Pretreatment with the beta-receptor blocker propranolol prevented the myocardial damage (Häggendal et al. 1982). Propranolol also prevented myocardial necrosis after experimental intracranial hemorrhage in the rat (Hunt and Gore 1972). Adrenalectomy did not preclude the myocardial changes resulting from stimulation of the mesencephalic reticular formation in cats, suggesting that local release of catecholamines from nerve terminals causes the damage (Greenhoot and Reichenbach 1969). This is supported by the finding of increased tissue catecholamines in the heart after experimental subarachnoid hemorrhage (Offerhaus and Van Gool 1969).

Increased Intracranial Pressure

Acute brain injury in dogs produced by epidural and subdural compression, cerebral injection of blood compressing the medulla, and cranial trauma all produce similar electrocardiographic changes. Immediately after injury, bradycardia, tachycardia, and supraventricular, nodal, and ventricular extrasystoles, and Wenckebach and AV blocks occurred, but never persisted beyond 15 min. Ventricular fibrillation only appeared after many hours of brain compression, usually preceded by repolarization defects. Changes in atrial and ventricular activation occurred either immediately or, more commonly, 2 h after the intracranial pressure was raised. Variation in the size and shape of the P-waves, the formation of ventricular complexes, bundle branch block, displacement of S-T segments, and characteristic deep wide negative T-waves occurred, probably through the direct or indirect stimulation of hypothalamic centers (Eichbaum et al. 1965).

Cardiac arrhythmias occurred in dogs even with modest increases of intracranial pressure, following injection of isoproterenol. Atropine and vagotomy prevented the arrhythmias induced by raised intracranial pressure, with or without injection of isoproterenol (Smith and Ray 1972).

Increased intracranial pressure increases plasma catecholamine levels in dogs (Richardson and Woods 1957). Graf and Rossi (1987) also found that a sharp increase of intracranial pressure in dogs caused tachycardia, systemic hypertension, and, within seconds, a 1200-fold increase in epinephrine, a 145-fold rise in norepinephrine, and a 35-fold augmentation in dopamine levels. They suggested that mechanical distortion of the brain stem as well as raised intracranial pressure may mediate these responses. Increased pressure in the third ventricle, leading to compression of the hypothalamus, may be the major cause of the autonomic effects of increased intracranial pressure.

Experimental Hemorrhagic Stroke

Myocardial damage and cardiac arrhythmias are amply documented after experimental intracranial hemorrhage (Weidler 1974). The mechanisms probably include damage or irritation of the frontocortical-brain stem pathway and raised intracranial pressure. Cats with vasospasm induced by subarachnoid hemorrhage and mechanical stimulation had a decrease in norepinephrine in the nerves to cerebral vessels ipsilateral and contralateral to the side of surgical operation (Rosenblum and Guilianti 1973). Interestingly, similar norepinephrine depletion also occurred in the nerves to mesenteric vessels of the experimental animals and in the nerves to cerebral vessels in sham-operated animals. These findings suggest that, in subarachnoid hemorrhage, a more generalized adrenergic disturbance occurs.

Experimental Ischemic Stroke

Cardiac arrhythmias occurred in cats following ligation of the left middle cerebral artery, the number of arrhythmias decreasing with infusion of atropine and propranolol (Weidler et al. 1976). Using a similar experimental stroke model, Hachinski et al. (1984, 1985) showed that somatosympathetic responses and plasma norepinephrine increase after middle cerebral artery occlusion, suggesting augmented sympathetic activity.

Myocardial necrosis produced by acute cerebral ischemia in the rabbit is prevented by the beta-receptor blocker pindolol (Heinrich and Muller 1974).

Clinical Evidence

Pool (1957) was impressed by ECG changes on the cardiac monitor (newly instituted after the introduction of surgical hypothermia) while operating on patients with subarachnoid hemorrhage. Bradycardia occurred most commonly, as well as extrasystoles and nodal tachycardia, with large T-waves and depressed ST segments on the ECG. These changes appeared and disappeared abruptly, on traction on the dura, and on handling the medial temporal, subfrontal, or cingulate gyri (i.e., the limbic system). The area most sensitive to traction was the circle of Willis, while manipulation of cortical arteries had no effect. He attributed these effects to increased "irritability" of vagal or hypothalamic areas due to extravasated blood. In one case, fatal ventricular fibrillation occurred during dissection of a saccular aneurysm.

Numerous anecdotal case series in the 1950s and 1960s reported ECG changes in patients with a variety of intracranial lesions, mainly subarachnoid hemorrhage and "stroke" but also head injuries, brain tumors, and meningitis. Most prominent were ST depression and large, often inverted T-waves (Hammermeister and Reichenbach 1969; Hersch 1964), prolonged Q-T intervals, and prominent U-waves (Burch et al. 1954). Explanations for these changes varied from vagal stimulation (Levine 1953), stimulation of frontal areas (Cropp and Manning 1960), to sympathetic stimulation (Burch et al. 1954). Less likely suggestions of etiology such as hypokalemia (Hersch 1964) and hypertension (Kreus et al. 1969) were soon discarded.

These changes were similar to myocardial infarction; yet autopsy examination of the heart, including microscopic sections, initially proved normal (Levine 1953; Cropp and Manning 1960; Wasserman et al. 1956). Subendocardial hemorrhages and focal myocytolysis in the presence of normal coronary arteries in patients with intracranial lesions were later documented (Smith and Tomlinson 1954; Schlesinger and Reiner 1955). In 1969 Hammermeister and Reichenbach correlated focal myocytolysis, ECG changes, and "neurogenic" pulmonary edema in subarachnoid hemorrhage patients. The spotty transmural pattern of these tiny foci of myocardial necrosis could explain the subendocardial pattern of cardiac damage seen on ECG. They suggested that sympathetic centers in the hypothalamus were stimulated by intracranial disease, and resulted in systemic (or possibly local, myocardial) release of catecholamines. This was clearly a different mechanism than the findings of Pool (1957), where ECG changes and arrhythmias started or stopped abruptly on intracranial stimulation. They rejected the notion that neurogenic pulmonary edema followed changes in the pulmonary capillaries, and suggested that myocardial damage had occurred to produce transient left ventricular failure. In the early era of heart transplants, they cautioned against the use of hearts "damaged" by intracranial catastrophes.

These cardiac lesions were not confined to cases of subarachnoid hemorrhage, and in a series of 231 autopsies including a variety of intracranial lesions varying from cerebral abscess, acute cerebral infarction, cerebral trauma, and brain tumor, 8% had focal myocytolysis, though by far the commonest cause was intracranial hemorrhage (Connor 1968). The intracranial lesions were acute in all cases, and both vagal stimulation and catecholamine release were suggested as the probable etiology.

Using sensitive histochemical techniques to detect myocardial fiber damage, there was a strikingly high and significant increase in myocardial lesions in patients dying from intracranial lesions compared with controls (Kolin and Norris 1984) (Fig. 10.2). The cardiac lesions were not seen in victims of sudden death, and signs of myocardial fiber damage appeared at 6 h, but not after 2 weeks. Patients dying from acute hypotensive shock such as circulatory failure showed similar myocardial changes, also suggesting a sympathetic or catecholamine effect. Myocardial damage was associated with intracranial lesions producing a sudden terminal rise in intracranial pressure, but rarely with lesions which were small or which produced gradual rises in intracranial pressure. The cardiac lesions were unrelated to intracranial pathology, which included cerebral infarction, intracerebral hemorrhage, brain abscess, and astrocytomas. The only residual trace of these transient cardiac micronecroses in survivors is mild interstitial myocardial fibrosis.

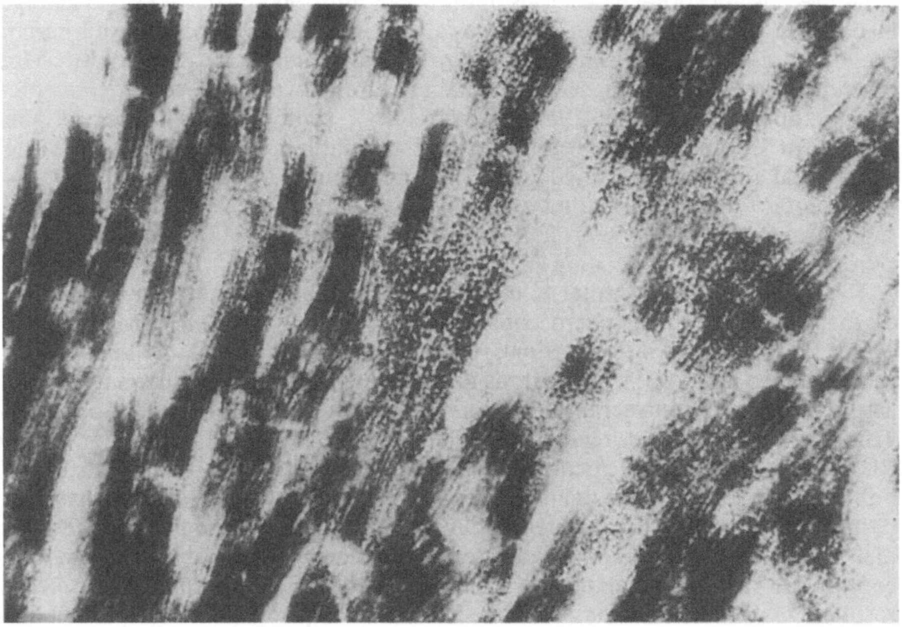

Fig. 10.2. Succinic dehydrogenase section showing coarse irregular granularity of myofibrils. Patient died of coning secondary to a glioma (Kolin and Norris 1984).

The causal role of catecholamines in pulmonary edema was first suggested in 1917 by Moutier, a French Army surgeon, who found acute and fatal pulmonary congestion in soldiers with head injuries. This explanation of acute intracranial lesions affecting cardiac function (Visscher et al. 1956) was later reinforced by experimental data from infusion of noradrenaline-like substances (Chappel et al. 1959; Lepeschkin et al. 1960), which produced myocardial lesions and cardiac arrhythmias.

The biochemical link between cardiac changes and subarachnoid hemorrhage was confirmed by urinary catecholamine assays (Tomomatsu et al. 1964). Both the increased incidence of ECG abnormalities and high urinary catecholamines were suggested as adverse prognostic factors in patients with subarachnoid hemorrhage, probably related to increased cerebral vasospasm (Cruickshank et al. 1974). Plasma noradrenaline levels are more sensitive indices of sympathetic tone, and Benedict and Loach (1978) found significantly higher levels in subarachnoid hemorrhage patients compared with controls (Fig. 10.3). Plasma noradrenaline levels were also significantly higher in patients with poor outcomes.

Hypothalamic damage secondary to cerebral vasospasm may explain the predominance of subarachnoid hemorrhage among other intracranial lesions producing cardiac dysfunction (Crompton 1963). ECG "ischemic" changes and focal myocytolysis were found in autopsied subarachnoid hemorrhage patients with hypothalamic infarction, but not in those with normal hypothalami (Doshi and Neil-Dwyer 1977). This mechanism does not explain the cardiac dysfunction

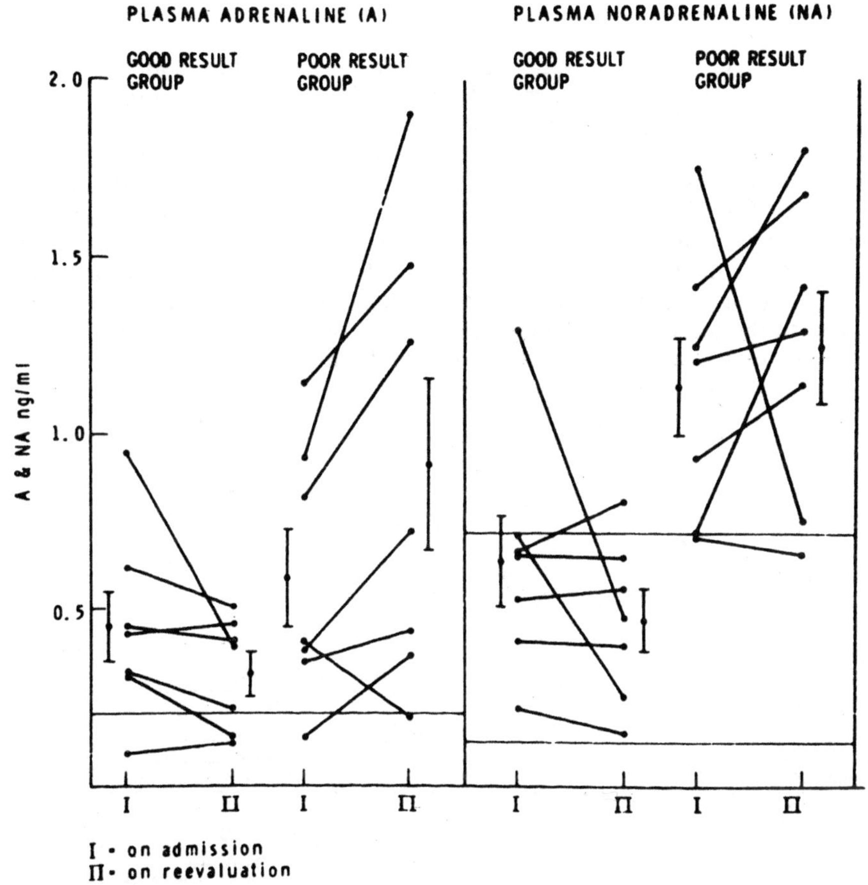

Fig. 10.3. Plasma adrenaline and noradrenaline concentrations related to prognosis in subarachnoid hemorrhage (Benedict and Loach 1978).

seen in other intracranial lesions, where some patients with ischemic stroke have superficial cortical lesions and no hypothalamic involvement (Myers et al. 1981).

Serum cardiac enzymes are sensitive markers of cardiac necrosis and, in 100 consecutive patients admitted to hospital with stroke compared with 100 controls with cancer of the colon, there was a seven- to tenfold increase in all types of ECG abnormalities in the stroke group, which correlated with an adverse outcome (Dimant and Grob 1977). Levels of serum cardiac enzymes (CK) correlated significantly with the ECG abnormalities, and could monitor progress in these patients. These findings were confirmed using the more specific electrophoretic assay for cardiac isoenzyme fraction (CK-MB) (Norris et al. 1979). There was a slow rise (4–7 days) and fall of serum CK-MB levels, quite unlike the acute necrosis of myocardial infarction and more in keeping with a smouldering low-grade necrosis such as focal myocytolysis. The incidence of cardiac arrhythmias and of S-T and T-wave abnormalities was significantly increased in the stroke patients with raised CK-MB levels.

Neurogenic Pulmonary Edema

Sudden and often fatal acute pulmonary edema may complicate subarachnoid hemorrhage and other acute intracranial catastrophes, such as head injury, brain tumor, or cerebral infarction (Hoff and Nishimura 1978; Harari et al. 1976). If severe, it is sometimes hemorrhagic, and it relates to the "severity" of the intracranial insult, i.e., the degree of raised intracranial pressure. In the autopsy series of Weir (1978), it occurred in 70% of cases of subarachnoid hemorrhage. Sudden coma was universal in his patients, and breathing difficulties began within minutes of the ictus. He ascribed it to the dramatic increase in intracranial pressure following aneurysmal rupture, triggering massive autonomic discharge. The speed of the increase in intracranial pressure was critical, an idea which is supported by experimental evidence (Hoff and Nishimura 1978).

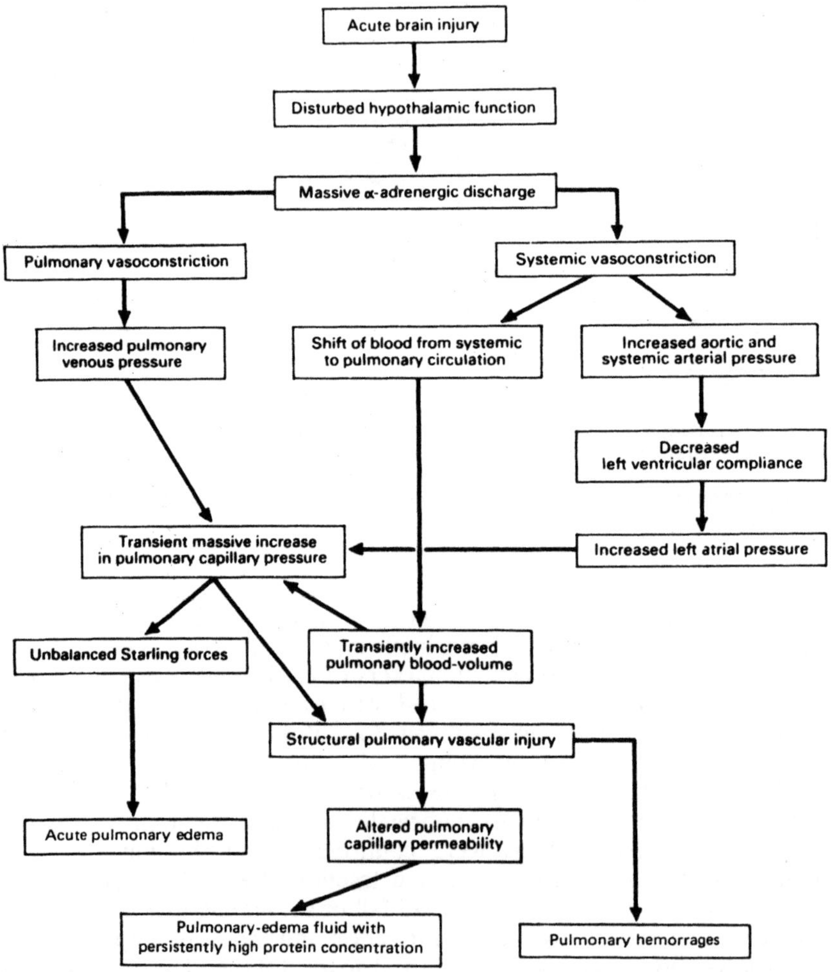

Fig. 10.4. Suggested mechanisms of pulmonary edema in acute cerebral lesions (Theodore and Robin 1975).

Neurogenic pulmonary edema appears rapidly and probably results from a massive centrally mediated sympathetic discharge producing intense systemic vasoconstriction. Blood shifts from the high-resistance systemic circulation to the low-resistance pulmonary circulation. Pulmonary edema follows from the hydrostatic effect of transiently increased pulmonary capillary pressure, and the pulmonary hypertension and ruptured pulmonary blood vessels produce lung hemorrhage. When it subsides, it leaves pulmonary edema with high protein content yet normal cardiac and hemodynamic function (Fig. 10.4), quite unlike the mechanism in left ventricular failure (Theodore and Robin 1975; Harari et al. 1976).

The dominant role of sympathetic discharge in neurogenic pulmonary edema is underlined by cases in which there is also a spectrum of changes with "neurogenic" ECG changes of subendocardial injury and focal myocytolysis at autopsy, suggesting both an immediate neurogenic effect and a later catecholamine cardiac micronecrosis (Hammermeister and Reichenbach 1969).

Cardiac Arrhythmias Secondary to Stroke

Cardiac monitoring in stroke patients produces ECG data so complex and controversial that it is difficult to distinguish between cause and effect. There is abundant evidence that the profuse variety of cardiac arrhythmias occurring in about half the patients does not just reflect the results of generalized atherosclerosis. Even when age and preexisting ischemic heart disease are taken into consideration, there is a significant increase in cardiac arrhythmias (Myers et al. 1982). Patients with acute intracerebral hemorrhage generate the same quantity and variety of cardiac arrhythmias as in those with acute ischemic stroke (Table 10.1) (Norris 1983). Initial reports from the intensive care stroke unit in Jerusalem suggested that the high incidence of cardiac arrhythmias reflecting associated cardiovascular disease had a direct causal role producing cerebral ischemia (Lavy et al. 1968). This view was later modified and the cardiac arrhythmias attributed to the cerebrovascular lesion were felt to cause further damage to ischemic brain (Lavy et al. 1974).

A clearer perspective of arrhythmias secondary to cerebral lesions (including stroke) is afforded by early clinical data and extrapolations from experimental studies. Pool's observations (1957) documented bradycardia and extrasystoles, nodal and ventricular tachycardia, and fibrillation. These were not the effects of early anesthetic procedures since the arrhythmias could be produced or arrested immediately by the surgical manipulation. Other acute arrhythmias reported in

Table 10.1. Incidence of cardiac arrhythmias (predominant arrhythmia for each patient) in patients admitted to an acute stroke unit. (Norris 1983)

	Arrhythmias			No.	
Cerebral lesion	Ectopics	A Fib	Misc	Arrhythmias	Total
Cerebral infarction	73	42	10	117	242
Cerebral hemorrhage	7	6	1	16	30
Controls (nonstroke)	12	8	0	70	90

intracranial hemorrhage and seen experimentally include wandering pacemaker, atrial fibrillation, and a variety of ectopic beats (Weidler 1974).

In the Toronto acute stroke unit, we have observed cardiac arrhythmias in patients with terminally raised intracranial pressure from acute ischemic and hemorrhagic stroke. Initial bradycardia, probably representing increased vagal tone, gives way to nodal escape rhythms, including ectopic beats, nodal tachycardia, or a combination (wandering pacemaker). When the atrioventricular node fails, idioventricular rhythms, ventricular ectopics, and ventricular fibrillation occur prior to death.

Therapeutic Implications

Experience in most acute stroke units indicates that cardiac arrhythmias are frequent but rarely serious or fatal (Norris and Hachinski 1976). Cardiac monitoring is useful to detect unsuspected arrhythmias such as wandering cardiac pacemaker or paroxysmal atrial fibrillation which may indicate an unsuspected source of cerebral embolism. Serious arrhythmias such as ventricular fibrillation are often terminal events due to raised intracranial pressure in patients with massive brain damage, and dramatic resuscitation measures in these patients are rarely indicated.

Cardiac arrhythmias occurring in patients with minor neurological deficits, such as subarachnoid hemorrhage, minor stroke (Silver et al. 1984), or transient ischemic attack, warrant more careful scrutiny. The exact figure is unknown, but sudden death in subarachnoid hemorrhage is frequently due to serious arrhythmias, possibly accounting for up to 15% of patients who die before reaching hospital (Estanol and Marin 1975). Cardiac monitoring in the acute stage in these patients is mandatory, since many potentially lethal cardiac arrhythmias can be promptly reversed. Both of Parizel's (1973) subarachnoid hemorrhage patients survived after electroshock and drug therapy, although they had paroxysms of supraventricular tachycardia, ventricular ectopics, ventricular tachycardia, and ventricular fibrillation.

As well as cardiac arrhythmias, the ECG changes seen in a variety of space-occupying intracranial lesions which raise intracranial pressure, including stroke, subarachnoid hemorrhage, subdural hematoma, and brain tumors (Lavy et al. 1974; Cruickshank et al 1974; VanderArk 1975; Burch and Phillips 1968), relate closely to the clinical management. Most of the changes, including Q-T prolongation, ST- and T-wave changes, represent delayed ventricular repolarization, presumably of neurogenic origin. Prolonged Q-T is especially dangerous, since it is unresponsive to most standard antiarrhythmic drugs and it predisposes to serious and potentially fatal arrhythmias such as ventricular flutter and fibrillation (Moss and McDonald 1971). It has been treated successfully in subarachnoid hemorrhage with beta-blockers, although repeated cardioversion or even left stellate ganglion block may be necessary (Carruth and Silverman 1980; Grossman 1976).

Attempts to relate adverse prognosis to the presence of neurogenic ECG changes in stroke (Lavy et al. 1974) or subarachnoid hemorrhage (Cruickshank et al. 1974) are unconvincing due to small numbers, though the hypothesis is credible. Monitoring CK-MB levels in stroke patients might be more helpful, since the cardiac isoenzyme is a sensitive index of the extent of myocytolysis and seems to relate to ECG abnormalities (Diamant and Grob 1977).

Human and experimental evidence for both cardiac dysfunction and neurogenic pulmonary edema indicates both massive sympathetic (Greenhoot and Reichenbach 1969; Weidler 1974; Ducker et al. 1968) and parasympathetic stimulation (Norris 1983). Combined alpha- and beta-blockade should represent the ideal treatment (except for the possible danger of systemic hypotension), and combined propranolol and phentolamine therapy had a cardioprotective effect in one study of subarachnoid hemorrhage patients (Neil-Dwyer et al. 1978), although there was difficulty distinguishing cardiac death from cerebral edema and recurrent subarachnoid hemorrhage. Also, all patients dying acutely (whether taking active drug or placebo) had perivascular hemorrhage or infarction of the hypothalamus.

Conclusion

Acute intracranial lesions (including stroke) often produce cardiac dysfunction, including cardiac arrhythmias, a "neurogenic" pattern of ECG abnormalities, acute pulmonary edema, and a specific cardiac pathological damage (focal myocytolysis) accompanied by increased blood levels of cardiac enzymes. The cerebral lesions always produce acute and usually rapid rises in intracranial pressure and the intracranial pathology is probably nonspecific. The high profile of subarachnoid hemorrhage in producing neurogenic cardiac dysfunction probably relates more to its role in producing dramatic, severe, and rapid increases in intracranial pressure, than to any effect of any substances released into the subarachnoid space.

Some of these secondary cardiac effects are life-threatening but reversible, and an awareness and detection of their presence in acute cerebrovascular disease is important in clinical management.

References

Aschenbrenner R, Bodechtel G (1938) Über EKG-Veränderungen bei Hirntumorkranken. Klin Wochenschr 17: 298–302

Benedict CR, Loach AB (1978) Clinical significance of plasma adrenaline and noradrenaline concentrations in patients with subarachnoid hemorrhage. J Neurol Neurosurg Psychiatr 41: 113–117

Burch GE, Meyers R, Abildskov JA (1954) A new electrocardiographic pattern observed in cerebrovascular accidents. Circulation 9: 719–723

Burch GE, Phillips JH (1968) The large upright T wave as an electrocardiographic manifestation of intracranial disease. South Med J 61: 331–336

Byer E, Ashman R, Toth LA (1947) Electrocardiograms with large upright T-waves and long Q-T intervals. Am Heart J 33: 796–806

Carruth JE, Silverman ME (1980) *Torsade de pointe*—atypical ventricular tachycardia complicating subarachnoid hemorrhage. Chest 78: 886–888

Chappel CI, Rona G, Balazs T, Gaudry R (1959) Comparison of cardiotoxic actions of certain sympathomimetic amines. Can J Biochem Physiol 37: 35–42

Connor RCR (1968) Heart damage associated with intracranial lesions. Br Med J 3: 29–31
Crompton MR (1963) Hypothalamic lesions following the rupture of berry aneurysms. Brain 86: 301–314
Cropp GJ, Manning GW (1960) Electrocardiographic changes simulating myocardial ischemia and infarction associated with spontaneous intracranial hemorrhage. Circulation 22: 25–38
Cruickshank JM, Neil-Dwyer G, Brice J (1974) Electrocardiographic changes and their prognostic significance in subarachnoid hemorrhage. J Neurol Neurosurg Psychiatr 37: 755–759
Dimant J, Grob D (1977) Electrocardiographic changes and myocardial damage in patients with acute cerebrovascular accidents. Stroke 8: 448–455
Doshi R, Neil-Dwyer G (1977) Hypothalamic and myocardial lesions after subarachnoid hemorrhage. J Neurol Neurosurg Psychiatr 40: 821–826
Ducker TB, Simmons RL, Anderson RW (1968) Increased intracranial pressure and pulmonary edema. Pt III. The effect of increased intracranial pressure on the cardiovascular hemodynamics of chimpanzees. J Neurosurg 29: 475–483
Eichbaum FW, Gazetta BH, Bissetti PC, Pereira CB (1965) Electrocardiographic disturbances following acute increase of intracranial pressure: Experiments in dogs. Z Ges Exp Med 139: 721–734
Estanol BV, Marin OS (1975) Cardiac arrhythmias and sudden death in subarachnoid hemorrhage. Stroke 6: 382–386
Estanol BV, Loyo MV, Mateos JH, Foyo E, Cornejo A, Guevara J (1977) Cardiac arrhythmias in experimental subarachnoid hemorrhage. Stroke 8: 440–446
Gillis RA (1971) Role of the nervous system in the arrhythmias produced by coronary occlusion in the cat. Am Heart J 81: 677–684
Graf CJ, Rossi NP (1978) Catecholamine response to intracranial hypertension. J Neurosurg 49: 862–868
Greenhoot JH, Reichenbach DD (1969) Cardiac injury and subarachnoid hemorrhage: a clinical, pathological and physiological correlation. J Neurosurg 30: 521–531
Grossman MA (1976) Cardiac arrhythmias in acute central nervous system disease. Successful management with stellate ganglion block. Arch Intern Med 136: 203–207
Hachinski VC, Norris JW (1985) The acute stroke. W Davis, Philadelphia
Hachinski VC, Ciriello J, Smith KE, Bihari F (1984) Changes in somatosympathetic reflexes after occlusion of the middle cerebral artery in the cat (abst). Soc Neurosci 10: 167
Hachinski VC, Ciriello J, Smith KE, Bihari F, Gibson C (1985) Changes in plasma catecholamines after occlusion of the middle cerebral artery in the cat (abst). Stroke 16: 136
Häggendal J, Johansson G, Jonsson L, Thoren-Tolling K (1982) Effect of propranolol on myocardial cell necrosis and blood levels of catecholamines in pigs subjected to stress. Acta Pharmacol Toxicol 50: 58–66
Hall RE, Livingston RB, Bloor CM (1977) Orbital cortical influences on cardiovascular dynamics and myocardial structure in conscious monkeys. J Neurosurg 46: 638–647
Hammermeister KE, Reichenbach DD (1969) QRS changes, pulmonary edema, and myocardial necrosis associated with subarachnoid hemorrhage. Am Heart J 78: 94–100
Harari A, Rapin M, Regnier B, Comoy J, Caron JP (1976) Normal pulmonary-capillary pressures in the late phase of neurogenic pulmonary oedema. Lancet 1: 494
Heinrich D, Muller W (1974) Focal myocardial necrosis in cases of increased intracranial pressure. Eur Neurol 12: 369–376
Hersch C (1961) Electrocardiography changes in head injuries. Circulation 23: 853–860
Hersch C (1964) Electrocardiographic changes in subarachnoid haemorrhage, meningitis, and intracranial space-occupying lesions. Br Heart J 26: 785–793
Hoff JT, Nishimura M (1978) Experimental neurogenic pulmonary edema in cats. J Neurosurg 18: 383–389
Hunt D, Gore J (1972) Myocardial lesions following experimental intracranial hemorrhage. Am Heart J 83: 232–236
Johansson G, Olsson K, Hággendal J, Jonsson L, Thoren-Tolling K (1982) Effect of stress on myocardial cells and blood levels of catecholamines in normal and amygdalectomized pigs. Can J Comp Med 46: 176–182
Kolin A, Norris JW (1984) Myocardial damage from acute cerebral lesions. Stroke 15: 990–993
Kreus KE, Kemila SJ, Takala JK (1969) Electrocardiographic changes in cerebrovascular accidents. Acta Med Scand 185: 327–334
Lavy S, Stern S, Herishianu Y, et al. (1968) Electrocardiographic changes in ischaemic stroke. J Neurol Sci 7: 409–415
Lavy S, Yaar I, Melamed E, Stern S (1974) The effect of acute stroke on cardiac functions as observed in an intensive stroke care unit. Stroke 5: 775–780

Lepeschkin E, Marchet H, Schroeder G, Wagner R, dePaula e Silva P, Raab W, Starcheska YK (1960) Effect of epinephrine and norepinephrine on the electrocardiogram of 100 normal subjects. Am J Cardiol 5: 594–603
Levine HD (1953) Non-specificity of the electrocardiogram associated with coronary artery disease. Am J Med 15: 344–354
Melville KI, Blum G, Shister HE, Silver MD (1963) Cardiac ischemic changes and arrhythmias induced by hypothalamic stimulation. Am J Cardiol 12: 781–791
Moss AJ, McDonald J (1971) Unilateral cerviocothoracic sympathetic ganglionectomy for the treatment of the long QT interval syndrome. N Engl J Med 285: 903–904
Myers MG, Norris JW, Hachinski VC, Sole MJ (1981) Plasma norepinephrine in stroke. Stroke 12: 200–204
Myers MG, Norris JW, Hachinski VC, Weingert ME, Sole MJ (1982) Cardiac sequelae of acute stroke. Stroke 13: 838–842
Nauta WJH (1964) Some afferent connections of the prefrontal cortex in the monkey. In: Warren JW, Akert K (eds) The frontal granual cortex and behavior. McGraw, New York, pp 327–396
Neil-Dwyer G, Walter P, Cruickshank JM, Doshi B, O'Gorman P (1978) Effect of propranolol and phentolamine on myocardial necrosis after subarachnoid haemorrhage. Br Med J 2: 990–992
Norris JW (1983) Effects of cerebrovascular lesions on the heart. Neurol Clin 1: 87–101
Norris JW, Hachinski VC (1976) Intensive care management of stroke patients. Stroke 7: 573–577
Norris JW, Hachinski VC, Myers MG, Callow J, Wong T, Moore RW (1979) Serum cardiac enzymes in stroke. Stroke 10: 548–553
Offerhaus J, Van Gool J (1969) Electrocardiographic changes and tissue catecholamines in experimental subarachnoid hemorrhage. Cardiovasc Res 3: 433–440
Parizel G (1973) Life-threatening arrhythmias in subarachnoid hemorrhage. Angiology 24: 17–21
Pool JL (1957) Vasocardiac effects of the circle of Willis. Arch Neurol Psychiatr 78: 355–368
Richardson JA, Woods EF (1957) The effects of increased intracranial pressure on plasma catecholamine levels, blood pressure and ventricular contractility (abst). J Pharmacol Exp Ther 119: 179
Rosenblum WI, Guilianti D (1973) Participation of cerebrovascular nerves in generalized sympathetic discharge: nonspecific release of norepinephrine in the presence or absence of subarachnoid hemorrhage and vasospasm. Arch Neurol 29: 91–94
Satinsky J, Kosowsky B, Lown B, (1971) Ventricular fibrillation induced by hypothalamic stimulation during coronary occlusion (abst). Circulation 44 [Suppl II]: 60
Schlesinger MJ, Reiner L (1955) Focal myocytolysis of heart. Am J Pathol 31: 443–459
Silver FL, Norris JW, Lewis AJ, Hachinski VC (1984) Early mortality following stroke: a prospective review. Stroke 15: 492–496
Skinner JE, Reed JC (1981) Blockade of frontocortical-brainstem pathway prevents ventricular fibrillation of ischemic heart. Am J Physiol 240: H156–H163
Smith M, Ray CT (1972) Cardiac arrhythmias, increased intracranial pressure, and the autonomic nervous system. Chest 61: 125–133
Smith OA, DeVitto JL (1984) Central neural integration for the control of autonomic responses associated with emotion. Ann Rev Neurosci 7: 43–65
Smith RP, Tomlinson BE (1954) Subendocardial haemorrhages associated with intracranial lesions. J Pathol Bacteriol 68: 327–334
Theodore J, Robin ED (1975) Pathogenesis of neurogenic pulmonary oedema. Lancet 2: 749–751
Tomomatsu T, Ueba Y, Matsumoto T (1964) Electrocardiographic observations and urinary excretion of catecholamines in cerebrovascular accidents. Jpn Circ J 28: 905–912
VanderArk GD (1975) Cardiovascular changes with acute subdural hematoma. Surg Neurol 3: 305–308
Visscher MB, Haddy FJ, Stephens G (1956) The physiology and pharmacology of lung edema. Pharmacol Rev 8: 389–434
Wasserman F, Choquette G, Cassinelli R, Bellet S (1956) Electrocardiographic observations in patients with cerebrovascular accidents. Am J Med Sci 231: 502–510
Weidler DJ (1974) Myocardial damage and cardiac arrhythmias after intracranial hemorrhage. A critical review. Stroke 5. 759–764
Weidler DJ, Das SK, Sodeman TM (1976) Cardiac arrhythmias secondary to acute cerebral ischemia: prevention by autonomic blockade (abst). Circulation 53 [Suppl II]: 102
Weir BK (1978) Pulmonary edema following fatal aneurysm rupture. J Neurosurg 49: 502–507

Chapter 11

Are Heart Attacks Really Brain Attacks?*

S. R. Levine, V. M. Patel, K. M. A. Welch, and J. E. Skinner

History and Perspective

In 1664, Thomas Willis recognized that the brain and the cardiovascular system are interdependent when he wrote *De Anatome Cerebri* (Willis 1664). For the relief of angina pain, Francois Franck, in 1899, proposed a cervicothoracic sympathectomy to interrupt the nociceptive cardiac efferents (Franck, cited by Danielopolu 1949). Through clinical and experimental work, a high thoracic sympathectomy was found to benefit angina (Leriche et al. 1931) and attenuate the tendency to ventricular fibrillation. Cox and Robertson (1936) reduced the incidence of acute cardiac deaths in dogs with stellate ganglionectomy following experimental coronary occlusion. Cannon (1931) hypothesized that the most highly encephalized parts of the brain should regulate both sensory input and autonomic output during an animal's response to a significant stimulus. Smith (1945) demonstrated that electrical stimulation of the cingulate cortex within the frontal lobe could temporarily stop the heart.

Thus from early times it has been clear that disorders of the CNS can alter cardiovascular function. This chapter reviews the experimental and clinical evidence for the brain-heart connection and the CNS link to sudden cardiac death. A theoretical model from which future research and rational therapy can be launched is proposed.

Anatomy of Central Cardiovascular Regulation: Neural Control of the Heart

Autonomic Anatomy

The heart is innervated by sympathetic and parasympathetic efferents. Afferent fibers arise from the myocardium, atrium, and blood vessels. Most preganglionic

* This work was supported in part by NIH grants #NS23393 to Dr. K.M.A. Welch and #HL31164 to Dr. James E. Skinner

sympathetic neurons are found in the intermediolateral cell column of the spinal cord. The spinal neurons are generally activated by the projections from the ventrolateral medulla. Preganglionic parasympathetic neurons involved in cardiovascular regulation are found largely in the dorsal motor nucleus of the vagus and the nucleus ambiguus, both also located in the medulla of the brain stem. All of the nerve components concerned mingle to some extent in the cardiac plexus, which consists of a superficial and deep portion. Extensions of this plexus along the coronary arteries are known as the right and left coronary plexus. The cardiac plexus includes numerous ganglia, all of which are parasympathetic. The sympathetic nerves of the heart include the superior, middle, and inferior cervical and thoracic sympathetic cardiac nerves. The superior cervical sympathetic cardiac nerve regularly arises from the superior sympathetic ganglion either as a single trunk or by several roots from the ganglion and one or more from the sympathetic trunk. The left superior cervical cardiac nerve joins the superficial cardiac plexus and other sympathetic cardiac nerves join the deep cardiac plexus. The parasympathetic innervation of the heart involves three branches of the vagus nerve on either side. On the left side, the inferior cervical carotid branch of the vagus joins the superficial cardiac plexus. On the right side, cardiac branches of the vagus join the deep cardiac plexus. It was originally thought that the cardiac auricle and atrioventricular bundle were supplied with both vagal and sympathetic fibers, whereas the ventricles were supplied only by the sympathetics. More recently, however, it has been shown that the sympathetic nerves project over the surface of the myocardium, whereas the parasympathetic projections dive into subendocardial layers at the base of the ventricles to distribute themselves widely to subendocardial regions (Zipes et al. 1984). Overlap between the two autonomic efferent classes seems to occur in the mesocardial layers of the ventricular tissue. The sinoauricular node is supplied mainly by the right vagus.

The nucleus tractus solitarius (NTS) of the medulla oblongata is the site of afferent fiber termination from cardiopulmonary and arterial baro- and carotid sinus receptors. Cells within this nucleus make extensive reciprocal connections with other suprasegmental nuclei which are also important in cardiovascular control. Axonal projections from the NTS terminate in the dorsal motor nucleus of the vagus, nucleus ambiguous, intermediolateral cell column of the spinal cord (ILC), serotonergic raphe nuclei, and ventolateral medullary reticular formations (Brodal 1981) (see Chap. 9).

The parabrachial nucleus of the pons and hypothalamus project axons directly to the intermediolateral cell column, but the ILC does not seem to receive projections from the cerebral cortex. However, there is an anatomical framework for cortical influences on sympathetic neurons through cortical-NTS, corticolimbic, corticohypothalamic, and corticoparabrachial nuclei connections. There are three major output pathways from the orbitofrontal cortex (Nauta 1964). One projects to the thalamus (inferior thalamic peduncle) and controls the sensory channels (Skinner and Yingling 1977); another projects to the temporal lobe and amygdaloid nuclei (uncinate faciculus) and has an unknown function; and the third projects through the subthalamus and dorsal hypothalamus to the brain stem (frontocortical-brain stem pathway) to control both visceral responses (Skinner and Yingling 1976) and cardiac vulnerability (Skinner and Reed 1981). This latter projection was noted to give off extensive collaterals to the hypothalamus. Some of the recipient cells in this hypothalamic region take up labeled amino acids and transport them to terminals located in brain stem cardiovascular control regions (i.e., NTS, cardiovascular motor nuclei, nucleus ambiguus) (Devito et al. 1979; Smith et al. 1980).

The hypothalamic and brain stem cells receiving input from the frontal cortex are also the recipients of axon terminals from the amygdala, via the stria terminalis and diagonal band (Galosy et al. 1981). Activation of the amygdala will result in defensive visceral reactions (Galosy et al. 1981), and stimulation of the rostral cingulate cortex results in an abrupt decrease in cardiac rate after a latent period of 1–2 s (Smith 1945) and even cardiac arrest (Ward 1948). These sources of autonomic activity may be held in check by the frontal cortex. Hierarchical control of limbic functions by higher telencephalic systems (e.g., frontocortical) is predicted by MacLean's triune theory of encephalization (MacLean 1970). In support of his proposition, Timms (1977) showed that electric stimulation of the frontal cortex inhibits the visceral defensive reactions elicited by stimulation of the amygdala.

To summarize, the frontal granular cortex has three principal subcortical projections: one that regulates the sensory input channels, one that directly regulates the viscera via the frontocortical-brain stem pathway, and one that regulates the viscera indirectly via the amygdala. Thus, an anatomic framework exists for coupling cardiovascular function to behavior, neuroendocrine function, and other autonomic activity.

Neural Mechanisms of Arrhythmogenesis

Cardiac Effects of Acute Intracranial Lesions: Arrhythmias

Acute intracranial events such as hemorrhages and infarctions have been associated with cardiovascular manifestations (Talman 1985, and see Chap. 10) that span electrocardiographic (EKG) changes including ventricular and supraventricular arrhythmias, blood pressure alterations, neurogenic pulmonary edema, cardiac enzyme elevation and autopsy evidence of myocardial damage, and, finally, sudden death itself. The evidence that acute intracranial events alter the functioning of the frontocortical-brain stem system will now be examined.

Byer et al. (1947) described a patient with subarachnoid hemorrhage who developed tall upright T-waves and a prolonged QT-interval on EKG. These EKG changes were subsequently attributed to subendocardial ischemia. Identical findings were reported by Levine (1953). At autopsy no cardiac changes were seen, leading to the speculation that the etiology may have been vagal stimulation, resulting in terminal asystole. A number of reports subsequently appeared, showing intracranial subarachnoid hemorrhage to be associated with a wide range of EKG changes, both in morphology and rhythm. These rhythm abnormalities included prolonged QTc, elevated or depressed ST-segments, deeply inverted or tall upright T-waves, large U-waves, increased amplitude of U-waves in postextrasystolic beats, Q-waves, notched T-waves, and ventricular tachycardia and fibrillation (Talman 1985, and see ref. within). Similar changes have been reported after spinal subarachnoid hemorrhage, in both lumbar (Yarnell and Clarke 1973) and cervical (McCarthy and Mitchell 1967) regions. Pathophysiologically, these acute conditions provide a remarkable glimpse into neurally mediated cardiovascular control. Hachinski and colleagues (1986) found the extent of myocardial damage to correlate with the circulating levels of serum catecholamines, suggesting that the increased catecholamine levels may cause the myocardial damage.

These electrocardiographic changes generally evolve over several days after the CNS insult, usually reverting to normal within 2 weeks (Fentz and Gormsen 1962). The changes occur most commonly in association with subarachnoid and intracerebral hemorrhage, ischemic cerebrovascular lesions, and head trauma. They have also been found less frequently in patients with cerebral neoplasia, meningitis or encephalitis, demyelinating disease, myelopathy, and hydrocephalus, and during neurosurgical procedures that involve the forebrain (Talman 1985; Finkelstein and Nigaglioni 1961; Hersch 1964; Millar and Abildskov 1968).

Cardiac Effects of Acute Intracranial Lesions: Myocardial Damage

Wasserman et al. (1956) described frank myocardial infarction during the evolution of subarachnoid hemorrhage. A wide variety of more subtle changes have been described subsequently including subendocardial hemorrhage, focal myocytolysis, and round cell infiltrates (Smith and Tomlinson 1954; Conner 1968; Norris et al. 1979). These changes are indistinguishable from "catecholamine cardiomyopathy" seen in patients dying from pheochromocytoma or in animals after intracoronary infusion of catecholamines. The earliest lesions are seen in patients dying within 6 h. Patients dying instantly appear to have normal hearts. If the patient survives long-term, then the acute lesions may reverse, leaving only traces in the form of stromal condensation and myocardial fibrosis (Reichenbach and Beneditt 1970).

Increased levels of circulating serum catecholamines have been demonstrated both in patients with subarachnoid hemorrhages (Peerless and Griffiths 1962; Marion and Segal 1986 for review) and ischemic stroke (Myers et al. 1981). A number of studies have shown that patients with acute cerebral lesions such as subarachnoid and intracerebral hemorrhage, ischemic brain infarction, cerebral contusion, and bacterial meningitis may have elevated creatine kinase (CK) levels. Cases with elevated cardiac CK isoenzyme (CK-MB) have a higher mortality as well as a greater incidence of cardiac arrhythmias (Dimant and Grob 1977; Kaste and Koutlinen 1978; Dubo et al. 1967). It is unclear whether or not the level of circulating catecholamines is high enough to evoke the cardiac damage directly or if neural release in the heart is of sufficient local concentration to produce the observed cardiac alterations. For an intravascular infusion of catecholamines to produce pathology, the injection must be into a coronary artery. This observation suggests that in patients with an intracranial insult the cardiac manifestations may be due to neural release directly into the heart, because the levels of circulating catecholamines cannot equal those required to produce direct pathology.

Hypothalamic and myocardial lesions were found in 42 of 54 patients dying after subarachnoid hemorrhage (Doshi and Neil-Dwyer 1977). Hypothalamic lesions were localized to the periventricular region, predominantly in the paraventricular and supraoptic nuclei.

In a double-blind randomized study of 88 patients with subarachnoid hemorrhage, a combination of phentolamine and propranolol normalized EKG changes (Neil-Dwyer et al. 1978). No necrotic myocardial lesions were seen at autopsy in treated patients. Despite the cardioprotective effect of the drugs, mortality was unaffected. Mortality appeared to be the result of recurrent brain hemorrhages in these cases.

Neurogenic Pulmonary Edema

Neurogenic pulmonary edema has also been reported with acute intracranial lesions (Cameron 1948; Richards 1963; Ciongoli and Poser 1972). Intense systemic vasoconstriction is postulated to shift blood to the low-resistance pulmonary circulation causing a massive increase in blood volume resulting in hydrostatic pulmonary edema. Pulmonary hypertension and hypervolemia causes vascular injury that produces increased capillary permeability, resulting in persistent pulmonary edema.

Pathophysiologic Considerations

Epidemiology

Reliable epidemiologic data concerning the incidence of sudden death in acute intracranial events is not available. According to one estimate (Estanol and Marin 1975), 15% of patients with subarachnoid hemorrhage die before reaching medical attention and a further 20% die in the next 24 h. To what extent specific organ system dysfunctions contribute to the terminal events that lead to death is unknown. Despite the fact that many patients die in monitored settings, detailed data concerning the mode of death (e.g., terminal cardiac arrhythmias) have not been reported.

The incidence of an abnormal EKG varies with the central process. For example, EKG abnormalities have been reported in 50%–70% of subjects with intracerebral hemorrhage, 15%–40% of individuals with nonhemorrhagic stroke, and 40%–70% of subjects with subarachnoid hemorrhage (Weidler 1974; Norris et al. 1978; Myers et al. 1982; Talman 1985). A poor prognosis has been associated with the presence of new EKG abnormalities in ischemic stroke (Lavy et al. 1974). A similarly poor prognosis occurs with combinations of four EKG findings in subarachnoid hemorrhage: peaked P-waves, short PR-intervals, prolonged acute QTc- and large U-waves (Cruickshank et al. 1974). In one series, 80% of the patients with ST-depression died after subarachnoid hemorrhage, in contrast to 33% of patients without ST depression (Hersch 1964). Yamour et al. (1980), in a retrospective study, found a higher incidence of EKG abnormalities such as QT-prolongation and "neurogenic" T-waves in those patients with frontal lobe spontaneous or traumatic hemorrhage compared with other cerebral areas. It is perhaps relevant that of the six cases with nontraumatic frontal lobe hemorrhages, those with EKG changes had lesions in the "dominant" frontal lobe. The one patient with a right-sided, nondominant lesion had no EKG changes.

Although ST-T changes associated with CNS disease are typical of those seen with myocardial injury or ischemia (Marriott 1977), vector cardiography has not suggested such an injury in affected individuals (Hugenholtz 1962). This result may be explained by the "spotty necrosis" seen in the heart following behaviorally induced stress cardiomyopathy (Johannson et al. 1974; Cebelin and Hirch 1980). The ischemic "islands" provide the ST-T changes, but do not significantly alter the conduction pathway of the depolarizing wavefront that travels between them in the nonischemic "sea."

Role of Cardiac Sympathetics (Stellate)

There are many studies linking the brain to myocardial injury and arrhythmias. Tachyarrhythmias will develop under appropriate intense stimulation of sympathetic cardiac nerves, by accelerating depolarization of the sinoatrial node (West et al. 1956). The opposite effect (bradycardia and bradyarrhythmias) results from aectylcholine application or vagal stimulation (West et al. 1956). Lepeschkin and coworkers (1960) infused norepinephrine or epinephrine intravenously into normal subjects and produced arrhythmias and conduction disturbances very much resembling "central" stimulation. Grossman (1976) showed the converse, namely, by interrupting sympathetic activity centrally mediated arrhythmias could be eliminated. In the cat, Weidler et al. (1976) showed that both atropine and propranolol together were required to stop life-threatening arrhythmias from cerebral ischemia. However, application of this information to clinical patients, at least with respect to beta-receptor blockade, could not be demonstrated in the case of a woman with subarachnoid hemorrhage and multifocal VPBs who did not respond to propranolol, but did respond to 1% lidocaine instilled into her left stellate ganglion (Grossman 1976).

Several experimental studies have shown a different physiologic effect for the left and right stellate ganglion. The left stellate ganglion has a greater arrhythmogenic effect (ventricular and supraventricular) when directly stimulated, not seen on right stellate ganglion stimulation (Schwartz et al. 1976). Similar arrhythmias can be produced by cooling the right stellate ganglion, giving a relative increase in activity of the left. A reduced ventricular refractory period is seen more frequently with stimulation of the left stellate ganglion, and this may be the reason for the increased risk of ventricular fibrillation with potentially profound clinical implications. Right stellectomy parodoxically results in a striking fall in the threshold.

Role of Cardiac Parasympathetics (Vagus)

The role of vagal activity in ventricular arrhythmogenesis is still unclear (Talman 1985). The traditional view that the vagus exerts little or no influence on ventricular electrical properties was challenged when Kent and Epstein (1976) reported that vagal stimulation significantly increased the threshold for ventricular fibrillation in both normal and ischemic myocardium. This protective effect was also seen when sympathetic activity was increased, but not seen when adrenergic input to the heart was largely prevented by beta-blockade. Recently, seven survivors of cardiac arrest were found to have significantly more abnormalities on tests of parasympathetic activity (severe vagal dysfunction) compared with controls (Sterman et al. 1986).

It appears from animal studies that the consequence of increasing vagal (cholinergic) activity to the heart depends on the time interval after the acute ischemic episode. Early (1st h) and late (6–24 h) dysrhythmias differ (Lazara et al. 1974; Scherlag et al. 1974; Corr and Gillis 1978). Early malignant dysrhythmias depend primarily on a reentrant mechanism whereas the relatively benign late dysrhythmias result from enhanced cardiac automaticity. Vagal stimulation during the 1st h after coronary occlusion has revealed: (1) mitigation or termination of the rhythm disturbance, (2) improved rate of rise of the ischemic zone electrogram, (3) increased ventricular fibrillation (VF) threshold, (4) reduced incidence of serious ventricular dysrhythmias, (5) decreased number of animals developing VF, and (6) increased time of onset to ventricular dysrhythmias (Corr and Gillis 1978; see refs. within). On the other hand, 24 h after coronary occlusion, vagal stimulation exacerbates ventricular dysrhythmias due to the unmasking of enhanced ventricular automaticity (Scherlag et al. 1974). Olson et al. (1974) in a preliminary study gave edrophonium to patients with acute myocardial infarctions in the first 24 h. This treatment failed to alter the incidence of total VPBs, although couplets and episodes of unsustained ventricular tachycardia were more frequent in the treated group. This deleterious effect was predicted by animal studies and supports the concept that only in early ischemia can a beneficial influence be expected. No clinical data currently exist from this early interval. Animal studies on the effect of bilateral vagotomy after coronary occlusion are conflicting, probably due to the natural differences in vagal tone after coronary occlusion in dogs and cats (Corr and Gillis 1978).

Role of the Diencephalon

Cardiovascular functions are also influenced by stimulation of the hypothalamus. Stimulation of the posterior lateral part of the hypothalamus produces an increase in blood pressure and heart rate (Garvey and Melville 1969; Pitts et al. 1981). Vasodilation and depressor responses have been seen chiefly from anterior hypothalamic stimulation (Korteweg et al. 1957).

Ranson et al. (1935) found only sympathetic responses to hypothalamic electrical stimulation. There is an almost immediate frequency-dependent increase in sympathetic activity in the inferior cardiac nerve with hypothalamic stimulation. Stimulation of the "cardioaccelerator center" of the posterior hypothalamus of dogs, performed by Lown and Verrier (1976), resulted in a lower threshold for VF in association with acute myocardial ischemia. Although cardiac arrhythmias following hypothalamic stimulation, in part, may be vagally mediated, at least three lines of evidence are inconsistent with this hypothesis. First, only sympathetic activity results from hypothalamic stimulation. Second, diencephalic stimulation elicits ventricular arrhythmias that are solely sympathetically mediated (Mauck et al. 1964; Hockman et al. 1966). Finally, the decreased VF threshold that follows hypothalamic stimulation was independent of vagal or adrenal function but was blocked by beta-adrenergic antagonists (Verrier et al. 1975). Garvey and Melville (1969) showed that lateral hypothalamic stimulation in dogs produced a marked increase in sympathetic activity with emergence of ST changes and arrhythmias. The arrhythmias were intensified by coronary artery ligation. If the stimulation was strong enough, it could produce VF in the nonligated heart. The sympathetic system as the only source of arrhythmias, however, is not supported by the work of Manning and Cotton (1962) or by Skinner et al. (1975). Manning and Cotton (1962) showed in cats that stimulation of the distal end of the cut vagus nerve resulted in a decrease in the sinus rate of the heart. Stimulation of the right stellate ganglion produced an increase in heart rate without producing arrhythmias. Stimulation of the fields of Forel produced multiple arrhythmias that were abolished by cooling the vagus nerve. Simultaneous stimulation of both parasympathetic and sympathetic systems produced arrhythmias similar to those evoked by diencephalic stimulation. Electric stimulation of the midbrain reticular formation and the posterior hypothalamus can produce sinus tachycardia, A-V dissociation, bigeminy, trigeminy, and unifocal or multifocal ventricular tachycardia (Talman 1985).

Role of the Cortex

The effects of cortical stimulation on the cardiovascular system have been reviewed (Delgado 1960; Weinberg and Fuster 1960; Talman 1985). The anterior half of the brain, including the tip of the frontal lobe, motor and premotor cortex, anterior part of the temporal lobe, insula, cingulate gyrus, and orbital frontal cortex, all contain specific pressor and depressor loci. The cortical specificity in evoking autonomic responses is underscored by the following: (1) separate pressor and depressor points are located within 3–4 mm of each other, (2) all vasomotor responses are abolished by local anesthesia of the cortex underlying the electrode, (3) the responses are eliminated by undercutting the cortex, and (4) when pathways degenerate after destruction of the overlying cortex no responses can be obtained. The autonomic pressure effects can be evoked by stimulation below the somatomotor threshold and they can be evoked in curarized animals.

Hall and colleagues (1977) drew attention to the observations that acute irritative lesions in the basal forebrain regions may lead to electrocardiographic changes and myocardial lesions. Multifocal myocardial lesions resembling those induced by coronary artery injection of catecholamines or by hypothalamic stimulation may be found at autopsy in patients with subarachnoid hemorrhage near the hypothalamus. Cropp and Manning (1960) reported that in patients with subarachnoid hemorrhage near the orbital cortex 3 of 15 had myocardial lesions at autopsy.

Significant stimulation along the trajectory of the frontocortical-brain stem pathway will produce cardiac arrhythmias of ventricular origin in the normal heart (Skinner and Reed 1981; see also refs within). Stimulation of the cingulate cortex of the frontal lobe can stop the heart (Smith 1945). Ventricular ectopy appears to be the result of the joint activation of both sympathetic and parasympathetic effectors (Manning and Cotton 1962; Skinner et al. 1975; Skinner et al. 1983). No cortical region has yet been found which can be regarded as influencing autonomic function only. To the contrary, all available evidence indicates that the "autonomic functions" of the cerebral cortex are subserved by areas which are also concerned with somatic activity.

The majority of these studies have demonstrated that increased sympathetic tone followed by arrhythmias results from CNS stimulation. However, CNS lesions are usually thought to be destructive rather than stimulative. That the vast majority of cases describing CNS-mediated cardiac arrhythmias involve either hemorrhagic (particularly subarachnoid hemorrhage) or potentially focally epileptogenic (trauma, surgery, or tumors) lesions is therefore notable. The common physiologic denominator could be neuronal excitation that increases the activation of sympathetic preganglionic neurons (Talman 1985). The common anatomic denominator appears to be the orbitofrontal cortex-hypothalamic-brain stem pathway.

Stress, Pain, and Emotion

Cannon (1931) developed the concept of a cerebral defense system and recognized that although the neural expression of emotion may be subcortical, cortical processes are much involved in the total behavioral-physiological reaction. For example, the difference in the response of an individual confronted by a real bear versus a stuffed bear is discrimination at the cortical level. This discriminatory process may subsequently trigger subcortical systems to carry out the complete emotional reaction. Cannon postulated that the response system consists of a priority controller (a discriminator) that regulates other component channels such as the sensory input, the behavioral motor effectors, and the appropriate autonomic support for the behavior. He argued that such a cerebral defense system must have important survival value and thus be a focus for natural selection.

Experimental Models

A number of experimental animal models have been developed to study the behavioral induction of cardiovascular changes, including arrhythmia and sudden death (Lown and Verrier 1976; Corr and Gillis 1978; Skinner et al. 1975; Malliana et al. 1980). Animals subjected to operationally defined environmental stresses within these models (e.g., novel surroundings, conditioned stimuli forewarning cutaneous shock or negative reinforcers) may produce autonomic changes, cardiac arrhythmias, and, if severe enough, VF.

The domestic pig appears to be the most satisfactory animal model. Pigs can be obtained with a known behavioral history, their cardiovascular system is more homologous to humans than other animals, and they are known to die from "transportation stress," a form of sudden death.

Skinner and colleagues (1975) examined the effect of psychologic stress on ventricular fibrillation-latency following temporary coronary-artery occlusion. The mere introduction of the pig to the unfamiliar laboratory environment results in arrhythmias, including VF, when associated with acute coronary artery occlusion. Following disocclusion and electrical cardioversion, the electrocardiogram became normal within minutes. The hearts of animals not subjected to occlusion for more than 20 min showed no histologic evidence of damage. Adaptation to the laboratory environment, however, markedly increased VF latency and even prevented its occurrence in all cases following 8 days of adaptation. This effect was reversed by the introduction of a novel stimulus in the form of a mild cutaneous shock. Animals with permanent coronary artery occlusion that were adapted to the laboratory did not develop VF for the subsequent 24 h.

Johanssen et al. (1974) studied stress in pigs using a short-acting muscle relaxant to produce restraint that, when combined with strong cutaneous shock, enhanced the stress. A variety of EKG changes, including ventricular arrhythmias, ST-T changes, and even lethal VF, were elicited. All animals subjected to stress showed acute cardiac cell damage resembling that produced by intracoronary artery injection of catecholamines. Thus, stressful stimuli can cause EKG changes and arrhythmias including VF. In contrast, in the laboratory animal adaptation to a stressful stimulus can prevent VF from occurring in the acutely ischemic heart.

"Thalamic Gating System"

In order for an individual to perceive stress, his or her attention must be drawn toward the stressful event. Neurophysiologic studies in the cat reveal that two systems are involved in the control of sensory input during attention (Skinner and Yingling 1977), the mesencephalic reticular formation (MRF) and the frontal cortex, both of which converge on the thalamic reticular nucleus. The latter acts as a switching mechanism that gates the ascent of sensory information through the thalamus to the primary receptive cortex. Stimulation at specific sites in the thalamic reticular nucleus attenuates the sensory evoked response for a specific sensory modality. Cryoblockade of part of the fibers that project from the frontal cortex to the thalamus will cause the enhancement of the evoked potential to a previously habituated stimulus. There is modality-specific organization in the frontocortical component of the system that regulates the sensory influx. Stimulation of the mesencephalic reticular formation, in contrast, produces an increase in the amplitude of all sensory evoked potentials to habituated stimuli. This latter effect indicates a nonspecific effect on the regulation of sensory input to the cerebral cortex. Skinner and Yingling (1977) concluded that the thalamic gating system is controlled by specific output from the frontal lobe, as well as nonspecific activity in the mesencephalic reticular formation, during the process of focusing attention to a meaningful stimulus.

The Cerebral Event-Related Slow Potential

The response of an individual to a stressful stimulus is associated with a negative-event-related slow potential (ERSP) in the frontal cortex. The ERSP is associated with norepinephrine release, cyclic AMP formation in the underlying tissue, and a decrease in K_0^+ (Skinner 1984a,b; Skinner and Molnar 1983; Skinner et al. 1976; Reed et al. 1978).

Recently, Skinner (1984b) showed that some neurons in the frontal cortex manifest slow changes in membrane potential when the conscious animal responded to a tone that forewarns cutaneous shock. This result, shown in Fig. 11.1, suggests that an extracellular ERSP is produced when the neurons manifest their slow event-related membrane potentials. A complex integrative mechanism involving a change in electrotonic structure is indicated by the lack of correlation between the slow membrane depolarization and the action potential frequency. If we knew more about this complex mechanism, we might then know how the event-related activity in the frontal cortex is converted into the deleterious autonomic outflow that increases cardiac vulnerability.

Stressors

The effects of stress on cardiac vulnerability may possibly be mediated by a specific brain system. Exposure to behaviorally defined states of stress or electric stimulation of peripheral neural structures will significantly enhance susceptibility of the heart to ventricular fibrillation. An understanding of a cerebral system that links the environmental stressors to the deleterious autonomic outflow is now much closer (see ref. in Skinner 1984b). In the normal heart electrical stimulation along a locus from the frontal cortex to the brain stem will produce both a variety of arrhythmias and cardiac myopathies (Talman 1985; Ulyanisky et al. 1977). The extreme effects include VF and myofibrillar degeneration. Lethal arrhythmias and permanent myocardial damage can also be produced by physical or psychologic stressors (Johansson et al. 1974; Corley et al. 1973). Stress cardiomyopathy has now been documented in humans (Cebelin and Hirsch 1980). Stressors specifically evoke electrical and chemical perturbations in the cerebral cortex (Skinner and Yingling 1976, 1977; Skinner et al. 1978a,b). This same cerebral system, when blocked physically, prevents the initiation of VF following acute coronary occlusions (Skinner and Reed 1981). Thus, defined environmental events evoke specific cerebral responses within a higher neural system that is known to regulate cardiac vulnerability.

Recently, a circadian variation in the frequency of onset of acute myocardial infarction has been found (Muller et al. 1985). This variation was not found in patients receiving beta-blockade and further suggests that central neural and/or neuroendocrine factors may play a role in initiating myocardial infarction.

Cardiac arrhythmias may be produced by anxiety through autonomic mechanisms. This was studied in 18 patients with heart disease: the mean heart rate increased during stress from 71 to 84 beats/min and the mean frequency of ventricular premature complexes increased from 2.96 to 6.62/min (Lown et al. 1978). In one patient with a history of recurrent episodes of ventricular tachycardia and fibrillation, ventricular tachycardia developed during psychologic stress. Paroxysmal ventricular tachycardia due to anxiety has been described in a young normal subject (Harvey and Levine 1952). Psychologic stress-induced cardiac arrhythmias have also been documented in animals (Lown et al. 1973). A man with episodic VF but no evidence of heart disease showed VPBs which were increased in frequency during psychologic stress or rapid eye movement sleep. The VPBs were abolished with propranolol or meditation (Lown et al. 1976). A study of 117 patients who presented with VF or symptomatic ventricular tachycardia not temporally associated with acute myocardial infarction showed that 25 had acute psychologic disturbances, usually anger, in the 24 h preceding onset of the dysrhythmia (Reich et al. 1981). These 25 patients were different from the rest of the series in having less severe structural heart disease.

Personality

Personality traits may predispose to heart disease, as described by Friedman and Rosenman (1959). They defined a section of the population (type A) with enhanced traits of aggressiveness, ambitiousness, competitive drive, primary work-orientation, and involvement with task subject to time restrictions. Subjects without such personality traits and behavioral characteristics were called type B. Type A behavior is associated with an increased risk of coronary heart disease (Friedman and Rosenman 1959; Rosenman et al. 1975). In a prospective study of 3154 middle-aged men, a type A behavior pattern was related to the incidence of coronary disease and was found to be independent of interrelationships of behavior patterns with other risk factors (Rosenman et al. 1975). The relative risk for men aged 39–49 years was 1.87 and for men aged 50–59 years of 2.16, as compared with type B subjects. This personality phenomenon has been confirmed (Jenkins 1976).

An increased response of plasma noradrenaline and adrenaline to psychologic stress can be seen in type A subjects (Friedman et al. 1975; Glass et al. 1980). They may also show increased cardiovascular reactivity, although results have been conflicting (Steptoe and Ross 1981). Myocardial damage or platelet aggregation could be directly caused by increased catecholamine secretion but such increases as have been documented are not completely explanatory. Type A subjects are prone to rapid alternation of active coping and giving up—or, in other words, hyperreactivity and hyporeactivity (Johnson et al. 1984)—and it has been suggested this could dispose to coronary disease (Glass 1977).

Type A subjects are probably vulnerable to the effects of psychologic and social stresses in producing myocardial infarction or sudden death (Johnson et al. 1984). There is evidence that myocardial infarction is frequently preceded by important life events (Theorell 1982). Depression is frequent in the period before myocardial infarction, more commonly in type A subjects (Folger and Appels 1982). They are most susceptible to reinfarction (Jenkins et al. 1976), which could in part be explained by the emotional stress of the first episode. In support of this, psychosocial stress in monkeys has been associated with increased arteriosclerotic disease (Kaplan et al. 1983).

Central Nervous System—Sudden Cardiac Death Link

Background

Sudden death accounts for approximately two-thirds of the 600 000 annual deaths that are attributable to coronary artery disease in the United States (Ruskin 1980). The World Health Organization defines sudden death as death occurring within 24 h of the onset of clinical signs and symptoms. Almost 50% of these individuals experience abrupt or "instantaneous" death within seconds or minutes of engaging in normal activity immediately prior to their collapse (Friedman et al. 1973). Instantaneous death in this population is almost always due to a catastrophic arrhythmia, most commonly ventricular tachycardia, which degenerates into ventricular fibrillation (Klein et al. 1979; Liberthson et al. 1974). Autopsy examinations in victims of instantaneous death only occasionally reveal evidence of acute occlusive coronary thrombosis, recent myocardial infarction, or both. In a majority of cases no evidence of acute infarction is discovered despite the presence of chronic atherosclerotic coronary artery disease (Ruskin 1980; Spain and Brades 1970). Thus it is a plausible hypothesis that sudden cardiac death is an electrical death as a result of VF in the absence of acute myocardial infarction.

The most common pathologic finding in patients with sudden cardiac death by far is coronary arteriosclerosis. Victims of sudden cardiac death have more severe and extensive obstructive coronary artery disease than comparable individuals dying accidentally. In addition to coronary artery disease, the presence of hypertension, cardiac enlargement, heart failure, ventricular hypertrophy, and chronic obstructive pulmonary disease have been identified as factors that are associated with an increased risk of sudden cardiac death (Ruskin 1980; Moss 1975).

Pathophysiology

To date, there has not been a specific structural lesion in the CNS related to the syndrome of sudden death, although there is considerable evidence that suggests a CNS mechanism is prominent in its genesis. Lown (1979) stated that, "the focus should be shifted from the heart as target to the brain as trigger."

Ventricular fibrillation, the presumed cause of most cases of sudden death, can be reproducibly elicited in the normal as well as the ischemic heart upon stimulation of cardiac sympathetic nerves as previously discussed (Talman 1985; Lown 1979; Schwartz et al. 1976; Verrier et al. 1974). It is less clear as to the mechanism by which the sympathetic nerves may be stimulated with sufficient specificity by the CNS. Stress, and an individual's particular response to it through the CNS, may play a role (Lown 1979; Light et al. 1983). The importance of genetic and developmental factors in the autonomic responses to stressful stimuli has been demonstrated (Ely 1981; Schwartz 1976). The type and extent of stress may be exceedingly important factors in the production of these arrhythmias. Stressful situations in which need for action is recognized, but which would be futile even if performed (no escape), are the most conducive to VF and sudden death (Engel 1976). This is supported by the observation of increased cardiac arrhythmias and sudden death in subjects exposed to a natural disaster (Trichopoulous et al. 1983; Vordis et al. 1983). Sudden death has been described in association with a voodoo spell ("sympathoadrenal" activation) by Cannon (1942).

Autonomic activation, especially if asymmetrically favoring the left side, can lead to VF (Schwartz et al. 1976; Armour et al. 1972; Hageman et al. 1973; Haws and Burgess 1978). The VF threshold in normal, and especially in ischemic, myocardium is lowered during the influence of sympathetic activation (Lown 1979; Schwartz et al. 1976). The level of autonomic tone is intimately related to behavioral events that are clearly under CNS control (Benson et al.

1974; Ekman et al. 1983; Gold and Cohen 1981). Psychologic stress can elicit pathologic autonomic discharges (Engel 1976; Cannon 1942; Johnsson and Hansson 1977; Obrist et al. 1974). Destroying the hypothalamus and its descending pathways normalizes the stress-induced decreased VF threshold (Skinner and Reed 1981). These studies support a causal role for a CNS mechanism in sudden cardiac death.

Stress

In a review of 275 examples of sudden death culled from the newspapers, Engel (1976) identified eight life settings: 21% died on the impact of news of the collapse or death of a close person, and 9% on the threat of imminent loss of such a person. Twenty percent died during the first 3 weeks of acute grief and 3% died during mourning or the anniversary of a death. Public humiliation or loss of self-esteem resulted in sudden death in 6%. Twenty-seven percent died suddenly in settings of extreme personal danger or upon threat of injury, whereas 7% died shortly after the danger had passed. Six percent collapsed during the excitement of reunion, triumph, or a happy ending. The common denominator to all these situations was that the circumstances were impossible for the victims to ignore and they responded with overwhelming excitation.

Myers and Dewar (1975) studied the circumstances prevailing at the time of sudden death in 100 males with coronary artery disease and found that 23% had significant psychologic stress in the 3 min before death and another 48% in the preceding 24 h.

Bereavement was associated with about 40% greater than expected death rate in widowers during the 6 months following the deaths of their wives (Parkes et al. 1969). Rahe et al. (1973) found that patients who develop myocardial infarction and sudden death have a significant increase in certain life events (e.g., bereavement, job insecurity, recently having moved) during the preceding 6 months.

Dangerous arrhythmias have been described in spectator sportsmen (Rose 1974), in patients with myocardial infarction during ward rounds (Jarvinen 1955), and in six patients who died suddenly while awaiting coronary artery surgery (Lewis and Gotsman 1974). The role of exertion and fright in precipitating sudden death in children with inherited QT prolongation is well documented (James 1969; Csaudy and Kiss 1973), as well as in members of families with a high incidence of unexplained sudden death (Green et al. 1969; McRae et al. 1974). Wellens et al. (1972) described a 14-year-old girl who, being awakened by a sudden loud voice, developed QT prolongation followed by premature ventricular complexes leading to ventricular fibrillation. During the initial episode, she had been suddenly awakened from sleep by a loud thunderclap.

Anorexia Nervosa

Patients with anorexia nervosa may exhibit bradycardia (Fohlin 1977), probably due to reduced sympathetic activity associated with starvation. However, patients with anorexia nervosa may also develop sinus tachycardia, prolonged

QT-interval, and S-T segment depression (Thurston and Marks 1974; Palossy and Oo 1977). Electrocardiographic abnormalities may be a specific feature of anorexia nervosa and are not associated with starvation due to other causes (Thurston and Marks 1974).

Sleep

Cardiovascular activation during rapid eye movement (REM) sleep may in some cases also act as an endogenous neurophysiologic trigger of malignant arrhythmias (Rosenblatt et al. 1973; Smith et al. 1972). Lown et al. (1973) found an increased incidence of arrhythmias during the late part of the nightly sleep period in acute myocardial infarction patients. During this interval the REM stage increases relative to non-REM sleep. This increased REM sleep, which occurs as a rebound from REM sleep deprivation or after withdrawal of drugs such as barbiturates, may be quite arrhythmogenic in those cases in which REM sleep is associated with increased arrhythmogenesis. During non-REM sleep, the QT-interval is prolonged compared with that observed during REM sleep (Rosenblatt et al. 1973; Smith et al. 1972) and prolonged QT-interval has been associated with increased vulnerability to arrhythmias (Schwartz and Wolf 1978). During non-REM sleep in pigs, VF onset is more rapid following coronary artery occlusion than the latency which occurs when the occlusion is made during REM sleep (Skinner et al. 1975). Abnormalities of autonomic control may be seen in other sleep disorders. A study of 53 patients with sleep apnea, sleep narcolepsy, or excessive drowsiness revealed marked increases in cardiac abnormalities associated with raised urinary and plasma catecholamine concentrations (Clarke et al. 1980).

Meditation

Over the years, conscious control of autonomic activity through meditation has been sought. Practitioners of transcendental meditation can reduce their heart rate, perspiration volume, and metabolism, the latter indicated by a fall in oxygen consumption and blood lactate (Wallace et al. 1971; Wallace and Benson 1972). Zen meditation may also produce similar physiologic changes (Woolfolk 1975). Meditation has generally been viewed as a state of deep physiologic relaxation (Johnson et al. 1984).

Epilepsy

A high incidence of sudden unexpected death occurs in epileptics with seizure-induced cardiac arrhythmias (Jay and Leestma 1981). Although this brain-heart effect is rare, it is most often seen in cases of temporal lobe epilepsy (Gastaut 1953). Ictal cardiac arrhythmias occurred in 52% of seizures in one recent study (Blumhardt et al. 1986). Vagal stimulation produced during an epileptic discharge might be so severe that cardiac arrest may occur, and a patient in whom episodic sinoatrial heart block was associated with a right temporal seizure focus has been described (Phizackerley et al. 1954). Ictal excessive sympathetic discharge during seizures (Simon et al. 1984) may also have a role in sudden unexpected death in epileptics (Terrence et al. 1981).

A left parasagittal meningioma causing seizures associated with transient atrial fibirillation has been described (Mathew et al. 1970). Another patient with a glioma and a seizure focus within the right frontal lobe presented with paroxysmal atrial tachycardia, dizziness, and faintness but with no loss of consciousness (Rush et al. 1977). Pritchett et al. (1980) reported two patients with episodes of paroxysmal supraventricular tachycardia with associated disturbance of consciousness. These spells were attributed to seizure foci in the temporal lobes as both patients showed epileptiform discharges on the electroencephalogram. Anticonvulsant therapy prevented cardiac arrhythmias in one.

Arrhythmias in association with epileptic discharges are presumably due to altered autonomic activity. A marked variability in cardiac sympathetic and parasympathetic neural discharge was seen with drug-induced seizures in cats (Lathers and Schraeder 1982). Increased seizure activity was associated with increased sympathetic neural firing. Cardiac autonomic neuronal activity did not always respond appropriately to changes in blood pressure, a possible factor in the hypertension which may accompany seizures.

Epilepsy may also induce hypoxic or ischemic cardiac damage. Falconer and Rajs (1976) studied nine patients at postmortem with epilepsy-related deaths, and found arterial wall fibrosis and interstitial scarring. Repeated hypothalamic stimulation in monkeys produced cardiac arrhythmias, an increase in arterial blood pressure, and structural myocardial damage (Chen et al. 1974). The cardiac lesions were similar to those induced by intracoronary catecholamines and were probably related to increased sympathetic discharge.

Sudden Infant Death Syndrome

The sudden infant death syndrome (SIDS) is the leading cause of death in Western countries among infants 1 week to 1 year old (Johnson et al. 1984). A possible mechanism involves an abnormality of cardiac autonomic control leading to a primary cardiac asystole or a lethal arrhythmia, such as VF (Froggatt and James 1973; Schwartz 1976; Matthews 1984). Abrupt sympathetic discharges through an asymmetrically developed sympathetic innervation of the heart with left-sided dominance has been one postulated mechanism. Another mechanism could be increased vagal activity provoking cardiac arrest. Abnormal autonomic control of the heart in an infant who subsequently died has been reported (Salk et al. 1974). Kahn et al. (1983) studied cardiac responses to ocular compression and showed a prolonged asystole greater than 2 s in 10 of 35 infants with near deaths from SIDS, and in none of the 69 normal control infants. Near death from SIDS has been shown in infants with prolongation of the Q-T interval, again possibly due to asymmetric cardiac sympathetic innervation (Schwartz 1976).

"Dual" Regulation Hypothesis

Psychosocial stress is clearly a contributor to the incidence of lethal arrhythmias and sudden death. Giving up in the face of emotional arousal and psychologic uncertainty are conditions felt to be conducive to vasodepressor syncope and sudden death (Engel 1978). In this setting it has been proposed that there may be simultaneous activation of two biologic emergency regulatory systems — flight-fight (sympathetic) and conservation-withdrawal (parasympathetic). The tonic situation is one in which vasodepressor syncope and benign cardiac arrhythmias and sudden death may develop. This dual regulation hypothesis has recently had further support. It has been shown in the psychologically stressed pig that when the heart spontaneously goes into the resting rate, heart-muscle phosphorylase-activity does not decline, as it does in the unstressed pig (Skinner et al. 1983). Phosphorylase, the rate-limiting enzyme controlling glycogenolysis, is thought to be activated by beta-receptor stimulation. Parasympathetic tone, however, must also be high, since cardiac work remains low. Further, during the stage of slow-wave sleep in a pig with a left ventricular infarction, ventricular ectopy is markedly higher than in the awake state, and the ectopy is immediately suppressed on entry into the REM sleep state. During the slow-wave sleep state, heart rate is kept constant by a combination of high parasympathetic and sympathetic tones (Skinner et al. 1975). Electrical stimulation of both the vagus nerve and the stellate ganglion together results in cardiac arrhythmias, whereas stimulation of either cardiac nerve alone does not (Manning and Cotton 1962). Thus, dual autonomic activation seems to be the mechanism by which cardiac vulnerability is increased, and this activation may arise under certain stressful conditions which in some cases may seem benign.

Long QT Syndrome: A Human Model of Neurogenic Sudden Death?

In 1957 an inherited syndrome of congenital deafness, prolongation of the QT-interval, syncope, and sudden death was described (Jorvell and Lange-Nielson 1957). A similar inherited syndrome without the deafness has also been reported (Mathews et al. 1972). Both autosomal recessive and autosomal dominant inheritance has been described in families with long QT-intervals. A few patients have had a long QT-interval and recurrent syncope on a sporadic (noninherited) basis (Moss and Schwartz 1979). The mechanism of syncope or sudden death, which has been documented in some cases, is ventricular tachycardia or fibrillation, respectively. The long QT-interval apparently represents a prolonged ventricular vulnerability period; a ventricular ectopic beat is thus more likely than usual to cause a ventricular tachyarrhythmia. The condition is usually diagnosed because of syncope between the ages of 2 and 6 years but may become apparent for the first time during adulthood. Why it is not more often apparent at birth is unclear (Langslit and Sorland 1975). The QT-interval may vary from time to time or even from complex to complex in the same patient. Although the reason for its prolongation is unknown, it is believed that it may be related to a disparity of right and left cardiac sympathetic activity, with the left side dominant (Moss and Schwartz 1979; Schwartz and Malliani 1975). Recent further study has found right-sided sympathetic deficiency manifested by a slower heart rate than controls in newborns and children up through 3 years of age (Vincent 1986). Since there was no difference from controls in older children or adults, the data were compatible with high sympathetic tone contributing to the resting heart rate during early years of life and primarily parasympathetic control of resting heart rate subsequently.

There is a high mortality in patients who are recognized because of syncope, but untreated. Syncope or sudden death often coincide with intense physical effort or emotional reaction (Schwartz et al. 1975). The incidence of syncope or death is greatly reduced by beta-adrenergic blockade (propranolol), which also reduces the QT-interval. If propranolol therapy alone does not completely eliminate episodes of syncope, phenytoin (dilantin) should be added, which further reduces the QT-interval (Schwartz et al. 1975). If syncope recurs, despite medical therapy, stellate ganglionectomy (usually left, but perhaps bilateral) has shortened the QT-interval and stopped recurrent syncope in several patients (Moss and Schwartz 1979; Schwartz et al. 1975). Prolongation of the QT-interval on the EKG associated with arrhythmias and ventricular sudden death may also occur under a wide variety of conditions including: myotonic dystrophy, phenothiazine or tricyclic amine administration, and certain stroke syndromes (Ruskin 1980).

The physiologic mechanisms responsible for alterations in the QT-interval during neurogenic and pharmacologic sympathetic stimulation of the heart remain undefined. Since all forms of sympathetic stimulation are known to reduce ventricular recovery times, the prolongation of the observed QT-interval, despite the decrease in recovery time with some types of sympathetic stimulation, appears to be a EKG effect (Abildskov 1976). Further evidence for a neural basis for the disorder has come from a pathologic study of eight patients with the prolonged QT syndrome and sudden death (James et al. 1978). Focal neuritis and neural degeneration in the sinus node, atrioventricular node, bundle of His, and ventricular myocardium were consistent findings.

The clinical observation that the syncopal episodes almost always follow an emotional or physical stress, such as fear or anger, is crucial for the understanding of the pathogenetic mechanisms. Although the most likely etiopathogenesis suggested by clinical and experimental data is a congenital imbalance between right and left cardiac sympathetic nerves with a right-sided deficiency, the basic defect may still be an unknown intracardiac abnormality decreasing electrical stability and sensitizing the myocardium to sympathetic discharges. The ventricular arrhythmias which lead these patients to death appear to depend on sudden increases in sympathetic activity, mostly through the dominant left stellate ganglion.

Theoretical Model for Brain Regulation of Cardiac Vulnerability

Our theoretical model of how the brain regulates cardiac vulnerability during psychologic stress is summarized in Fig. 11.1. A stressor (EVENT) is transduced, projected through the thalamus to the primary cortex, and then relayed to the frontal cortex where a cellular process (P) occurs. Correlated with, but not identical to, this process P, are a set of event-related electrochemical responses. The event may or may not be perceived as stressful, depending upon the neural transactions that govern process P. Humans with recent frontal lobe damage both verbally report and behaviorally demonstrate

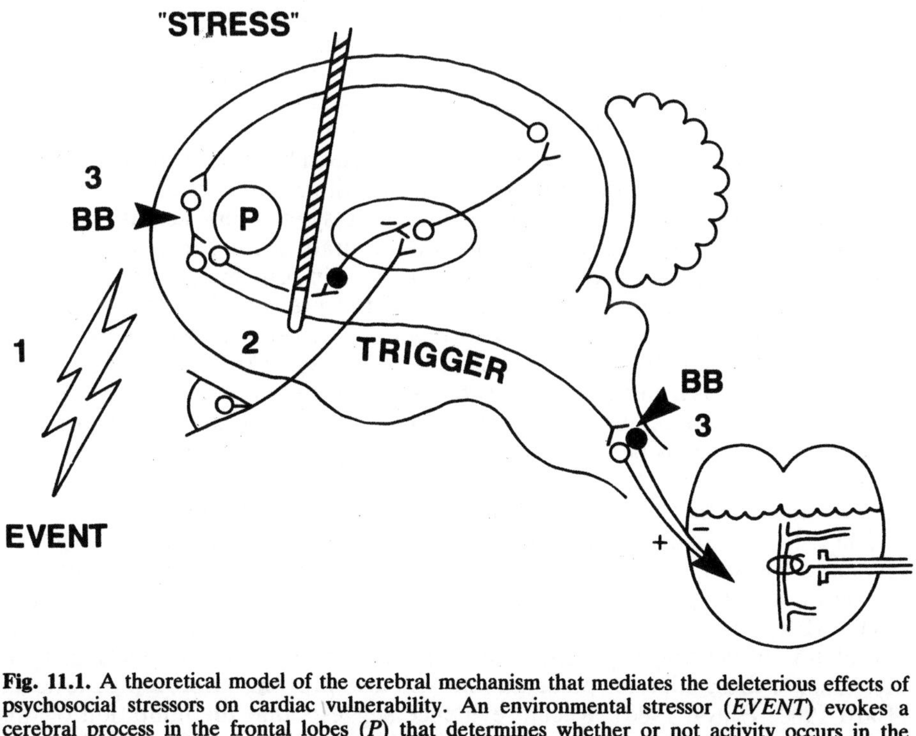

Fig. 11.1. A theoretical model of the cerebral mechanism that mediates the deleterious effects of psychosocial stressors on cardiac vulnerability. An environmental stressor (*EVENT*) evokes a cerebral process in the frontal lobes (*P*) that determines whether or not activity occurs in the frontocortical-brain stem pathway (*TRIGGER*). The activity in this pathway results in dual autonomic outflow (±) and inhibits homeostatic reflexes. The projected autonomic activity, either alone or in combination with myocardial ischemia, triggers the initiation of ventribular fibrillation. Three independent interventions can prevent the lethal consequence of coronary artery occlusion in the psychologically stressed pig: (1) behavioral adaptation to the stressful event, (2) cryogenic blockade of the frontocortical-brain stem pathway, and (3) the intracerebral injection of a beta-blocker (*BB*); the latter can inhibit known noradrenergic transactions at either the origin or termination of the trigger pathway. During process *P*, the frontal lobes also gate sensory inputs through the thalamus and control limbic activities via the amygdala.

(Teuber 1964) that they no longer have "stress"; these patients also show a complete lack of autonomic responsiveness to all psychologically meaningful stimulus-events (Rockstrob et al. 1982; Heilman et al. 1978). Emphasis should be placed upon this observation that "stress" is a cerebral reaction of a particular individual to a stimulus-event and is not an inherent feature of the stressor itself (STRESS). Depending upon the state of acquisition or adaptation to the event, process P then may (or may not) lead to the initiation of activity in the output pathway that controls the pattern of autonomic projection to the heart. The mechanism by which the event-related electrochemical correlates of the stressor evoke activity in this descending pathway (i.e., process P) is unknown, and probably highly complex, but there can be little doubt that experience-dependent modifications occur within the linkages that are associated with noradrenergic transactions. Stimulation of A1 and A5 CNS noradrenergic neurons appears to diminish sympathetic activity (Blessing et al. 1982; Loewy and McNeil 1981), as does activation of noradrenergic and adrenergic receptors within the nucleus tractus solitarius (Coote and McLeod 1974; Zandberg et al. 1979). Stimulation of C1 adrenergic neurons appears to increase sympathetic tone (Ross et al. 1984), suggesting that CNS neurons lying close together may have different—even opposite—effects on sympathetic activity. An increase in the VF threshold occurs with an increase in global CNS catecholamine activity caused by tyrosine given intravenously (Scott et al. 1981). This suggests that decreased CNS catecholamine receptor stimulation may help mediate cardiac arrhythmias produced by CNS lesions. An increase in brain serotonin appears to reduce cardiac sympathetic activity (Baum and Shropshire 1975) and increase VF threshold. More recently, however, increased sympathetic activity has been demonstrated following direct stimulation of brain stem serotonergic fibers (McCall 1984), suggesting that the role of serotonin remains unclear.

Experience-dependent neuronal activity of the prefrontal cortex—based on the "behavioral relevance" of the environmental event—has been demonstrated in monkeys (Furster 1973; Kubota et al. 1980; Kojima 1980; Thorpe et al. 1983). Therefore, there is a cortical neural substrate for different reactions to identical physical or environmental stimuli—dependent on context and past experience (Mesulam 1986). This behavioral flexibility of higher species including humans that allows for far greater autonomy from the environment may have the same neural substrate that is capable of triggering sudden cardiac death.

The activity in the frontocortical-brain stem pathway represents a trigger of increased cardiac vulnerability, because its functional blockage or electric activation will, respectively, prevent or evoke ventricular fibrillation (Fig. 11.1, TRIGGER). The presentation of a behavioral stressor or the direct electric stimulation of the trigger pathway will evoke dual autonomic outputs (Fig. 11.1, ±). Each of these stimulus presentations will also prevent baroreceptor reflexes (Bard 1960; Hilton 1980). Recent evidence suggests that the inhibition of this homeostatic reflex is a significant sign of the increased state of vulnerability of the ischemic heart to VF (Billman et al. 1982; Schwartz et al. 1984). Thus, the occurrence of dual autonomic regulation and baroreceptor inhibition, each of which is predictive of the increased state of cardiac vulnerability, may be produced by a common higher cerebral influence upon the brain stem.

Therapeutic Implications

Attempts to reduce the incidence of life-threatening arrhythmias in patients at high risk of sudden cardiac death should be directed against those factors which may induce or increase cardiac electrical instability. The overwhelming evidence pointing to the crucial role of the cardiac innervation as the precipitating factor implies that measures which prevent or antagonize sympathetic or parasympathetic effects might prove beneficial.

Beta Blockade

Beta-adrenergic-blocking drugs have gained wide clinical acceptance as antiarrhythmic agents. Similarly, surgical ablation of the cardiac sympathetics has been suggested as a possible therapeutic procedure.

The reason that beta-blockers, and perhaps other antiarrhythmic drugs, are not remarkably effective in reducing cardiac vulnerability may be related to undesirable side effects that occur with increasing dosage. It is reported that most persons taking racemic propranolol experience a 30-min period of confusion immediately following each ingestion of the drug (Goodman and Gilman 1970). It has also been reported (Solomon 1983) that persons taking this beta-blocker have a 30% reduction in short-term memory recall. Thus higher levels of the peripherally administered beta-blockers, which may be more efficacious in reducing cardiac vulnerability because of the increased cerebral concentration, may not be tolerated by cardiac patients because of the incapacitating effect on their memory mechanisms. How then does one deal with this tolerance problem? The solution is likely to appear when we have a better understanding of the cerebral mechanisms that underlie the stress reactions of the brain.

The fact that peripheral blockade of sympathetic beta-receptors is not completely successful in preventing stress-evoked increases in measures of cardiac vulnerability may be related to the dual autonomic outflow. Although the intravenous injection of beta-blockers alone prevents some stress-induced increases in vulnerability (Matta et al. 1976), intravenous propranolol has no effect on the prevention of ischemia-induced VF in the pig model of acute coronary artery occlusion. The *intracerebral* injection of *l*-propranolol (0.01 mg/kg), however, does significantly retard the occurrence of VF (Skinner 1984b). This observation in the psychologically stressed pig implies that the antiarrhythmic property of propranolol may in fact be due to its cerebral action, and not to its peripheral affect upon the cardiac beta-receptors.

A similar conclusion about the central action of other antiarrhythmic drugs has been drawn following a study in cardiac patients. In this double-blind, randomized-crossover, placebo-controlled study (Skinner et al. 1982), morizine (Ethmazine) or disopyramide (Norpace) reduced ventricular ectopic rates, as expected, but additionally either drug was noted to reduce the amplitude of the cerebral event-related slow potential (ERSP), a potential previously noted to be specific for frontal lobe functioning in both animals and humans (Knight et al. 1980). The ERSP and ventricular arrhythmia-rate were found to have a statistically significant linear correlation over the three drug conditions. In a subsequent study the two measures were varied between individual patients; the slope of the correlation-coefficient found in the latter experiment was the same as that observed in the within-subject drug-study. These findings imply a tight coupling between a specific cerebral potential (i.e., the ERSP) and cardiac vulnerability to arrhythmogenesis.

Inhibitory Neuropeptides

A new approach to pharmacologic intervention in the mechanism of sudden cardiac death may be at hand. Instead of reducing cardiac vulnerability with intracerebral beta-blockers, whose receptors are widely distributed throughout the brain, inhibitory neuropeptides may be found that are specific to the output cells in the frontal cortex (i.e., the neurons mediating process P in Fig. 11.1). It is reasonable to expect this specificity of action, because it has been demonstrated for at least some of the 10 000 brain peptides (e.g., the relatively low abundance hypothalamic neuropeptide P7) that target receptors are located on as few as 100 neurons (Skinner 1984b)]. Thus, if a specific inhibitory neuropeptide can be identified that acts on the output cells forming the frontocortical-brain stem pathway, then it may be possible to invent a cerebrally acting peptidergic compound which will prevent stress-evoked arrhythmogenesis without interfering with the learning and memory mechanisms that are mediated by noradrenergic processes distributed widely throughout the brain.

Cardiac Sympathectomy

An alternative procedure for preventing or limiting sympathetic arrhythmogenic influences upon the heart is cardiac sympathectomy. Evidence from animal experiments that we have summarized above clearly shows that beneficial results can be obtained even when cardiac sympathectomy is limited to the left side by left stellectomy. Left stellectomy reduces the incidence of ventricular arrhythmias associated with short-lasting coronary occlusion and it produces a marked increase in the threshold for ventricular fibrillation. It prolongs the ventricular refractory period and increases the capability of the coronary bed to dilate. Cardiac performance is not reduced during exercise following cardiac sympathectomy. Reduction in the incidence of ventricular fibrillation associated with acute ischemia in conscious dogs with a previous myocardial infarction is also seen.

In cats and dogs the majority of sympathetic outflow to the heart is relayed via the stellate ganglia. Man requires a more extensive surgical procedure effectively to interrupt the cardiac sympathetic innervation. The left sympathetic chain must be ablated down to the fourth to fifth thoracic segment in order to provide effects comparable to those obtained in left stellate ganglionectomized dogs. On the other hand, the cephalic pole of the stellate ganglion should be left intact so as to avoid the Bernard-Horner syndrome. Thus, in man an appropriate terminology for the surgical intervention could be "high thoracic left sympathectomy" (HTLS) (Malliani et al. 1980).

High thoracic left sympathectomy, an extrapleural surgical procedure, practically has no risk, provided the locally anesthetized nerves are carefully manipulated. A possible limitation of this surgical procedure may be that sympathetic influences to the heart are largely but not completely interrupted, because fibers from the right side, though quantitatively and possibly qualitatively less important than the left fibers, remain untouched. This, however, can also be viewed as a positive aspect, as the cardiac pump would not be entirely deprived of adrenergic support (Malliani et al. 1980).

High thoracic left sympathectomy has so far been performed as a preventive procedure against lethal arrhythmias only in the rather limited number of young patients suffering from the long QT syndrome. This favorable experience, though restricted to a relatively rare syndrome, may be applied as an alternative or as a supplement to pharmacologic beta-blockade in the population of patients at risk for lethal arrhythmias consequent to cardiac ischemia.

Conclusions and Future Directions

Stimulation of the orbital frontal cortex, hypothalamus, or midbrain (prerubral fields of Forel) produces a number of cardiovascular changes, including ventricular arrhythmias and cardiomyopathy. Stimulation of both parasympathetic and sympathetic outflows together appears important in the genesis of arrhythmias. It may be the case that the central loci of stimulations that are effective in producing ventricular arrhythmias evoke simultaneously both sympathetic and parasympathetic outflows to the heart. This is most likely due to the spread of the stimulating current to specific sympathetic and parasympathetic zones, as weak currents do not evoke the arrhythmias, and it is known that the zones are close to one another anatomically. How the dual outflows are produced behaviorally remains unknown, but they do occur naturally, during sleep and certain types of stress.

There are three cerebral manipulations that will prevent the lethal consequence of acute myocardial ischemia in a psychologically stressed pig: (1) learned behavioral adaptation to the stressor event, (2) physical blockade of a trigger pathway that arises from a frontocortical site and projects to the brain stem cardioregulatory centers, and (3) intracerebral injection of a beta-blocker. The latter intervention may (1) operate directly on the mechanism by which initiation of activity occurs in the trigger pathways (i.e., process P), (2) prevent the relay of the initiated information in the trigger pathway into the dual autonomic outputs, or (3) do both. It is concluded that psychologic stressors in the environment evoke a learning-related noradrenergic process in the frontal cortex (process P) that determines whether or not activity is relayed via the frontocortical-brain stem pathway into the cardioregulatory centers; the relayed activity leads to dual autonomic outflow, an action which increases the vulnerability of the myocardium to arrhythmogenesis.

What significance the dual regulation hypothesis has for the cardiac mechanism by which VF is initiated, either directly or in combination with acute ischemia, is not yet understood. Clearly there exist local interactive mechanisms between cardiac sympathetic and parasympathetic channels (e.g., through the regulatory proteins) (Watanabe 1983). Biochemical and electrical studies of this interaction could be expected to show how the dual activation of the heart leads to the lethal electrical instability. The study of the set of event-related electrochemical responses of the cerebral cortex ("STRESS") to the initiation of deleterious autonomic outflow (process P) may eventually provide an understanding of the complete cerebral mechanism by which a stressful stimulus-event is transformed into increased cardiac vulnerability. As coronary artery occlusion is neither necessary nor sufficient to cause VF the clinical reversal of ischemic heart disease may not actually solve the problem of sudden cardiac death, as we are accustomed to believing. The combined studies of the central stress-reaction, process P, and the peripheral dual-regulation, however, may eventually lead to a pharmacologic intervention that will have a significant impact upon the alleviation of sudden cardiac death—an impact more than the 22% reduction in mortality that has been reported (Beta-blocker Heart Attack Trials Research Group 1982) for the peripheral administration of beta-blockers.

In summary, both acute intracranial events (e.g., hemorrhage, infarction) and cerebral reactions to psychosocial stressors may induce a variety of cardiovascular effects in susceptible individuals, including malignant arrhythmias and sudden death. Considerable evidence has accumulated that delineates how cardiac vulnerability is regulated by a specific neural pathway that arises in the orbital frontal cortex and projects to the brainstem cardioregulatory centers. The activation of this pathway is known to arise following the presentation of a psychosocial stressor or direct electric activation, and it may arise following an intracranial insult. This review has served to provide a unifying theoretical model to explain how several diverse actions on the nervous system provoke lethal arrhythmias and sudden death. Present-day cardiac monitoring and invasive electrophysiologic techniques may further clarify "neurogenic arrhythmogenesis" (Reichek 1985) in patients with primarily neurologic disease. Future research based on the proposed model should probe the complex pathophysiologic processes that are involved in the activation of the frontocortical-brain stem system, triggering the "brain-heart attack."

Acknowledgments. The authors wish to thank Hally Phelps for preparing the manuscript.

References

Abildskov JA (1976) Adrenergic effects of the Q-T interval of the electrocardiogram. Am Heart J 92: 210–216

Armour JA, Hageman GR, Randall WC (1972) Arrhythmias induced by local cardiac nerve stimulation. Am J Physiol 223: 1068–1075

Bard P (1960) Anatomical organization of the central nervous system in relation to control of the heart and blood vessels. Physiol Rev 40 (Suppl 4): 3–26

Baum T, Shropshire AT (1975) Inhibition of efferent sympathetic nerve activity by 5-hydroxytryptophan and centrally administered 5-hydroxytryptamine. Neuropharmacology 14: 227–233

Benson H, Rosner BA, Marzetta BR, Klemchuk HM (1974) Decreased blood pressure in

pharmacologically treated hypertensive patients who regularly elicited the relaxation response. Lancet i: 289–291
Beta-blocker Heart Attack Trials Research Group (1982) A randomized trial of propranolol in patients with acute myocardial infarctions. JAMA 247: 1707–1714
Billman GE, Schwartz PJ, Stone HL (1982) Baroreceptor reflex control of heart rate: a predictor of sudden cardiac death. Circulation 66: 874–880
Blessing WW, Sved AF, Reis DJ (1982) Destruction of noradrenergic neurons in rabbit brain stem elevates plasma vasopression, causing hypertension. Science 217: 661–663
Blumhart LD, Smith PEM, Owen L (1986) Electrocardiographic accompaniments of temporal lobe epileptic seizures. Lancet i: 1051–1055
Brodal A (1981) Neurological Anatomy, 3rd edn. Oxford University Press, New York, pp 210, 461, 704
Byer E, Ashman R, Toth LA (1947) Electrocardiograms with large, upright T-waves and long Q-T intervals. Am Heart J 33: 796–906
Cameron G (1948) Pulmonary edema. Br Med J 1: 1965
Cannon WB (1931) Again the James-Lange and the thalamic theories of emotion. Psychol Rev 38: 281–295
Cannon WB (1942) "Voodoo" death. Ann Anthropologist (new series) 44: 169–181
Cebelin MS, Hirsch CS (1980) Human stress cardiomyopathy: myocardial lesions in victims of homicidal assaults without internal injuries. Human Pathol 11: 123–132
Chen HI, Sun SC, Chai CY, Kau SL, Kon C (1974) Encephalogenic cardiomyopathy after stimulation of the brain stem in monkeys. Am J Cardiol 33: 845–852
Ciogoli AK, Poser CM (1972) Pulmonary edema secondary to subarachnoid hemorrhage. Neurology 22: 867–870
Clark RW, Boudoulas H, Schaal SF, Schmidt HS (1980) Adrenergic hyperactivity and cardiac abnormality in primary disorders of sleep. Neurology 30: 113–119
Connor RCR (1968) Heart damage associated with intracranial lesions. Br Med J 3: 29–31
Coote JH, Macleod VH (1974) The influence of bulbospinal monoaminergic pathways on sympathetic nerve activity. J Physiol (Lond) 241: 453–475
Corley KC, Shiel FO'M, Mauck HP, Greenhoot J (1973) Electrocardiographic and cardiac morphological changes associated with environmental stress in squirrel monkeys. Psychosom Med 35: 361–366
Corr PB, Gillis RA (1978) Autonomic neural influences on the dysrhythmias resulting from myocardial infarction. Circ Res 43: 1–9
Cox WV, Robertson HF (1936) The effect of stellate ganglionectomy on the cardiac function of intact dogs and its effect on the extent of myocardial infarction and on cardiac function following coronary artery occlusion. Am Heart J 12: 285–300
Cropp GJ, Manning GW (1960) Electrocardiographic changes simulating myocardial ischemia and infarction associated with spontaneous intracranial hemorrhage. Circulation 22: 25–38
Cruickshank JM, Neil-Dwyer G, Brice J (1974) Electrocardiographic changes and their prognostic significance in subarachnoid hemorrhage. J Neurol Neurosurg Psychiatr 37: 755–759
Csaudy M, Kiss Z (1973) Heritable QT prolongation without congenital deafness (Romano-Ward Syndrome). Chest 64: 359–362
Danielopolu D (1949) Etat actuel du traitement chirurgical de l'angine de poitrine, Cardiologia 14: 45
Delgado JMR (1960) Circulatory effects of cortical stimulation. Physiol Rev 40 (Suppl 4): 146–171
DeVito J, Smith O, Stein J, Walsh K (1979) Autoradiographic analysis of hypothalamic area controlling cardiovascular response to emotion. Abstr Soc Neurosci 5: 230 (abstract)
Dimant J, Grob D (1977) Electrocardiographic changes and myocardial damage in patients with acute cerebrovascular accidents. Stroke 8: 448–455
Doshi R, Neil-Dwyer G (1977) Hypothalamic and myocardial lesions after subarachnoid hemorrhage. J Neurol Neurosurg Psychiatr 40: 821–826
Dubo H, Park DC, Pennington RJT, Kalbag RM, Walton JN (1967) Serum creatine kinase levels in cases of stroke, head injury and meningitis. Lancet ii: 743–748
Ekman P, Levenson RW, Frieson WV (1983) Autonomic nervous system activity distinguishes among emotions. Science 221: 1209–1210
Ely DL (1981) Hypertension, social rank, and aortic atherosclerosis in CBA/J mice. Physiol Behav 26: 655–661
Engel GL (1976) Psychologic factors in instantaneous cardiac death. New Engl J Med 294: 664–665
Engel GL (1978) Psychologic stress, vasodepressor (vasovagal) syncope and sudden death. Ann Intern Med 89: 403–412

Estanol BV, Martin OSW (1975) Cardiac arrhythmias and sudden death in subarachnoid hemorrhage. Stroke 6: 382–386
Falconer B, Rajs I (1976) Post-mortem findings of cardiac lesions in epileptics: a preliminary report. Forensic Science 8: 63–71
Fentz V, Gormsen J (1962) Electrocardiographic patterns in patients with cerebrovascular accidents. Circulation 25: 22–28
Finkelstein D, Nigaglioni A (1961) Electrocardiographic alterations after neurosurgical procedures. Am Heart J 66: 772–784
Fohlin L (1977) Body composition, cardiovascular and renal function in adolescent patients with anorexia nervosa. Acta Paeditrica Scand Suppls 268: 7–19
Folger P, Appels A (1982) Psychological risk factors over the life course of myocardial infarcted patients. Adv Cardiol 29: 132–139
Friedman M, Byers O, Diamant J, Rosenman RH (1975) The plasma norepinephrine response of coronary prone subjects (type A) to a specific challenge. Metabolism 24: 205–210
Friedman M, Manwaring JH, Rosenman RH, Donlon G, Ortega P, Grube SM (1973) Instantaneous and sudden deaths. Clinical and pathological differentiation in coronary artery disease. JAMA 225: 1319
Friedman M, Rosenman RH (1959) Association of specific overt behavior pattern with blood and cardiovascular findings. JAMA 169: 1286–1296
Froggatt P, James TN (1973) Sudden unexpected death in infants. Evidence on a lethal cardiac arrhythmia. Ulster Med J 42: 136–152
Furster JM (1973) Unit activity in prefrontal cortex during delayed-response performance: neural correlates of transient memory. J Neurophysiol 36: 61–63
Galosy RA, Clarke LK, Vasko MR, Crawford IL (1981) Neurophysiology and neuropharmacology of cardiovascular regulation and stress. Neurosci Biobehav Revs 5: 137–175
Garvey JL, Melville KI (1969) Cardiovascular effects of lateral hypothalamic stimulation in normal and coronary ligated dogs. J Cardiovas Surg 10: 377–385
Gastaut H (1953) A propos des functions "non olfactive" du rhinencaphale. Journal de Physiologie (Paris) 45: 117–120
Glass DC, Krakoff LR, Contrada R, Hilton WF, Kehoe K, Mannucci EG, Collins C, Snow B, Elting E (1980) Effect of harassment and competition upon cardiovascular and plasma catecholamine reponses in type A and type B individuals. Psychophysiology 17: 453–463
Glass DC (1977) Stress, behavior patterns, and coronary disease. Am Sci 65: 177–187
Gold MR, Cohen DH (1981) Modification of the discharge of vagal cardiac neurons during learned heart rate change. Science 214: 345–347
Goodman LS, Gilman A (1970) The pharmacologic basis of therapeutics. MacMillan, New York, p 569
Green JR, Korovetz MJ, Shanklin DR, Devito JJ, Taylor WJ (1969) Sudden unexpected death in three generations. Arch Intern Med 124: 359–364
Grossman MA (1976) Cardiac arrhythmias in acute central nervous system disease: successful management with stellate ganglion block. Arch Intern Med 136: 203–207
Hachinski VC, Smith KE, Silver MD, Gibson CJ, Ciriello J (1986) Acute myocardial and plasma catecholamine changes in experimental stroke. Stroke 17: 387–390
Hageman GR, Goldberg JM, Armour JA, Randall WC (1973) Cardiac dysrhythmias induced by autonomic nerve stimulation. Am J Cardiol 82: 823–830
Hall RE, Livingston RR, Bloor MD (1977) Orbital cortical influences on cardiovascular dynamics and myocardial structure in conscious monkeys. J Neurosurg 46: 630–647
Harvey WP, Levine SA (1952) Paroxysmal ventricular tachycardia due to emotion. Possible mechanism of death due to fright. JAMA 150: 479–480
Haws CW, Burgess MJ (1978) Effects of bilateral and unilateral stellate stimulation on canine ventricular refratory periods at sites of overlapping innervation. Circ Res 42: 195–198
Heilman KM, Schwartz HD, Watson RT (1978) Hypoarousal in patients with the neglect syndrome and emotional indifference. Neurology 28: 229–232
Hersch C (1964) Electrocardiographic changes in subarachnoid hemorrhage, meningitis, and intracranial space-occupying lesions. Br Heart J 26: 785
Hilton SM (1980) Inhibition of the baroreceptor reflex by the brainstem defense centre. In: Sleight P (ed) Arterial baroreceptors and hypertension. Oxford University Press, Oxford, pp 318–323
Hockman CH, Mauck HP Jr, Hoff EC (1966) ECG changes resulting from cerebral stimulations: II. A spectrum of ventricular arrhythmias of sympathetic origin. Am Heart J 71: 695–700
Hoff EC, Green HD (1936) Cardiovascular reactions induced by electrical stimulation of the cerebral cortex. Am J Physiol 117: 411–422

Hugenholtz PG (1962) Electrocardiographic abnormalities in cerebral disorders. Report of six cases and review of the literature. Am Heart J 63: 451–461
James TN (1969) QT prolongation and sudden death. Mod Concepts Cardiovasc Dis 38: 35–38
James TN, Froggatt P, Atkinson WJ Jr, Lurie PR, McNamara DG, Miller WW, Schloss GT Carroll JF, North AL (1978) Observations on the pathophysiology of the long Q-T syndromes with special reference to the neuropathology of the heart. Circulation 57: 1221–1231
Jarvinew KAS (1955) Can ward rounds be a danger to patients with myocardial infarction? Br Med J 1: 318–320
Jay GW, Leestma JE (1981) Sudden death in epilepsy. Acta Neurologica Scand 63 (suppl 82): 11–16
Jenkins CD (1976) Recent evidence supporting psychologic and social risk factors for coronary disease. New Engl J Med 294: 987–994
Jenkins CD, Zyzanski SJ, Rosenman RH (1976) Risk of new myocardial infarction in middle-aged men with manifest coronary heart disease. Circulation 53: 342–347
Jervell A, Lange-Nielson F (1957) Congenital deaf-mutism. Functional heart disease with prolongation of the Q-T interval, and sudden death. Am Heart J 54: 59
Johansson G, Johnsson L, Lannek N, Blomgren L, Lindberg P, Pouph O (1974) Severe stress-cardiopathy in pigs. Am Heart J 87: 451–457
Johnson RH, Lambie DG, Spalding JM (eds) (1984) Neurocardiology, vol 13 in major problems in Neurology, chap 6: Emotion and pain. Saunders, London, p 66
Johnsson A, Hansson L (1977) Prolonged exposure to a stressful stimulus (noise) as a cause of raised blood-pressure in man. Lancet i: 86–87
Kaplan JR, Manuck SB, Clarkson TB, Lusso FM, Taub DM, Miller EW (1983) Social stress and atherosclerosis in normocholesterolemic monkeys. Science 220: 733–736
Kahn A, Riazi J, Blum D (1983) Oculocardiac reflex in near miss for sudden infant death syndrome infants. Pediatrics 71: 49–52
Kaste SH, Kouttinen A (1978) Heart type creatine kinase isoenzyme (CKMB) in acute cerebral disorders. Br Heart J 40: 802–805
Kent KM, Epstein SE (1976) Neural basis for the genesis and control of arrhythmias associated with myocardial infarction. Cardiology 61: 71–74
Klein RC, Amsterdam EA, Grehl T, Hurley E, Lee G, Bommer WJ, Demaria AN, Mason DT (1979) Emergency surgery in acquired ventricular septal defect: successful repair with anterior but no inferior acute myocardial infarction. Clin Res 1979, 27: 7A
Knight RT, Hillyard SA, Woods DL, Neville HJ (1980) The effects of frontal and temporal-parietal lesions on the auditory evoked potential in man. Electroenceph Clin Neurophysiol 50: 112–124
Kojima S (1980) Prefrontal unit activity in the monkey: relation to visual stimuli and movements. Exp Neurol 69: 110–123
Korteweg GCJ, Boeles JTF, Ten Cate J (1957) Influence of stimulation of some subcortical areas on the electrocardiogram. J Neurophysiol 20: 100–107
Kubota K, Tonoike M, Mikami A (1980) Neuronal activity in the monkey dorsolateral prefrontal cortex during a discrimination task with delay. Brain Res 183: 29–42
Langslit A, Sorland SJ (1975) Sudocardiac syndrome of Jervell and Lange-Nielsen with prolonged Q-T interval present at birth and severe anemia and syncopal attacks in childhood. Br Heart J 37: 830
Lathers CM, Schraeder PL (1982) Autonomic dysfunction in epilepsy: characterization of autonomic cardiac neural discharge associated with pentylenetetrazol-induced epileptogenic activity. Epilepsia 23: 633–647
Lavy S, Yaar I, Melamed E, Stern S (1974) The effect of acute stroke in cardiac functions as observed in an intensive stroke care unit. Stroke 5: 775–780
Lazarra R, El-Sherif N, Scherlag BJ (1974) Early and late effects of coronary artery occlusion on canine Purkinje fibers. Circ Res 35: 391–399
Lepeschkin E, Marchet H, Schroeder G, Wagner R, De Paula e Silva P, Raab W (1960) Effect of epinephrine and norepinephrine on the electrocardiogram of 100 normal subjects. Am J Cardiol 5: 594–603
Leriche R, Herman L, Fontaine R (1931) Ligature de la coronaire gauche et fonction de colur apès enervation sympathique. C.R. Soc Biol (Paris) 107: 547–548
Levine HO (1953) Nonspecificity of the electrocardiogram associated with coronary heart disease. Am J Med 15: 344–355
Lewis BS, Gostman MS (1974) Sudden death in patients awaiting coronary artery surgery. Thorax 29: 209–214
Liberthson RR, Nagel EL, Hirschman JC, Nussenfeld SR (1974) Prehospital ventricular defibrillation: prognosis and followup course. New Engl J Med 291: 317–321

Light KC, Koepke JP, Obrist PA, Willis PW (1983) Psychological stress induces sodium and fluid retention in men at high risk for hypertension. Science 220: 429–431
Loewy AD, McNeill JJ (1981) The role of descending monoaminergic systems in central control of blood pressure. Fed Proc 40: 2778–2785
Lown B (1979) Sudden cardiac death: the major challenge confronting contemporary cardiology. Am J Cardiol 43: 313–328
Lown B, DeSilva RA, Lesnon R (1978) Roles of psychologic stress and autonomic nervous system changes in provocation of ventricular premature complexes. Am J Cardiol 41: 979–985
Lown B, Temte JV, Reich P, Gaughan C, Regestein Q, Hai H (1976) Basis for recurring ventricular fibrillation in the absence of coronary heart disease and its management. New Engl J Med 294: 623–629
Lown B, Tykocinski M, Garfein A, Brooks P (1973) Sleep and ventricular remature beats. Circulation 48: 691–701
Lown B, Verrier RL (1976) Neural activity and ventricular fibrillation. New Engl J Med 294: 1165–1170
Lown B, Verrier RL, Corbalan R (1973) Psychologic stress and threshold for repetitive ventricular response. Science 182: 834–836
MacLean PD (1970) The triune brain, emotion and scientific bias. In: Schmitt FO (ed) The neurosciences, second study program. Rockefeller University Press, New York, pp 336–348
Malliana A, Schwartz PJ, Zanchetti A (1980) Neural mechanisms in life-threatening arrhythmias. Am Heart J 100: 705–715
Manning JW, Cotton MDeV (1962) Mechanism of cardiac arrhythmias induced by diencephalic stimulation. Am J Physiol 203: 1120–1124
Marion DW, Segal R, Thompson ME (1986) Subarachnoid hemorrhage and the heart. Rev Neurosurg 18: 101–106
Marriott HJ (1977) Practical electrocardiography, 6th edn. Williams and Wilkins, Baltimore
Mathew NT, Taori GM, Mathai, K, Chanoy J (1970) Atrial fibrillation associated with seizure in a case of frontal meningioma. Neurology 20: 725
Mathews EC Jr, Blount AW Jr, Townsend JI (1972) QT prolongation and ventricular arrhythmias with and without deafness in the same family. Am J Cardiol 29: 702
Matta RJ, Lawler JE, Lown B (1976) Ventricular electrical instability in the conscious dog. Effects of psychologic stress and beta adrenergic blockade. Am J Cardiol 38: 594–598
Matthews TG (1984) Is autonomic control a factor in some causes of sudden infant death. Lancet i: 744
Mauck HP Jr, Hockman CH, Hoff EC (1964) ECG changes resulting from cerebral stimulation I. Anomalous atrioventricular excitation elicited by electrical stimulation of the mesencephalic reticular formation. Am Heart J 68: 98–101
McCall RB (1984) Evidence for a serotonergically-mediated sympathoexcitatory response to medullary raphe stimulation. Neurosci Abst 10: 300
McCarthy DS, Mitchell J (1967) Multiple transient electrocardiographic changes associated with dysfunction of the cervical sympathetic outflow. J Irish Med Assoc 60 (366): 469–471
McRae JR, Wagner GS, Roges MC, Canent RV (1974) Paroxysmal familial ventricular fibrillation. J Pediatr 84: 515–518
Mesulam MM (1986) Frontal cortex and behavior. Ann Neurol 19: 320–325
Millar K. Abildskov JA (1968) Notched T waves in young persons with central nervous system lesions. Circulation 37: 597–603
Moss AJ (1975) Profile of high risk in people known to have coronary heart disease. A review. Circulation 52 (Suppl III): 147
Moss AJ, Schwartz PJ (1979) Sudden death and the idiopathic long Q-T syndrome. Am J Med 66: 6–7
Muller JE, Stone PH, Zoltan GT, Rutherford JD, Czeisler CA, Parker C, Poole WK, Passamani E, Roberts R, Robertson T, Sobel BE, Willerson JT, Braunwald E (1985) Circulation variation in the frequency of onset of acute myocardial infarction. New Engl J Med 313: 1315–1322
Myers A, Dewar HA (1975) Circumstances attending 100 sudden deaths from coronary artery disease with coroner's necropsies. Br Heart J 37: 1133–1143
Myers MG, Norris JW, Hachinski VC, et al. (1981) Plasma norepinephrine in stroke. Stroke 12: 200–204
Myers MG, Norris JW, Hachinski VC, Wingert ME, Sole MJ (1982) Cardiac sequelae of acute stroke. Stroke 13: 838–842
Nauta WJH (1964) Some afferent connections of the prefontral cortex in the monkey. In: Warren JW, Akert K (eds) The frontal granular cortex and behavior. McGraw-Hill, New York, pp 372–396

Neil-Dwyer G, Walter P, Cruickshank JM, Doshi R, O'Gorman P (1978) Effect of propranolol and phentolamine on myocardial necrosis after subarachnoid hemorrhage. Br Med J 2: 990–992
Norris JW, Froggatt GM, Hachinski VC (1978) Cardiac arrhythmias in acute stroke. Stroke 9: 392–396
Norris JW, Hachinski VC, Myers MG, Callow J, Moore RW (1979) Serum cardiac enzymes in stroke. Stroke 10: 548–553
Obrist PA, Lawler JE, Howard JL, et al. (1974) Sympathetic influences on cardiac rate and contractility during acute stress in humans. Psychophysiology 11: 405–427
Olson HG, Miller RR, DaSilva O, Amsterdam EA, Mason DT (1974) Vagal stimulation in patients with acute myocardial infarction: antiarrhythmic and hemodynamic effects of edrophenium. Circulation 1974 (Suppl III) 50: 33
Pa'lossy B, Oo M (1977) ECG alterations in anorexia nervosa. Adv Cardiol 1: 280–282
Parkes CM, Benjamin G, Fitzgerald RG (1969) Broken heart: a statistical study of increased mortality among widowers. 1: 740–743
Peerless SJ, Griffiths JC (1962) Plasma catecholamines following subarachnoid hemorrhage. Ann Roy Col Phys Surg Can 5: 48
Phizackerley PJR, Poole EW, Whitty CWM (1954) Sino-auricular heart block as an epileptic manifestation. Epilepsia 3: 89–91
Pitts RF, Larrabee MG, Bronk DW (1981) An analysis of hypothalamic cardiovascular control. Am J Physiol 134: 359–383
Pratt CM, Skinner JE, Evans MB (to be published) Covariation of ventricular arrhythmia rates and cerebral event-related slow potentials during 24-hour ambulatory monitoring in cardiac patients with high ectopy.
Pritchett ELC, McNamara JO, Gallagher JJ (1980) Arrhythmogenic epilepsy: an hypothesis. Am Heart J 100: 683–688
Rahe RH, Bennett L, Romo M, Seltanen P, Arthur RS (1973) Subjects recent life changes and coronary heart disease in Finland. Am J Psychiatr 130: 1222–1226
Ranson SW, Kabat H, Magoun HW (1935) Autonomic responses to electrical stimulation of hypothalamus, preoptic region and septum. Arch Neurol Psychiatr 33: 467–477
Reed JC, Skinner JE, Welch KMA, Nell JH (1978) Correlated changes in cortical 3′, 5′-adenosine monophosphate level and extracellular slow potential amplitude evoked by psychological and physical stress in the conscious rat. In: George JW, Ignaro LJ (eds) Advances in cyclic nucleotide research. Raven, New York, p 747
Reich P, DeSilva RA, Lown B, Murawski BJ (1981) Acute psychological disturbances preceding life-threatening ventricular arrhythmias. JAMA 246: 233–235
Reichek N (1985) Head and heart (editorial). Ann Neurol 18: 13
Reichenbach DD, Beneditt EP (1970) Catecholamines and cardiomyopathy. The pathogenesis and potential importance of myofibrillar degeneration. Hum Pathol 1: 125–130
Richards P (1963) Pulmonary edema and intracranial lesions. Br Med J 2: 83–170
Rockstrob B, Elbert T, Birbaumer N, Lutzenberger W (1982) Slow brain potentials and behavior. Urban and Schwarzenberg, Baltimore, pp 128, 169
Rose K (1974) The post coronary patient as a spectator sportsman. In: Eliot RL (ed) Stress and the heart. Futura, New York, pp 207–218
Rosenblatt G, Hartman E, Zwilling GR (1973) Cardiac irritability during sleep and dreaming. J Psychosomat Res 17: 129–134
Rosenman RH, Jenkins CD, Brand RJ, Friedman M, Straus R, Wurm M (1975) Coronary heart disease in the western collaborative group study: a final follow-up experience of 8.5 years. JAMA 233: 872–877
Ross CA, Rugglero DA, Park DH, Joh TH, Sved AF, Fernandez-Pardal J, Saavedra JM, Reis DJ (1984) Tonic vasomotor control by the rostral ventrolateral medulla: effect of electrical or chemical stimulation on the area containing C1 adrenaline neurons on arterial pressure, heart rate, and plasma catecholamines and vasopressin. J Neurosci 4: 474–494
Rush JL, Everett BA, Adams AH, Kusske JA (1977) Paroxysmal atrial tachycardia and frontal lobe tumor. Arch Neurol 34: 578–580
Ruskin JN, Johnson RA, Haber E, Austen WG (eds) (1980) Ventricular arrhythmias. In: The practice of cardiology, Chap 6, 1st edn. Little, Brown, Boston, pp 153–200
Salk L, Grellong BA, Dietrich J (1974) Sudden infant death: normal cardiac habituation and poor autonomic control. New Engl J Med 291: 219–222
Scherlag BJ, El-Sherif N, Hope R, Lazarra R (1974) Characterization and localization on ventricular arrhythmias resulting from myocardial ischemia and infarction. Circ Res 35: 372–383
Schwartz PJ (1976) Cardiac sympathetic innervation and the sudden infant death syndrome. Am J Med 60: 161–172

Schwartz PJ, Malliana A (1975) Electrical alteration of the T-wave: clinical and experimental evidence of its relationship and the sympathetic nervous system and with the long Q-T syndrome. Am Heart J 89: 45–50

Schwartz PJ, Wolf S, (1978) QT-interval prolongation as predictor of sudden death in patients with myocardial infarction. Circulation 57: 1074–1977

Schwartz PJ, Periti M, Malliani A (1975) The long Q-T syndrome. Am Heart J 89: 378–390

Schwartz PJ, Stone HL, Brown AM (1976) Effects of unilateral stellate ganglion blockage on the arrhythmias associated with coronary occlusion. Am Heart J 92: 589–599

Schwartz PJ, Billman GE, Stone HL (1984) Autonomic mechanisms in ventricular fibrillation induced by myocardial ischemia during exercise in dogs with healed myocardial infarction. Circulation 69: 790–800

Scott NA, DeSilva Ra, Lown B, Wurtman RJ (1981) Tyrosine administration decreased vulnerability to ventricular fibrillation in the normal canine heart. Science 211: 727–729

Simon RP, Aminoff MJ, Benowitz NL (1984) Changes in plasma catecholamines after tonic-clonic seizures. Neurology 34: 255–257

Skinner JE (1984) Central gating mechanisms that regulate event-related potentials and behavior. In: Elbert T, Rockstroh B et al. (eds) Self-regulation of the brain and behavior. Springer, Berlin Heidelberg New York, pp 42–58

Skinner JE (1984b) Psychosocial stress and sudden cardiac death: brain mechanisms. In: Bequish RE, Singal PK, Dhalla NS (eds) Stress and heart disease. Martinus Nihoff Publishing, University of Manitoba, pp 44–59

Skinner JE, Beder SD, Entman ML (1983) Psychological stress activates phosphorylase in the heart of the conscious pig without increasing heart rate and blood pressure. Proc Nat Acad Sci USA 80: 4513–4517

Skinner JE, Reed JC (1981) Blockage of a frontocortical-brainstem pathway prevents ventricular fibrillation of the ischemic heart in pigs. Am J Physiol 240: H156–H163

Skinner JE, Yingling CD (1976) Regulation of slow potential shifts in nucleus reticularis thalami by the mesencephalic reticular formation and the frontal cortex. Electroencephalogr Clin Neurophysiol 40: 288–296

Skinner JE, Yingling CD (1977) Central gating mechanisms that regulate event-related potentials and behavior: a neural model for attention. In: Desmedt JE (ed) Progress in clinical neurophysiology, vol 1. Karger, Basel, pp 30–69, 70–96

Skinner JE, Lie JT, Entman ML (1975) Modification of ventriculation fibrillation latency following coronary artery occlusion in the conscious pig: the effects of psychological stress and beta-adrenergic blockade. Circulation 51: 656–667

Skinner JE, Mohr DN, Kellaway P (1975) Sleep-stage regulation of ventricular arrhythmias in the unanesthetized pig. Circ Res 37: 342–349

Skinner JE, Reed JC, Welch KMA, Nell JH (1976) Correlated shifts in a surface-negative slow potential and a reduction in 3′, 5′-adenosine monophosphate in the cortex of conscious rats. In: Neurosci Abstracts, 6th annual meeting. Bethesda, Maryland. Society for Neuroscience, vol II, part 1, p 590

Skinner JE, Welch KMA, Reed JC, Nell JH (1978a) Psychological stress reduces cyclic 3′, 5′-adenosine monophosphate level in the parietal cortex of the conscious rat. J Neurochem 30: 691–698

Skinner JE, Reed JC, Welch KMA, Nell JH (1978b) Cutaneous shock produces correlated shifts in slow potential amplitude and cyclic 3′, 5′-adenosine monophosphate level in the parietal cortex of the conscious rat. J Neurochem 30: 699–704

Skinner JE, Montaŕon MF, Pratt CM (1982) The efficacy of antiarrhythmic drugs in cardiac patients in proportion to their ability to reduce the amplitude of the cerebral event-related slow potential. Soc Neurosci Abstr 8: 428

Skinner JE, Molnar M (1983) Event-related extracellular potassium in activity changes in the frontal cortex of the conscious cat. J Neurophysiol 49: 204–215

Smith OA, Astley CA, DeVito JL, Stein JM, Walsh KE (1980) Functional analysis of hypothalamic control of the cardiovascular responses accompanying emotional behavior. Fed Proc 39: 2487–2494

Smith R, Johnson L, Rothfeld D, Zir L, Tharp B (1972) Sleep and cardiac arrhythmia. Arch Intern Med 130: 751–753

Smith RP, Tomlinson BE (1954) Subendocardial hemorrhages associated with intracranial lesions. J Path Bacteriol 68: 327–334

Smith WK (1945) The functional significance of the rostral cingulate cortex as revealed by its responses to electrical excitation. J Neurophysiol 8: 241–255

Solomon S (1983) Long Island Jewish-Hillside Medical Center. In: Graedon J (ed) Does drug cause loss of memory? The Houston Post, September

Spain DM, Bradess VA (1970) Sudden death from coronary heart disease. Survival time, frequency to thrombi, and cigarette smoking. Chest 58: 107–110

Steptoe A, Ross A (1981) Psychophysiological reactivity and the prediction of cardiovascular disorders. J Psychosom Res 25: 23–31

Sterman AB, Vlay S, Panasci D (1986) Autonomic dysfunction in cardiac arrest survivors: evidence of severe vagal dysfunction. Ann Neurol 20: 158 (abstract)

Talman WT (1985) Cardiovascular regulation and lesions of the central nervous system. Ann Neurol 18: 1–12

Terrence CF, Rao GR, Perper JA (1981) Neurogenic pulmonary edema in unexpected, unexplained death of epileptic patients. Ann Neurol 9: 458–464

Teuber HL (1964) Some effects of frontal lobotomy in man. In: Warren JM, Akert K (eds) The frontal granular cortex and behavior. McGraw Hill, San Francisco, pp 332–333

Theorell TGT (1982) Review of research on life events and cardiovascular illness. Adv Cardiol 29: 140–147

Thorpe SJ, Rolls ET, Maddison S (1983) The orbitofrontal cortex: neuronal activity in the behaving monkey. Exp Brain Res 49: 93–115

Thurston J, Marks P (1974) Electrocardiographic abnormalities in patients with anorexia nervosa. Br Heart J 36: 719–723

Timms RJ (1977) Cortical inhibition and facilitation of the defense reaction. J Physiol 266: 98–99

Trichopoulous D, Katsouyanni K, Zavitsanos X, Tzonov A, Dalla-Vorgia P (1983) Psychological stress and fatal heart attacks: the Athens earthquakes natural experiment. Lancet 1983: i: 441–443

Ulyanisky LS, Stepanyan EP, Krymsky IP (1977) Cardiac arrhythmias of hypothalamic origin in sudden death. In: Proceedings USA-USSR joint symposium on sudden death. DHEW No., (NIH) 78–1472, Washington, D.C. U.S. Government Printing Office, pp 417–429

Verrier RL, Calvert A, Lown B (1975) Effect of posterior hypothalamic stimulation on ventricular fibrillation threshold. Am J Physiol 228: 923–927

Verrier RL, Thompson P, Lown B (1974) Ventricular vulnerability during sympathetic stimulation: role of heart rate and blood pressure. Cardiovasc Res 8: 602–610

Vincent OM (1986) The heart rate of Romano-Ward syndrome patients. Am Heart J 112: 61–64

Vordis EM, Mallios KD, Papantonia TM (1983) Holter monitoring during 1981 Athens earthquake. Lancet i: 1281–1282

Wallace RK, Benson H (1972) The physiology of meditation. Sci Am 226: 85–90

Wallace RK, Benson H, Wilson AF (1971) A wakeful hypometabolic physiologic state. Am J Physiol 221: 795–799

Ward AA (1948) The cingulate gyrus: area 24. J Neurophysiol 11: 13–23

Wasserman F, Choquette G, Cassinelli R, Bellet S (1956) Electrocardiographic observations in patients with cerebrovascular accidents. Report of 12 cases. Am J Med Sci 231: 502–510

Watanabe A (1983) Cholinergic agonists and antagonists. In: Rosen MR, Hoffman BF (eds) Cardiac therapy. Martinas Nijhoff, Boston, pp 95–144

Weidler DJ (1974) Myocardial damage and cardiac arrhythmias after intracranial hemorrhage. A critical review. Stroke 5: 759–764

Weidler DJ, Das SK, Sedeman TM (1976) Cardiac arrhythmias secondary to acute cerebral ischemia: prevention by autonomic blockade. Circulation 53: 54: II–102

Weinberg SJ, Fuster, JM (1960) Electrocardiographic changes produced by localized hypothalamic stimulation. Ann Intern Med 53: 332–341

Wellens HJ (1972) Ventricular fibrillation occurring on arousal from sleep by auditory stimuli. Circulation 46: 661–665

West TC, Falk G, Cervoni P (1956) Drug alteration of transmembrane potentials in atrial pacemaker cells. J Pharmacol Exp Thes 117: 245–252

Willis T (1664) The anatomy of the brain. In: The remaining medical works of Dr. Thomas Willis, vol 2 S.P. Esq, London

Woolfolk RL (1975) Psychophysiological correlates of meditation. Arch Gen Psychiatr 32: 1326–1333

Yamour BJ, Sridhakan MR, Rice JR, Floers WG (1980) Electrocardiographic changes in cerebrovascular hemorrhage. Am Heart J 99: 294–300

Yarnell PR, Clark G (1973) EKG changes after spinal subarachnoid hemorrhage. Stroke 4: 156–159

Zandberg P. DeJong W, DeWied D (1979) Effect of catecholamine receptor stimulating agents on blood pressure after local application in the nucleus tractus solitarii of the medulla oblongata. Eur J Pharmacol 55: 43–56

Zipes DP, Barber MJ, Takahashi N, Gilmour RF Jr (1984) Recent observations on autonomic innervation of the heart. In: Zipes DP, Jalife J (eds) Cardiac electrophysiology and arrhythemias. Grune-Stratton, Orlando, pp 181–189

Section C

GLOBAL BRAIN ISCHEMIA

Chapter 12

Anoxic Encephalopathy Following Resuscitation from Cardiopulmonary Arrest

R. E. Jackson

Introduction

Cardiopulmonary-cerebral resuscitation (CPCR), defined as the institution upon a pulseless, breathless individual of artificial ventilation, artificial circulation, intravenous drugs administration, and electrical defibrillation, is without question an important and successful life-saving procedure. The purpose of CPCR is to provide artificial circulation of oxygenated blood to the vital organs, especially the heart and brain, in an attempt to halt the destructive processes associated with ischemia and anoxia until spontaneous circulation can be restored. Goldberg (1974) stated that "The goal of CPR is to prevent irreversible cerebral anoxic damage after the cardiac arrest."

With the numbers of patients undergoing resuscitation increasing, and with earlier and more sophisticated interventions, more and more are being resuscitated and admitted to hospital (Eisenberg et al. 1980). The advent of widespread, aggressive treatment of victims of cardiac arrest has created a new problem: anoxic encephalopathy. Much of the initial enthusiasm over the ability to successfully restore circulation has been supplemented by the sobering reality of brain dead or severely damaged individuals. The physical, emotional, and economic impact of the brain dead patient on family members and society is tragic and immeasurable. The focus of this review, therefore, is the etiology, prognosis, prevention, and treatment of anoxic encephalopathy complicating CPCR.

Epidemiology of Cardiac Arrest and Anoxic Encephalopathy

The total number of out-of-hospital cardiac arrests and attempted resuscitations in the United States yearly is unknown. These rates probably are fairly constant in most urban areas. In King County, where detailed records are kept, during a 30-month period among a population of 598 000 there were 927 cardiac arrests in which there was an Emergency Medical Services (EMS) response, an incidence of 6.2/100 000 population per year (Eisenberg et al. 1979).

Definitions are important when discussing epidemiologic data on resuscitation. "Successful defibrillation" simply means the restoration of an organized heart rhythm for at least a short period. "Successful resuscitation" can mean anything from the temporary restoration of a pulse and blood pressure, to discharge alive from hospital. Survival is typically reported as the number of alive patients discharged from the hospital. The ultimate definition of a successful resuscitation should be the discharge from hospital of an intact, functioning human being. Important issues in many of the studies discussed below are whether the arrests were witnessed or unwitnessed, and if the anoxic-ischemic times were accurately noted. These are crucial factors in interpreting the data on resuscitation.

Determinants of Resuscitability

The most important variable affecting the ability to successfully resuscitate an individual is the amount of time from the onset of the arrest to the restoration of circulation. Many other factors have an impact on the eventual outcome of the arrest and resuscitation, but the most important of these is the initial rhythm. Ventricular fibrillation and tachycardia have much better outcomes than do bradycardia, electrical-mechanical dissociation (normal QRS complexes without pulses), pulseless idioventricular rhythms (wide QRS without a pulse), and asystole. In a study in which all arrests were witnessed and EMS was summoned immediately and arrived within 4 min, 62% of the patients were found to be in ventricular fibrillation, 7% in ventricular tachycardia, and 31% in bradycardiac arrest. With ventricular tachycardia, 88% were successfully resuscitated and admitted to hospital, with 67% discharged alive. Forty percent of the patients with ventricular fibrillation were admitted alive and 23% discharged alive from the hospital; with bradycardiac arrests 9% were admitted to the hospital and none survived the hospitalization (Myerberg et al. 1982). Over a 12-year experience only 1% of patients found in an asystolic arrest survived (Weaver et al. 1985).

The maximum amount of anoxia/ischemia time that can be tolerated is variable between patients, but if a spontaneous pulse and pressure can be established within 8 min of collapse, then the likelihood of a successful outcome is improved (Eisenberg et al. 1979). Lund (Lund and Skulberg 1976) noted that if anoxia time was less than 1 min then the percentage survival was 61% whereas if the anoxic time was greater than 10 min the survival was less than 1%.

The impact of standard closed-chest massage on the outcome of out-of-hospital arrests is not clear in the literature, with conflicting results in different studies. Lund (Lund and Skulberg 1976) noted that bystander CPR improved outcome, but any difference in anoxic times between the CPR and no-CPR groups was not reported. Similarly others have reported that CPR does indeed improve survival and neurologic outcome (Copley et al. 1977; Thompson et al. 1979; Tweed et al. 1980; Gudjonsson et al. 1982; Vertesi et al. 1983; Guzy et al. 1979), but these studies neither critically looked at witnessed arrests with ventricular fibrillation nor documented anoxic-ischemic times accurately and consistently. However, Pionkowski et al. (1983) in a study from Milwaukee noted that in patients with witnessed arrests whose initial rhythm was ventricular fibrillation that the shorter the amount of time of the resuscitation the better the outcome; after 20 min of resuscitative efforts and survival rate was significantly diminished. He did not observe any benefit from bystander CPR. This study suggests that standard closed-chest massage does not impact on the outcome of arrests. Kowalski et al. (1984) noted that among patients with *witnessed* arrest whose initial rhythm upon arrival of the paramedics was ventricular fibrillation and in whom the initial treatment was defibrillation, that bystander CPR had no effect on outcome and that the major factor determining successful resuscitation was the time to defibrillation. Roth et al. (1984) reported that of 252 out-of-hospital arrests only 55 (21%) were resuscitated and only 18 (7%) were discharged alive from the hospital. No mention was made of the eventual neurologic outcome.

Prolonged closed-chest massage does not even have the ability to maintain an initial favorable rhythm. In a study of out-of-hospital arrests with basic EMS response, Holter monitors were applied to 21 arrested patients. Fifteen of these patients initially had a predominantly favorable rhythm (ventricular tachycardia or fibrillation, or supraventricular tachycardia), but after a mean of 22 min of closed-chest massage only five had a favorable rhythm and only one was resuscitated (Tweed et al. 1980).

Prolonged resuscitation is associated with poor outcome (Eisenberg et al. 1980; Pionkowski et al. 1983; Kowalski et al. 1984; Enns et al. 1983; Abramson et al. 1982; Mahoney and Mirick 1983). Anoxia/ischemia time is also crucial for the neurologic outcome. Jorgensen and Malchow-Moller (1978) noted that unless the resuscitation is successful in less than 20 min, the chance for full cerebral and circulatory recovery is less than 5%.

The expected neurologic outcome after prolonged resuscitation from cardiac arrest is dismal. Of 117 people admitted after an out-of-hospital cardiac arrest, only 53 were discharged alive, and of these only 11 (9.4% of the resuscitated patients) were able to return to their previous jobs (Earnest et al. 1980). Only two patients (1.7%) had no neurologic deficits, while six (5%) had a minimal deficit (Earnest et al. 1980). Bates et al. (1977) noted that only 2 of 60 patients who were comatose after 6 h postresuscitation had a good neurologic outcome 1 year later. In another study, only 10% of patients who were comatose after arrest had a good neurologic recovery 1 year later (Levy et al. 1985). Therefore, the prospects of surviving a cardiac arrest and subsequent resuscitation as an intact, functioning human being are dim unless definitive action is taken almost immediately to restore an effective spontaneous circulation. It is also clear that current resuscitative efforts are unable to sustain the mechanism of life for more than a short time.

Resuscitation-Related Brain Damage

Certain areas in the CNS demonstrate selective vulnerability to global ischemia (Adams et al. 1966; Brierley et al. 1969; Brierley 1970). The pyramidal cells in the third and fifth layers of the cerebral cortex (laminar necrosis), Sommers sector in the hippocampus, and the cerebellar Purkinje cells can be damaged even with brief ischemia/anoxia. The amygdala, basal ganglia, thalamus, lateral geniculate body, substantia nigra, and inferior colliculus are affected by moderate ischemia/anoxia. More diffuse CNS injury often occurs with prolonged cardiac arrest.

The range of neurologic deficits seen after resuscitation has been reviewed by Caronna and Finklestein (1978). Neurologic abnormalities have been correlated with outcome following cardiac arrest (Levy et al. 1985; Snyder et al. 1977; Snyder et al. 1980; Snyder et al. 1981). Survival is rare in adults with coma persisting beyond 24 h after arrest, especially when associated with absent brain stem reflexes. Patients with neocortical death may evolve into a persistent vegetative state associated with relatively "normal" sleep/wake cycles and roving eye movements, but without evidence of higher brain function (Brierly et al. 1971).

Watershed zones between the areas of supply of the major cortical vessels are particularly vulnerable to global ischemia (Torvik 1984). The parietal-occipital watershed zone is most vulnerable and infarction here can produce cortical blindness. Other watershed syndromes include paraparesis and proximal arm weakness (man-in-the-barrel syndrome).

Anoxic leukoencephalopathy is a peculiar type of delayed injury affecting cerebral white matter. It occurs in approximately 2 out of 1000 cardiac arrests and is characterized by a period of recovery from the insult followed by progressive deterioration to coma and death (Plum et al. 1962).

Pathophysiology of Anoxic Encephalopathy

Simplistically, the pathogenisis of anoxic encephalopathy is the deprivation of oxygen from neurons for a period as short as 4–6 min (Heymans 1950; Weinberger et al. 1940). However, there is some evidence that neurons are more resistant to ischemia than previously believed. Ames (1963) demonstrated extended retinal survival in anoxic tissue baths. Hossman (1976) found recovery of high-energy metabolism, enzymatic functions, and generation of action potentials after 60 min of global ischemia in cats. The cellular processes involved in the development of anoxic encephalopathy are complex and poorly understood, and are not simply related to the deprivation of oxygen, but rather involve complex interactions between subcellular and membrane functions which include ionic fluxes, acid-base interactions, and generation of free radicals. These interactions alter the energy-producing and -regulating mechanisms of the cell, leading to cell death. A short review of these potential mechanisms of neuronal cell death will be presented; however, a detailed analysis and discussion is beyond the scope of this review. There are a number of recent excellent reviews of this subject (Siesjo 1981; Winegar and White 1983).

The development of ischemic-anoxic cellular injuries has been divided into two phases: the anoxic-ischemic phase and the reperfusion phase.

Anoxic-Ischemic Injury

During the anoxic-ischemic phase of cellular injury, the alteration of cellular energy dynamics leads to loss of cellular integrity by the accumulation of lactic acid, loss of membrane integrity, deterioration of ionic gradients, and cellular and mitochondrial edema. The production of ATP in neuronal cells is dependent upon a continuous delivery of oxygen. However, there is evidence that cerebral blood flow rates 30% of normal can maintain normal ATP levels in neuronal cells by stimulation of anaerobic metabolism (DeCree et al. 1979; Paschen et al. 1981). If the flow rates are diminished further to the range of 15%–30% of normal flow, cellular ATP content declines. Lactic acid begins to accumulate which results in further decrease of ATP production by inhibition of phosphofructokinase (PFK), the rate-limiting enzyme in glycolysis (Kubler and Spieckermann 1970). Lactate accumulation increases cellular osmolality and is partially responsible for ischemic cellular edema. Lactate accumulation has been correlated with irreversible neuronal injury (Rehnchrona et al. 1979, 1981). Prolonged exposure of cells to flow rates of 15%–30% will deplete them of ATP and will lead to irreversible cellular injury even if circulation is restored to normal. With flow rates of 10%–15% or less there is a rapid decrease in the levels of ATP and the development of the "ischemic freeze" (Hossman and Kleihues 1973).

Restoration of normal perfusion with normal substrate and oxygen delivery may result in the structural and functional recovery of neuronal cells if the level of perfusion was maintained at 30% or higher. With lower perfusion rates, cellular dysfunctions may or may not resolve, or may be exacerbated during reperfusion. The outcome is ultimately determined by the degree and duration of the ischemic injury.

Maintenance of ionic gradients is a major, energy-dependent function of neuronal cell membranes. Without sufficient ATP, sodium and potassium equilibrate between the cytosol and the interstitial fluid (Nicholson 1980; Robbins and Cotran 1979; Seimkowics and Hansen 1981; Vskocil et al. 1972), which leads to cellular edema (Robbins and Cotran 1979). Cellular calcium entry also occurs (Strosnajder 1980; Harris et al. 1981) during low flow states. Once in the cytosol, calcium is actively sequestered in the mitochondria, with the uncoupling of oxidative phosphorylation. Also calcium entry activates proteases (Dayton and Schollenmeyer 1980) and phospholipases (Weglicki et al. 1972) which destroy cell membranes. Free fatty acid byproducts of membrane destruction accumulate in neurons during ischemia (Nemoto et al. 1983) and act as detergents which further disrupt both cellular and mitochondrial membranes and lead to further reduction of ATP synthesis (Harris 1977; Katz and Messineo 1981; Kuwashima et al. 1987; Lazarewics et al. 1972) and more ionic fluxes (Messineo 1983). The loss of the cellular control of calcium homeostasis has been implicated as the trigger in a cascade of consumptive events which leads to cell death (Siesjo 1981; White et al. 1983a,b). Increase in intracellular "free" iron has also been noted as a possible catalyst in the development of free radicals, which also degrade cellular membranes (White et al. 1984).

Reperfusion Injury

The restoration of circulation does not necessarily restore cellular function and integrity and may even accelerate the reactions of cell death. Reperfusion of neurons with already compromised membrane integrity and a reduced cellular energy state may result in further decay of ionic gradients, increased cellular calcium and edema (Naylor 1980; Shen 1972), and further reduction in ATP synthesis (Grinwald and Naylor 1981). Calcium influx and the accumulation of cytotoxic substances such as prostaglandins (Gaudet and Levine 1979) and free radicals (Siesjo 1981) have been hypothesized to contribute to cell damage with reperfusion.

Cerebral Blood Flow and CPCR

No Flow Versus Low Flow

The relative impact of varying levels of blood flow to the brain on the ischemic-anoxic insult during cardiac arrest is a topic that has yet to be resolved (Newberg 1984; White 1984). In cats, Hossmann (1973) found that 30 min of no flow resulted in a better functional recovery than 30 min of 10% flow. The reasons for this paradoxical observation are uncertain. With a low flow state, cells may be provided with enough oxygen and substrates for some oxidative phosphoprylation and free radical formation to occur combined with anaerobic glycolysis. Loss of cellular membrane integrity follows and depletion of energy stores allows sodium and calcium flux into the cell. Lactate accumulates (Rehnchrona 1981) and mitochondrial function is irreversibly injured (Rehnchrona 1979).

In models of global brain ischemia fasted animals do better than nonfasted animals. With increased glucose delivery during low flow compared with zero flow there is increased production of lactic acid intracellularly (Siesjo 1981; Newberg 1984).

White (1985), looking at mitochondrial function after a 15-min arrest and subsequent resuscitation using three different methods of CPR which are known to generate different levels of CBF, noted that with no flow there was minimal injury to brain mitochondrial oxygen consumption. Subsequent resuscitation with a method (interposed abdominal compression CPR) which is thought to produce between 13% (Voorhees 1984) and 51% (Walker 1984) of prearrest CBF resulted in severe inhibition of mitochondrial oxygen utilization. With open-chest massage, which is known to produce excellent cerebral blood flows (Jackson 1984), there was no additional mitochondrial injury. The issue of whether low flow is more detrimental than no flow has yet to be resolved. However, it is clear that low cerebral blood flow (less than 30% of pre-arrest) is not beneficial.

Cerebral Blood Flow During Resuscitation

The critical objective of closed-chest massage is to provide adequate blood flow to the brain and heart. The evidence cited above, concerning the critical levels of blood flow to these organs which either delay or exacerbate ischemic-anoxic injury, provides an objective basis by which to judge the efficacy of different forms of artificial circulation in providing cerebral blood flow.

During standard closed-chest massage, only meager carotid blood flows are produced. Compared with prearrest flow values, 8% flows have been demonstrated in small dogs (Bircher and Safar 1981), with 4% and 17% in larger dogs during closed chest massage (Chandra et al. 1981a,b). Other investigators have observed flows of less than 10% of control values (Ditchey et al. 1982; Lee et al. 1981; Niemann et al. 1981; Redding 1971). Closed-chest massage does not provide adequate carotid artery flows.

Cerebral blood flow during standard closed chest massage is also low. Using the double thermistor method, regional cerebral blood flow during closed chest massage after a 3-min cardiopulmonary arrest was found to be 9.8% of the control value (Jackson et al. 1984). With the radioactive microsphere technique, cerebral blood flows with closed chest massage were found to be 11% (Walker et al. 1984), 12% (Luce et al. 1983), and 4% (Brown et al. 1985) of the prearrest flows. Ischemic-anoxic time prior to resuscitative efforts decreases the eventual cerebral blood flow produced (Michael et al. 1984). Sharff (1984) found that if closed-chest massage is instituted immediately after arrest that the cerebral blood flow initially is excellent, 92%, but deteriorates after 10 min to 26%. The low level of cerebral blood flow generated by standard closed-chest massage is not in the range (minimum 30%) needed to preserve cellular integrity for any length of time. As outlined above, this low flow state might even exacerbate the production of cellular injury.

Poor perfusion of the brain during closed-chest massage can be improved with two types of maneuvers: one, by increasing the aortic diastolic pressure with epinephrine, and two, by increasing the aortic systolic pressure by maneuvers which increase the intrathoracic pressure.

Role of Epinephrine in Resuscitation. Since 1906, epinephrine has been an essential drug in resuscitation (Crile and Dolley 1906). In the doses used during resuscitation, epinephrine not only exhibits the properties of a beta-adrenergic agonist, but also that of a potent alpha-adrenergic agonist. It is this alpha-agonist effect which is important in resuscitation of the heart and brain.

During standard closed-chest massage, the aortic diastolic pressure is low, ranging from 10 to 30 mmHg (Jackson and Freeman 1983) at the onset of chest compressions, but soon falls to 10–15 mmHg (Sharff et al. 1984; Crile and Dolley 1906). The diastolic pressure is critical because it is the driving force for coronary blood flow during closed-chest massage. Without prompt restoration of normal hemodynamics, there is little chance for cerebral salvage. The determinants of myocardial perfusion during closed-chest massage are: diastolic coronary perfusion pressure; intracoronary resistance whether it is fixed or spastic; and intramyocardial flow resistance. Little is known of the tone of the coronary vasculature during arrest. During ventricular fibrillation, the intramyocardial flow resistance increases especially in the endocardium because fibrillation acts as a persistent disordered systole. In vitro studies of fibrillating hearts show that a gradient of compression in the endocardium ranges from 28 to 50 mmHg (Baird et al. 1975; Downey et al. 1979). The diastolic coronary perfusion pressure (diastolic aortic pressure—right atrium diastolic pressure) is 4–16 mmHg during standard closed-chest massage (Niemann 1984). It is clear that closed-chest massage does not provide the diastolic coronary perfusion pressure to overcome the intramyocardial flow resistance during ventricular fibrillation. It has been observed that aortic diastolic pressures of 30–40 mmHg must be attained in order to assure a chance of resuscitation of the heart (Crile and Dolley 1906; Ralston et al. 1984). Epinephrine, by its alpha-agonist properties, augments the aortic diastolic pressure, increasing the coronary perfusion pressure and myocardial blood flow in a linear fashion (Chandra et al. 1981; Ditchey et al. 1982; Michael et al. 1984; Ralston et al. 1984).

Cerebral blood flow is also augmented with the use of epinephrine. Using a high dose of continuous epinephrine (30 μg/kg per minute) during standard closed-chest massage, cerebral blood flow increased from 10% of the prearrest value to 36% of the pre-arrest value (Jackson et al. 1984). With a 38- to 45-μg/kg bolus and a subsequent infusion of 4 μg/kg per minute, cerebral blood flow was 38% of the pre-arrest flow (Michael et al. 1984). Epinephrine increases cerebral blood flow not only by increasing the cerebral perfusion pressure (mean carotid pressure—intracranial pressure) but also by redistributing the carotid blood flow from the facial structures to the central nervous system (Michael et al. 1984).

The current recommended dose of epinephrine used in resuscitation of humans is 0.5–1.0 mg, which in a 70-kg man is a dose of 7.1–14.3 μg/kg, repeated every 5 min (Standards and Guidelines for Cardiopulmonary Resuscitation and Emergency Cardiac Care 1980). This dose was determined empirically. Using 15, 45, 75, and 150 μg/kg during standard closed-chest massage in dogs after a 3-min arrest, Kosnik et al. (1985) determined that the 15-μg/kg dose did not augment the aortic diastolic pressure for more than 2 min, and that the 45-μg/kg dose was effective for 5 min. Larger doses did not augment the maximal change in the diastolic pressure but did increase the duration of effect. Using 20 μg/kg and 200 μg/kg epinephrine in standard closed-chest massage in swine following a 10-min arrest, Brown et al. (1985) determined that the lower dose was ineffective in augmenting cerebral cortical blood flow over that of closed-chest massage, whereas the higher dose increased the cerebral cortical blood flow to 53% of the pre-arrest value. This amount of blood flow in theory would prevent the rapid deterioration of intracellular processes associated with lower flows.

Therefore, the use of epinephrine, or any agent with potent alpha-adrenergic agonist action, during closed-chest massage has potential for augmenting cerebral blood flow in humans. The optimal dose and method for delivery of epinephrine during closed-chest resuscitation in humans has yet to be determined. Whether increased dosing will augment cerebral blood flow in humans and result in improved neurologic outcome is an area which demands exploration.

Intrathoracic Pressure Modulation and Cerebral Blood Flow. When closed-chest massage was reintroduced to the medical community in 1960 by Kouwenhoven et al. (1960) blood flow was hypothesized to result from a pressure gradient which developed between the arterial system and the venous system by the actual compression of the heart between the sternum and spine. Competent cardiac valves are an essential component of this theory. However, Weale and Rothwell-Jackson (1962) found that during closed-chest massage in dogs the iliac artery and vein pressures were equal during compression. They concluded that blood flow was generated by a generalized increase in intrathoracic pressure and not by direct cardiac compression. MacKenzie et al. (1964), with similar results in humans, suggested that "it is very likely that much if not the major portion of the pressure pulse recorded is due to direct transmission of the extrathoracic compression applied to the aorta." That an intrathoracic-extrathoracic pressure gradient (thoracic pump) not a left heart-right heart pressure gradient (cardiac pump) is developed during compression is supported by evidence that all intrathoracic pressures (left ventricle, right ventricle, superior vena cava, thoracic inferior vena cava, esophageal, aortic and pleural) are equal during the compression phase (Jackson and Freeman 1983; Rudikoff et al. 1980). Without demonstrating a pressure difference between the left ventricle and right atrium, it is highly unlikely that direct heart compression provides the impetus for flow.

Two-dimensional ultrasonography in humans undergoing closed-chest massage and cineangiography of dogs shows no change in left ventricular dimensions during compression and incompetent aortic and mitral valves (Niemann et al. 1981; Rich et al. 1981; Werner et al. 1981; Niemann et al. 1981b). Also demonstrated were competent jugular venous valves at the thoracic inlet, which prevent the transmission of the increased thoracic pressure to the venous outflow of the brain. The thoracic pump mechanism generates blood flow by creating an intrathoracic-extrathoracic pressure gradient. With prevention of the transmission of the intrathoracic pressure to the venous side of the central nervous system vasculature, maneuvers which increase intrathoracic pressure in theory should increase carotid and cerebral blood flow.

The most dramatic form of cardiopulmonary resuscitation which takes advantage of the thoracic pump mechanism is Cough-CPR, first described by Criley in 1976. This form of CPR consists of rhythmic coughing (every 1–3 s) by the patient. Consciousness during ventricular fibrillation has been maintained for up to 92 s using this method (Criley et al. 1976; Niemann et al. 1980). Cineangiograms during Cough-CPR show that blood flows primarily cephalad, starting from the descending aorta and then from the left ventricle. The aortic valve remains incompetent (Rosborough et al. 1981).

There are a number of adjunctive methods to closed-chest massage which increase the magnitude of intrathoracic pressure generated in experimental animals. Inflating the lungs during chest compression, instead of during the relaxation phase, augments intrathoracic pressure. This method is called simultaneous ventilation compression CPR or SVC-CPR. This method does not change the aortic diastolic pressure but does increase the aortic and carotid systolic pressures and cerebral perfusion pressure. Cerebral blood flow (CBF) also increases with SVC-CPR; 32% of the prearrest CBF has been generated after 2 min of SVC-CPR started immediately upon arrest compared with 6% with standard closed-chest massage (Luce 1983; Luce 1984). Koehler et al. (1983) also demonstrated a similar CBF with SVC-CPR. Combining this method of CPR with epinephrine further improves CBF and the fall in CBF over time is prevented with epinephrine infusion (Michael et al. 1974). However, this improvement in cerebral blood flow did not improve neurologic or overall outcome after arrest and 30 min of SVC-CPR (Sanders 1982; Bircher 1984).

The use of abdominal binding, by preventing the descent and eversion of the diaphragm, increases intrathoracic pressure by changing the compliance of the thorax (Ducas et al. 1981). This method has been shown to increase carotid blood flow (Chandra et al. 1981a; Rudikoff et al. 1980) and has been used experimentally with SVC-CPR to augment intrathoracic pressure and carotid blood flow (Chandra et al. 1981; Chandra et al. 1980). The MAST garment which sometimes is used during CPR may work by increasing intrathoracic pressure (Guerci et al. 1981).

Interposed abdominal compression CPR involves compressing the abdomen and chest alternately. This form of artificial circulation has been shown to increase cardiac output in experimental animals (Voorhees et al. 1984; Ralston et al. 1982). The data on augmentation of cerebral blood flow are not clear at this time with values of 13% (Voorhees et al. 1982) to 51% (Walker et al. 1984) of control values.

One method of artificial circulation which is effective is direct massage of the heart either manually or mechanically. Manual open-chest cardiac massage generates superior hemodynamic values to those of closed-chest massage (Jackson and Freeman 1983). Cerebral blood flow is normal during open-chest massage (Jackson et al. 1984; Arai et al. 1984; Stajduhar et al. 1983). The applicability of this method is limited since it requires highly skilled individuals in a controlled situation. Currently, this is the only method of artificial circulation which fulfills the goal of providing adequate blood flow to the brain.

The effect of different methods of artificial circulation on outcome was demonstrated most dramatically in a study by Bircher et al. (1984). Thirty-two dogs were divided into four groups and each underwent different forms of resuscitation. The control group was immediately defibrillated and resuscitated and developed no neurologic deficits. Of the eight dogs in the group which received 30 min of standard closed-chest massage, six were resuscitated and one survived 24 h with a severe neurologic deficit. Of the eight dogs in the group which received SVC-CPR, only five were resuscitated and none survived 24 h. All of the dogs that received open-chest massage were resuscitated and survived for 24 h with minimal neurologic deficits. This study emphasizes the critical importance of good cerebral perfusion during resuscitation.

Measures such as epinephrine and augmentation of intrathoracic pressure do increase cerebral blood flow during resuscitation. However, whether this increase is to a level which prevents or diminishes the insult to the brain is not known at this time.

Postresuscitation Cerebral Blood Flow

Following a cardiopulmonary arrest and resuscitation with restoration of circulation, CBF may not return to normal. Often there ensues a short period of hyperemia, followed by a progressive decrease in CBF and increase in cerebral vascular resistance. This phenomenon, sometimes referred to as "no-reflow," but more accurately defined as "post-ischemic hypoperfusion" (Ames 1963), has been documented in many experiments using different arrest times and types of resuscitation (White et al. 1983b; Kagstrom et al. 1983; Newberg et al. 1984; Tintinalli et al. 1985; Rehncrona et al. 1979; Snyder et al. 1975; Nemoto et al. 1981). Postischemic hypoperfusion occurs concomitantly with the development of brain hypermetabolism (Hossman 1983) and the resultant ischemic insult may determine the neurologic outcome. The minimum arrest time needed to prevent this phenomenon is unknown, but CBF of 30%–40% during resuscitation may prevent postischemic hypoperfusion (Kagstrom et al. 1983). Interestingly, in models of absolute global brain ischemia, with the remainder of the body well perfused, postischemic hypoperfusion may not occur (Hossman 1983). This again supports the hypothesis that no flow is better than low flow during resuscitation.

The pathogenesis of postischemic hypoperfusion has been postulated to be sludging of blood, intravascular clotting, or rise in intracranial pressure. White (1982) speculated that it is secondary to vascular spasm resulting from calcium influx that occurs during arrest and subsequent recirculation. The use of calcium channel blockers after 15 min of complete arrest and subsequent open-chest massage in dogs prevented postischemic hypoperfusion (White et al. 1982; Edmonds et al. 1985) and improved neurologic outcome (Edmonds et al. 1985; Vaagnees et al. 1984; Winegar et al. 1983; Vaagnees et al. 1984; Waquier 1982). However, calcium channel blockers did not improve CBF postarrest in another model of total cerebral ischemia (Dean et al. 1984). The use of 5 mg/kg naloxone postarrest did not prevent postischemic hypoperfusion (Tintinalli et al. 1985).

Postresuscitative Treatment of Anoxic Encephalopathy

In the experimental animal, calcium channel blockers seem to ameliorate some of the neurologic deficits seen postresuscitation (Winegar et al. 1983). However, White (1984) has reported that the effects are transient. In a multicenter trial, thiopental loading did not substantially improve the neurologic outcome among CPR survivors (BRCT 1986). Other potential therapies are targeted at preventing the intracellular development and actions of free radicals (White et al. 1984).

Based on current knowledge and state-of-the-art expertise in postresuscitation treatment, the most beneficial intervention that might prevent anoxic encephalopathy remains rapid restoration of normal hemodynamics. Ventricular tachycardia and fibrillation are rhythms with the best prognosis and can be electrically converted to an organized rhythm. Early defibrillation has been reported to improve neurologic recovery (Weaver et al. 1984). Development of advanced paramedic systems are expensive but effective (Eisenberg et al. 1980). Currently, a number of automatic, portable, computer-operated defibrillators and pacemakers are being tested. These can be operated with little instruction and could be an effective, readily available means of converting a chaotic rhythm quickly, potentially increasing survival (Weaver et al. 1985). Until substantial advances have been made in postresuscitative measures to protect the brain, efforts that will shorten the ischemic-anoxic time will have the most impact on decreasing the incidence of anoxic encephalopathy.

References

Abramson N, Safar P, Detre K, Monroe J, Kelsey S, Reinmuth O, Snyder J, Mullie A, Hedstrandu, Tammisto T, Lund I, Breivik H, Lind B, Jastremski M (1982) Long term follow-up of cardiac arrest survivors (abstr). Crit Care Med 10: 215

Brain Resuscitation Clinical Trial Study Group (1986) Randomized clinical trial of thiopental loading in comatose survivors of cardiac arrest. New Engl J Med 314: 395–403

Adams JH, Brierley JB, Connor RCR, Treip CS (1966) The effects of systemic hypotension upon the human brain. Clinical and neuropathological observations in 11 cases. Brain 89: 235–268
Ames A, Guarian BS (1963) Effects of glucose deprivation on function of isolated mammalian retina. J Neurophysiol 26: 617
Arai T, Dote K, Tsukahara I, Nitta K, Nagaro T (1984) Cerebral blood flow during conventional, new and open-chest cardio-pulmonary resuscitation in dogs. Resuscitation 12: 147–154
Baird RJ, Dutka F, Okumori M (1975) Surgical aspects of regional myocardial blood flow and myocardial pressure. J Thoracic Cardiovasc Surg 69: 17–29
Bates D, Caronna JJ, Cartlidge NEF, Knill-Jones RP, Levy DE, Shaw DA, Plum F (1977) A prospective study of nontraumatic coma: methods and results. Ann Neurol 2: 211–220
Bircher N, Safar P (1981) Comparison of standard and "new" closed-chest CPR and open-chest CPR in dogs. Crit Care Med 9: 384–385
Bircher N, Safar P (1984) Preserving the brain during cardiopulmonary resuscitation in dogs (abstr). Crit Care Med 12: 251
Borgers M, Thone F, Van Reempts J, et al. (1983) The role of calcium in cellular dysfunction. Am J Emerg Med 1: 154
Brierley JB (1970) Systemic hypotension—neurological and neuropathological aspects. In: Williams D (ed) Modern trends in neurology—5, chap 9. Butterworths, London, pp 164–177
Brierley JB, Brown AW, Excell BJ, Meldrum BS (1969) Brain damage in the rhesus monkey resulting from profound arterial hypotension. I: its nature, distribution and general physiological correlates. Brain Res 13: 68–100
Brierley JB, Adams JH, Graham DI, Simpson JA (1971) Neocortical death after cardiac arrest. Lancet I: 560–565
Brown CG, Werman RL, Hamlin RL, et al. (1985) Effect of high-dose epinephrine on regional blood flow during CPR in a porcine model. Ann Emerg Med (abstr) 14: 506
Caronna JJ (1983) Acute management of severe brain anoxia. In: Earnest MP (ed) Neurologic emergencies. Churchill Livingstone, New York, pp 413–438
Caronna JJ, Finkelstein S (1978) Neurological syndromes after cardiac arrest. Stroke 9: 517–520
Chandra N, Rudikoff MT, Weisfeldt ML (1980) Simultaneous chest compression and ventilation at high airway pressure during cardiopulmonary resuscitation. Lancet 1980 (1): 175–178
Chandra N, Tsitlik J, Weisfeldt ML (1981a) Optimization of carotid flow during CPR in arrest dogs. Crit Care Med 9: 379
Chandra N, Weisfeldt ML, Tsitlik J, Vaghaiwala F, Snyder LD, Hoffecker M, Rudikoff MT (1986) Augmentation of carotid flow during cardiopulmonary resuscitation by ventilation at high airway pressures simultaneous with chest compressions. Am J Cardiol 98: 1053–1063
Copley DP, Mantle JA, Rogers WJ, Russell RO, Rackley CE (1977) Improved outcome for prehospital cardiopulmonary collapse with resuscitation by bystanders. Circulation 56: 901–905
Crile G, Dolley DH (1906) Experimental research into resuscitation of dogs killed by anesthetics and asphyxia. J Exp Med 8: 713–720
Criley JM, Blkaufuss AH, Kissel GL (1976) Cough-induced cardiac compression: self-administered form of cardiopulmonary resuscitation. JAMA 236: 1246–1250
Dayton WR, Schollenmeyer JV (1980) Isolation from porcine cardiac muscle of a Ca^{+2}-activated protease that partially degrades myofibrils. J Mol Cell Cardiol 12: 533
Dean JM, Hoehner PJ, Rogers MC, Tratstman RJ (1984) Effect of lidoflazine on cerebral blood flow following twelve minutes total cerebral ischemia. Stroke 15: 531–535
DeCree J, De Cook W, Geukens M, DeClerck F, Beerens M, Verhaegen H (1979) The rheological effects of cinnarizine and flunarizine in normal and pathological conditions. Angiology 30: 505–515
Ditchey RV, Winkler JV, Rhodes CA (1972) Lack of coronary blood flow during closed-chest resuscitation. Circulation 66: 297–302
Downey JM, Chagrasulis RW, Hemphill V (1979) Quantitative study of intramyocardial compression in the fibrillating heart. Am J Physiol 237: H191–196
Ducas J, Roussas C, Karardis C, Angle M, Magder S (1981) Factors affecting the intrathoracic pressure during CPR. Circulation 64 [Suppl IV]: 302
Earnest MP, Yarnell PR, Merrill SL, Knapp GL (1980) Long-term survival and neurologic status after resuscitation from out-of-hospital cardiac arrest. Neurology 30: 1298–1302
Edmonds HL, Waquier A, Melis W, et al. (1985) Improved short-term neurologic recovery with flunarizine in a canine model of cardiac arrest. Am J Energ Med 3: 150–155
Eisenberg MS, Bergner L, Hallstrom (1979) Cardiac resuscitation in the community: importance of rapid provision and implication for program planning. JAMA 241: 1905–1907
Eisenberg MS, Copass MK, Hallstrom A, et al. (1980) Management of out-of-hospital cardiac arrest: failure of basic emergency medical technician services. JAMA 243: 1049–1051

Enns J, Tweed WA, Donen N (1983) Prehospital cardiac rhythm deterioration in a system providing only basic life support. Ann Emerg Med 12: 478–481
Harris EJ (1977) The uptake and release of calcium by the heart mitochondria. Biochem J 168: 447
Harris RJ, Symon L, Bronston NM, et al. (1981) Changes in extracellular calcium activity in cerebral ischemia. J Cereb Blood Flow Metab 1: 203
Heymans C (1950) Survival and revival of nervous tissue after arrest of circulation. Physiol Rev 30: 375
Hossman KA (1976) Development and resolution of ischemic brain swelling. In: Pappius H, Feindel W (eds) Dynamics of brain edema. Springer, Berlin Heidelberg New York, pp 219–227
Hossman KA (1983) Neuronal survival and revival during and after cerebral ischemia. Am J Emerg Med 1: 191
Hossman KA, Kleihues P (1973) Reversibility of ischemic brain damage. Arch Neurol 29: 375
Gaudet RJ, Levine L (1977) Transient cerebral ischemia and brain prostaglandins. Biochem Biophys Res Commun 6: 893
Goldberg AH (1974) Cardiopulmonary arrest. N Engl J Med 290: 381–384
Grinwald PM, Naylor WG (1981) Calcium entry in the calcium paradox. J Mol Cell Cardiol 13: 867
Gudjonsson H, Baldvinsson E, Oddsson G, Asgeirsson E, Krist Jansson H, Hardarson T (1982) Results of attempted cardiopulmonary resuscitation in patients dying outside the hospital in Reykjavik and the surrounding area, 1976–1979. Acta Med Scand 212: 247–251
Guerci A, Chandra N, Levin H, Koehler RC, Tsitlik JE, Traystman RJ, Rogers MC, Weisfeldt ML (1981) Hemodynamic determinants of intercranial pressure during resuscitation. Circulation 64 [Suppl IV]: 304
Guzy PM, Pearce ML, Greenfield S (1979) The survival benefit of bystander cardiopulmonary resuscitation in a paramedic-serviced metropolitan area. Am J Public Health 69: 30–38
Jackson RE, Freeman SB (1983) Hemodynamics of cardiac massage. N A Clin Emerg Med 1: 501–513
Jackson RE, Joyce K, Danosi SF, White BC, Vigor D, Hoehner TJ (1984) Blood flow in the cerebral cortex during cardiac resuscitation in dogs. Ann Emerg Med 13: 657–659
Jorgensen EO, Malchow-Moller A (1978) Cerebral prognostic signs during cardiopulmonary resuscitation. Resuscitation 6: 217–225
Kagstrom E, Smith M-L, Siesjo BK (1983) Recirculation in the rat brain following incomplete ischemia. J Cereb Blood Flow Metab 3: 183–192
Katz AM, Messineo FC (1981) Lipd-membrane interactions and the pathogenesis of ischemic damaged in the myocardium. Circ Res 48: 1
Koehler RC, Michael JR, Guerci AD, Shi AY, Tsitlik J, Chandra N, Rogers MC, Travstman RJ, Weisfeldt ML (1983) Effect of epinephrine on cerebral blood flow during cardiopulmonary resuscitation in dogs. Anesthesiology 59 [Suppl]: A94
Kouwenhoven WB, Jude JR, Knickerbocker CG (1960) Closed chest cardiac massage. JAMA 173: 1064–1067
Kosnik JW, Jackson RE, Keats S, Tworek RM, Freeman SB (1985) Dose-related response of centrally administered epinephrine on the change in aortic diastolic pressure during closed-chest massage in dogs. Ann Emerg Med 14: 204–208
Kowalski R, Thompson BM, Horowitz L, Aprahamian C, Darin JC (1984) Bystander CPR in prehospital course ventricular fibrillation. Ann Emerg Med 13: 1016–1020
Kubler W, Spieckermann PG (1970) Regulation of glycolysis in the ischemic and anoxic myocardium. J Mol Cell Cardiol 1: 351
Kuwashima J, Nakamura K, Fujitani B, et al. (1987) Relationship between cerebral energy failure and free fatty acid accumulation following prolonged brain ischemia. Jpn J Pharmacol 28: 277
Lazarewics JW, Strosznajder J, Gromek A (1972) Effects of ischemia and exogenous fatty acids on the energy metabolism in brain mitochondria. Bull Acad Polish Sci Biol 20: 599
Lee HR, Wilder RJ, Downs P, Massion W, Blank WF (1981) MAST augmentation of external cardiac compression: role of changing intrapleural pressure. Ann Emerg Med 10: 560–565
Lehninger AL (1974) Role of phosphate and other proton donating cations in respiration-coupled transport of CA^{+2} by mitochondria. Proc Nat Acad Sci 71: 1520
Levy DE, Caronna JJ, Singer BH, Lapinski RH, Frydman H, Plum F (1985) Predicting outcome from hypoxic-ischemic coma. JAMA 253: 1420–1426
Luce JM, Ross BK, O'Quin RJ, Culver BH, Sivarajan M, Amory DW, Niskanen RA, Alferness CA, Kirk WL, Pierson LB, Butler J (1983) Regional blood flow during cardiopulmonary resuscitation in dogs using simultaneous and nonsimultaneous compression and ventilation. Circulation 67: 258–265
Luce JM, Rizk NA, Niskanen RA (1983) Regional blood flow during cardiopulmonary resuscitation in dogs. Crit Care Med 12: 874–878

Lund I, Skulberg A (1976) Cardiopulmonary resuscitation by lay people. Lancet (2): 702–705
MacKenzie GJ, Taylor SH, McDonald AH, Donald KW (1964) Hemodynamic effects of external cardiac compression. Lancet (1): 1342–1345
Mahoney BD, Mirick MJ (1983) Efficacy of pneumatic trousers in refractory prehospital cardiopulmonary arrest. Ann Emerg Med 12: 8–12
Messineo FC (1983) The possible role of endogenous amphiphiles in the membrane abnormalities of ischemic and reperfused myocardium. Am J Emerg Med 1: 162
Micheal JR, Guerci AD, Koehler RC, Shi AY, Tsitlik J, Chandra N, Niedermeyer E, Rogers MC, Traystman RJ, Weisfeldt ML (1984) Mechanism by which epinephrine augments cerebral and myocardial perfusion during cardiopulmonary resuscitation in dogs. Circulation 69: 822–835
Myerberg RJ, Kessler KM, Zaman L, Conde CA, Castellanos A (1982) Survivors of prehospital cardiac arrest. JAMA 247: 1485–1490
Naylor WG, Ferrari R, Williams A (1980) Protective effect of pretreatment with verapamil, nifedipine and propranolol on mitochondrial function in the ischemic and reperfused myocardium. Am J Cardiol 46: 242
Nemoto EM, Hossmann KA, Cooper HK (1981) Post-ischemic hypermetabolism in cat brain. Stroke 12: 666
Nemoto EM, Shui GK, Nemmer JP, et al. (1983) Free fatty acid accumulation in the pathogenesis and therapy of ischemic anoxic brain injury. Am J Emerg Med 1: 175
Newberg LA: Cerebral resuscitation (1984) Advances and controversies. Ann Emerg Med 13: 853–855
Newberg LA, Steen PA, Milde JH, Michenfelder JD (1984) Failure of flunarazine to improve cerebral blood flow or neurologic recovery in a canine model of complete cerebral ischemia. Stroke 15: 666–671
Nicholson C (1980) Measurment of extracellular ions in the brain. Trends Neurosci 3: 216
Niemann JT (1984) Differences in cerebral and myocardial perfusion during closed-chest resuscitation. Ann Emerg Med 13: 849–852
Niemann JT, Rosborough J, Hausnecht M (1980) Cough-CPR. Crit Care Med 8: 141–146
Niemann JT, Rosborough J, Hausnecht M, Garner P, Criley JM (1981a) Pressure-synchronized cineangiography during experimental cardiopulmonary resuscitation. Circulation 64: 985–991
Niemann JT, Rosborough J, Hausnecht M, Ung S, Criley JM (1981b) Blood flow without cardiac compression during closed chest CPR. Crit Care Med 9: 380–381
Paschen W, Djuricic B, Bosma HL, et al. (1981) Regional blood flow and regional distribution of biochemical substrates in experimental stroke in gerbils. J Cereb Blood Flow Metab [Suppl] 1: 174
Pionkowski RS, Thompson BM, Gruchon HW, Aprahamian C, Darin JC (1983) Resuscitation time in ventricular fibrillation—a prognostic indicator. Ann Emerg Med 12: 733–738
Plum F, Posner JB, Hain RF (1962) Delayed neurological deterioration after anoxia. Arch Int Med 110: 18–25
Ralston SH, Babbs CF, Niebauer MJ (1982) Cardiopulmonary resuscitation with interposed abdominal compression in dogs. Anesth Analg 61: 645–651
Ralston SH, Voorhees WD, Babbs CF (1984) Intrapulmonary epinephrine during prolonged cardiopulmonary resuscitation: improved regional blood flow and resuscitation in dogs. Ann Emerg Med 13: 79–86
Ralston SH, Showen L, Carter A, Tacker WA (1985) Comparison of endotracheal and intravenous epinephrine dosage during CPR in dogs. Ann Emerg Med (Absrt) 14: 494
Redding JS (1971) Abdominal compression in cardiopulmonary resuscitation. Anesth Analg 50: 668–675
Rehnchrona S, Mela L, Siesjo BK (1979) Recovery of brain mitochondrial function in the rat after complete cerebral ischemia. Stroke 10: 437
Rehncrona S, Abdul-Rahman A, Siesjo BK (1979) Local cerebral blood flow in the post ischemic period. Acta Neurol Scand 60 [Suppl]: 294
Rehchrona S, Rosen I, Siesjo BK (1981) Brain lactic acidosis and cell damage. Biochemistry neurophysiology. J Cereb Blood Flow Metab 1: 297
Rich S, Wix HL, Shaporo EP (1981) Clinical assessment of heart chamber size and valve motion during cardiopulmonary resuscitation by two-dimensional echocardiography. Am Heart J 102: 368–373
Robbins SL, Cotran RS (eds) (1979) Cell injury and death. In: Pathologic basis of disease, 2nd edn. Saunders, Philadelphia, pp 22–54
Rosborough J, Hausnecht M, Niemann JT (1981) Cough supported circulation. Crit Care Med 9: 371–372
Roth R, Stewart RD, Rogers K, Cannon GM (1984) Out-of-hospital cardiac arrest: factors associated with survival. Ann Emerg Med 13: 237–243

Rudikoff MT, Maughan WL, Effron M, Freund P, Weisfeldt ML (1980) Mechanisms of blood flow during cardiopulmonary resuscitation. Circulation 61: 345–352
Sanders AB, Ewy GA, Alferness CA, Taft T, Zimmerman M (1982) Failure of one method of simultaneous compression, ventilation and abdominal binding during CPR. Crit Care Med 10: 509–513
Seimkowics E, Hansen AL (1981) Brain extracellular ion composition and EEG activity following 10 minutes ischemia in normo and hyperglycemic rats. Stroke 12: 236
Sharff JA, Pantley G, Noel E (1984) Effect of time on regional organ perfusion during two methods of cardiopulmonary resuscitation. Ann Emerg Med 13: 649–656
Shen AC, Jenning RB (1972) Kinetics of calcium accumulation in acute myocardial ischemic injury. Am J Pathol 67: 441
Siesjo BK (1981) Cell damage in the brain: a speculative synthesis. J Cereb Blood Flow Metabol 1: 155–185
Snyder JV, Nemoto EM, Carrol RG, Safar P (1975) Global ischemia in dogs: intracranial pressure, brain blood flow and metabolism. Stroke 6: 21–27
Snyder BD, Ramirez-Lassepas M, Lippert DM (1977) Neurologic status and prognosis after cardiopulmonary arrest: I. A retrospective study. Neurology (Minn) 27: 807–811
Synder BD, Loewenson RB, Gummit RJ, Hauser WA, Leppik IE, Ramirez-Lassepas M (1980) Neurologic prognosis after cardiopulmonary arrest. II Level of consciousness. Neurology (NY) 30: 52–58
Synder BD, Gummit RJ, Leppik IE, Hauser WA, Loewenson RB, Ramirez-Lassepas M (1981) Neurologic prognosis after cardiopulmonary arrest: IV. Brainstem reflexes. Neurology 31: 1092–1097
Stajduhar K, Steinberg R, Sotosky M, Safar P, Stezoski SW (1983) Cerebral blood flow and common carotid blood flow during open chest cardiopulmonary resuscitation in dogs. Anesthesiology 59: A117
Standards and Guidelines for Cardiopulmonary Resuscitation and Emergency Cardiac Care (1980) JAMA 244: 453–572
Strosnajder J (1980) Role of phospholipids in calcium accumulation in brain mitochondra from adult rat after ischemia-anoxia and hypoxic-hypoxia. Bull Acad Polish Sci Biol 27: 683
Thompson RG, Hallstrom AP, Cobb LA (1979) Bystander-initiated cardiopulmonary resuscitation in the management of ventricular fibrillation. Ann Intern Med 90: 737–740
Tintinalli JE, Zwanger M, Koster K (1985) Effect of naloxone on cerebral blood flow postarrest. Ann Emerg Med 14: 507
Torvik A (1984) The pathogenesis of watershed infarcts in the brain. Stroke 15: 221–223
Tweed WA, Bristow G, Donen N (1980) Resuscitation from cardiac arrest: assessment of a system providing only basic life support outside the hospital. Can Med Assc J 122: 297–300
Vaagnees P, Cantadore R, Safar P, Moosy J, Rao G, Diven W, Alexander H, Stezoski W (1984a) Amelioration of brain damage by Lidoflazine after prolonged ventricular fibrillation cardiac arrest in dogs. Crit Care Med 12: 846–855
Vaagnees P, Cantadore R, Safar P, Alexander H (1984) The effect of Lidoflazine and Verapamil on neurologic outcome after 10 minutes ventricular fibrillation cardiac arrest in dogs. Crit Care Med 12: 228
Vertesi L, Wilson L, Glick N: Cardiac arrest (1983) Comparison of paramedic and conventional ambulance services. Can Med Assoc J 128: 809–813
Voorhees WD, Ralston SH, Babbs CF (1984) Regional blood flow during cardiopulmonary resuscitation with abdominal counterpulsation in dogs. Am J Emerg Med 2: 123–128
Vskocil F, Kritz N, Bures J (1972) Potassium selective microelectrodes used for measuring brain potassium during spreading depression and anoxic depolarization in rats. Brain Res 39: 255
Walker JW, Bruestle JC, White BC, Evans AT, Indreri R, Bialek H (1984) Perfusion of the cerebral cortex by use of abdominal counterpulsation during cardiopulmonary resuscitation. Am J Emerg Med 2: 391–393
Waquier A (1982) Brain protective properties of Etomidate and Flunarazine. J Cereb Blood Flow Metabol 2 [Suppl I]: S53–56
Weale FE, Rothwell-Jackson RL (1962) The efficacy of cardiac massage. Lancet (1): 990–992
Weaver WD, Copass MK, Bufi D, Ray R, Hallstrom AP, Cobb LA (1984) Improved neurologic recovery and survival after early defibrillation. Circulation 69: 943–948
Weaver WD, Cobb LA, Copass MK, Hallstrom AP, Emery M (1985) Enhancing survival after cardiac arrest—the effect of initial rhythm and a new strategy in emergency care. Ann Emerg Med (abstr); 14: 511
Weglicki WB, Owens K, Urschell CW, et al. (1972) Hydrolysis of myocardial lipids during acidosis

and ischemia. In: Dhalla NS (ed) Recent advances of studies on cardiac structure and metabolism. University Park Press, Baltimore, pp 781–793

Weinberger LM, Gibbon MH, Gibbon JH (1940) Temporary arrest of the circulation to the central nervous system: I. Physiologic effects. Arch Neurol Psych 40: 615

Werner JA, Greene HL, Janko CL, Cobb LA (1981) Visualization of the cardiac valve motion in man during external chest compression using two-dimensional echocardiography. Implication regarding the mechanism of blood flow. Circulation 63: 1417–1421

White BC, Hoehner PJ, Wilson RF (1980) Mitochondria O2 use and ATP synthesis: kinetic effect of Ca^{+2} and HPO4-2 modulated by glucocorticoids. Ann Emerg Med 9: 396

White BC, Gadzinski DS, Hoehner PJ, Krome C Hoehnner T, White JD, Trombley JH Jr (1982) Effect of flunarizine on canine cerebral cortical blood flow and vascular resistance post cardiac arrest. Ann Emerg Med 11: 119–126

White BC, Winegar CD, Jackson RE, et al. (1983a) Cerebral cortical perfusion during and following resuscitation from cardiac arrest in dogs. Am J Emerg Med 1: 128–138

White BC, Winegar CD, Henderson O, Jackson RE, Krause G, O'Hara T, Goodin T, Vigor DN (1983b) Prolonged hypoperfusion in the cerebral cortex following cardiac arrest and resuscitation in dogs. Ann Emerg Med 12: 414–417

White BC, Aust SD, Arfors KE, Aronson LD (1984) Brain injury by ischemic anoxia—hypothesis extension: a tale of two ions? Ann Emerg Med 13: 862–867

White BC, Hildebrandt JF, Evans AT, Aronson L, Indrieri RJ, Hoehner T, Fox L, Huang R (1985) Prolonged cardiac arrest and resuscitation in dogs: brain mitochondrial function with different artificial perfusion methods. Ann Emerg Med 14: 383–388

Winegar CD, White BC (1983) Physiology of resuscitation. N A Clin Emerg Med 1: 179–199

Winegar CD, Henderson O, White BC, Jackson RE, O'Hara T, Krause GS, Vigor DN, Kontry R, Wilson W, Shelby-Lane C (1983) Early amelioration of neurologic deficit by lidoflazine after fifteen minutes of cardiopulmonary arrest in dogs. Ann Emerg Med 12: 471–477

Chapter 13

Orthostatic Hypotension: Circulatory Dynamics and Clinical Spectrum

F. M. Fouad and J. D. Maloney

Introduction

The hemodynamic responses to upright posture have been studied extensively and are fairly well defined (Tarazi and Fouad 1983; Rushmer 1976). As one stands up, about 500 ml blood gets trapped in the distensible veins below the level of the heart. This peripheral relocation of intravascular volume results in a reduction in cardiac output. Sympathetic system activation is rapidly induced by two separate routes. The first is the classical high-pressure baroreceptor reflex and the second involves the diminished stretch of sensors in the low-pressure cardiopulmonary receptor area. The renin-angiotensin system is also activated in the upright posture and increased angiotensin II levels may play a role in the immediate response of blood pressure (Schatz 1984). When these compensatory mechanisms fail to occur, orthostatic hypotension follows. Syncope is the most dramatic clinical expression of the phenomenon (see Chap 14).

Orthostatic hypotension can be due to autonomic failure, but a significant reduction in arterial pressure on standing or following dynamic exercise can occur in many other nonneurogenic conditions. The differentiation between these various causes will depend to a large extent on an accurate determination of the hemodynamic changes provoked by upright posture.

Definition of Orthostatic Hypotension

The fall in arterial pressure with upright posture can either involve the systolic and diastolic levels or be restricted to systolic levels. No agreement exists as to the normal range of these postural changes. Normal values in our laboratory were obtained from 26 normal volunteers; blood pressure was 119±4 (SE)/71±3 mmHg in the supine position and 116±3/80±3 mmHg during head-up tilt (60° for 10 min). Myers et al. (1978) reported that similar values apply to all subjects up to 99 years old.

The blood pressure should be measured in the supine position and after 2 min standing if tolerated. A graded tilt test, however, is more useful for quantification of the results. A stimulus response curve can be drawn for the heart rate, diastolic blood pressure, total peripheral resistance, and plasma norepinephrine level. Comparison of responses among patients and at different times in the same patient can be made in relation to both the duration of tilt and the response of the indices to the same degree of tilt.

An orthostatic fall restricted to the systolic blood pressure is more likely to be due to a nonneurogenic hemodynamic disturbance. The orthostatic hypotension of autonomic failure involves both the systolic and diastolic levels. We believe that an orthostatic fall in diastolic blood pressure greater than 10 mmHg warrants a full clinical evaluation even if the patient remains asymptomatic. Further evaluation is also indicated when blood pressure fall with upright posture is intermittent since the course of autonomic failure may be variable (Ibrahim et al. 1975).

Classification of Orthostatic Hypotension

The range of neurohumoral and circulatory responses to upright posture has been recently reviewed (Tarazi and Fouad 1983; Campese et al. 1980). The following discussion will therefore only highlight some aspects that are particularly relevant to clinical problems.

Neurogenic Hypotension

Neurogenic orthostatic hypotension (autonomic failure) is best classified according to the anatomic site of the disorder, which may be in the afferent or efferent pathway of the baroreceptor arc, or in the central nervous system connections (Table 13.1). The natural course of these illnesses can range from an easily tolerable, relatively stable condition lasting many years to a progressive and severe deterioration of cardiovascular and autonomic nervous system function.

Baroreceptor Arc

Diseases which interfere with initiation of the baroreceptor feedback loop are more commonly encountered than previously thought and include alteration in elasticity of carotid sinus and aortic arch walls, degenerative changes (atherosclerotic) in these areas, or interruption of afferent pathways of the baroreceptor reflex as in diabetes mellitus (Sharpey-Schafer and Taylor 1960), chronic alcoholism (Barraclough and Sharpey-Schafer 1960), tabes dorsalis (Barraclough and Sharpey-Schafer 1960), and Holmes-Adie syndrome (Johnson et al. 1971). Most cases of neurogenic orthostatic hypotension, however, involve lesions of efferent pathways among which are lesions of sympathetic ganglia in diabetes mellitus (Hilsted 1982) and chronic alcoholism (Appenzeller and

Table 13.1. Causes of autonomic failure. (modified from Johnson 1976)

I. Lesions of afferent pathway of baroreceptor reflex
  1. Change in elastic properties or degenerative changes in carotid sinus or aortic arch
  2. Interruption of afferent fiber activity
     - Diabetes mellitus
     - Chronic alcoholism
     - Tabes dorsalis
     - Holmes-Adie syndrome

II. Lesions of efferent pathway of baroreceptor reflex
  1. Ganglionic lesions
     - Diabetes mellitus
     - Chronic alcoholism
  2. Acute sensory motor neuropathy (Guillain-Barré' syndrome)
  3. Chronic postganglionic neuropathy
     - Diabetes mellitus
     - Chronic alcoholism
     - Neoplasms (pancreas, bronchus)
     - Porphyria
     - Primary amyloidosis
  4. Deficient release of catecholamines from postganglionic nerves
     - Anorexia nervosa
     - Drugs (reserpine)
  5. Idiopathic (IOH)

III. Central (brain stem) lesions
     - Shy-Drager syndrome
     - Familial dysautonomia
     - Multiple infarcts
     - Parkinsonism
     - Tumors of posterior fossa
     - Craniopharyngioma
     - Postsurgery to brain stem
     - Centrally acting drugs (clonidine, methyldopa)

IV. Selective vagal neuropathy
     - Diabetes mellitus

Richardson 1966), peripheral sensorimotor neuropathy as in the acute Guillain-Barré syndrome, or the chronic neuropathy of diabetes mellitus and chronic alcholism or in association with malignant neoplasm (Siemson and Meister 1963). Autonomic neuropathy with orthostatic hypotension has also been described in association with porphyria (McLeod 1983) and primary amyloidosis (Kyle et al. 1966). Sensorimotor neuropathy may occur in the Guillain-Barré syndrome without evidence of autonomic dysregulation; conversely, pure autonomic dysfunction may be the only presenting abnormality in this disease (Young et al. 1975). Finally, efferent baroreflex dysfunction may be due to deficient release of catecholamines from postganglionic nerves such as occurs in anorexia nervosa (Schatz 1984).

Central Nervous System Lesions

Shy-Drager Syndrome. In addition to peripheral autonomic failure, this disorder involves lesions of the central autonomic nervous system including the corticobulbar, corticospinal, and cerebellar systems (Shy and Drager 1960; Hohl et al. 1965; Schwarz 1967). A Parkinson-like syndrome is usually present, although orthostatic hypotension may be the initial and only sign for a long period.

The differentiation between central (Shy-Drager syndrome) and peripheral autonomic insufficiency (idiopathic orthostatic hypotension, IOH) was attempted by some investigators on the basis of differences in plasma norepinephrine levels (Polinsky et al. 1981; Ziegler et al. 1977). In our experience, however, seven out of seven patients with Shy-Drager syndrome and four out of nine IOH patients had normal plasma catecholamines at rest and stimulated normally during head-up tilt; the remaining five IOH patients had supine plasma norepinephrine equal to or less than 100 ng/liter and had a rather blunted response to upright tilt. Thus, the reports by Polinsky et al. (1981) and Ziegler et al. (1977) that plasma norepinephrine is normal in multiple-system atrophy (Shy-Drager syndrome) patients and low in idiopathic orthostatic hypotension patients was not confirmed in our studies. On the other hand, the use of tyramine to differentiate between the two groups of patients (Ibrahim et al. 1979) was supported by the recent report by Glassman et al. (1979).

Other CNS Lesions. Since integrated structures in the brain are necessary for proper control of circulatory reflexes, conditions such as familial dysautonomia, multiple cerebral infarcts, Wernicke's encephalopathy, tumors of posterior fossa, or craniopharyngioma can be associated with autonomic disturbances because of involvement of the hypothalamus, midbrain, and fourth ventricular nuclei (Schatz 1984). Some degree of orthostatic drop in blood pressure is commonly seen in patients with idiopathic parkinsonism (Gross et al. 1972), the exact mechanism of which is still unknown, but which has been attributed to inactivity, the use of dopaminergic drugs, and defective bioregulatory reflexes.

Parasympathetic Dysfunction. Apart from abnormalities of the sympathetic nervous system, some disorders with autonomic neuropathy are characterized predominantly by interruption of *vagal* activity, e.g. diabetes mellitus. In these patients resting tachycardia is usually present, but orthostatic hypotension may not always be a feature (Watkins 1973; Wheeler and Watkins 1973).

Nonneurogenic Hypotension

Inadequate Cardiac Filling

The vast majority of cases of nonneurogenic orthostatic hypotension result from inadequate cardiac filling either because of absolute or relative hypovolemia or because of some interference with venous return. Diminished cardiac performance on the other hand is not a common cause of orthostatic hypotension. Patients with congestive heart failure are known to tolerate head-up tilt quite well, presumably because of their hypervolemia (Abdelmann and Fareeduddin 1969), but orthostatic hypotension may become a problem following overtreatment with diuretics and/or converting enzyme inhibitors (Cody et al. 1981).

Other Causes

Other causes of nonneurogenic orthostatic hypotension cover a wide variety of illnesses including diminished aortic compliance, pacemaker syndrome, serious cardiac arrhythmias as well as physical deconditioning, aging, and pharmacologically induced reactions.

Aortic Compliance and Orthostatic Hypotension. The aorta and large vessels play a major hemodynamic role in dampening the pressure fluctuations due to sudden changes in aortic volume (Windkessel effect) (Sleight 1976). It is commonly accepted that reduced compliance of the aorta and its large branches results in isolated systolic hypertension (Koch-Wieser 1973; Tarazi et al. 1975) because of the difficulty in accommodating the sudden ejection of each stroke volume. Conversely, the same aortic pathology will lead to a marked fall in systolic pressure and pulse pressure when stroke volume is reduced on standing up. Diastolic pressure is usually unchanged. The relation between the reduction in stroke volume and the orthostatic fall of systolic pressure in these patients is less well documented in relation to their symptoms. In our experience 9 of 12 patients with systolic orthostatic hypotension became symptomatic (light-headedness, dizziness, weakness, shakiness) during tilt, suggesting the need for treatment of this disease (Table 13.2). Correlation of cerebral flow with systolic as opposed to mean levels of arterial pressure is needed to establish the connection firmly. Clinically, improvement of stroke volume by measures increasing venous return has often proven successful in controlling symptoms. In some cases, the patient's problems are compounded by a reduction in baroreceptor sensitivity associated with age (Gribbin et al. 1971) and atherosclerosis; the initial systolic hypotension is then made worse by failure of the baroreceptor mechanism.

Table 13.2. Symptoms associated with systolic hypotension

Patient	Supine blood pressure	Blood pressure during maximum tilt	Symptoms
1	174/97	134/96	Light-headedness
2	150/77	126/80	Dizziness
3	146/60	102/62	Light-headedness
4	140/70	118/76	Light-headedness
5	200/84	110/60	Light-headedness "chest pounding" "warm"
6	142/60	122/68	None
7	163/83	98/72	Weakness and shakiness
8	122/75	104/80	Light-headedness
9	143/91	118/92	"Warmth"
10	128/72	100/70	None
11	138/98	116/96	None
12	150/84	110/80	Light-headedness

Pacemaker Syndrome. Hypotension with lightheadedness and near syncope can occur in patients during effective ventricular pacing, particularly when the ventricular pacing is intermittent and associated with retrograde ventriculoatrial conduction (Alicandri et al. 1978; Erbel et al. 1977). The mechanism(s) underlying this fall in arterial pressure is not the simple reduction in cardiac output consequent to loss of a properly timed atrial contraction (Braunwald et al. 1961). As similar reduction in output could be easily compensated for by moderate vasoconstriction, the paradoxical lack of response of compensatory peripheral resistance is related temporarily to the cannon waves in the atrial tracing (Fig. 13.1). This lack of peripheral vasoconstriction (or development of inappropriate vasodilatation) is even more noticeable when there is 1:1 retrograde conduction. These observations led to the suggestion that the abnormal resistance response was related to a reflex originating from the sudden distention of the atria, pulmonary veins, and/or vena cava (Alicandri et al. 1978). In that respect, Kahl et al. (1974) found that inflation of a balloon in the left atrium led to renal artery vasodilatation. Incomplete heart block and irregularly occurring cannon A waves produced by atrial systole when atrial contraction occurs with the tricuspid valve closed by ventricular systole result in intermittent transient atrial distention. Patients with sick sinus syndrome receiving ventricular demand pacemakers are even more vulnerable to this reflex response whereby periods of ventricular pacing are usually associated with 1:1 retrograde VA conduction and atrial contraction during the time of ventricular contraction. Frequently, the atrial descent associated with atrial contraction is associated with simultaneous AV valve insufficiency which further augments stretch and distension of the atria and associated venous inflow. In contrast, decreases in cardiac output due to occlusion of the superior vena cava led to full and compensatory increases in total peripheral resistance. Although this reflex response is common to all patients, its relative severity varies greatly from patient to patient and in relationship to other parameters such as

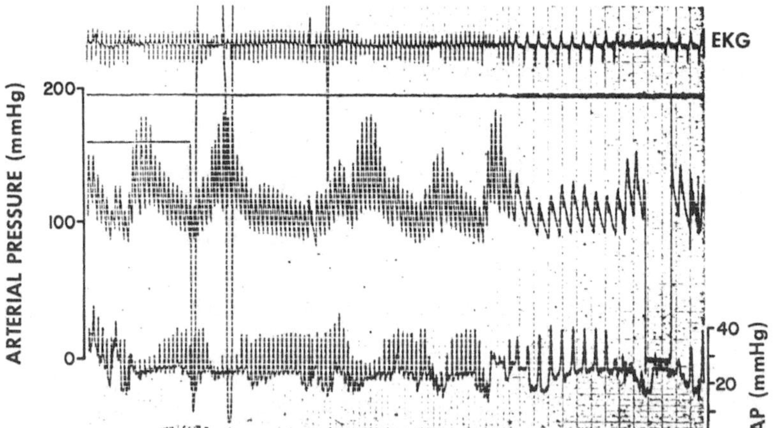

Fig. 13.1. Pacemaker syndrome showing fluctuating blood pressure with lower levels occurring during activation of demand pacemaker either spontaneously or during carotid sinus massage. Note cannon waves in the right atrial pressure tracing (*RAP*) during activation of the pacemaker

cardiopulmonary blood volume, relative vagal tone, demand pacing, and others. Pacemaker syndrome orthostatic hypotension is of clinical significance because it is an iatrogenic problem, more frequently encountered in patients being paced for sick sinus syndrome, and may be minimized or avoided by more physiologic modalities of pacing and/or minimizing the need for pacing by reducing the demand rate.

Prolonged Bed Rest. The deconditioning associated with prolonged bed rest or loss of gravity (astronauts after prolonged space flights) may result in brief episodes of orthostatic hypotension in response to inadequate arterial and venous constriction (Schatz 1984).

Effect of Aging. Aging causes slowing of postural reflexes so that a substantial percentage of subjects older than 65 years have postural hypotension (Caird et al. 1974). Studies by Gribbin et al. (1971) have demonstrated a diminished sensitivity of the high-pressure arterial baroreceptors to sudden rises in blood pressure induced by pharmacologic agents (phenylephrine). This can be further accentuated in the presence of loss of Windkessel function of the large arteries (arteriosclerosis, hypertension, etc.). Such patients could be at risk when the abnormality becomes accentuated after prolonged bed rest or after the administration of sedatives. Prolonged straining associated with prostatism may add a risk in this population.

Pharmacologic Causes of Orthostatic Hypotension. Any agent that interferes with peripheral sympathetic or catecholamine activity or that reduces blood volume may induce orthostatic hypotension. This includes guanethidine, reserpine, prazosin, most diuretics, and centrally acting antihypertensive agents (Reid and Dollery 1976); peripheral sympatholytics are more potent than centrally acting agents in this respect (Barnett and Cantor). Antidepressants, narcotics, and sedatives may at times be responsible for hypotension (Sleight 1976). Venodilators such as nitrites may be also responsible (Weiss et al. 1937). Occasionally gold preparations have been shown to reduce the baroreflex sensitivity and induce postural hypotension associated with abnormal Valsalva (Fig. 13.2). Although these drugs may induce orthostatic hypotension on their

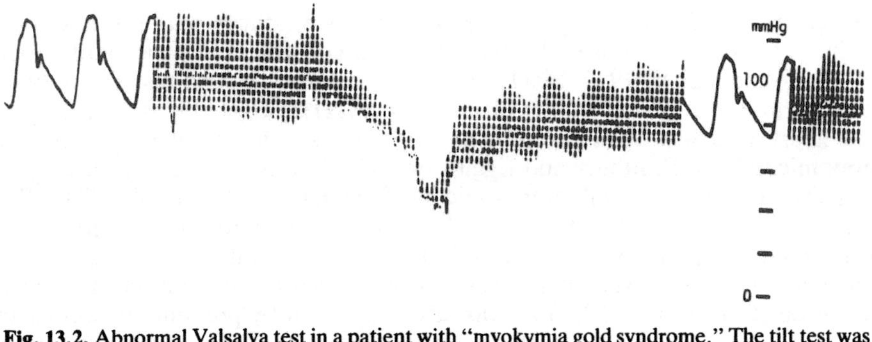

Fig. 13.2. Abnormal Valsalva test in a patient with "myokymia gold syndrome." The tilt test was also abnormal (BP 124/78 mmHg supine, 88/66 mmHg at 35° for 2 min, HR 108 and 114 bpm respectively. Four months after discontinuance of gold therapy, the tilt test was normal (BP 150/84 supine, 136/94 at 60° for 10 min, HR 94 and 11 bpm, respectively).

own, they might also act by exacerbating the abnormal response in predisposed patients.

Of clinical importance is the differentiation between orthostatic hypotension (related to posture) and exercise hypotension described in obstructive valvular heart disease such as severe aortic or pulmonary stenosis (Weissler and Warren 1966).

Hemodynamic Abnormalities in Orthostatic Hypotension

Head-up tilt is associated with reduction in cardiac output that averages 15% and rarely exceeds 20% of supine levels in normal individuals (Frohlich et al. 1967; Tuckman and Shillingford 1966; Weissler et al. 1962). Total peripheral resistance increases normally by 25% and may rise higher if needed to maintain arterial pressure (Frohlich et al. 1967).

In patients with hypovolemia the left ventricular filling pressure is insufficient to stretch myocardial fibers adequately during diastole, thus resulting in a decrease in cardiac output unless excessive venous constriction (sympathetic stimulation) takes place to maintain the cardiopulmonary volume. In the upright posture the hemodynamic hallmark is a marked increase in resistance attempting to compensate for the fall in cardiac output; the rise in systemic vascular resistance will at first maintain the diastolic blood pressure with a resultant narrowing of pulse pressure; tachycardia is usually marked in these patients. With prolonged standing further reduction in venous return initiates afferent vagal reflexes from the strongly contracting atria or ventricles (Epstein et al. 1968), with resultant peripheral vasodilation and fall in blood pressure (vasovagal attack). Although of neurogenic origin, this sudden hypotension is not due to autonomic failure, but is more correctly related to activation of some depressor reflexes (Greene et al. 1961).

Hemodynamic Aspects of Autonomic Failure

The fall in blood pressure with *upright posture* in these patients has been conclusively linked to failure of reflex arteriolar constriction (Tarazi and Fouad 1983; Stead and Ebert 1974; Maclean and Allen 1940; Hickam and Pryor 1951; Bickelmann et al. 1961; Ibrahim et al. 1974; Magrini et al. 1976). Although a fixed heart rate has been traditionally viewed as a hallmark of progressive autonomic failure (Bradbury and Eggleston 1926; Ewing et al. 1980), this sign is often absent in patients with autonomic insufficiency (Ibrahim et al. 1974). The close correspondence we have found between the chronotropic effects of atropine in these patients and acceleration of their heart rate on tilt suggests that cardiac acceleration in such cases was mostly related to modulation of residual vagal tone (Fouad et al. 1985) as was also supported by preliminary studies of parasympathetic control of heart rate in our laboratory. Thus, the absence of change of heart rate favors autonomic insufficiency, but the presence of heart rate change does not rule it out.

A mirror image of this abnormality was found in studies of *head-down tilt* (Magrini et al. 1976). In response to the increase of cardiac output produced by this maneuver, total peripheral resistance did not fall as would have occurred in normal subjects; as a result blood pressure increased markedly in patients with autonomic insufficiency in this posture. This failure of adjustment of the peripheral resistance to accommodate an increased flow suggested the possibility of treating these patients with blood volume expanders.

In contrast with the uniformly low arterial pressure found on head-up tilt, the blood pressure in the *supine position* can vary widely among patients with progressive autonomic failure from hypotension to definitely hypertensive levels (Magrini et al. 1976; Niarchos et al. 1978). Supine hypertension was found to be related to spontaneous fluctuations in systemic vascular resistance without significant changes in cardiac output (Niarchos et al. 1978). It is of interest that such swings in resting resistance are not transcribed to life-threatening stresses in these patients such as standing or head-up tilt.

The *cardiac aspects* of autonomic failure have been appreciated more fully in recent years. Both systolic performance and diastolic filling of the heart showed signs of impairment in patients with adrenergic dysfunction. Stroke volume was reduced on head-up tilt more than could be accounted for by the fall in cardiopulmonary volume (Ibrahim et al. 1974; Magrini et al. 1976). In addition, Fouad et al. (Fouad et al. 1985) recently reported a significant prolongation in left ventricular relaxation time in patients with efferent adrenergic dysfunction. This diminished cardiac performance is probably due to defective sympathetic innervation of the heart rather than an abnormality of the myocardium. However, surgical denervation of the heart in experimental animals did not produce significant variations in cardiac performance at rest (Noble 1972). Differences in extent or duration of sympathetic denervation, or species differences, might explain the discrepancy between our observations and experimental reports. The changes reported were, however, subtle and were not associated with clinical evidence of heart failure.

Evaluation of Orthostatic Hypotension

Because of the multiple etiologic factors in orthostatic hypotension, it is necessary to approach these patients in a way which reaches the proper diagnosis in a cost effective manner. Our long-term experience with the hemodynamic evaluation of patients with orthostatic hypotension has led to the development of the approach outlined in Table 13.3. A screening graded tilt test, blood volume determination, and noninvasive hemodynamic evaluation form the basic minimum requirement for the workup. The latter evaluation includes determination of cardiac output and cardiopulmonary volume in the supine position and during head-up tilt to 60° or as tolerated by the patient with subsequent calculation of changes in total peripheral resistance. Plasma catecholamines are measured in the supine position and during head-up tilt. Specific tests are planned thereafter according to the suspected diagnosis. In patients with suspected autonomic insufficiency or in whom a diagnosis is not confirmed, intraarterial blood pressure recording with autonomic reflex testing (Tarazi et al.

1985; Fouad et al. 1985; Ibrahim et al. 1985) is performed. This includes the Valsalva maneuver, a cold pressor test, and pharmacologic baroreflex testing (phenylephrine IV and/or amylnitrite inhalation). In cases of suspected pacemaker syndrome, the tilt test is repeated with the pacemaker off (if safe and feasible) or with the pacemaker turned down as low as 30–40 bpm in order to test the response of the underlying cardiac rhythm. In cases of suspected vasovagal syncope, the tilt test is repeated after sublingual atropine or transdermal scopolamine. In cases with documented hypovolemia, the tests are repeated after blood volume expansion (Fouad et al. 1985), acutely with human serum albumin or long term with alpha fluorohydrocortisone and high salt diet. In cases of peripheral venous pooling during head-up tilt, the test is repeated with support hose.

Table 13.3. Evaluation of orthostatic hypotension

A. Screening tests
   1. Graded tilt test
   2. Blood volume determination
   3. Noninvasive hemodynamics

B. Specific tests
   1. Autonomic reflex testing for autonomic insufficiency
   2. Repeat tilt test at a low pacing rate (or deactivate pacemaker) for pacemaker syndrome
   3. Repeat tilt test postsublingual atropine or transdermal scopolamine for vasovagal syncope
   4. Repeat tilt test post blood volume expansion for hypovolemia syndrome
   5. Repeat tilt test with lower limb compression for excess venous pooling

Treatment of Orthostatic Hypotension

The treatment of orthostatic hypotension depends largely on the underlying cause:

Shy-Drager Syndrome and Idiopathic Orthostatic Hypotension

These conditions are very difficult to treat. Several approaches have been tried including: (a) blood volume expansion, by administration of alpha fluorohydrocortisone and Florinef (fluorocortisone acetate) (0.1 mg qd or bid) associated with high salt intake and (b) vasoconstrictor agents. Several vasoconstrictor agents have been utilized including ephedrine, vasopressin, and dihydroergotamine (Fouad et al. 1981; Jennings et al. 1974). Propranolol as well as pindolol has been tried to induce blockade of the peripheral beta$_2$ receptors allowing an uninhibited alpha receptor vasoconstrictor action (Man in't Veld and Schalekamp 1981). Clonidine has been claimed to produce an agonist vasoconstriction in patients with impaired autonomic function (Robertson et al. 1974); results could not be confirmed in our laboratory. Recently, midodrine, a synthetic alpha adrenergic agonist, has been tried rather successfully in many centers (Schirger et al. 1981). Although midodrine has been helpful in some of our patients for periods as long as 2 years, it has not cured the disease and the improvement was classified as moderate.

These various therapeutic approaches share the problem of inducing supine hypertension in some of the treated patients. Blood pressure control could then be achieved pharmacologically by administration of hydralazine or mechanically by "taking advantage of the disease," i.e., avoiding the recumbent position and use of the vascular position whenever the patient lies down.

Idiopathic Hypovolemia

Long-term treatment with Florinef (0.4–1.0 mg/day) and a high-salt diet has met limited success in our patients. Although initial evidence of plasma volume expansion and weight gain was observed, maintenance of fluid retention was difficult to achieve in these patients except with the use of large doses. In general, these patients have not responded well to beta blockers (contrary to patients in a hyperbeta adrenergic state). A few patients have responded successfully to the central alpha adrenergic agonist, clonidine; the mechanism of action of clonidine in this syndrome is not well understood.

Peripheral Venous Pooling

Physiotherapy to develop muscle tone as well as support hose has been successful to variable degrees in different patients. Venoconstrictors such as midodrine and dihydroergotamine have also been used.

Pacemaker Syndrome

The advent of AV sequential pacemakers (DVI, DDD, DDI) has reduced the incidence of pacemaker syndrome. In those patients with a ventricular pacemaker (VVI) and orthostatic hypotension due to the pacemaker syndrome, symptoms can frequently be reduced by minimizing unnecessary ventricular pacing associated with VA conduction (using lower demand rates of 50–60 beats/min, utilizing historesis thereby also decreasing the relative activation of the demand pacemaker, and avoiding the use of VVI pacing systems in patients with intact retrograde VA conduction). Other methods of decreasing the symptomatology of pacemaker syndrome include: avoiding hypovolemia due to diuretics and other medications. At times, medications can be used to impede retrograde VA conduction. This is acceptable in unusual circumstances, but is generally not a preferred approach by us. If symptoms are significant in pacemaker syndrome and cannot be easily managed, then upgrading the pacemaker system to one that maintains AV synchrony is appropriate. In selected patients, this can be done by using the AAI pacing system but the treatment of choice is upgrading the single-chambered pacing device to a dual-chambered device that provides AV synchrony as well as rate responsiveness. The ventricular demand pacing system induced "pacemaker syndrome" is best managed by avoidance. Patients with extrinsic sick sinus syndrome (carotid sinus hypersensitivity, vasovagal bradyarrhythmias, etc.) are most prone to pacemaker syndrome. These patients are best managed with pacing modalities other than standard ventricular devices.

Vasovagal Syncope (see Chap. 14)

Sublingual atropine (and atropine-like drugs), reassurance and education, aminophylline, permanent pacing, and other modalities have been utilized with varying degrees of success for patients with infrequent episodes of vasovagal syncope. Sublingual atropine has been utilized successfully in patients with infrequent episodes and a relatively pronounced prodromal aspect to their vasovagal syncope. The sublingual drug can be utilized as soon as the premonitory manifestations are noticed. Proper patient selection is critical. Long-term treatment with transdermal scopolamine is currently under study; the preliminary results are encouraging (Table 13.4). In some severe cases of vasovagal syncope, frank loss of consciousness is associated with dramatic peripheral vasodilatation in combination with prolonged asystolic episodes. Treatment may have to be directed toward both aspects of the syndrome, that is, control of peripheral vasomotor tone plus prevention of cardiac asystole with a pacing system.

Table 13.4. Vasovagal syncope. Response to scopolamine ($\bar{x}\pm SE$)

	Prescopolamine		Transdermol scopolamine	
	Supine	Maximum tilt	Supine	Maximum tilt
SBP (mmHg)	116±5.26	83± 9.86	112±4.10	114±8.30
DBP (mmHg)	74±3.03	39±13.45	71±4.83	80±8.44
HR (bpm)	65±3.82	54± 6.12	60±3.08	81±7.15
Maximum tilt	60° for 10.6±3.20 min		60° for 22.3±1.69 min	

n=6

Acknowledgment. The authors acknowledge the assistance of Tammie Lee in the preparation of this manuscript.

References

Abdelmann WH, Fareeduddin K (1969) Increased tolerance of orthostatic stress in patients with heart disease. Am J Cardiol 23: 354–363

Alicandri C, Fouad FM, Tarazi RC, Castle L, Morant V (1978) Three cases of hypotension and syncope with ventricular pacing, possible role of atrial reflexes. Am J Cardiol 42: 137–142

Appenzeller O, Richardson ET (1966) The sympathetic chain in patients with diabetic and alcoholic polyneuropathy. Neurology 16: 1206–1209

Barnett AJ, Cantor S (1968) Observation on the hypotensive action of Catapres (St 155) in man. Med J Aust I: 87–91

Barraclough MA, Sharpey-Schafer EP (1963) Hypotension from absent circulatory reflexes: effects of alcohol, barbiturates, psychotherapeutic drugs and other mechanisms. Lancet 1: 1121–1126

Bickelmann AG, Lippschutz EJ, Branjes CF (1961) Hemodynamics of idiopathic orthostatic hypotension. Am J Med 30: 26–38
Bradbury S, Eggleston C (1926) Postural hypotension: a report of three cases. Am Heart J 1: 73–86
Braunwald E, Frahm CJ (1961) Studies on Starling's law of the heart. IV. Observation of the hemodynamic functions of the left atrium in man. Circulation 24: 633–642
Caird FI, Andrews GR, Kennedy RD (1974) Effect of posture on blood pressure in the elderly. Br Heart J 35: 527–531
Campese VM, Romoff M, Dequattro V, Massry SG (1980) Relationship between plasma catecholamines, plasma renin activity, aldosterone, and arterial pressure during postural stress in normal subjects. J Lab Clin Med 95: 927–933
Cody RJ Jr, Bravo EL, Fouad FM, Tarazi RC (1981) Cardiovascular reflexes during long-term converting enzyme inhibition and sodium depletion. The response to tilt in hypertensive patients. Am J Med 71: 422–426
Epstein SE, Stampfer M, Beiser GD (1968) Role of the capacitance and resistance vessels in vasovagal syncope. Circulation 37: 524–533
Erbel R, Schweizer P, Fleischmann D, Meyer J (1977) Zur Bedeutung der Vorhofkontraktion fuer die Funktion des Herzens 9: 549–554
Ewing DJ, Campbell IW, Clarke BF (1980) Assessment of cardiovascular effects in diabetic autonomic neuropathy and prognostic implications. Ann Intern Med 92: 308–312
Fouad FM, Tarazi RC, Bravo EL (1981) Dihydroergotamine in idiopathic orthostatic hypotension: short-term intramuscular and long-term oral therapy. Clin Pharm Ther 30 (6): 782–789
Fouad FM, El-Sanadi N, Hanson MR, MacIntyre WJ, Tarazi RC (1985a) Diastolic properties of the left ventricle in patients with autonomic dysfunction. Clin Res 33: 185A
Fouad FM, Tarazi RC, Bravo EL (1985b) Orthostatic hypotension. Cleveland Clin Q 52: 561–568
Fouad FM, Tadena-Thome L, Bravo EL, Tarazi RC (1985c) Idiopathic hypovolemia. Ann Int Med
Frohlich ED, Tarazi RC, Ulrych M, Dustan HP, Page IH (1967) Tilt test for investigating a neural component in hypertension. Its correlation with clinical characteristics. Circulation 36: 387–393
Glassman AH, Giardina EV, Perel JM, Bigger Jr JT, Kantor SJ, Davis M (1979) Clinical characteristics of imipramine-induced orthostatic hypotension. Lancet I: 468–472
Greene MA, Boltax AJ, Ulberg RJ (1961) Cardiovascular dynamics of vasovagal reactions in man. Circ Res 9: 12
Gribbin B, Pickering TG, Sleight P, Peto R (1971) Effect of age and high blood pressure on baroreflex sensitivity in man. Circulation 29: 424–431
Gross M, Bannister R, Godwin-Austen R (1972) Orthostatic hypotension in Parkinson's disease. Lancet 1: 174–176
Hickman JB, Pryor WW (1951) Cardiac output in postural hypotension. J Clin Invest 30: 401–405
Hilsted J (1982) Pathophysiology in diabetic autonomic neuropathy. NY State J Med 82: 892–902
Hohl RD, Frame B, Schatz IJ (1965) The Shy-Drager variant of idiopathic orthostatic hypotension. Am J Med 39: 134–141
Ibrahim MM (1975) Localization of lesion in patients with idiopathic orthostatic hypotension. Br Heart J 37: 868–872
Ibrahim MM, Tarazi RC, Dustan HP, Bravo EL (1974) Idiopathic orthostatic hypotension: circulatory dynamics in chronic autonomic insufficiency. Am J Cardiol 34: 288–294
Ibrahim MM, Tarazi RC, Dustan HP (1975) Fundamentals of clinical cardiology. Am Heart J 90: 513–520
Ibrahim MM, Tarazi RC, Shafer WH, Bravo EL, Dustan HP (1979) Unusual tyramine responsiveness in idiopathic orthostatic hypotension. Med J Cairo Univ 47: 49–55
Jennings G, Esler M, Holmes R (1974) Treatment of orthostatic hypotension with dihydroergotamine. Br Heart J 4: 288–294
Johnson RH, McLellan DL, Love DR (1971) Orthostatic hypotension and the Holmes-Adie syndrome. J Neurol Neurosurg Psychiatr 34: 562–570
Kahl FR, Flint JF, Azidon JP (1974) Influence of left atrial distention on renal vasomotor tone. Am J Physiol 226: 240–246
Koch-Weser J (1973) Correlation of pathophysiology and pharmacology in primary hypertension. Am J Cardiol 32: 399–410
Kyle RA, Kottke BA, Schirger A (1966) Orthostatic hypotension as a clue to primary systemic amyloidosis. Circulation 34: 883–888
Maclean AR, Allen EF (1940) Orthostatic hypotension and orthostatic tachycardia. J Am Med Ass 155: 2162–2167
McLeod JG (1983) Distal autonomic neuropathy. In: Bannister R (ed) Autonomic failure. Oxford University Press, pp 543–573

Magrini F, Ibrahim MM, Tarazi RC (1976) Abnormalities of supine hemodynamics in idiopathic orthostatic hypotension. Cardiology 61 [Suppl 1]: 125–135
Man in't Veld AJ, Schalekamp MADH (1981) Pindolol acts as beta-receptor agonist in orthostatic hypotension: therapeutic implications. Br Med J 282: 929–931
Myers MG, Kearns PM, Kennedy DS, Fisher RH (1978) Postural hypotension and diuretic therapy in the elderly. Can Med Assoc J 119: 581–584
Niarchos AP, Magrini F, Tarazi RC, Bravo EL (1978) Mechanism of spontaneous supine blood pressure variations in chronic autonomic insufficiency. Am J Med 65: 547–552
Noble MJ (1972) Left ventricular performance in the conscious dog with chronically denervated hearts. Cardiovasc Res 6: 457–477
Polinsky RJ, Kopin IJ, Ebert MH, Weise V (1981) Pharmacologic distinction of different orthostatic hypotension syndromes. Neurology (Ny) 31: 1–7
Reid JL, Dollery CT (1976) Central and peripheral catecholamine mechanisms in circulatory control. Cardiology 61 [Suppl 1]: 113–124
Rushmer RF (1976) Effects of posture, part 1: circulatory response to arising. In: Rushmer RF (ed) Cardiovascular dynamics, 4th edn. Saunders, Philadelphia. pp 363–384
Robertson D, Goldberg MR, Hollister AF, Wade D, Robertson RM (1974) Clonidine raises blood pressure in severe idiopathic orthostatic hypotension. Am J Med 74(2): 193–200
Schatz IJ (1984) Orthostatic hypotension. Arch Intern Med 144: 773–777
Schirger A, Sheps SG, Thomas JE, Fealey RD (1981) Midodrine. A new agent in the management of idiopathic orthostatic hypotension and Shy-Drager syndrome. Mayo Clin Proc 56: 429–433
Schwarz GA (1967) The orthostatic hypotension syndrome of Shy-Drager syndrome: diagnosis and treatment of cholinergic dysfunction. Arch Neurol 16: 123–139
Sharpey-Schafer EP, Taylor PJ (1960) Absent circulatory reflexes in diabetic neuritis. Lancet 1: 559–562
Shy DM, Drager GA (1960) A neurological syndrome associated with orthostatic hypotension: a clinical-pathologic study. Arch Neurol 2: 511– 527
Siemson JK, Meister L (1963) Bronchogenic carcinoma associated with severe orthostatic hypotension. Ann Intern Med 58: 669–676
Sleight P (1976) Neurophysiology of the carotid sinus receptors in normal and hypertensive animals and man. Cardiology 61 [Suppl 1]: 31–45
Stead EA, Ebert RV (1974) Postural hypotension: a disease of sympathetic nervous system. Arch Intern Med 67: 546–562
Tarazi RC, Fouad FM (1983) Circulatory dynamics in progressive autonomic failure. In: Bannister R (ed) Autonomic failure. A textbook of clinical disorders of the autonomic nervous system. Oxford University Press, pp 96–114
Tarazi RC, Magrini F, Dustan HP (1975) The role of aortic distensibility in hypertension. In: Milliez P, Safar M (eds) Recent advances in hypertension. Boehringer Ingelheim, Reims, pp 133–142
Tuckman J, Shillingford J (1966) Effect of different degrees of tilt on cardiac output, heart rate, and blood pressure in normal man. Br Heart J 28: 32–39
Watkins PJ (1973) Facial sweating after food: a new sign of diabetic autonomic neuropathy. Br Med J I: 583–587
Weiss S, Wilkins RW, Haynes FW (1937) Nature of circulatory collapse induced by sodium nitrite. J Clinic Inves 16: 73–84
Weissler AM, Roehl W II, Peeler RG (1962) Effect of posture on the cardiac response to increased peripheral demand. J Lab Clin Med 59: 1000–1007
Weissler AM, Warren JV (1966) Syncope, shock and sudden death. In: Hurst JW, Logue RB (eds) The heart. New York, McGraw-Hill, p 356
Wheeler T, Watkins PJ (1973) Cardiac denervation in diabetes. Br Med J IV: 584–586
Wiggers CJ (1949) Physiology in health and disease. Lea & Febiger, Philadelphia
Young RR, Asbury AK, Corbett JL, Adams RD (1975) Pure pan-dysautonomia with recovery. Description and discussion of diagnostic criteria. Brain 98:613–635
Ziegler M, Lake C, Kopin I (1977) The sympathetic nervous system defect in primary orthostatic hypotension. N Engl J Med 296: 293–297

Chapter 14

Syncope: A Practical Diagnostic Approach

F. M. Abi-Samra, F. M. Fouad, P. J. Sweeney, and J. D. Maloney

Introduction

History records that in ancient Rome those afflicted with periodic loss of consciousness, whatever its cause, were often venerated as special individuals. One can easily understand such mysticism regarding this occurrence: a previously healthy individual suddenly became almost lifeless, as if dead, yet complete recovery occurred. Indeed, some of the older literature referred to death as "permanent syncope."

Syncope ranks as one of the most dramatic symptoms which elicits considerable concern in those who suffer from it and hence prompts them to seek diagnostic answers and therapeutic relief. Unfortunately, the diagnostic workup for syncope may represent a formidable task. This is partly due to the fact that the symptomatology is intermittent, often elusive, and is commonly unassociated with abnormalities that are identified during the "remission" period. Hence, the yield of a workup of recurrent syncope is quite variable and is attended by financial, social, and legal ramifications which frustrate not only the patient but the physician as well. Another complicating and unfortunate factor relates to the confusion that has surrounded the definition of syncope.

The term "syncope" derives from the Greek "synkope," meaning a cessation or a pause, literally a pause in one's conscious state. Even in the recent past, it has been an omnibus term. This is illustrated in several series, especially Wayne's (Wayne 1961) large study, wherein diagnostic entities which today would be considered separately (epilepsy, hysteria, migraine) were offered as causes of syncope. In short, imprecision in definition of terms and lack of a sound conceptual framework for approaching the clinical symptom complex of syncope has confounded many discussions of syncope. Historically, this conceptual framework has evolved slowly. Morgagni attempted to differentiate sanguineous apoplexy (acute cerebral vascular congestion) from fatal syncope in his *Third Letter* published in 1761 (Morgagni 1761). He pondered "syncope that would proceed from the head, and not from the heart," and states "when sudden death happens without any manifest cause, then it is always palsy of the heart." Morgagni's *Ninth Letter* probably describes the first case of heart block. In 1827

Robert Adams, an Irish surgeon, described a man with not less than 20 epileptic attacks who proved to have classic Stokes- Adams attacks (Adams 1827). In 1846 William Stokes (Stokes 1846) referred to Adams' case and reported several other cases of cardiovascular syncope which he classified into two forms: "in one, the systole of the heart is broken up, as it were, into a number of slight and irregular contractions, giving a permanently irregular and rapid pulse . . . in the second form, the contractions are complete, and with long intervals." He concludes his report with a statement that is still applicable today: "The preceding observations are published with a view of drawing the attention of the profession to a combination of cerebral and cardiac phenomena, of which our knowledge is still imperfect."

While its mechanisms and etiologies are complex, syncope can be defined as a brief, sudden, and transient loss of consciousness which subsides spontaneously without treatment and without localizing neurological deficit. It is best considered a clinical "symptom complex" that results from acute transient global cerebral hypoperfusion and/or global cerebral cellular hypoxemia. The instability may be so brief that consciousness is diminished, but not lost (presyncope, near syncope), or it may be so prolonged that it results in sudden death or aborted sudden death. Of course when sudden death supervenes, the diagnosis of syncope is masked. A more gradual onset and prolonged loss of consciousness resulting from cardiogenic shock or hypoglycemia should be differentiated from syncope.

The Syncopal History: A Testing Dilemma

Syncope is a common event with up to 20% of all adults experiencing it by age 75. Further, syncope accounts for about 3% of all emergency room visits and about 1% of all hospital admissions (Stults 1986). Bearing in mind that the etiologies of syncope are myriad and range from the relatively benign vasovagal attacks to the ominous ventricular tachycardias, these data underscore the staggering economical and ethical burdens that a full diagnostic investigation would pose.

As in all other aspects of medicine, the first order of investigation is a careful, detailed, and perceptive history. While the patient's recall is invariably incomplete, his prelude activities, feelings, and symptoms may be important. The first important goal of historical interrogation is to substantiate that the problem is indeed syncope and not epilepsy, hysteria, etc. Several seconds of nonspecific lightheadedness or dizziness coupled with a gradual loss of vision are often characteristic presyncopal symptoms; alternatively, specific sensory or motor auras suggest the problem may be a seizure.

The Syncopal History: Situational Syncope

The history alone will usually not identify the etiology of syncope except for certain characteristic "situational" syncope syndromes. By definition, situational syncope syndromes are syncopal events that occur in association with (following) a specific activity or circumstance. The relationship is consistent, but not necessarily constant (i.e., syncope occurs only after the specific activity, but the said activity does not always elicit syncope). Examples are vasovagal syncope secondary to phobic stimuli, cough syncope, and micturition syncope.

Emotional Syncope

Precipitating emotional circumstances with pain, fear, abhorring sights (trauma, blood, etc.), nausea, diaphoresis, etc. all suggest common vasodepressor or vasovagal syncope. "After the prodrome, which may last for 10–20 s, the patient collapses to the floor pale, diaphoretic, with a slow feeble pulse, and mydriatic pupils. Usually no movements are noted during unconsciousness, but when they occur they are mainly tonic extensor spasms, often opisthotonic" (Gastaut 1957). Not infrequently, injury may be incurred in the fall. Usually the patient awakens within 10–60 s after the horizontal position is reached. Residual nervousness, dizziness, nausea, and diaphoresis are common. Sometimes a desire to defecate is reported.

Cough Syncope

Although "cough syncope" is a fairly uncommon occurrence, the history is rather typical: presyncopal and syncopal symptoms occur moments after a bout of strenuous, repetitive coughing usually in a patient with chronic pulmonary disease. Pathophysiological and hemodynamic mechanisms underlying cough syncope include impairment to venous return by the increased intrathoracic pressure (and subsequent fall in blood pressure) (McIntosh 1956), transmission of large pressure transients from the chest to the aorta and great vessels (with subsequent baroreceptor stimulation and reflex vasodilation), and posttussive cerebrospinal pressure gradients that produce a downward sucking effect on the cerebellar tonsils (William 1976). Since syncope of any etiology could theoretically occur coincidentally with cough, the diagnosis of true cough syncope cannot be made with confidence unless several episodes have been noted. Moreover, any episode of syncope that does not follow a period of increased intrathoracic pressure cannot be classified as cough syncope and another or a second etiology has to be invoked.

Carotid Sinus Syncope

Although an abnormal response to carotid sinus massage is not infrequently seen (especially in the elderly) (Sigler 1933; Brown 1980), the incidence of true carotid sinus syncope syndrome is rare. The history should elicit presyncopal and syncopal symptoms that are temporally related to the incidental application of pressure on the carotid sinus (e.g., shaving, resting the phone headset at the angle of the jaw, and tight collars). The history alone, however, cannot assure the underlying pathophysiology of carotid hypersensitivity as it cannot differentiate between the vasodepressor type, the cardioinhibitory type, and the mixed type.

Micturition Syncope

The history attending micturition syncope is also quite characteristic: The condition is said to affect males almost exclusively. Typically, an elderly man wakes up during the night or at dawn, goes to the bathroom, attempts to void, and suddenly develops presyncopal or syncopal symptoms. Syncope may actually occur after voiding (Donker 1972). The loss of consciousness is transient and the patient wakes up shortly after falling. Injuries attending the episodes are rather frequent (Proudfit 1959). Pathophysiologically, the event may involve a combination of decreased venous return, sleep-related bradycardia and hypotension, and vasodepressive reflexes (Donker 1972).

The Syncopal History: Relationship to Pathophysiological Mechanisms

As described above, the history may be quite useful. However, even in the most characteristic cases, complicating factors may be present and the exact pathogenetic mechanisms and contributing factors cannot be determined by history alone. Since adequate treatment may heavily depend on it, it is essential whenever possible to delineate pathophysiological mechanisms ultimately leading to syncope. For instance, pacemaker therapy may be beneficial for patients with the cardioinhibitory form of carotid sinus hypersensitivity, but inappropriate for the vasodepressor type of the syndrome. When cough syncope is associated with increased intracranial pressure and cerebellar herniation, surgery may be beneficial (Corbett 1976; Larson 1974). In micturition syncope, prostatectomy may not be beneficial since the Valsalva maneuver may not be part of the events that lead to loss of consciousness (Donker 1972).

The Diagnostic Approach to Syncope

Obviously, the framework by which the practitioner can logically approach a patient with syncope will vary from case to case and will be heavily modulated by the usefulness of the history and clinical background. Patients with syncope present to the physician in five or more major ways: (1) The patient presents with a classical history (situational syncope); (2) the patient is undergoing evaluation for other cardiovascular disease complexes and is found to have syncope as a manifestation of that disorder (aortic stenosis, idiopathic hypertrophic subaortic stenosis, varying degrees of heart block, WPW syndrome, etc.); (3) the patient presents with a previously diagnosed rhythm disorder and new onset syncope (prior anteroseptal myocardial infarction with left ventricular aneurysm formation developing syncope 2 years later); (4) the patient presents to the neurologist with the presumptive diagnosis of a convulsive disorder; and (5), finally, the patient presents with syncope and historical data that do not suggest a likely mechanism (syncope of unknown etiology). In any one of the first three presentations, further workup is directed by the history and the clinical background while syncope of unknown etiology requires the broadest diagnostic workup. When epilepsy has been erroneously diagnosed, one first has to substantiate the presence of true syncope before further diagnostic tests are performed.

The conceptual framework for the investigative workup of syncope can be structured along the following lines: (1) neurological considerations, (2) "metabolic" considerations, (3) cardiac obstructive lesions, (4) arrhythmias, and (5) anomalies of peripheral blood pressure control. This scheme is organized in a roughly increasing order of etiological relevance as current knowledge differentiates syncope from loss of consciousness secondary to neurological and metabolic disturbances, while arrhythmias and disturbances of blood pressure control are very important causes of syncope.

Neurological Considerations

The importance of a neurological assessment in the diagnostic workup of syncope lies mainly in discriminating between true syncope and other neurological manifestations of impaired consciousness, such as convulsive disorders. Primary cerebrovascular disease is rarely, if ever, the cause of isolated syncope.

The literature is much more a chorus than a debate in indicating the futility of multiple, sophisticated neurological tests in diagnosing syncope. Large studies in the past decade have dispelled the notion that isolated syncope can be a manifestation of transient ischemic attacks (TIAs). Bousser et al. reported that none of their 557 patients with TIA presented with syncope. In contrast, syncope occurred in 4%–8% of patients with established cerebrovascular accidents (CVAs) as defined by localizing neurological symptoms lasting for at least 24 h (therefore, none of these cases had isolated syncope) (Bousser 1981). Kapoor's seminal study (Kapoor 1982) found, in a review of 121 patients, that the definitive cause of syncope was discovered in only 13 of the patients after extensive testing! The final cost was staggering: the average hospitalization was 9 days at a cost of $2563 per patient (in 1976–1980). Looked at another way, the cost per definitive diagnosis was in excess of $23 000! The need for a more cost effective approach to this patient population was emphasized. In terms of specific neurological studies, Kapoor's data are revealing: EEGs, skull X-rays, CT, glucose tolerance tests, lumbar punctures, and even cerebral angiography did not aid in establishing a cause of the syncope!

The usefulness of EEGs lies mainly in helping discriminate between true epileptic syndromes and the postsyncopal tonic stiffening that frequently occurs as a result of global cerebral hypoxemia. If the period of reduced cerebral blood flow is sufficient, it may trigger myoclonic jerks or a generalized seizure as a result of hypoxia. This erroneously suggests seizure as the primary disorder causing unconsciousness. This has been termed "convulsive syncope" (Li 1982). Waking and sleep EEG studies in patients with "convulsive syncope" have invariably been normal. Because of this, the "seizure" or convulsive-like movements have been interpreted as a brain stem "release" phenomenon secondary to generalized cerebral anoxia. Sequential EEG changes, from bilateral slow waves to flattened activity coinciding with the development of convulsive movements, have been demonstrated (Gastaut 1957).

Cataplexy, part of the narcoleptic tetrad, may suggest syncope and loss of consciousness. However, careful questioning will reveal preserved consciousness and an association with highly charged emotional states together with a history of excessive daytime sleepiness.

Vertebral basilar insufficiency can also give rise to diagnostic uncertainty when it presents as so-called "drop attacks." Here too, there is no true alteration of consciousness. Finally, especially in the young, conversion reactions and hysteria can mimic unconsciousness and "fainting."

On occasion, syncope secondary to cardiac disease and arrhythmia with global hypoperfusion can result in focal brain infarction. Most often, the resulting clinical picture is asymmetrical in terms of deficits. The neural pathology of these cases reveals laminar necrosis or "watershed" zones of infarction (Torvik 1984). Alternatively, hypoperfusion may lead to focal brain infarction as a consequence of preexisting high-grade stenosis of major arteries in the involved territory (Ruff 1981). The exception notwithstanding, cardiac dysrhythmias which produce transient hypotension and syncope seldom result in focal brain deficits (Reed 1973; Price 1977). Therefore, it probably is neither medically appropriate nor cost effective to launch into a detailed angiographic assessment of the cerebrovascular tree in the elderly patient with unexplained syncope.

"Metabolic" Considerations

Although disorders such as hypoglycemia, chronic anemia, and electrolyte imbalances may cause changes in consciousness, they rarely cause true syncope. Here, the development of symptoms is gradual (minutes) and their resolution is protracted and often needs therapeutic intervention (such as administration of intravenous glucose). Occasionally, true syncope may occur with these disorders, but this is usually related to orthostatic hypotension and vasovagal phenomena enhanced by the presence of hypovolemia (see later). Metabolic or endocrine disturbances may lead to reduction in plasma volume, to alteration in sympathetic control, or to intermittent vasodilatation. Hypovolemia is seen in association with salt-wasting nephritides, hypoaldosteronism, and pheochromocytoma (Williams 1972; Strecten 1972). Tumors secreting epinephrine, bradykinins, or vasoactive peptides may cause circulatory instability (e.g., pheochromocytoma, carcinoid, etc.). Finally, disturbances causing inhibition of the renin angiotensin axis may cause hypotension and impaired consciousness.

Although a definitive diagnosis of hypoaldosteronism or vasoactive peptide secreting tumors may be difficult and time-consuming, a rapid screening may be quite helpful to exclude these possibilities. For instance, the absence of hyperkalemia strongly contradicts the diagnosis of hypoaldosteronism, which can be established with a simple ACTH stimulation test. Normal levels of properly sampled serum catecholamines are strong evidence against the presence of pheochromocytoma. When in doubt, a clonidine suppression test is indicated. In a positive test, catecholamine levels will remain elevated and comparable to the control levels throughout the study despite decreases in blood pressure and heart rate (Bravo 1981).

Since these conditions are fairly rare causes of syncope, an extensive endocrinological workup should not be performed unless the clinical index of suspicion is very high. Moreover, even when one such metabolic derangement is diagnosed, it is often hard to prove a causal relationship to syncope as methods for provocative testing and symptom reproduction are not available.

Obstructive Cardiac Lesions and Syncope

The list of possible cardiac lesions causally related to syncope is large (Table 14.1). These include both left-sided and right-sided lesions. The most common anatomical lesions associated with syncope are aortic stenosis and obstructive subaortic stenosis. Less commonly, prosthetic valve malfunction, atrial myxoma, mitral valve prolapse, mitral stenosis, cardiac tamponade, and aortic dissection may contribute to or produce syncopal symptoms (Schwartz 1969; Hickler 1979). Pulmonary stenosis, pulmonary emboli, primary pulmonary hypertension, tetralogy of Fallot, and Eisenmenger syndrome are "right-sided" causes of syncope (Dressler 1952; Noble 1971). Except for pulmonary embolic disease, the diagnosis of these structural lesions is fairly straightforward, requiring a careful history and physical examination usually supplemented with electrocardiographic and echocardiographic studies. However, even when a specific anatomical obstructive lesion is diagnosed, it is often difficult to assess its relevance to syncopal symptoms, especially when these symptoms are not related to effort. This is for several reasons: First, the incidence of syncope in association with these disorders is often low. Second, few or no data are available to relate the severity of specific lesions to the likelihood of occurrence of syncopal attacks. Third, syncopal attacks often go unwitnessed, and even when witnessed by the treating physician, concomitant hemodynamic data are frequently unavailable. For instance, syncope related to aortic stenosis may be secondary to mechanical obstruction, reflex peripheral vasodilation (Johnson 1971), ventricular tachycardia or complete AV block alone or in combination (Flamm 1967). Clearly, to make a definitive pathophysiological link between a cardiac lesion and the syncopal symptoms, one needs to observe the syncopal attack and record the heart rhythm and the blood pressure. This frequently requires some form of provocative testing such as reproducing syncope by giving amyl nitrate to patients with hypertrophic obstructive cardiomyopathy. Lastly, in any one patient a cardiac structural lesion may coexist with another totally unrelated cause of syncope. Overall, cardiac obstructive lesions are relatively infrequent causes of syncope.

Arrhythmic Syncope

Arrhythmias are probably the most important, and maybe the most frequent, cause of syncope. Table 14.1 lists the specific bradyarrhythmias and tachyarrhythmias that commonly underlie syncopal symptoms. Even though both clinical and electrocardiographic manifestations of "arrhythmic syncope" are intermittent, cardiac syncope carries a very serious prognosis. Recent studies by Kapoor and others (Kapoor 1983) list the 1-year mortality as 25%–30%. About two-thirds to three-quarters of this mortality rate was due to sudden, presumably arrhythmic, death. Although the salutary effect of specific therapies is still somewhat unsettled, it is imperative in a syncopal patient to make every effort to rule out a potentially lethal arrhythmic condition. To that end, both passive

Table 14.1. Causes of syncope

1. "Metabolic"
   - Salt-wasting nephritides
   - Hypoaldosteronism
   - Pheochromocytoma
   - Bradykinin-secreting tumors
   - Vasoactive peptide secreting tumors

   Cardiac—obstructive
   - a) "Left heart"
     - Aortic stenosis
     - IHSS
     - Prosthetic valve malfunction
     - Mitral stenosis
     - Mitral valve prolapse
     - Atrial myxoma
     - Cardiac tamponade
   - b) "Right heart"
     - Pulmonary stenosis
     - Pulmonary emboli
     - Primary pulmonary hypertension
     - Tetralogy of Fallot
     - Eisenmenger syndrome
3. Cardiac—arrhythmic
   - a) Sick sinus syndrome
   - b) AV nodal complete heart block
   - c) His-Purkinje heart block
   - d) Supraventricular tachycardias (atrial, AV nodal, WPW, etc.)
   - e) Ventricular tachycardia
4. Disorders of BP regulation
   - a) Situational syncope (emotional, cough, etc.)
   - b) Vasovagal/vasodepressor syncope
   - c) Pacemaker syndrome
   - d) Autonomic dysfunction

observation and provocative testing are widely available and safely performed. ECG and transtelephonic and Holter recordings offer a valuable opportunity to record cardiac events during spontaneous symptoms, while exercise testing and electrophysiologic procedures allow provocative testing and systematic analysis of the cardiac electrical system.

In the following paragraphs we will discuss the merits of these techniques, their yield, and the significance of some of the anomalies they uncover. Generally after an extensive electrical investigation, one of three situations is encountered:

No Causative Arrhythmia Can Be Identified. This is not uncommon even after a thorough investigation (20%–60% of cases) (Akhtar 1983; Hess 1982; Teichman 1985). Although such a negative investigation leaves the main question unanswered (i.e., What is the specific cause of syncope?), it provides very important information as only a very small possibility persists that tachyarrhythmias, conduction disease, or sinus node disease are in fact responsible for recurrent syncope (but are simply not detectable by available methods). Bearing in mind that nonarrhythmic syncope carries a much better prognosis than its arrhythmic counterpart, a negative arrhythmic investigation is probably a desirable result.

A Symptomatic Arrhythmia Is Recorded. Generally, the diagnosis is considered definitive when an arrhythmia (complete AV block, SVT, VT, etc.) is electrocardiographically successfully recorded during a clinical episode of syncope. When syncope is reproduced in the electrophysiological laboratory, the interpretation of the significance of the responsible arrhythmia is less straightforward and is modulated by the sensitivity and specificity of the methods used for induction.

An Asymptomatic Arrhythmia Is Recorded. This situation is very frequent and provides a clinical dilemma. Because multiple arrhythmias may coexist, one needs to be confident that other symptomatic arrhythmias have not been missed. Also, under certain circumstances some so-called arrhythmias (sinus bradycardia, AV nodal Wenckebach) may only represent variations of normal or clinically nonsignificant anomalies. On the other hand, the recording of a dysrhythmia that carries a high statistical correlation with syncope (such as infra-Hisian block or sustained ventricular tachycardia) should prompt therapeutic intervention even in the absence of accompanying symptoms.

The 12-Lead Electrocardiogram

Limitations of the 12-lead ECG are obvious and relate to the short span of recording. Although generally nondiagnostic, ECG recordings may offer valuable indirect and circumstantial clues that could channel further diagnostic efforts. It is probably most informative when it reveals evidence for preexcitation and significant prolongation of the QT interval. Helpful but less diagnostic abnormalities are bifascicular or trifascicular blocks as well as the presence of ischemic changes. Standard 12-lead ECGs are generally less helpful in uncovering the diagnosis of sick sinus syndrome, intermittent heart block, or paroxysmal supraventricular or ventricular tachycardias. However, when one has the opportunity to obtain electrocardiographic recordings of a sustained paroxysmal tachycardia, every effort should be made to record all 12 leads before suppressing it. At least one should attempt to obtain a vectorial recording of the tachycardia (i.e., leads I, AVF, and V1). This information may become crucial later in the course of events if and when electrophysiological studies are performed.

Ambulatory ECG Monitoring

Ambulatory ECG recordings are of particular value in the evaluation of syncope in patients with frequent symptoms. In general, the longer the recording the more enhanced our ability to detect intermittent tachyarrhythmias and bradyarrhythmias. Electrocardiographic abnormalities which may be diagnostic if associated with syncope include severe intermittent sinus bradycardia, long sinus pauses, advanced degrees of atrioventricular block, rapid supraventricular tachycardias, or sustained ventricular tachycardia. The most important limitation of long-term ECG monitoring is that the recorded arrhythmias are not always associated with symptoms. In one study, only 13% of 371 patients had concurrent symptoms and arrhythmias, whereas in 34% typical symptoms occurred without any concomitant arrhythmia. Finally, 86% of patients with tachycardias were asymptomatic at the time (Kola 1982; Clark 1980; Zeldis 1980). It is very important to establish a firm temporal relationship between a syncopal episode and supraventricular tachycardia. This is probably less crucial when sustained ventricular tachycardia is recorded. Again, establishing a temporal relationship may be of paramount importance in the presence of certain bradycardias. For instance, young healthy athletes commonly have significant sinus bradycardia (at times as low as 30 beats/min) and may show long sinus pauses up to 2.8 s. They also display a high (up to 40%) incidence of type I second-degree AV block which frequently occurs during sleep and is most often a benign finding (Talan 1982; Brodsky 1977). Resting heart rates of 50 beats/min or lower are also found in more than 10% of asymptomatic elderly patients (Camm 1980). Also, high-grade frequent PVCs and infrequent short runs of nonsustained ventricular tachycardia are commonly seen in the asymptomatic elderly and, by themselves, do not require treatment (Viitasalo 1982; Fleg 1982).

In patients suffering from infrequent spells, it is unlikely that an episode of syncope will be recorded by any of the methods described. In these patients, an event recorder may be helpful. The technology for transtelephonic electrocardiographic monitoring was originally developed for pacemaker follow-up. Generally the device consists of a small ECG transmitter carried by the patient, which, when activated and connected to a telephone, transmits a single-channel electrocardiogram to a central receiving station. Although useful, this technology suffers from a number of limitations. First, technically adequate electrocardiograms are not always obtained. Second, the unit or the telephone may not be readily available to the patient when symptoms occur. Third, precious time may be lost while setting up the system for transmission. However, units are available that have an intrinsic memory which may record and keep events for later transmission and analysis. Fourth, because arrhythmic syncope is generally so sudden, the patient will often simply not be able to activate the device before passing out.

Newer implantable permanent pacemakers have additional telemetry and storage capabilities that allow prolonged intracardiac ECG montoring. These devices may be valuable in the management of patients afflicted with a combination of ventricular tachycardia and pacemaker-requiring bradyarrhythmia, and in patients who persist with syncope despite pacemaker insertion for a previously recognized or assumed bradyarrhythmia.

Exercise Testing

Despite its low yield, exercise testing is a provocative test and as such is an essential part of the investigation of effort syncope. Although probably contraindicated in patients with severe aortic stenosis (Council on Scientific Affairs 1981), it may reveal hypotension related to dynamic outflow obstruction (hypertrophic cardiomyopathy) or to severe left ventricular dysfunction (triple-vessel coronary artery disease, dilated cardiomyopathy) or to neuroregulatory dysfunction.

Both supraventricular and ventricular arrhythmias may be induced by exercise testing. The surge of catecholamines associated with exercise may be pathogenetically related to the occurrence of automatic atrial tachycardia. Increasing numbers of PACs may trigger paroxysms of atrial fibrillation or flutter. In patients with Wolff-Parkinson-White syndrome, the ventricular response to atrial fibrillation is of crucial importance as antegrade conduction down the accessory bypass tract may be extremely rapid and may result in syncope and even sudden death. The increased oxygen demand of exercise may induce ventricular tachycardia in patients with ischemic heart disease. In addition, exercise testing may uncover ventricular tachycardias in otherwise apparently healthy individuals. The mechanism here is not fully understood, but probably relates to the direct effect of catecholamines.

On a different level, exercise testing may help evaluate the significance of arrhythmias documented by Holter monitoring or induced by electrophysiological testing. Apparently profound but asymptomatic sinus bradycardia can thus be further evaluated. A slow but otherwise normal sinus node mechanism will increase its rate in relation to the level of exercise. Supraventricular tachycardia for instance with atrial rates of 200 beats/min occurring at rest may elicit an asymptomatic ventricular response of 100 beats/min due to 2:1 AV block. On the other hand, symptoms, including syncope, may develop when catecholamines facilitate AV conduction and thus allow a very rapid ventricular response that does not sustain adequate left ventricular filling and stroke volume. Exercise testing can help recognize the rare cases of Wenckebach AV block secondary to His-Purkinje system disease (Narula 1970a; Mangiardi 1982). More commonly, it may help localize the site of delay in patients with 2:1 AV block. As mentioned previously, AV nodal conduction is enhanced by exercise and therefore resting AV Wenckebach or 2:1 block will be expected to improve if the delay is occurring at the level of the AV node. On the other hand, conduction properties of the His-Purkinje system may be stressed more as AV nodal conduction is improved and more impulses are allowed distally.

Electrophysiological Testing

When syncope occurs with a documented tachycardia or bradycardia, further electrophysiological assessment may be needed and should be directed toward the primary cardiac arrhythmia in question. In a significant number of patients, however, an arrhythmia is suspected but has eluded the diagnostic recording attempts previously described. Such patients are also candidates for electrophysiological testing. Although invasive, the study carries a very low incidence of complications and virtually no mortality. It is also a provocative test that can theoretically condense several days or even weeks of passive electrocardiographic recordings into 2 or 3 h of laboratory study. However, concerns about sensitivity and specificity have tempered the usefulness of some of the techniques utilized during these studies (Wellens 1985; Brugada 1984). Moreover, the prognostic significance of certain inducible arrhythmias remains controversial (Swerdlow 1983; Wit 1970; Damato 1969). Nevertheless, a keen analysis of electrophysiological testing in light of accompanying symptomatology, clinical picture, and the attendant cardiac structural anomalies makes electrophysiological study a very powerful tool in the diagnostic investigation of syncope (Teichman 1985; Olshansky 1985; Morady 1984).

The basic diagnostic concepts and intracardiac electrophysiological techniques used to characterize rhythm disorders are similar for patients with syncope of undetermined etiology; however, the task is more formidable because the electrophysiologist must rule out the syncope potential for all forms of bradycardia, tachycardia, and other possible causes. We, therefore, generally limit invasive electrophysiological testing to those patients with recurrent syncope, and perform it only after noninvasive cardiac assessment has been completed. In nonselected cases, the diagnostic yield from electrophysiological study in patients with syncope of unknown etiology is quite small (DiMarco 1981); however, in patients with documented structural heart disease or in patients with electrocardiographic abnormalities that suggest vulnerability to tachycardia or bradycardia, a presumptive mechanism can be documented in approximately two-thirds of patients (Akhtar 1983).

Techniques of Intracardiac Electrophysiological Testing

Intracardiac electrical signals are usually obtained with multipolar electrode catheters. Amplification and filtration are necessary to display and record these signals for diagnostic purposes. The His bundle deflection can be reliably obtained by filtering out signals with frequencies below 30 Hz and above 500 Hz. The frequency of some of the ventricular signals approaches 1000 Hz.

From one to six multipolar electrode catheters are used in electrophysiological studies, usually three or four. The catheters are placed percutaneously by the Seldinger technique or may be inserted by standard cutdown techniques in the peripheral veins or arteries. The arterial approach is limited to use in left ventricular stimulation and mapping. Our standard approach for testing patients with syncope of undetermined etiology would include three catheters inserted through the right femoral vein. One catheter is positioned with its most distal electrodes in the atrial appendage and with a semicircular curve so the more proximal electrodes approach the sinus node region. The second catheter is positioned close to the tricuspid valve in the region of the His bundle, and the third catheter is positioned in the right ventricular apex. It is our custom to use quadripolar catheters for the atrium and ventricle, and a tripolar catheter for the His bundle recording. In patients suspected of having preexcitation, a quadripolar catheter is also placed in the coronary sinus to record left atrial and left ventricular depolarization (Fig. 14.1). This catheter is usually introduced percutaneously through the antecubital, internal jugular, or subclavian vein.

Fig. 14.1. **a** X-ray demonstrating electrode catheter placement for recording and stimulation during routine diagnostic electrophysiological test. Quadripolar catheter is placed in high right atrial-atrial appendage location, tripolar catheter is placed in the low right atrium-His bundle region, third catheter is placed via a subclavian venipuncture in the mid coronary sinus, and fourth catheter is a bipolar lead placed in the right ventricular apex. **b** Recordings obtained from the same electrode catheters in a teenager with recurrent syncope associated with palpitations secondary to Wolff-Parkinson-White syndrome. Pacing from CS increases degree of preexcitation and conceals the His bundle deflection within ventricular depolarization. *HRA*, high right atrium; *His*, low right atrial His bundle region recording; *CS*, coronary sinus; *V*, *I*, *AVF*, standard surface electrocardiogram recordings. **c** Standard electrocardiogram recorded when rapid atrial pacing produces 1:1 antegrade conduction down an accessory pathway with rates exceeding 214 beats/ min. This reproduced near syncope in a 62-year-old female.

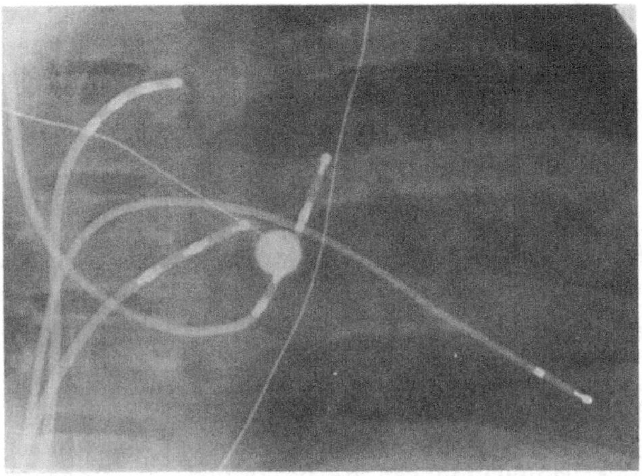

a

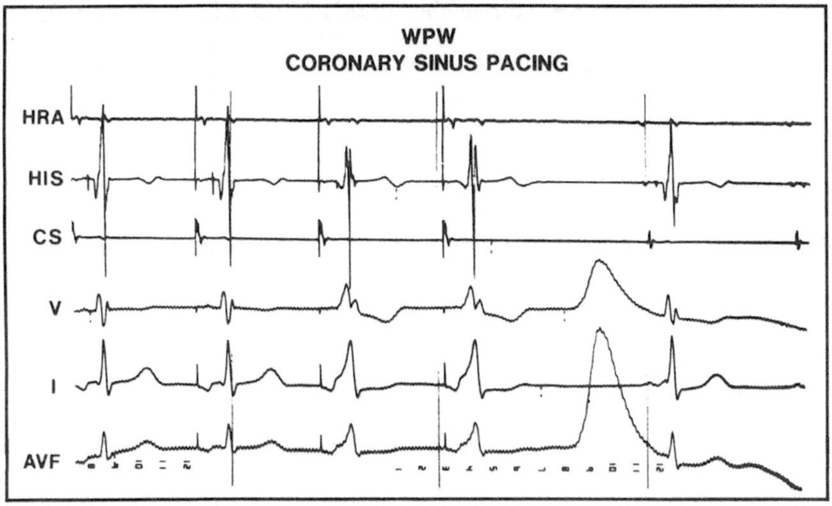
WPW
CORONARY SINUS PACING
HRA
HIS
CS
V
I
AVF

b

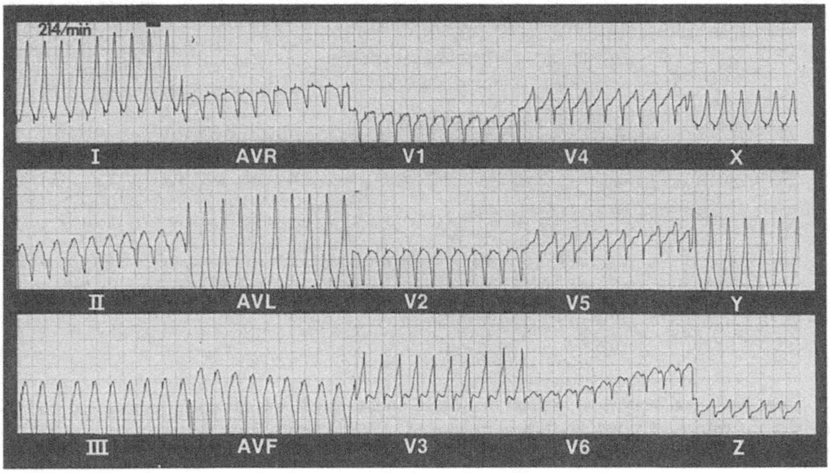
214/min
I
AVR
V1
V4
X
II
AVL
V2
V5
Y
III
AVF
V3
V6
Z

c

Catheter positioning is monitored through fluoroscopic observation and appropriate electrogram recordings. As the study progresses, these catheters may be moved to various positions in the heart, including the right ventricular outflow tract, various right atrial mapping positions, and across a patent foramen ovale.

The proximal electrode pins are connected to a junction box for recording, and to a programmed stimulator for various pacing techniques. Three simultaneous electrocardiographic leads are used (I, AVF, V1). This permits vectorial assessment of the surface electrocardiogram. The signals are then observed and recorded using an electrostatic analogue printing system. For most clinical studies, paper speeds of 100 mm/s are accurate to within 5 ms as long as precise time signals are recorded.

Patients undergoing electrophysiological testing are without food for 4–6 h, receive mild sedation at the time of the procedure, and receive heparin when two or more catheters are passed through the inferior vena cava or when the left ventricle is entered. Cardiac stimulation can be performed by temporary pacemakers; however, for most studies the stimulator must be more complex to allow for programmed intracardiac stimulation that is able to induce a variety of timed multiple extra stimuli at 10-ms intervals or less. The commonly used stimulators have a constant current source, and are usually set at twice the stimulation threshold (Fig. 14.1).

Protocol of Electrophysiological Studies

In evaluating patients that present with syncope of undetermined etiology, we

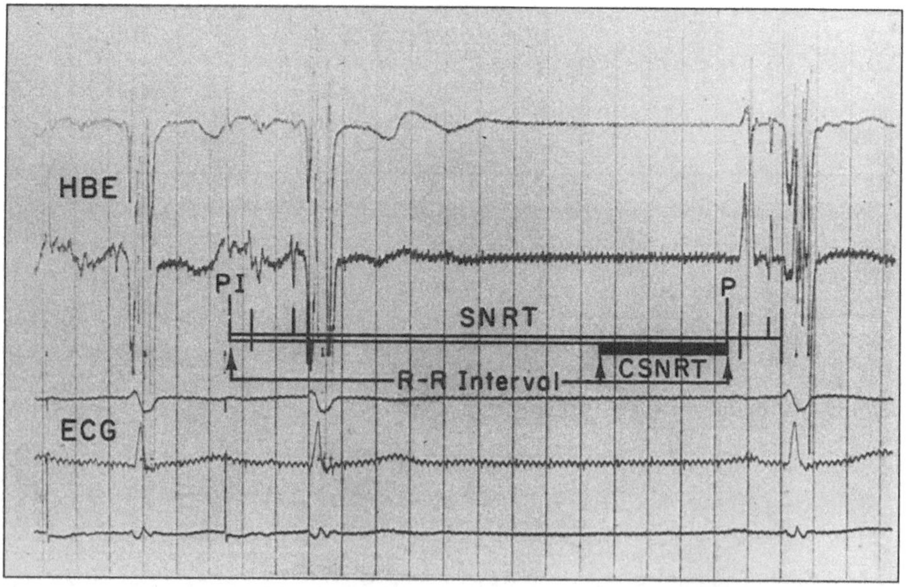

Fig. 14.2. Sinus node recovery time. Atrial overdrive pacing for 30 s is abruptly terminated and the time required for return of sinus rhythm is measured. *SNRT*, sinus node recovery time; *CSNRT*, corrected sinus node recovery time; see text.

thoroughly evaluate sinus node function, AV nodal transmission, His-Purkinje conduction, and vulnerability to tachycardia induction. The latter is first attempted in the atrium and then in the ventricle.

The typical electrophysiological study in our laboratory includes the following: (1) recording baseline intervals, (2) performing multiple sinus node recovery times, (3) determining Wenckebach cycle length during progressively more rapid atrial pacing, (4) assessing AV nodal conduction characteristics and refractory periods by programmed atrial stimulation, (5) characterizing the presence or absence of ventriculoatrial conduction during various ventricular pacing cycle lengths, (6) performing programmed ventricular stimulation to determine VA and ventricular refractory periods, (7) paroxysmal tachycardia induction using atrial and/or ventricular stimulation techniques, and (8) atrial and ventricular endocardial mapping to characterize the sequence of depolarization and tachycardia circuits. Response to various drug interventions requires repetition of one or more of the above steps.

Assessment of Sinus Node Function. Atrial bradyarrhythmias are frequently encountered as a cause of syncope or lightheadedness and are usually referred to as abnormalities of sinus node function, more commonly termed the *sick sinus syndrome*. The syndrome is associated with sinus bradycardia and abnormal sinoatrial impulse formation and conduction, plus depressed atrial, junctional, and ventricular escape mechanisms. These abnormalities may be due to intrinsic disorders of sinoatrial electrical activity or may result from extrinsic neuroregulatory reflex mechanisms. Although more frequent in the elderly, sick sinus syndrome can occur in patients of all ages (Shaw 1978; Scott 1976). Invasive electrophysiological testing generally assesses sinus node function through indirect techniques. These techniques include assessment of sinus node recovery time, sinoatrial conduction time, and chronotropic competence (intrinsic heart rate). A direct recording of sinus node activity can be attained using special techniques.

Table 14.2. Normal values for sinus node electrophysiological function tests

SNRT	<1600 ms
CSNRT	<550 ms
TSNRT	<5 s
SACT	50–125 ms
IHR	$\geqslant(117.2 - (0.53 \times \text{age})) \pm 10$ bpm
Postatropine HR	>90 bpm or 1.25 control HR
SNERP	250–380 ms

a) *Sinus Node Recovery Time.* Overdrive suppression of spontaneous sinus node depolarization following atrial pacing rates greater than the spontaneous atrial rhythm is normal. However, prolonged overdrive suppression correlates with depressed automaticity of the sinus node and is a characteristic of sick sinus syndrome (Mandel 1971; Delius 1976). Sinus node recovery time (SNRT) is defined as the interval from the last atrial paced beat until the first spontaneous beat (Fig. 14.2). In our laboratory 30 s of overdrive atrial pacing is performed at a constant cycle length from a site near the sinus node. This is repeated at several cycle lengths (600, 500, 450, 400, 350, and 300 ms). In patients with sinus dysfunction, the peak recovery time usually occurs at pacing rates longer than 450 ms, although this response is variable and must be measured following multiple pacing rates. Pauses greater than 1600 ms (Kulbertus 1975; Delius 1976) are abnormal but do vary according to the resting heart rate. To correct for this variation in baseline heart rate, sinus node recovery time is corrected by subtracting the baseline heart rate from the sinus node recovery time. SNRT minus baseline heart rate equals CSNRT (Table 14.2).

A corrected sinus node recovery time greater than 550 ms is abnormal (Narula 1972; Josephson 1979c). Patients with intrinsic sinus node dysfunction frequently demonstrate suppressed atrial activity following the initial recovery atrial depolarization. The secondary pauses should also be considered evidence of sinus node dysfunction (Bigger 1973; Benditt 1976). The total sinus node recovery time (TSNRT) incorporates assessment of primary and secondary pauses. Normal patients should have a return to a stable baseline rhythm within 5 s of overdrive atrial pacing (Delius 1976; Josephson 1979c). The relative value of sinus node recovery time for assessing patients with sick sinus syndrome is somewhat controversial (Li 1978; Reiffel 1977; Gupta 1974). Abnormal SNRTs and CSNRTs have a strong correlation with resolution of syncope by pacing; however, a normal sinus node recovery time does not exclude the possibility of intermittent sinoatrial arrest as the cause of syncope in an individual patient.

b) *Sinoatrial Conduction Time*. Sinoatrial conduction time (SACT) is an indirect method to assess impulse transmission from the sinus node to the atrium and from the atrium to the sinus node. Two methods for indirectly calculating sinoatrial conduction times have been forwarded. Strauss' method involves measuring the response of the sinus cycle length to programmed atrial stimulation (Strauss 1973) while Narula utilizes atrial pacing several beats faster than sinus node and assesses the pause following the last paced beat (Narula 1978). Neither one of these techniques have helped us enhance the clinical assessment of sinus node dysfunction.

c) *Effect of Atropine*. The "Response to Atropine" is the most frequently used method of assessing the effect of the parasympathetic tone on the sinus node and AV node. After baseline electrophysiological assessment, 1–3 mg atropine sulfate (0.04 mg/kg) is administered intravenously and the heart rate response is noted (Breithardt 1978). A normal response is a rise in heart rate to greater than 90 beats/min or an increase of greater than 25% over the control rate. A small percentage of patients with sick sinus syndrome show a blunted heart rate response to this atropine test. SNRT is usually shortened after atropine; however, in a small percentage of patients with sinus node dysfunction, there may be a paradoxical increase in SNRT. This reflects improvement in sinoatrial entrance during atrial overdrive pacing (Reiffel 1975).

d) *Intrinsic Heart Rate*. Complete autonomic blockade with a beta blocker and atropine provide measurement of intrinsic heart rate (IHR). This is achieved by intravenous administration of 0.04 mg/kg atropine sulfate and 0.2 mg/kg propranolol (Jose 1970). Theoretically, exposing the intrinsic heart rate to atrial overdrive pacing will more clearly identify intrinsic sinus node dysfunction from so-called extrinsic sinus node dysfunction (increased vagal tone, vagotonia).

e) *Sinus Node Effective Refractory Period* (SNERP). By observing return cycles after atrial premature beats during paced rhythm, sinus node refractoriness can be assessed in about 80% of patients. SNERP is defined as the longest premature interval that results in the interpolation of the premature beat (i.e., when the recovery cycle shortens abruptly and becomes equal to the basic sinus rate). Limited observations indicate that an SNERP of 500 ms or more is associated with sick sinus syndrome (normal 250–380 ms) (Kerr 1983). Further studies are needed to substantiate the usefulness of SNERP in uncovering diseases of the sinus node.

f) *Monophasic Action Potential-Like Recordings.* Monophasic action potential recordings can be obtained from the area of the sinus node when the catheter is properly positioned at the junction of the superior vena cava and the right atrium. Although this technique is still considered experimental (Reiffel 1981), we have been able to obtain stable recordings during clinical diagnostic electrophysiological studies. For the best results, silver/silver chloride electrodes should be used (as larger signal amplitudes can be obtained), but regular platinum electrode catheters can also be successfully used. Signal filtering is different and is bracketed between 1 and 1000 Hz. This technique theoretically allows differentiation between disorders of sinus impulse formation (automaticity) and disorders of sinoatrial conduction (sinus exit block) (Reiffel 1981; Gang 1985). Further studies are needed to assess the clinical usefulness and predictive power of this technique.

Although each of these tests have significant limitations, when used in combination they do give a fairly good picture of sinus node function. In general, these tests have a better specificity than sensitivity. Unfortunately, syncope is rarely reproduced by any of these tests. Therefore, the crucial temporal relationship between symptoms and the arrhythmia at hand is rarely confirmed.

Assessment of Carotid Sinus Hypersensitivity. Carotid sinus syncope is a syndrome mediated by a bradyarrhythmia resulting from mild inadvertent pressure applied through normal head motion to the carotid sinus baroreceptors. Bending or turning the head to the side, pressure from a tight collar, enlarged glands or tumors may elicit the reflex and cause syncope. A slight touch of the carotid sinus may suffice to induce cardiac standstill (Heron 1965; Hutchinson 1960).

Carotid sinus hypersensitivity exists as an exaggerated response to carotid sinus massage (Sigler 1963; Thomas 1969). This test can be evaluated at the bedside or in the electrophysiological laboratory. Carotid massage must be relatively vigorous and usually applied in a massaging manner, for approximately 5 s to one carotid bulb at a time. The maneuver should be performed with caution, particularly in patients with carotid artery bruits or a history of cerebral vascular disease. An abnormal response is arbitrarily defined as a sinus pause of greater than 3 s or the development of high-grade AV block (Thomas 1969). Slowing of the sinus mechanism and/or development of AV block is secondary to the cardioinhibitory vagal effects of carotid sinus pressure. Also, part of the normal response to carotid sinus massage is the vasodepressor response (Thomas 1969). The heart rate response is usually initiated within the first 1.5 s of massage while the drop in blood pressure is slower in onset, longer in duration, and may be relatively independent of the heart rate response. In a prospective study (Brown 1980), we found more than 30% of patients coming to cardiac catheterization had an exaggerated response to carotid massage. This was not associated with clinical occurrences of syncope. Thus, a positive response to carotid sinus massage is common and may be totally unrelated to the particular etiology of syncope in a specific patient. Marked variations in response to carotid sinus massage and other vagal maneuvers are also typical of normal and abnormal physiology.

Assessment of Atrioventricular (AV) Nodal Function (Table 14.3). Depressed impulse transmission through the AV node may be a contributor to syncope in patients with sick sinus syndrome, paroxysmal supraventricular tachycardias, drug-induced AV block, high-grade heart block associated with inferior myocardial infarction, and primary conduction system disease.

Table 14.3. Normal values for atrioventricular conduction system (AVCS) function tests

	AV Node	HPS
AH	60–130 ms	H duration ≤25 ms HV = 35–55 ms
ERP[a]	<430 ms	<450 ms
Atrial pacing rate at which block occurs	>100 bpm	>150 bpm

[a] ERP, effective refractory period.

Anatomically, heart block is defined as supra-His (AV nodal), intra-His, and/or infra-His. Current techniques do not permit direct recordings from the AV node. AV node conduction is thus reflected on the His bundle electrogram by the A–H interval (the time from low right atrial depolarization to the His potential). Normal A–H intervals range between 60 and 130 ms (Damato 1969; Narula 1970b). Intra-Hisian conduction is reflected by the duration of the His potential itself, which should not exceed 25 ms (Narula 1970a). Infra-His conduction is reflected by the HV interval (normal from 35 to 55 ms) (Schuilenburg 1972; Puech 1971). In addition to the resting intervals, conduction properties are assessed by (1) incremental atrial pacing, (2) programmed electrical stimulation of the atrium (whereby premature atrial depolarizations are introduced during sinus or paced rhythm and are progressively shortened until refractoriness is met), and (3) the response to drugs such as atropine or Pronestyl. There techniques will act as "stressors" of the conduction system at its different levels. Normally during incremental atrial pacing, block first develops at the level of the AV node (Wenckebach) and occurs at pacing rates greater than 120 beats/min. Intra- or infra-His bocks do not normally occur at pacing rates slower than 150 beats/min (H_1–H_1 intervals of 400 ms or more) (Josephson 1979b). However, when AV nodal conduction is enhanced (1:1 conduction during atrial pacing above 200 beats/min), the first site of block may be normally seen below the AV node (Damato 1973). Alternatively, when AV nodal conduction is delayed, it may not be possible adequately to study the His-Purkinje system as the pacing stress at this level may be too mild. When it is due to vagotonia, AV nodal delay may be minimized by the administration of atropine.

Programmed electrical stimulation allows assessment of effective refractory periods (the point at which an impulse does not capture a specific tissue). Prolonged effective refractory periods of the AV node (normal <430 ms)

(Akhtar 1975) and/or the His-Purkinje system (normal <450 ms) (Akhtar 1975; Josephson 1979b) are indicative of abnormal conduction properties. Procainamide administration directly affects conduction times across the His-Purkinje system, causing marked prolongation of the HV interval in susceptible individuals. This test has been used with some success to uncover otherwise undiagnosed His-Purkinje system block (Scheinman 1974a; Tonkin 1978).

The site of block can be easily localized by using the techniques described above (Fig. 14.3). Such localization has significant therapeutic implications, as any degree of intra- or infra-His block associated with syncope provides a good indication for pacemaker insertion. Indeed, even in the absence of symptoms, the demonstration of second- or third-degree intra- or infra-Hisian block should be treated with permanent pacing (Josephson 1979b). Even asymptomatic first-degree Hisian block carries a significant risk of progression to complete heart block when the HV interval is 80 ms or more (Narula 1975; Scheinman 1977). When the HV interval is 70–95 ms, careful follow-up is recommended. On the other hand, asymptomatic AV nodal block of any degree does not require pacing. For instance, patients with congenital heart block are usually asymptomatic and demonstrate adequate heart rate in response to exercise or isoproterenol administration (Michaelson 1972; Thilenius 1972). Mobitz type II or third-degree block at the level of the AV node requires permanent pacing when associated with symptoms such as syncope. Treatment of inappropriate AV nodal Wenckebach is more controversial. Until recently, only observation was recommended, but this has been questioned (Shaw 1985).

In addition to antegrade conduction properties, retrograde conduction characteristics should be assessed when selecting various modes of bradycardia pacing. This helps define the optimal settings for rate responsiveness in dual chamber pacemakers while still providing adequate protection from pacemaker-mediated tachycardia. For example, a long VA time of 400 ms would indicate that the upper rate response of the pacemaker should be limited to approximately 100 beats/min (as the postventricular atrial refractory period should be extended beyond 400 ms and as the usual programmed AV interval is 150–200 ms). Finally, whenever possible, atrial or dual chamber pacing is recommended over simple ventricular pacing. Although dual chamber pacemakers are somewhat more expensive and atrial sensing problems may sometimes be frustrating, atrial (or dual chamber) pacing has many hemodynamic and electrophysiological advantages. First, it provides rate responsive pacing; second, it is not associated with pacemaker syndrome; and third, compared with VVI pacing it is not associated with an increased incidence of atrial fibrillation (Rosenguist 1986).

Supraventricular Arrhythmias. All forms of supraventricular tachycardias can result in syncope. The occurrence of syncope depends on the rate of the tachycardia, the status of AV nodal conduction, and the presence of accessory tracts. All of these determine the ventricular response to the arrhythmia. Electrophysiological techniques are very effective in inducing, localizing, and terminating supraventricular tachycardias. Sinoatrial reentry tachycardia, paroxysmal atrial tachycardia, and AV nodal reentry tachycardia are all relatively easily induced by programmed electrical stimulation. In susceptible patients, the induction of atrial tachycardias can be expected in at least 80% of cases (Wellens 1971). Occasionally atropine has to be administered to enhance the effectiveness of atrial stimulation. When induced, these arrhythmias are usually clinically relevant. However, in patients with recurrent syncope, they cannot be assumed to be the cause of the syncope unless the symptoms are reproduced or at least a significant decrease in blood pressure is observed. The latter may be enhanced by head up tilting. Induction of sustained atrial flutter or fibrillation is also clinically significant when the inducing stress is minimal (such as a single PAC). On the other hand, short periods of atrial fibrillation or flutter (<30 s) (Haft 1968) can be induced in almost everyone when high-rate atrial pacing is performed. Such a finding is obviously nonspecific.

Automatic atrial tachycardia is not inducible with programmed electrical stimulation; however, they may be enhanced with the administration of Isuprel. Typically, this type of tachycardia shows some overdrive suppression following cessation of atrial pacing. Using mapping techniques, the focus of an automatic atrial tachycardia can then be localized to a discrete portion of the atrium (Goldreyer 1973; Scheinman 1974b; Gillette 1977).

Atrioventricular nodal reentry tachycardia and atrioventricular circus movement tachycardias (WPW, concealed bypass tract) are reliably induced and terminated during electrophysiological testing (Wellens 1971).

Tachycardia mechanisms can be examined and bypass tracts can be localized, thus delineating possible therapeutic manipulations which may include antiarrhythmic drugs (all tachycardias), antitachycardia devices (reentrant arrhythmias), and electrical or surgical ablations (bypass tract, AV node, automatic focus).

Ventricular Arrhythmias. A crucial role of electrophysiological testing is to rule out ventricular tachycardia as the cause of syncope. Recurrent sustained ventricular tachycardia associated with chronic coronary artery disease can be reliably induced with programmed electrical stimulation of the ventricle (Hartzer 1977; Vandepol 1980; Livelli 1982; Josephson 1978) (Fig. 14.4) The sensitivity, specificity, and clinical significance of inducible ventricular tachycardia has been extensively debated (Brugada 1984a; Wellens 1985; Morady 1984;

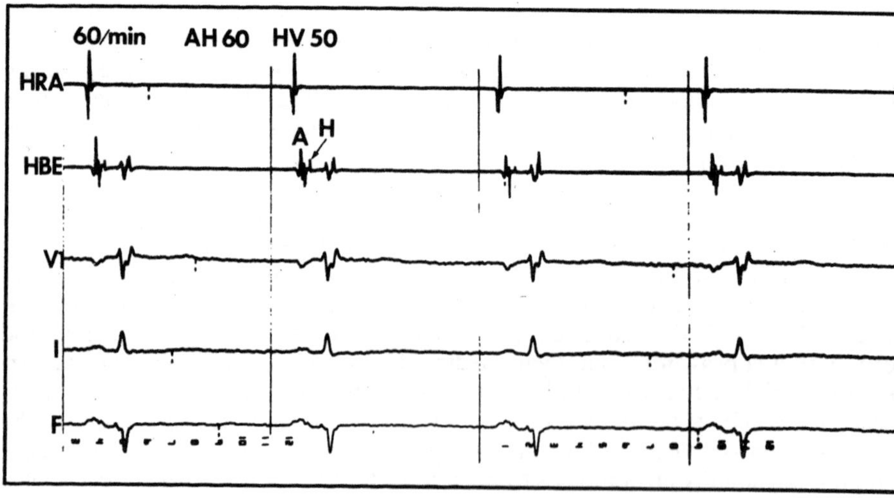

a

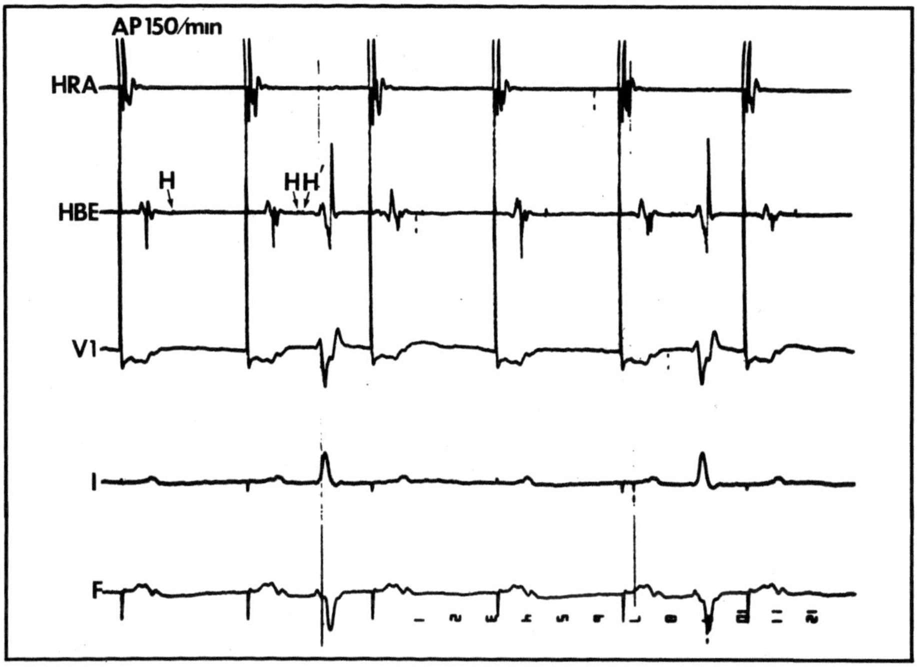

b

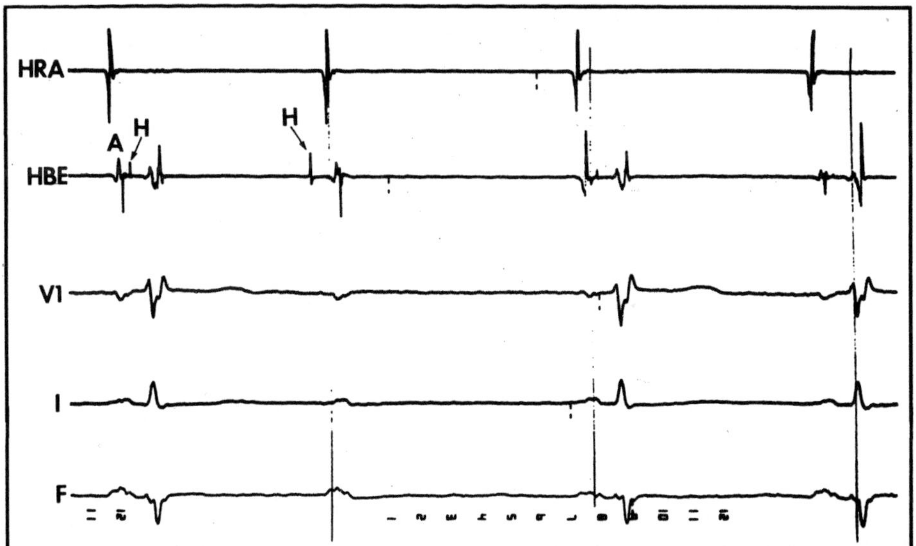

c

Fig. 14.3a–c. Tracings during complete electrophysiological testing obtained from a 60-year-old female presenting with recurrent syncope of approximately 2 years duration. The resting 12-lead electrocardiogram was normal; however, cardiac rhythm slowed abruptly during advanced stages of exercise testing. **a** Normal intracardiac electrograms and intervals at rest with a heart rate of 60 beats/min. **b** Atrial pacing at 150 beats/min induces advanced heart block. The second paced beat is conducted with intra-Hisian delay (split His potential). A small His potential is produced after each nonconducted atrial paced beat, confirming the diagnosis of intra-His block. **c** A "His extra systole" with retrograde conduction to the atrium and absence of antegrade conduction to the ventricle further supports the diagnosis of intra-His disease.

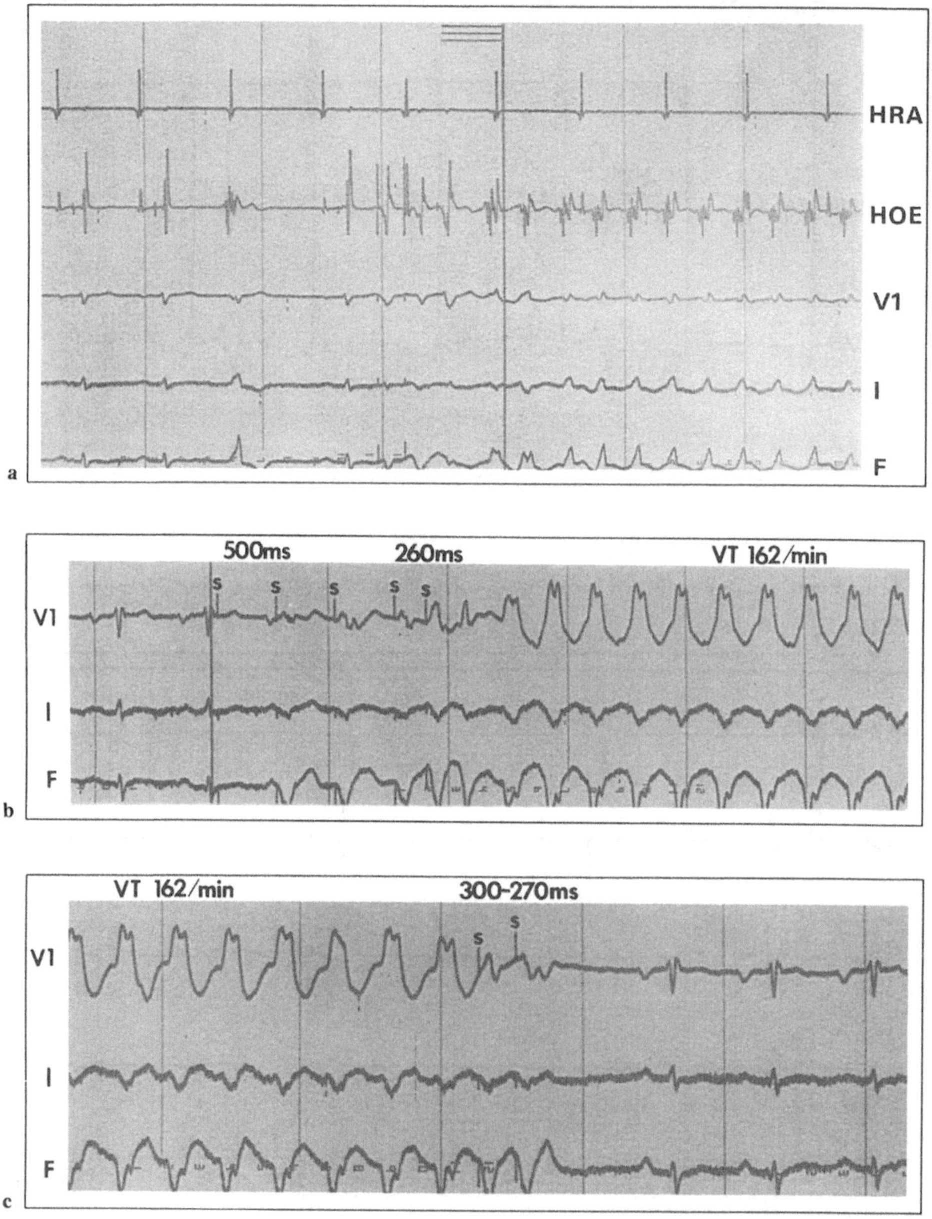

Fig. 14.4a–c. Electrophysiological tracing taken from an elderly female with a history of recurrent syncope, seizures, and aborted sudden death. **a** Recordings obtained at the time of complete electrophysiological study. Ventricular tachycardia (rate 165 beats/min) was induced by paired ventricular stimuli coupled by 370/280 ms to the preceding QRS complex in sinus rhythm. *HRA*, high right atrium; *HBE*, recording from the region of the His bundle; *V1*, *I*, *F*, standard electrocardiographic leads. **b** Induction of ventricular tachycardia in the coronary care unit during serial drug testing. A single premature stimulus coupled by 260 ms to a ventricular paced rhythm of 500 ms cycle length induced ventricular tachycardia (rate 162 beats/min). **c** Same tachycardia as **b**. Tracing illustrates termination of ventricular tachycardia by two consecutive ventricular stimuli coupled at 300/270 ms.

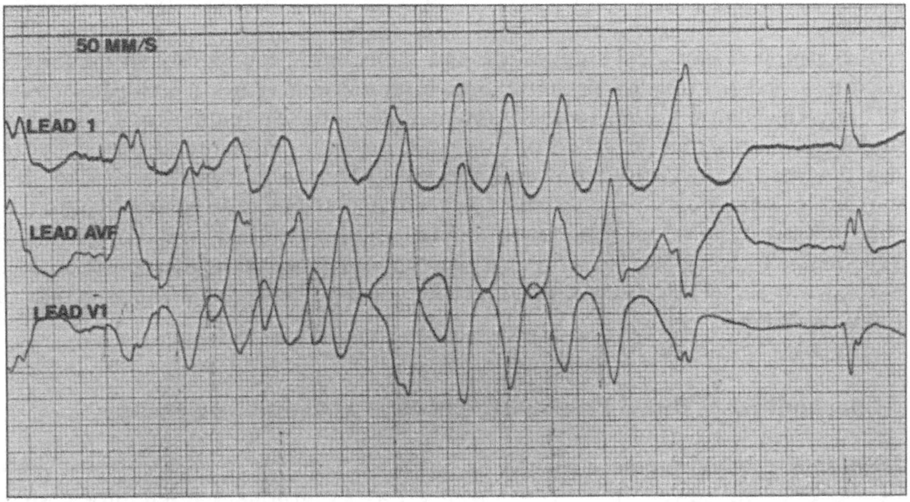
50 MM/S
LEAD 1
LEAD AVF
LEAD V1

documented sustained ventricular tachycardia approaches 100% (Brugada 1984b).

Programmed electrical stimulation and tachycardia induction can be serially used to assess the efficacy of therapeutic interventions (Ruskin 1980; Josephson 1979a; Abi-Samra 1986e) (which may include antiarrhythmic drugs, electrical endocardial ablation, cryoablation, surgical resection, implantable antitachycardia devices, and cardioverter defibrillators). It is important to realize that current understanding of programmed ventricular stimulation is largely based on the investigation of patients with documented sustained and nonsustained ventricular tachycardia. Nevertheless, current electrophysiological practice does extend the same interpretive approach to patients suffering from syncope of unknown origin.

Abnormalities of Blood Pressure Regulation as Causes of Syncope

Disorders of blood pressure regulation have classically been neglected as causes of syncope and have often been advanced as exclusionary possibilities when general diagnostic workups were negative. This is partially due to the assumed benignity of these disorders and to the lack of relevant standarized provocative investigative techniques.

Besides the fact that they are not always physically benign, these disorders causing recurrent syncope often impart very heavy psychosocial stress on the affected individual and, thus, are worthy of proper diagnostic identification and treatment. In our laboratory, head up tilt testing has proven invaluable in evaluating patients with unexplained syncope. Our methodology is described in

Table 14.4. Possible BP and HR abnormalities observed during head up tilt

SBP	DBP	HR	Condition
↓↓	Normal	↑↑	Loss of aortic compliance Hypovolemia Venous pooling
↓/	Normal	↑↑	Hypovolemia Venous pooling
↑/	Normal	↑↑↑	Hyperbeta adrenergic state/syndrome
↓↓	↓		Autonomic dysfunction
Normal	Normal		"Chronotropic insufficiency"

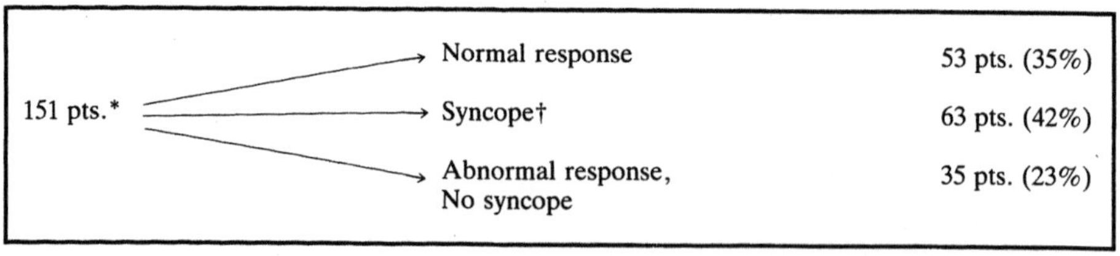

Fig. 14.6. Overall response to head up tilt in 154 patients three with syncope of unknown origin. *, additional patients could not finish the test because of leg pain; †, syncopal attacks occurred within 11.7 ± 6.1 min of 60° head up tilt (range = 1–20 min)

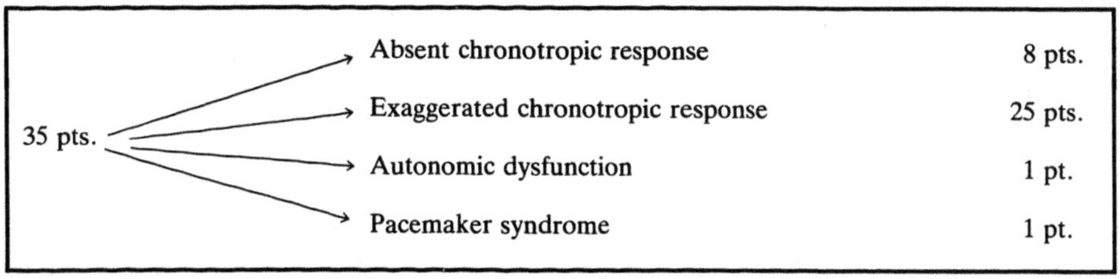

Fig. 14.7. Findings in patients with abnormal but nonsyncopal response to head up tilt.

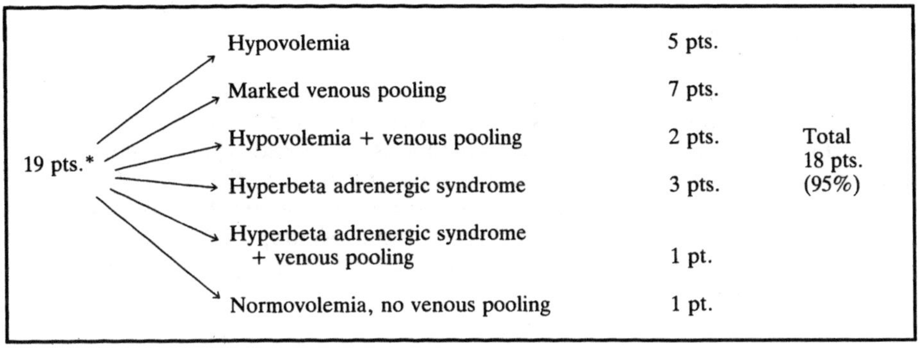

Fig. 14.8. Mechanisms underlying an exaggerated chronotropic response to head up tilt. *, 19/25 patients fully investigated as outlined above (see text).

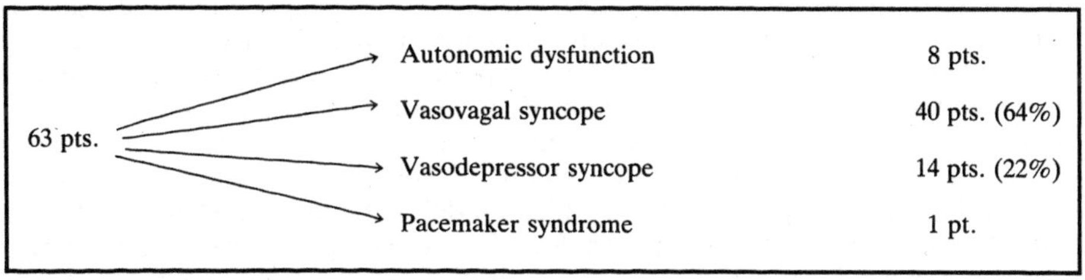

Fig. 14.9. Specific mechanisms of syncope during head up tilt.

detail in Chap. 13 and a summary of the possible abnormalities detected is given in Table 14.4.

The Cleveland Clinic Experience

We have studied 154 patients with unexplained syncope (78 males, 76 females, mean age 56 years). Three patients could not finish the tilt test because of arthritic problems in their knees. Fifty-three patients (35%) had a normal response to tilt. Of the remaining 98 patients, 63 (42%) developed a syncopal attack during tilt (Fig. 14.6). The other 35 patients (23%) had an abnormal response that potentially could explain the syncopal symptoms, but no induced syncope (Fig. 14.7). In the group with an exaggerated chronotropic response to tilt, an abnormality of volume or volume distribution was present in 15 patients.

Three patients had hyperbeta adrenergic syndrome (Fig. 14.8). Of the 63 patients with induced syncope during tilt, 54 had vasovagal or vasodepressor syncope. One fainted because of pacemaker syndrome (Abi-Samra 1986a; Abi-Samra 1986b) (Fig. 14.9).

In contrast, when 15 normal volunteers without a history of syncope (eight males, seven females; age 19–53) were studied with head up tilt carried out for a total 60° tilt time of 30 min, none developed syncope. These results suggest that head up tilt test is a sensitive and specific provocative test for induction of vasovagal/vasodepressor syncope in susceptible patients.

Vasovagal and Vasodepressor Syncope

Vasovagal syncope is defined as syncope occurring secondary to a sudden marked drop in blood pressure associated with, but not necessarily preceded by, marked bradycardia. Vasodepressor syncope is diagnosed when syncope occurs following a sudden marked decrease in blood pressure without an appreciable decrease in heart rate. Since even in vasodepressor syncope there is no increase in heart rate when the sudden hypotension occurs, both vasovagal and vasodepressor syncope can be thought of as having an inappropriate "bradycardic" component.

Clinical Considerations

Clinically, the two conditions are often lumped together and represent what is often referred to as the common faint. Classically, vasovagal attacks are said to occur in younger patients. Typically, syncope or presyncope is triggered by unpleasant physical and psychological experiences. Loss of consciousness is preceded by a wide variety of premonitory symptoms including lightheadedness, blurring of vision, dizziness, nausea, abdominal cramps, pallor, and cold sweats. These preliminary symptoms are usually of sufficient duration as to allow assumption of the supine position, which modifies the attack. This condition is considered to be quite benign with few, if any, complications. Furthermore, patients are said to "outgrow" the condition as the frequency of attacks decreases with advancing age.

Although such a clinical picture is frequently seen, it certainly does not occur in every, and maybe not in most, patients with vasovagal syncope who seek medical attention. For example, most of our patients with vasovagal or vasodepressor syncope were middle-aged (mean age 56 years) and had relatively recent onset of symptoms. A history of benign syncope in childhood was common. In addition, many had experienced devastating, potentially lethal complications prior to their presentation to our center.

One of the reasons that such potential seriousness is overlooked stems from the clinical belief that vasovagal syncope is benign. Unheralded syncope is appropriately attributed to dangerous ventricular arrhythmias or heart block until proven otherwise. Unfortunately, when these arrhythmias are not documented, no specific diagnosis may be made, and adequate diagnostic or provocative testing for vasovagal and vasodepressor syncope is omitted. Sometimes an epileptic disorder is assumed and anticonvulsant therapy may be inappropriately administered for years.

Although our population is selected, only a minority had typical warning signs of sufficient duration that would theoretically allow them to abort attacks. Most had sustained various musculoskeletal injuries related to their syncopal episodes. More ominously, there were several episodes of motor vehicle accidents and brain concussions. The psychosocial impact of these symptoms was quite marked: multiple hospitalizations for diagnostic purposes, prolonged absenteeism, and even forced unemployment occurred frequently. Patients reacted to their symptoms with severe anxiety and most exhibited at least a moderate degree of social dependency, such as inability to drive, avoidance of social gatherings, or even fear of being left alone at any time.

Pathophysiological Considerations

With this in mind, it is clear that effective therapeutic interventions are indicated in selected patients who suffer from multiple attacks of vasovagal syncope. Such therapeutic manipulations may be difficult to delineate and should be based on a clear understanding of the precipitating factors and the exact pathophysiological events leading to loss of consciousness. In this regard, it is important to realize that vasovagal and vasodepressor syncope are not diseases by themselves but merely the product of exaggerated reflexes and that they are often a mere manifestation of an underlying "metabolic" or "hemodynamic" disorder, such as hemorrhage and venous pooling.

It is apparent from observations made during tilt testing that hypotension almost always precedes bradycardia. Bradycardia was observed prior to hypotension in only one patient, while in seven patients both changes occurred simultaneously. Hence, hypotension preceded bradycardia in most patients. Furthermore, when events preceding the syncopal attack were analyzed, most patients had had an exaggerated chronotropic response to tilt (as defined by an increase of at least 20 beats/min or 30% above control heart rate). When further hemodynamic workup was performed, abnormalities of blood volume and blood volume distribution were uncovered in most patients who had an exaggerated chronotropic response (while marginal volume abnormalities were found in only two patients who had normal heart rate response to tilt) (Abi-Samra 1986a).

Further observations using serum catecholamines (as measurement of sympathetic nerve activity) and variation of the heart period (as measurement of basal parasympathetic tone) have suggested that patients who develop a vasovagal attack during head up tilt testing have higher basal parasympathetic tone than those patients who do not. On the other hand, catecholamines sampled immediately after the syncopal attack do not differ significantly from those sampled at 10 min of head up tilting (Abi-Samra 1986c). Although these data have to be interpreted with caution, they suggest that the sympathetic system is adequately stimulated during provoked vasovagal or vasodepressor attacks. In other words, we were not able to document sympathetic "withdrawal" during vasovagal syncope. Alternatively, it is conceivable that this may actually represent insufficient sympathetic stimulation in the face of a rapidly falling blood pressure. Moreover, catecholamine values measured at the time of syncope could be spuriously high due to insufficient wash out between onset of syncopal events and sampling time.

These observations allow us to construct the following pathophysiological scheme: As hypovolemia or venous incompetence accentuate the degree of diminution of venous return during head up tilt, left ventricular filling is diminished and sympathetic stimulation results in tachycardia and increased inotropy. In other words, a situation is occurring whereby the ventricle is strongly contracting around an empty cavity. This causes inappropriate stimulation of the afferent C fibers in the left ventricle, thus releasing an efferent parasympathetic inhibitory discharge (Mark 1983).

In the hyperbeta adrenergic syndrome, a similar pathogenesis may apply even though venous pooling may not be exaggerated. In this case, reduction in left ventricular filling occurs secondary to the marked tachycardia and its attendant decrease in diastolic filling time. Similarly, observations made during vasovagal syncope that is precipitated by phobic stimuli reveal that a state of sympathetic overactivity almost always precedes the syncopal attack.

Although there is a large body of circumstantial evidence that appears to substantiate the validity of this pathophysiological mechanism, it does not offer a valid representation of events in all patients. For instance, the scheme would not apply to patients who develop vasovagal syncope without the preceding tachycardia and hyperadrenergic state (although hypercontractility might occur as an isolated response to rises in catecholamines—especially in patients who suffer from so-called chronotropic insufficiency). Obviously, all these responses are heavily modulated by cerebrocortical as well as hypothalamic influences.

Therapeutic Considerations

Bearing in mind the above pathophysiological mechanisms and associated conditions, multiple therapeutic options can be considered. One can attempt to break the cycle of events at any step along the cascade leading to syncope. For instance, hydrofluorocortisone and supplemental salt can be administered in cases of essential hypovolemia; waist-high support hose with or without volume expansion can be prescribed for patients with venous pooling; beta blockers are very effective in the treatment of patients with the hyperbeta adrenergic syndrome; anticholinergic drugs can be administered in the hope of preventing the final efferent vagal stimulation; biofeedback inhibition may be useful in cases where the emotional or phobic overlay is considerable, etc.

Although most of these therapeutic manipulations can be quite successful, they are frequently cumbersome and sometimes accompanied by significant side effects that make them unacceptable. Therefore, the decision to treat vasovagal or vasodepressor syncope has to be made only after close consultation with the patient, keeping in mind that patient education and reassurance are probably one of the most important aspects of the overall management of vasovagal syncope.

Patients with Typical Common Faint (Benign Vasovagal/Vasodepressor Syncope). Generally, if the patient has infrequent symptoms and if loss of consciousness is always preceded by pathognomonic warning signs that last for at least 30 s, we will simply instruct the patient to abort the attacks by assuming the supine position and/or vigorous repetitive coughing. In addition, we will recommend biofeedback inhibition which teaches them how to respond to premonitory symptoms and modulate vasovagal attacks using breathing exercises and mental conditioning. We also recommend that they avoid phone booths and similar environments which prevent them from lying down or, if syncope occurs, falling to the floor. This educational process should be extended to the family.

Patients with Vasovagal/Vasodepressor Syncope and the Hyperbeta Adrenergic Syndrome. Although syncope is an unusual manifestation of the hyperbeta adrenergic state, presyncopal symptoms are relatively frequent. In this group of people who usually are young, healthy women with recurrent symptoms of palpitations from inappropriate sinus tachycardia occurring in response to the slightest physiological stress (i.e., standing, mild anxiety, etc.) and with apparent emotional lability, beta blockers are the mainstay of management and are generally well tolerated (Frohlich 1969). It is also of paramount importance to educate these patients as to the nature of the hyperbeta adrenergic syndrome and the availability of specific treatment. Such education will in most cases rebuild self-esteem as they are often accused of hypochondriasis or emotional instability.

Patients with Vasovagal/Vasodepressor Syncope and Hypovolemia. In our series, cases of hypovolemia (as diagnosed by blood volume measurement that is 2 SDs lower than the mean for the general population) have not generally been associated with hyponatremia or with a specific endocrinological defect such as hypoaldosteronism (aldosterone was routinely measured when hypovolemia was observed). In some cases, diuretic intake was the cause of the hypovolemia and in these instances the first step is to discontinue the drug. After an adequate waiting period, the tilt test is repeated and further management will depend on the results of the test. When no cause for hypovolemia can be uncovered, it is labeled "idiopathic" (Fouad 1985) and patients are treated with salt supplementation and mineralocorticoids. Serious side effects such as hypertension are not generally seen since these patients often have relatively low baseline blood pressures. Patients will generally add weight and often feel edematous. Occasionally, marked fluid retention can occur (as measured by an increase in body weight) without the expected significant increases in blood volume. Presumably, these patients are accumulating fluids in their extravascular extracellular space.

Patients with Vasovagal/Vasodepressor Syncope and Exaggerated Venous Pooling. The treatment of marked venous pooling includes the use of exercise to tone up leg and abdominal muscles. Although the effect of such conditioning has not been systematically studied, there are limited data to suggest that individuals with poor abdominal muscle tone are more prone to develop syncope during provocative tilt testing than well-conditioned, sex- and age-matched controls (Henry 1943; Lee 1966). These patients should be fitted with thick waist-high support hose (Jobsts). Although effective, support hose are often cosmetically unacceptable to young women and difficult to apply for the older patient. Volume expansion with salt supplementation and mineralocorticoid administration can be a useful adjunctive therapy for the nonhypervolemic pooler.

The Use of Scopolamine. For patients with vasovagal syncope without preceding sympathetic overstimulation or volume abnormalities, treatment with parasympatholytic agents appears to be the most attractive solution. Similarly, a parasympatholytic agent may be helpful as adjunctive treatment even for patients with vasovagal syncope and detectable volume abnormalities. It may even be used as a single treatment when volume expansion or support hose result in unacceptable side effects.

Clinically, we have used multiple anticholinergic agents including sublingual and oral atropine, Robinul, and Pamine. However, we have been most impressed by our experience with transcutaneous scopolamine (Abi-Samra 1986d).

We have studied ten patients with head up tilt before and during scopolamine treatment. There were four men and six women, ranging in age from 21 to 67 years. Their clinical presentation was variable with a duration of recurrent symptoms ranging from 2 weeks to 20 years. The estimated frequency of syncope over the past 6 months ranged from once a month to twice a day. Only three patients had typical warning signs that would theoretically allow them to abort the attacks. All patients were otherwise healthy.

Scopolamine was administered as a transcutaneous patch to be changed every other day. Follow-up included repeat tilt testing while on scopolamine. Scopolamine did not significantly affect baseline heart rate or the chronotropic response to head up tilt in these patients. On the other hand, tolerance to tilt was markedly improved by transderm scopolamine in all ten patients, including the two who fainted during their follow-up study. The head up tilt data correlate well with the clinical results as nine patients remained free of symptoms for as long as they were on scopolamine. One patient continued to have recurrent but less frequent symptoms. In addition, she began to have helpful preliminary warning signs. In all patients, the psychosocial impact of the symptoms appeared to be markedly dampened during the treatment.

Side effects from scopolamine included dry mouth, drowsiness, diplopia, photophobia, anisocoria, and localized eczematous reactions. These were transient in some and well tolerated by all except two patients who discontinued treatment. After stopping transderm scopolamine, both patients have had frequent severe recurrent symptoms.

The exact mechanism of action of scopolamine is unclear. Although its parasympatholytic effects may be important, administration of atropine failed to prevent induction of syncope by head up tilt. Moreover, at the doses administered, scopolamine did not induce a significant change in baseline heart rate. Contrary to atropine, scopolamine has a central depressant effect (Clissold 1985) and it is quite conceivable that its efficacy in vasovagal syncope may be related to modulation of cerebral autonomic outflow.

Use of Pacemakers in the Treatment of Vasovagal/Vasodepressor Syncope. No discussion of treatment of vasovagal syncope is complete without mentioning pacemakers. The efficacy of artificial pacing in the prevention of vasovagal syncopal attacks is a matter of controversy and published clinical results are quite variable (McLaran 1986; Sutton 1986).

Our observations suggest that bradycardia is rarely the precipitating factor in hypotension and syncope, although it certainly makes things worse when it occurs. The efficacy of pacemakers would thus be limited and contingent on the contribution of bradycardia to hypotension. At best, one would hope for prevention of actual loss of consciousness with the expectation that presyncopal symptoms will not be eliminated. We limit the use of pacemakers to patients who have failed other forms of therapy or as adjunctive therapy to patients who develop long periods of cardiac standstill during their vagal episodes. In this regard, there are several reasons for the preferential use of dual chamber demand pacers (DDD) rather than simple ventricular demand units (VVI). Firstly, in a state of such diminished cardiac output and poor venous return, restoration of AV synchrony may become of paramount importance as it allows for more consistent (timing) and better (atrial kick) ventricular filling. Second, a sequential AV contraction would obviate the possibility of activating vasodepressor atrial stretch receptors (due to atrial contraction against closed AV valves). Obviously, such vasodepression would compound the original problem. Third, in the presence of hypotension there are sympathetic discharges that attempt to cause vasoconstriction and an increase in sinus rate. Restoration of a heart rate by an artificial pacemaker can theoretically modulate and partially inhibit these corrective reflexes. It would therefore be logical to have a P-wave responsive pacer that tracks the natural compensatory changes (while still providing baseline low rate protection) rather than a fixed rate VVI unit. Last but not least, if symptoms are not well controlled with pacing, a ventricular single chamber unit will always leave room for the possibility of a pacemaker syndrome. This may lead to performance of difficult diagnostic studies as well as reoperation for system "upgrade" to a dual chamber unit.

References

Abboud FM, Eckberg DL, Johannsen UJ, Mark AL (1979) Carotid and cardiopulmonary baroreceptor control of splanchnic and forearm vascular resistance during venous pooling. J Physiol (London) 286: 173–184

Abi-Samra FM, Maloney JD, Fouad FM, Castle LW (1985) Vasovagal and vasodepressor syncope: abnormalities in blood-volume and its distribution. Circulation 72 (II): 251

Abi-Samra FM, Fouad FM, Maloney JD, Castle LW (1986a) Clinical characterization of pathogenetic mechanisms in vasovagal and vasodepressor syncope. Clin Prog Electrophysiol Pacing 4: 57

Abi-Samra FM, Fouad FM, Maloney JD, Castle LW (1986b) The role of hemodynamic testing in the investigation of syncope of unknown origin. Clin Progr Electrophysiol Pacing 4: 62

Abi-Samra FM, Fouad FM, Maloney JD, Bravo EL, Castle LW (1986c) Vasovagal syncope: vagal overtone or lack of stimulation sympathetic withdrawal? Circulation 14 [Suppl II]: 727

Abi-Samra F, Maloney J, Castle L (1986d) Usefulness of transderm scopolamine in the treatment of severe recurrent vasovagal syncope. PACE 9: 289

Abi-Samra FM, Simmon TW, Maloney JD, Sterba R, Castle LW, Morant VA (1986e) The role of electrophysiologic testing during Amiodarone therapy for sustained ventricular tachycardia. Clin Progr Electrophysiol Pacing 4: 62

Adams R (1827) Cases of diseases of the heart accompanied with pathological observations. Dublin Hosp Rep 4: 353–453

Akhtar M, Damato AN, Batsford WP, Ruskin JN, Ogunkelu JB (1975) A comparative analysis of antegrade and retrograde conduction patterns in man. Circulation 52: 766–778

Akhtar M, Shenasa M, Denker S, Gilbert CJ, Rizwi N (1983) Role of cardiac electrophysiologic studies in patients with unexplained recurrent syncope. PACE 6: 192–201

Alicandri C, Fouad FM, Tarazi RC, Castle L, Morant V (1978) Three cases of hypotension and syncope with ventricular pacing: possible role of atrial reflexes. Am J Cardiol 42: 137–142

Benditt DG, Strauss HC, Scheinman MM, Behar VS, Wallace AG (1976) Analysis of secondary pauses following termination of rapid atrial pacing in man. Circulation 54: 436–441

Bigger JT Jr, Strauss HC (1973) The evaluation of sinoatrial function in man. Med Coll Va Q 9: 77

Bousser MG, Dubois B, Castaigne P (1981) Transient loss of consciousness in ischaemic cerebral events. A study of 557 ischaemic strokes and transient ischaemic attacks. Ann Med Interne 132: 300–305
Bravo EL, Tarazi RC, Fouad FM, Vidt DG, Gifford RW Jr (1981) Clonidine suppression test: a useful aid in the diagnosis of pheochromocytoma. New Engl J Med 305: 623–626
Breithardt G, Seipel L (1978) Influence of drugs on the relationship between sinus node recovery time and calculated sinoatrial conduction time in man. Basic Res Cardiol 73: 68–76
Brodsky M, Wu D, Denes P, Kanakis C, Rosen KM (1977) Arrhythmias documented by 24 hour continuous electrocardiographic monitoring in 50 male medical students without apparent heart disease. Am J Cardiol 39: 390–395
Brown KA, Maloney JD, Smith CH, Haritzler GO, Ilstrup DM (1980) Carotid sinus reflex in patients undergoing coronary angiography: relationship of degree and location of coronary artery disease to response to carotid sinus massage. Circulation 62: 697–703
Brugada P, Green M, Abdollah H, Wellens HJ (1984a) Significance of ventricular arrhythmias initiated by programmed ventricular stimulation: the importance of the type of ventricular arrhythmia induced and the number of premature stimuli required. Circulation 69: 87–92
Brugada P, Wellens HJJ (1984b) Programmed electrical stimulation of the human heart. In: Josephson ME (ed) Tachycardias. Lea and Febiger, Philadelphia, p 61–89
Buxton AE, Waxman HL, Marchlinski FE, Untereker WJ, Waspe LE, Josephson ME (1984) Role of triple extrastimuli during electrophysiologic study of patients with documented sustained ventricular tachyarrhythmias. Circulation 69: 532–540
Camm AJ, Evans KE, Ward DE, Martin A (1980) The rhythm of the heart in active elderly subjects. Am Heart J 99: 598–603
Clark PI, Glasser SP, Spoto E (1980) Arrhythmias detected by ambulatory monitoring. Chest 77: 722–725
Clissold SP, Heel RC (1985) Transdermal hyoscine (scopolamine). A preliminary review of its pharmacodynamic properties and therapeutic efficacy. Drugs 29: 189–207
Corbett JJ, Butler AB, Kaufman B (1976) Sneeze syncope, basilar invagination and Arnold-Chiari type I malformation. J Neurol Neurosurg Psychiatr 39: 381–384
Council on Scientific Affairs (1981) Indications and contraindications for exercise testing. J Am Med Assoc 246: 1015–1018
Damato AN, Lau SH, Helfant R, Stein E, Patton RD, Scherlag BJ, Berkowitz WD (1969) A study of heart block in man using His bundle recordings. Circulation 39: 297–305
Damato AN, Lau SH, Patton RD, Steiner C, Berkowitz WD (1969) A study of atrioventricular conduction in man using premature atrial stimulation and His bundle recordings. Circulation 40: 61–69
Damato AN, Varghese PJ, Caracta AR, Akhtar M, Lau SH (1973) Functional 2:1 A–V block within the His-Purkinje system. Simulation of type II second-degree A–V block. Circulation 47: 534–542
Delius W, Witzfeld A (1976) Significance of sinus node recovery time in sick sinus syndrome. In Lųderitz B (ed) Cardiac pacing: diagnostic and therapeutic tools. Springer, Berlin New York, p 25
DiMarco JP, Garan H, Harthorne JW, Ruskin JN (1981) Intracardiac electrophysiologic techniques in recurrent syncope of unknown cause. Ann Intern Med 95: 542–548
Donker DNJ, Robles de Medina EO, Kieft J (1972) Micturition syncope. Electroenceph Clin Neurophysiol 33: 328–331
Dressler W (1952) Effort syncope as an early manifestation of primary pulmonary hypertension. Am J Med Sci 223: 131–143
Flamm MD, Braniff BA, Kimball R, Hancock EW (1967) Mechanism of effort syncope in aortic stenosis. Circulation 36 (suppl II): 109
Fleg JL, Kennedy HL (1982) Cardiac arrhythmias in a healthy elderly population: detection by 24-hour ambulatory electrocardiography. Chest 81: 302–307
Furman S (1973) Therapeutic uses of atrial pacing. Am Heart J 86: 835–840
Gang ES, Oseran DS, Mandel WJ, Peter T (1985) Sinus node electrogram in patients with the hypersensitive carotid sinus syndrome. J Am Coll Cardiol 5: 1484–1490
Gastaut H, Fischer-Williams M (1957) Electroencephalographic study of syncope: its differentiation from epilepsy. Lancet 2: 1018–1025
Gauer OH, Thron HL (1965) Postural changes in the circulation. In: Hamilton WF (ed) Handbook of physiology, Sect. 2: Circulation, vol. III Am Physiol Soc, Washington DC, p 2409–2439
Gillette PC, Garson A Jr (1977) Electrophysiologic and pharmacologic characteristics of automatic ectopic atrial tachycardia. Circulation 56: 571–575
Goldreyer BN, Gallagher JJ, Damato AN (1973) The electrophysiologic demonstration of atrial ectopic tachycardia in man. Am Heart J 85: 205–215

Haft JI, Lau SH, Stein E, Kosowsky BD, Damato AN (1968) Atrial fibrillation produced by atrial stimulation. Circulation 37: 70–74

Hammill SC, Holmes DR, Wood DL, Osborn MJ, McLaran C, Sugrue DD, Gersh BJ (1984) Electrophysiologic testing in the upright position: improved evaluation of patients with rhythm disturbances using a tilt table. J Am Coll Cardiol 4: 65–71

Hartzer GO, Maloney JD (1977) Programmed ventricular stimulation in management of recurrent ventricular tachycardia. Mayo Clin Proc 52: 731–741

Henry F (1943) Functional test IV: vasomotor weakness and postural fainting. Res Q 14: 144

Heron JR, Anderson EG, Noble IM (1965) Cardiac abnormalities associated with carotid sinus syndrome. Lancet ii: 214–216

Hess DS, Morady F, Scheinman MM (1982) Electrophysiologic testing in the evaluation of patients with syncope of undetermined origin. Am J Cardiol 50: 1309–1315

Hickler RB, Howe JP III (1979) Syncope: its etiology, pathophysiology, management. Primary Cardiol 5: 46–51

Hutchinson EC, Stock JPP (1960) Carotid sinus syndrome. Lancet ii: 445–449

Ibrahim MM (1975) Localization of lesion in patients with idiopathic orthostatic hypotension. Br Heart J 37: 868–872

Johnson AM (1971) Aortic stenosis, sudden death, and the left ventricular baroceptors: Br Heart J 33: 1–5

Jose AD, Collison D (1970) The normal range and determinants of the intrinsic heart rate in man. Cardiovasc Res 4: 160–167

Josephson ME, Horowitz LN, Farshidi A, Kastor JA (1978) Recurrent sustained ventricular tachycardia. 1. Mechanisms. Circulation 57: 431–440

Josephson ME, Horowitz LN (1979a) Electrophysiologic approach to therapy of recurrent sustained ventricular tachycardia. Am J Cardiol 43: 631–642

Josephson ME, Seides SF (1979b) Intraventricular conduction disturbances. In: Josephson ME, Seides SF (eds) Clinical cardiac electrophysiology: techniques and interpretations. Lea and Febiger, Philadelphia, pp 103–118

Josephson ME, Seides SF (1979c) Sinus node function. In: Josephson ME, Seides SF (eds) Clinical cardiac electrophysiology: techniques and interpretations. Lea and Febiger, Philadelphia, pp 61–78

Kala R, Viitasalo MT, Toivonen L, Eisalo A (1982) Ambulatory ECG recording in patients referred because of syncope or dizziness. Acta Med Scand [Suppl] 668: 13–19

Kapoor WN, Karpf M, Maher Y, Miller RA, Levey GS (1982) Syncope of unknown origin: the need for a more cost-effective approach to its diagnostic evaluation. J Am Med Assoc 247: 2687–2691

Kapoor WN, Karpf M, Wieand S, Peterson JR, Levey GS (1983) A prospective evaluation and follow-up of patients with syncope. N Engl J Med 309: 197–204

Kenny RA, Ingram A, Bayliss J, Sutton R (1986) Head up tilt—useful test in identification of vasovagal syndrome as cause of unexplained syncope. PACE 9: 288

Kerr CR, Strauss HC (1983) The measurement of sinus node refractoriness in man. Circulation 68: 1231–1237

Kulbertus HE, de Leval-Rutten F, Mary L, Casters P (1975) Sinus node recovery time in the elderly. Br Heart J 37: 420–425

Larson SJ, Sances A, Baker JB, Riegel DH (1974) Herniated cerebellar tonsils and cough syncope. J Neurosurg 40: 524–528

Lee TD Jr, Lindeman RD, Yiengst MJ, Shock NW (1966) Influence of age on the cardiovascular and renal responses to tilting. J Appl Physiol 21: 55–61

Levenson JA, Safar ME, London GM, Simon AC (1980) Haemodynamics in patients with phaeochromocytoma. Clin Sci 58: 349–356

Lin JT, Ziegler DK, Lai CW, Bayer W (1982) Convulsive syncope in blood donors. Ann Neurol 11: 525–528

Livelli FD, Bigger JT, Reiffel JA, Gang ES, Patton JN, Noethling PM, Rolnitzky LM, Gliklich JI (1982) Response to programmed ventricular stimulation: sensitivity, specificity, and relation to heart disease. Am J Cardiol 50: 452–458

Mandel W, Hayakawa H, Danzig R, Marcus HS (1971) Evaluation of sinoatrial node function in man by overdrive suppression. Circulation 44: 59–66

Mangiardi LM, Bonamini R, Conte M, Gaita F, Orzan F, Presbitero P, Brusca A (1982) Bedside evaluation of atrioventricular block with narrow QRS complexes: usefulness of carotid sinus massage and atropine administration. Am J Cardiol 49: 1136–1145

Mark AL (1983) The Bezold-Jarisch Reflex revisited: clinical implications of inhibitory reflexes originating in the heart. J Am Coll Cardiol 1: 90–102

McIntosh HD, Estes EH Jr, Warren JV (1956) The mechanism of cough syncope. Am Heart J 52: 70–82
McLaran CJ, Gersh BJ, Osborn MJ, Wood DL, Sugrue DD, Holmes DR Jr, Hammill SC (1986) Increased vagal tone as an isolated finding in patients undergoing electrophysiological testing for recurrent syncope: response to long-term anticholinergic agents. Br Heart J 55: 53–57.
Michaelsson M, Engle MA (1972) Congenital complete heart block: an international study of the natural history. Cardiovasc Clin 4: 85–101
Morady F, DiCarlo L, Winston S, Davis JC, Scheinman MM (1984) A prospective comparison of triple extrastimuli and left ventricular stimulation in studies of ventricular tachycardia induction. Circulation 70: 52–57
Morady F, Higgins J, Peters RW, Schwartz AB, Shen EN, Bhandari A, Scheinman MM, Sauve MJ (1984) Electrophysiologic testing in bundle branch block and unexplained syncope. Am J Cardiol 54: 587–591
Morgagni JB (1761) The seats and causes of disease. In: Major HH (ed) Classic descriptions of disease (1948) p 346
Narula OS, Samet P (1970a) Wenckebach and Mobitz type II AV block due to block within the His bundle and bundle branches. Circulation 41: 947–965
Narula OS, Cohen LS, Samet P, Lister JW, Scherlag B, Hildner FJ (1970b) Localization of A–V conduction defects in man by recording of the His bundle electrogram. Am J Cardiol 25: 228–237
Narula OS, Samet P, Javier RP (1972) Significance of the sinus-node recovery time. Circulation 45: 140–158
Narula OS, Gann D, Samet P (1975) Prognostic value of H–V intervals. In: Narula OS (ed) His bundle electrocardiography and clinical electrophysiology. Davis, Philadelphia, pp 437–449
Narula OS, Shantha N, Vasquez M, Towne WD, Linhart JW (1978) A new method for measurement of sinoatrial conduction time. Circulation 58: 706–714
Noble RJ (1977) The patient with syncope. J Am Med Assoc 237: 1372–1376
North American Society of Pacing and Electrophysiology (1984) Policy conference on ventricular tachycardia.
Ogawa S, Dreifus LS, Shenoy PN, Brockman SK, Berkovits BV (1978) Hemodynamic consequences of atrioventricular and ventriculoatrial pacing. PACE 1: 8–15
Olshansky B, Mazuz M, Martins JB (1985) Significance of inducible tachycardia in patients with syncope of unknown origin: a long-term follow-up. J Am Coll Cardiol 5: 216–223
Peuch P, Grolleau-Raoux R (1971) Les blocs auriculo-ventriculaires. Classification basee sur l'enregistrement de l'activite du tissu de conduction. Coeur Med Interne 10: 615–638
Price TR, Gotshall RA, Poskanzer DC, Haerer AF, Swanson PD, Calanchini PR, Conneally PM, Dyken ML, Futty DE (1977) Cooperative study of hospital frequency and character of transient ischemic attacks. VI. Patients examined during an attack. J Am Med Assoc 238: 2512–2515
Proudfit WL, Forteza ME (1959) Micturition syncope. New Engl J Med 260: 328–331
Reed RL, Siekert RG, Merideth J (1973) Rarity of transient focal cerebral ischemia in cardiac dysrhythmia. J Am Med Assoc 223: 893–895
Reiffel JA, Bigger JT, Giardina EG (1975) "Paradoxical" prolongation of sinus node recovery time after atropine in the sick sinus syndrome. Am J Cardiol 36: 98–104
Reiffel JA, Gang E, Livelli F Jr, Gliklich J, Bigger JT Jr (1981) Clinical and electrophysiologic characteristics of sinoatrial entrance block evaluated by direct sinus node electrography: prevalence, relation to antegrade sinoatrial conduction time, and relevance to sinus node disease. Am Heart J 102: 1011–1014
Rosenqvist M, Brandt J, Schuller H (1986) Atrial versus ventricular pacing in sinus node disease: a treatment comparison study. Am Heart J 111: 292–297
Ruff RL, Talman WT, Petito F (1981) Transient ischemic attacks associated with hypotension in hypertensive patients with carotid artery stenosis. Stroke 12: 353–355
Ruskin JN, DiMarco JP, Garan H (1980) Out-of-hospital cardiac arrest: electrophysiologic observations and selection of long-term antiarrhythmic therapy. New Engl J Med 303: 607–613
Samet P, Castillo C, Bernstein WH (1966) Hemodynamic sequelae of atrial, ventricular, and sequential atrioventricular pacing in cardiac patients. Am Heart J 72: 725–729
Scheinman MM, Weiss AN, Shafton E, Benowitz N, Rowland M (1974a) Electrophysiologic effects of procaine amide in patients with intraventricular conduction delay. Circulation 49: 522–529
Scheinman MM, Basu D, Hollenberg M (1974b) Electrophysiologic studies in patients with persistent atrial tachycardia. Circulation 50: 266–273
Scheinman MM, Peters RW, Modin G, Brennan M, Mies C, O'Young J (1977) Prognostic value of infranodal conduction time in patients with chronic bundle branch block. Circulation 56: 240–244

Schuilenburg RM, Durrer D (1972) Conduction disturbances located within the His bundle. Circulation 45: 612–628

Schwartz LS, Goldfischer J, Sprague GJ, Schwartz SP (1969) Syncope and sudden death in aortic stenosis. Am J Cardiol 23: 647–658

Scott O, Macartney FJ, Deverall PB (1976) Sick sinus syndrome in children. Arch Dis Child 51: 100–105

Shaw DB, Kekwick CA, Veale D, Gowers, J, Whistance T (1985) Survival in second degree atrioventricular block. Br Heart J 53: 587–593

Shaw DB, Kekwick CA (1978) Potential candidates for pacemakers. Survey of heart block and sinoatrial disorder (sick sinus syndrome). Br Heart J 40: 99–105

Sigler LH (1933) Clinical observations on the carotid sinus reflex. II. The response to carotid sinus pressure at various ages and heart rates and rhythms. Am J Med Sci 186: 118–124

Sigler LH (1963) The cardioinhibitory carotid sinus reflex: its importance as a vagocardio-sensitivity test. Am J Cardiol 12: 175–183

Stevenson WG, Brugada P, Waldecker B, Zehender M, Wellens HJ (1986) Can potentially significant polymorphic ventricular arrhythmias initiated by programmed stimulation be distinguished from those that are specific? Am Heart J III: 1073–1080

Stokes W (1846) Observations on some cases of permanently slow pulse. Dublin Quarterly J Med Sci 2: 73–85

Strauss HC, Saroff AL, Bigger JT Jr, Giardina EG (1973) Premature atrial stimulation as a key to the understanding of sinoatrial conduction in man. Presentation of data and critical review of the literature. Circulation 47: 86–93

Stryjer D, Freidensohn A, Schlesinger Z (1982) Carotid sinus hypersensitivity: diagnosis of vasodepressor type in the presence of cardioinhibitory type. PACE 5: 793–800

Stults BM, Gandolfi RJ (1986) Diagnostic evaluation of syncope. West J Med 144: 234–238

Swerdlow CD, Winkle RA, Mason JW (1983) Prognostic significance of the number of induced ventricular complexes during assessment of therapy for ventricular tachyarrhythmias. Circulation 68: 400–405

Talan DA, Bauernfeind RA, Ashley WW, Kanakis C Jr, Rosen KM (1982) Twenty-four hour continuous ECG recordings in long-distance runners. Chest 82: 19–24

Tarazi RC (1985a) Blood volume. Europ Heart J 6 (suppl C): 41–42

Tarazi RC (1985b) Pulmonary blood volume. Europ Heart J 6 (suppl C): 43

Teichman SL, Felder SD, Matos JA, Kim SG, Waspe LE, Fisher JD (1985) The value of electrophysiologic studies in syncope of undetermined origin: report of 150 cases. Am Heart J 110: 469–479

Thilenius OG, Chiemmongkoltip P, Cassels DE, Arcilla RA (1972) Hemodynamics studies in children with congenital atrioventricular block. Am J Cardiol 30: 13–18

Thomas JE (1969) Hyperactive carotid sinus reflex and carotid sinus syncope. Mayo Clin Proc 44: 127–139

Tonkin AM, Heddle WF, Tornos P (1978) Intermittent atrioventricular block: procainamide administration as a provocative test. Aust NZ J Med 8: 594–602

Torvik A (1984) The pathogenesis of watershed infarcts in the brain. Stroke 15: 221–223

Untereker WJ, Waxman HL, Waspe LE, Marchlinski FE, Buxton AE, Groh WC, Martin JL, Josephson ME (1982) Programmed electrical stimulation in patients without clinical ventricular tachycardia. Circulation 66 (suppl II): 147

Vandepol CJ, Farshidi A, Spielman SR, Greenspan AM, Horowitz LN, Josephson ME (1980) Incidence and clinical significance of induced ventricular tachycardia. Am J Cardiol 45: 725–731

Viitasalo MT, Kala R, Eisalo A (1982) Ambulatory electrocardiographic recording in endurance athletes. Br Heart J 47: 213–220

Wayne HH (1961) Syncope, physiological considerations and an analysis of the clinical characteristics in 50 patients. Am J Med 30: 418–438

Wellens HJJ (1971) Electrical stimulation of the heart in the study and treatment of tachycardias. University Park Press, Baltimore

Wellens HJ, Brugada P, Stevenson WG (1985) Programmed electrical stimulation of the heart in patients with life-threatening ventricular arrhythmias: what is the significance of induced arrhythmias and what is the correct stimulation protocol? Circulation 72: 1–7

Williams B (1976) Cerebrospinal fluid pressure changes in response to coughing. Brain 99: 331–346

Wit AL, Weiss MB, Berkowitz WD, Rosen KM, Steiner C, Damato AN (1970) Patterns of atrioventricular conduction in the human heart. Circ Res 27: 345–359

Zeldis SM, Levine BJ, Michelson EL, Morganroth J (1980) Cardiovascular complaints. Correlation with cardiac arrhythmias on 24-hour electrocardiographic monitoring. Chest 78: 456–461

Section D

STROKE AND OPEN HEART SURGERY

Chapter 15

Central Nervous System Complications Related to Open Heart Surgery

A. J. Furlan and S. C. Jones

Introduction

Brain dysfunction is a major cause of morbidity and occasional mortality complicating many forms of heart surgery requiring cardiopulmonary bypass (CPB), including pediatric cardiovascular surgery (Becker 1982), cardiac transplantation (Hotson and Pedley 1976), and artificial heart implantation. This chapter focuses on the CNS complications associated with coronary artery bypass graft (CABG) surgery since it is the most common procedure utilizing CPB. In the United States over 150000 patients undergo CABG surgery annually and of these at least 5000 patients will suffer a stroke and perhaps 30000 more will experience a diffuse encephalopathy. Although CABG surgery and CPB pose many potential embolic, hemodynamic, and metabolic threats to the brain, the cause of neurologic dysfunction often remains obscure in the individual patient.

Cardiac Catheterization

Central nervous system complications are rare during heart catheterization (Dawson and Fischer 1977). In the course of over 30000 catheterizations done at the Cleveland Clinic during a 5-year period, we are aware of 35 patients who sustained a focal deficit (carotid 15, vertebral-basilar 20) (Lockwood et al. 1983). Diffuse encephalopathy occurs somewhat more frequently, especially in elderly dehydrated patients who receive large volumes of contrast material. Among our patients with a focal neurologic complication, the deficit resolved within 48 h in 19 patients. In 16 patients the deficit persisted, and 2 patients died as a result of stroke sustained during catheterization. The etiology of the focal cerebral event was embolism or systemic hypotension in six patients; in two patients a vertebral artery was inadvertently injected with contrast. No clear etiology was identified in the remaining patients, although many had a past history of stroke, documented cerebrovascular disease, or potential cardiac embolic risk factors such as ventricular hypokinesia, mural thrombus, or valvular disease.

Percutaneous Transluminal Coronary Angioplasty

Widespread clinical application of percutaneous transluminal coronary angioplasty (PTCA) followed innovations in catheter design (Gruntzig and Hopff 1974). The National Heart, Lung, and Blood Institute (Dorros et al. 1983) reported the complications seen among 1500 patients undergoing PTCA. Five patients suffered a CNS complication including one cerebrovascular accident, three transient neurologic deficits, and one anoxic encephalopathy. Among 1829 patients undergoing PTCA at the Cleveland Clinic, 4 suffered a central nervous system complication (Galbreath et al. 1985). Two patients experienced a left cerebral hemisphere infarct, one patient suffered a right hemisphere transient ischemic attack, and one patient experienced a rostral brainstem infarct. In two cases the symptoms appeared while the ascending aorta was being "scraped" with the stiff guiding catheter in search of a saphenous bypass graft ostium. In one case a small quantity of air was injected through the guiding catheter, and the last complication was related to hypotension after a successful PTCA.

Complications of CABG/CPB Surgery

Brain Infarction

In the setting of open heart surgery, "stroke" generally refers to focal brain infarction in a specific vascular territory. This risk has decreased since the 1960s partly as a result of improved monitoring and surgical techniques, along with the introduction of membrane oxygenators and in-line filtration which decrease the release of microaggregates into the circulation. Since the 1970s there has been little change in the stroke rate, which ranges between 2% and 5% in various studies (Table 15.1).

In a prospective study (Breuer et al. 1983), we found a 5% rate of focal brain or ocular infarction among 421 patients undergoing CABG surgery. Only 2% suffered major neurologic disability. In our institution the risk of stroke and encephalopathy during bypass surgery did not differ significantly from other forms of cardiac surgery (Table 15.2).

Etiology of Brain Infarction

We were unable to correlate a large number of preoperative, intraoperative, and postoperative variables with the risk of stroke during CABG surgery. A prior history of stroke was the only preoperative variable which approached a statistically significant correlation. Such factors as age, duration of pump time, fluctuations in blood pressure, type of oxygenator, and carotid bruits could not be correlated with the risk of focal brain infarction. However, probable causes for stroke could be identified in individual patients (Table 15.3). Subsequently, left ventricular mural thrombus was found to be associated with a twofold increase in risk of stroke during open heart surgery, presumably because of an increased risk of embolization (Breuer et al. 1981). Small left ventricular thrombi are frequently not removed at the time of surgery. Although transient postoperative atrial fibrillation occurs in up to 30% of patients undergoing open heart surgery, we found that this dysrhythmia does not significantly increase the risk of stroke (O'Neill et al. 1983).

Since major stroke occurs in less than 2% of all patients undergoing open heart surgery, from a statistical standpoint it would be extremely difficult to demonstrate that one variable significantly alters that risk. Nonetheless, extracranial carotid artery disease is often suggested as an important cause of stroke during open heart surgery. This theory proposes that infarction may occur ipsilateral to a severely stenosed internal carotid artery (ICA) if there is a drop in blood pressure during surgery. The logic is deceptively persuasive, but the evidence suggests that extracranial ICA stenosis is a relatively insignificant factor in causing stroke during heart surgery (Hart and Easton 1983; Furlan et al. 1985).

Despite the lack of convincing data, it is common practice in some hospitals to perform a "prophylactic" carotid endarterectomy in asymptomatic patients discovered to have a hemodynamically significant ICA stenosis prior to open heart surgery. Whether there is a group of patients who might benefit from such surgery requires further study. Presently there is no evidence that staged or combined endarterectomy improves stroke risk during open heart surgery (see Chaps. 16, 17).

Atheromatous embolization from the aorta is a potential risk during CABG surgery. During CABG surgery atherosclerotic plaques are frequently seen in the aorta, although the aorta is considered "unclampable" in only one patient/1000 (L. R. Golding, personal communication). Our surgeons avoid cannulating or clamping obviously diseased segments of aorta; yet an audible crunch is sometimes heard as the aortic cross-clamp is applied.

Thurlbeck and Castleman (1957) speculated that turbulence proximal to an aortic cross-clamp would tend to "churn up" atheromatous material and predispose to embolism. How often this occurs during CABG surgery and whether such factors as anticoagulation modify this risk is unknown. Multiple atheromatous brain emboli are rarely found in large series of open heart surgery cases coming to autopsy (Hill et al. 1969; Aguilar et al. 1971). Subtle neuropsychiatric disturbances after open heart surgery have been ascribed to microembolism (i.e., <20 μm) of air, fat, particulate matter, and platelet/fibrin clumps generated during cardiopulmonary bypass, but have not been linked with atheromatous emboli. Atheromatous emboli tend to be larger (i.e., >50 μm) and produce multiple cerebral infarcts, often in a watershed distribution. We, and others (McKibbin et al. 1976; Price and Harris 1970), have documented multiple atheromatous emboli ("embolic shower") from the aorta as one cause of coma complicating open heart surgery (see next section). It is much more difficult to demonstrate the source of a single atheromatous embolus since these patients often have widespread atherosclerotic disease.

Table 15.1. Summary of recent data on CNS complications of open heart surgery. (Modified from Breuer et al. 1983)

	Authors	Year[a]	Study design	Type of OHS	No. of patients	% with CNS deficit		Method of ascertainment
1.	Hill et al.	1968	Pathologic analysis autopsy cases	Mixture	133	[b] (fat emboli in 62% brains non-fat emboli in 31% brains)	[b]	Pathologic analysis of brains
2.	Heller et al.	1969	Prospective	Mixture	100	[b] 24% had postoperative delirium)	9%	Psychiatric interview, psychologic testing
3.	Javid et al.	1969	Prospective	Mixture	100	13+%	35%	Clinical exam, psychologic testing
4.	Tufo et al.	1969	Prospective	Mixture	100	13+%	43%	Clinical exam, psychologic testing
5.	Branthwaite	1970	Retrospective % prospective	Mixture	417	9.4%	10.1%	Chart review, clinical exam
6.	Hansotia et al.	1972	Prospective	Mixture	177	[b] (51% with persistently abnormal EEG at discharge. Includes 11 patients who died)	[b]	Serial EEG
7.	Cannon et al.	1972	Retrospective	Mixture	400	1%[c]	[b]	Chart review
8.	Hutchinson et al.	1972	Retrospective	CABG alone	376	0.3%[c]	[b]	Chart review
9.	Branthwaite	1973	Prospective	Mixture	140	[b] (7.1% had clinical neurologic damage)	[b]	Intraoperative use of cerebral function monitor
10.	Branthwaite	1973	Retrospective	Mixture	538	3%	4.8%	Chart review
11.	Hodgman et al.	1974	Retrospective	Mixture	100	[b] (20% had minor psychiatric problems)[c]	[b]	Chart review
12.	Kolkka et al.	1977	Prospective	Mixture	204	2.9%	17.2%	Clinical exam
13.	Lee et al.	1978	Retrospective	Mixture	943	0.7%	[b]	Chart review
14.	Gonzalez-Sacrano et al.	1978	Retrospective case control	CABG alone	1427	1%	0.4%	Chart review
15.	Loop et al.	1978	Retrospective	CABG alone	8741	[c] 1.3%–2%	[b]	Chart review, computerized cardiovascular information registry

Table 15.1. *(continued)*

16.	Muraoka et al.	1979	Prospective	Congenital heart disease	57	0% (10.5% had persistent CT scan changes)	0%	Chart review
17.	Turnipseed et al.	1979	Prospective	CABG alone	170	4.7%	[b]	Clinical exam
18.	Breuer et al.	1980	Prospective	CABG alone	421	5.2% (total) 2% (severe)	11.6%	Clinical exam
19.	Coffey et al.	1981	Retrospective	CABG alone	1669	0.8%	3.4%	Chart review

[a] Latest year patients in study underwent surgery reflecting technology of that time (i.e., not year study published)
[b] No clinical examination data available
[c] These retrospective studies are largely devoted to analyses of nonneurologic issues and complications and mention CNS dysfunction

Table 15.2. Central nervous system complications in patients undergoing various types of open heart surgery. (Furlan and Breuer 1984)

% with	CABG (*n* =421)	Left heart valves (*n*=80)	Ventricular aneurysm (*n*=19)	Valves + aneurysms (*n*=99)
Stroke	5	8	0	6
Encephalopathy	12	10	5	9
Death	2	9	0	7

Table 15.3. Myocardial revascularization: possible etiology of focal CNS deficits[a] (Furlan and Breuer 1984)

Cause	No. of patients
Cardiac arrhythmia intra/perioperatively	6
Internal carotid artery atherosclerosis	5
Air embolism from left ventricle	2
Carotid artery trauma during internal jugular vein cannulation	1
Aortic atherosclerosis at site of clamping	1
Prolonged intraoperative blood pressure decrease	1

[a] Cause identified in 16 of 22 patients (73%)

Other causes of brain dysfunction after open heart surgery must be considered. Both Halothane and Ethrane may produce alterations in neuronal microtubules and thereby alter axonal transport (Hinkley 1976). Ethrane may produce occult seizures unwitnessed during general anesthesia, resulting in a prolonged postical encephalopathy in some patients (Fariello 1980). Complement activation during bypass (Chendweth et al. 1981), complement-induced granulocyte aggregation (Jacobs et al. 1980), or altered thromboxane synthesis with effects on platelet function during extracorporeal circulation (Addonizio et al. 1980) may also play a role in producing some central nervous system dysfunction. However, since all patients undergo anesthesia and all have their blood exposed to the surfaces of the disposable plastic extracorporeal tubing, yet only a few develop CNS dysfunction, other factors must be involved.

Failure to Awaken After CABG Surgery

Nonmetabolic coma is a rare complication of open heart surgery, occurring in less than 1% of patients. Over a 4-year period, during which more than 12 000 procedures were performed at the Cleveland Clinic, our Stroke Service was asked to see 34 patients who failed to awaken after open heart surgery. The causes of coma in this group are given in Table 15.4. These cases illustrate that failure to awaken after open heart surgery is not synonymous with intraoperative hypotension and global brain ischemia/hypoxia. Two of the patients with massive hemispheric infarction and herniation had severe ipsilateral internal carotid artery disease documented postmortem. One of these cases had an internal carotid occlusion with fresh thrombus and distal embolization to the middle cerebral artery (Fig. 15.1). One of the patients with multiple embolic infarcts underwent cross-clamping of an extremely brittle aorta and had multiple arteriolar emboli in the brain and other organs at postmortem (Fig. 15.2). All of the patients with diffuse neuronal damage at postmortem sustained significant intraoperative hypotension. Three of these patients demonstrated watershed infarctions on CT (Fig. 15.3). No definite etiology for coma could be documented in 16 patients, and despite coma the CT scan was normal in 5 cases. It is possible that some of the patients with normal CT had cortical laminar necrosis as the cause of coma. The prognosis in this group of patients is very poor; 85% of our patients died. Four evolved into a persistent vegetative state or had serious neurologic residua, and only one patient had a useful neurologic recovery.

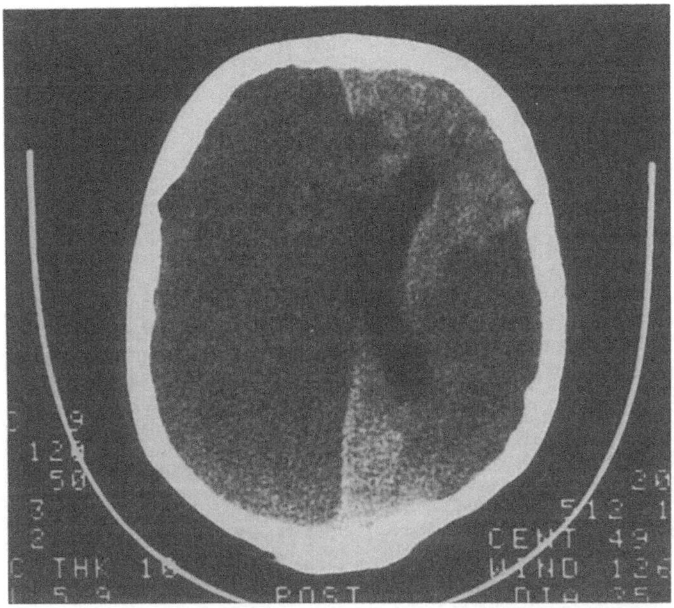

Fig. 15.1. Coma after OHS. CT shows massive left hemisphere and smaller right hemisphere infarcts with herniation. At postmortem the left internal carotid artery was occluded by fresh thrombus and there was distal embolization to the left middle cerebral artery.

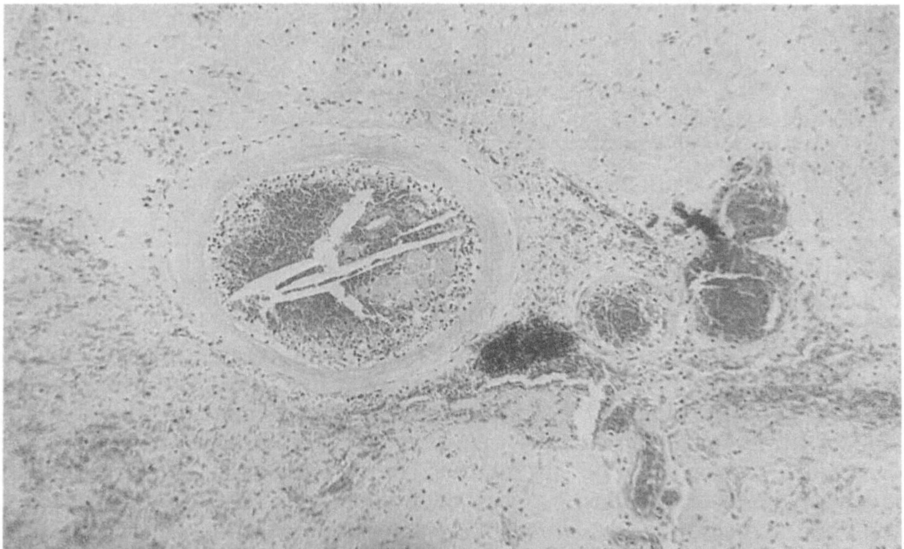

Fig. 15.2. Coma after OHS. Cholesterol embolus in a brain arteriole. Patient underwent cross-clamping of a very brittle aorta. There were numerous cholesterol emboli in the brain and other organs at postmortem.

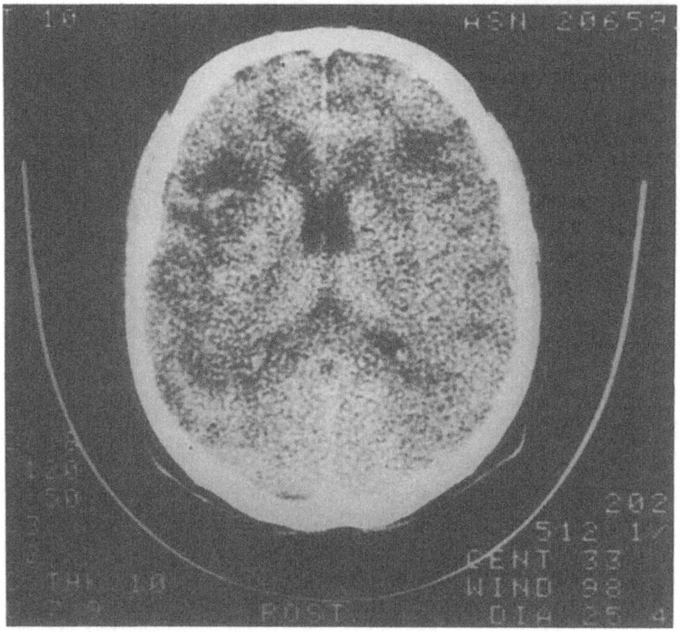

Fig. 15.3. Coma after OHS. CT shows patchy watershed infarcts in a patient who sustained intraoperative hypotension.

Table 15.4. Causes of prolonged coma after open heart surgery. (Furlan and Breuer 1984)

Cause	No. of patients
Uncertain	19
Global ischemia/hypoxia	7
Hemisphere infarct with herniation	5
Multifocal infarcts	3
Total	34

Intracranial Hemorrhage

Epidural and subdural hematoma, intracerebral hemorrhage, and subarachnoid hemorrhage have been reported following open heart surgery (Hungxi et al. 1982; Humphreys et al. 1975). Subdural and epidural hematoma, although rare, appear to occur more frequently than other types of intracranial hemorrhage. Lateralizing signs may be absent, and the predominant clinical picture is decrease in level of consciousness or frank coma. The preponderance of subdural and epidural hematomas has led to speculation that shrinkage of the brain substance and reduction of brain volume as a result of hypertonic perfusion may result in tearing of dural bridging veins. The bleeding tendency may then be augmented by the state of anticoagulation associated with open heart surgery.

We have seen two cases of intracerebral hemorrhage following heart transplantation which were probably related to a sudden increase in cerebral perfusion pressure induced by a relatively high cardiac output (Fig. 15.4). Postmortem studies also indicate a high rate of brain hemorrhage complicating cardiac transplantation (Montero and Martìnez 1986).

Pituitary Apoplexy

Hemorrhage into or ischemic necrosis of a previously silent pituitary tumor can occur during CPB. The initial sign in such cases may be a dilated and fixed pupil which can lead to a misdiagnosis of brain herniation if the patient is not yet fully awakened from anesthesia. Precipitating factors include tissue edema, hypotension, and anticoagulation during CPB (Cooper et al. 1986).

Neuropsychiatric Disturbances and Global Encephalopathy

Clinically detectable diffuse encephalopathy occurs in at least 12% of patients undergoing CABG/CPB surgery (Breuer et al. 1983). Postsurgical encephalopathy is often multifactorial and can be related to postanesthetic effect, drugs, intensive care psychosis, metabolic derangements, hemodynamic instability, and a host of other factors acting alone or in combination. In our prospective study, a

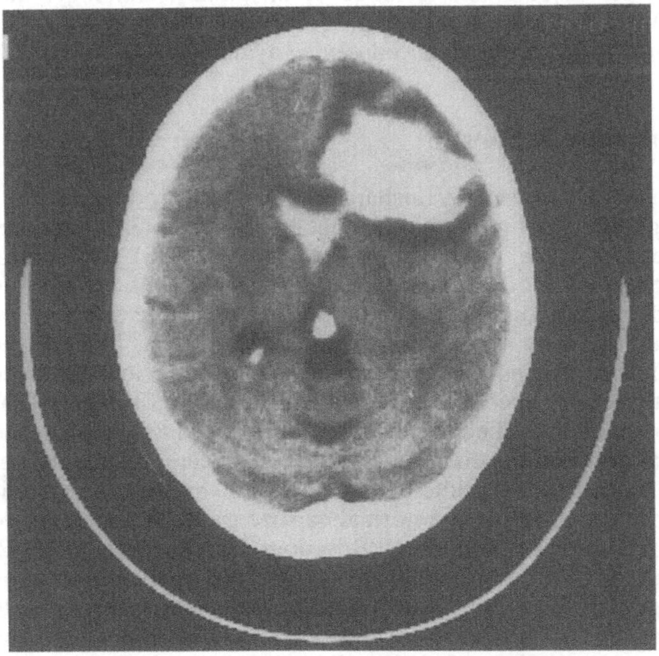

Fig. 15.4. Intracerebral hemorrhage complicating cardiac transplantation. The patient is a 24-year-old woman with cardiomyopathy. The posttransplant cardiac index increased fivefold.

decrease in blood pressure was the only factor we could statistically correlate with the risk of developing encephalopathy. This suggests that a decrease in cerebral blood flow above the frank infarction threshold can result in altered mentation in some patients (see below).

More subtle changes in mental functioning detectable by psychometric testing may occur in up to 30% of patients undergoing CABG/CPB surgery (Sotaniemi et al. 1986). The etiology of long-term changes in mental status and memory function following such surgery is unknown. Lowering mean blood pressure to accepted levels for routine CPB may be a neglected cause of diffuse brain ischemia in patients with arteriolar cerebrovascular disease and defective autoregulation of cerebral blood flow (Stockard et al. 1973; Furlan and Breuer 1984; Henriksen 1984). Alternatively, multiple microemboli have been proposed as a mechanism for diffuse encephalopathy (Henriksen et al. 1983; Brennan et al. 1971).

Effect of Cardiopulmonary Bypass Technology Development on Neurologic Complications

Since the introduction of CPB procedures in 1953 (Given 1954), the frequency of stroke during the procedure has decreased. This is partly due to the development and refinement of the techniques used for CPB. These developments include improved oxygenation techniques, filtration technology, and continuous display hemodynamic monitoring. Presently, the polypropylene hollow fiber oxygenator is the most advanced device available.

Pulsatile Versus Nonpulsatile Flow

Bypass pumps have remained essentially unchanged since the introduction of the roller pump. Although the roller pump has not been replaced, pulsatile pumps have been advocated by some investigators (Marvoudis 1978) for several reasons. The advantages of a roller pump include simplicity of set up and operation, and blood compatibility. Pulsatile pumps are available but have no clear advantages over the most recent nonpulsatile technology. Indeed, the interpretation of different studies that compare pulsatile perfusion has been complicated by exactly how to specify the amount of pulsatility (Taylor 1982).

Pulseless perfusion has been evoked to explain cerebral dysfunction as a result of CPB surgery. Areas between the distribution of the main cerebral arteries, or "watershed zones," might be susceptible to low perfusion without the systolic pressure pulse that is present during the normal cardiac cycle. A series of two studies compared nonpulsatile to pulsatile CPB in dogs (Sanderson et al. 1972; Wright and Sanderson 1972). Cerebral damage was assessed by the observation of ischemic cell change. In the first study, diffuse cell changes were attributed to nonpulsatile flow and other complicating factors. Focal lesions were found and were thought to be due to embolism of blood cell aggregates and/or air emboli. In the second study, diffuse nerve cell changes were not present in the pulsatile group, but were present in the nonpulsatile roller pump group. However, focal damage was present in both studies. These early studies are difficult to interpret because current CPB techniques have resulted in improved survival; in the second study only 5 of our 20 dogs survived for over 1 week.

A greater increase in brain-specific creatine kinase isoenzymes in the cerebrospinal fluid of dogs during pulseless perfusion compared with pulsatile perfusion has been reported (Taylor et al. 1980). However, for a CPB procedure of typical duration there does not seem to be an advantage to pulsatile perfusion. Indeed, long-term nonpulsatile perfusion has been shown to be well tolerated (Golding et al. 1980). The controversy regarding pulsatile versus nonpulsatile flow may be summarized by stating that currently there is no evidence that nonpulsatile bypass is detrimental (Edmunds 1982).

Filtration and Microemboli

Blood filtration technology has improved CPB procedures. Microemboli (Taylor 1982) could consist of air, silicone from antifoaming agents (Orenstein et al. 1982), fat, platelet aggregates, and fibrin. Blood filtration can be used to remove particles in excess of 25 μm. This can still allow particles into the systemic circulation that can obstruct the brain microcirculation. Filtration of blood down to 10 μm or less would be necessary to prevent capillary obstruction, but this is not technically feasible because of the pressure drop across such a fine filter. Also, emboli from the left ventricle or aorta could be introduced into the circulation during reperfusion for which a filter in the perfusion circuit would not be effective (Buris 1979).

Attempts have been made to reduce microemboli production as well as to eliminate them by filtration. The membrane oxygenator was proposed as a way of reducing microemboli production. The use of platelet activation inhibitor substances such as prostacyclin have been advocated to prevent microemboli (Pokar et al. 1982).

Continuous monitoring of intraoperative hemodynamic parameters has also improved the procedure because it allows operating room personnel to respond to a hypotensive episode immediately and in unison.

Cerebral Blood Flow During Cardiopulmonary Bypass

Two concepts regarding the control of the cerebral circulation are important for assessing the maintenance of the cerebral circulation during cardiopulmonary bypass.

1. *Autoregulation* is defined as the capacity of the normal cerebral circulation to maintain a constant level of CBF over the blood pressure range of 50–160 mmHg. Thus if the cerebral perfusion pressure is between these limits, CBF remains constant and is independent of cerebral perfusion pressure. Cerebral perfusion pressure (CPP) is controlled by three components: central venous pressure (VP), intracranial pressure (ICP), and arterial blood pressure (BP): CPP=BP–VP–ICP. If arterial blood pressure falls or intracranial pressure rises, cerebral perfusion pressure falls. The venous pressure is negligible in almost all cases.

2. The sensitivity of CBF to *arterial carbon dioxide tension* (PCO_2) is a well-documented phenomenon. There is a roughly linear response of CBF with a slope of 3%/mmHg within the PCO_2 range of 25–60 mmHg.

These two factors are important during CPB because typical perfusion pressures are near the normal lower autoregulatory limit of 50 mmHg. Below this level of arterial blood pressure, any drop in BP produces a drop in CBF. A rise in ICP can also cause a drop in CPP and a subsequent fall in CBF. The maintenance of PCO_2 above 25 mmHg is important to minimize any further drop in CBF. Both of these factors could be influenced by anesthesia and hypothermia. Also, there is an interaction between the two; for instance, hypotension to 50 mmHg can abolish CO_2 sensitivity. The effect of hypothermia on CO_2 sensitivity and autoregulation has not been fully elucidated.

Animal Models

Using a magnetic flowmeter technique, Halley et al. (1958) made early attempts to measure cerebral blood flow in a dog model of extracorporeal circulation. These investigators did not recognize the phenomenon of cerebral blood flow autoregulation, and this study is mainly of historical interest. Brennan et al. (1971) measured cortical cerebral blood flow in a dog model of CPB using the Kety-Schmidt method modified for the use of ^{85}Kr. Using a bubble oxygenator, they found that cortical CBF fell by an average of 25% in animals perfused with unfiltered blood. The cerebral metabolic rate for O_2 ($CMRO_2$) fell 45% and CMRgl fell 60% in animals subjected to unfiltered bubble oxygenator bypass. Measurements were repeated in dogs after interposing a 25-μm wire mesh filter in the arterial bypass line. There was no decrease in cerebral blood flow in animals undergoing filtered bypass, and in this group $CMRO_2$ and CMRgl transiently fell by only 4% and 16% respectively. Brennan et al. (1971) speculated that microembolism was the cause of depressed global cerebral blood flow, and oxygen and glucose metabolism in patients undergoing unfiltered bypass.

A study by Fox et al. (1984) of extreme hypothermic CPB in monkeys demonstrated that CBF decreased during hypothermia to 20°C as a function of perfusion flow rate. Regional CBF was determined with labeled microspheres at four different perfusion flow rates. Although CBF was low because of the profound hypothermia, adequate cerebral perfusion was demonstrated because brain oxygen consumption was maintained even at the lowest perfusion rate of 0.5 liters/m^2 per minute.

Human Studies

There have been very few studies which examine the effects of CPB on CBF in man. Early measurements of global CBF during CPB in man using the Kety-Schmidt method were made by Wollam et al. (1966) and Branthwaite (1974). More recent studies have measured regional CBF during CPB using modern isotope clearance techniques.

Henriksen et al. (1981) and Henriksen et al. (1983) measured regional CBF during CPB using the intraarterial xenon-133 injection technique. After sternotomy but prior to initiation of CPB, mean CBF was 38.3 ml/100 g per minute. This modest apparent (i.e., preanesthesia CBF not measured) decrease in CBF could be attributed to hypothermia and hypocarbia. During the 1st min of CPB, mean CBF fell by 33%. During steady state hypothermic CPB, CBF unexpectedly increased to a mean of 64 ml/100 g per minute. Upon rewarming to a steady state temperature, CBF returned to 42 ml/100 g per minute. CBF measured within 30 min of terminating CPB in two patients was 40 and 41 ml/100 g per minute. Of note, CBF fell in nine patients during CPB. In these patients the mean arterial pressure averaged 45±7 mmHg compared with a mean arterial pressure of 57±14 mmHg in 15 patients in whom CBF increased during CPB, suggesting to the authors that the lower limit of autoregulation had been reached. The authors speculated that the increase in CBF seen in some patients during CPB could reflect reactive hyperemia induced by microemboli. The perfusion circuit for these studies consisted of a bubble oxygenator without a filter and there is the possibility that microemboli were introduced into the circulation. Another explanation for the high CBF values observed during CPB could be the use of enflurane as the anesthetic agent. No clinical correlations were made.

In another group of patients, Henriksen (1984) measured regional cerebral blood flow before and after CPB using single photon emission computed tomography (SPECT) and ^{133}Xe inhalation. Mean cerebral blood flow fell from 53.5 to 44.7 ml/100 g per minute following CPB. Eleven patients investigated 1 year after CPB still showed slightly reduced cerebral blood flow (50.5 ml/100 g per minute). Although statistically significant, the decrease in CBF demonstrated with SPECT is small and certainly above the ischemic threshold. Furthermore, these SPECT changes were not correlated with clinical outcome. Thus, the significance of these results is uncertain.

Govier et al. (1984) measured regional CBF using the ^{133}Xe injection clearance technique. They found no correlation between CBF and mean arterial blood pressure when these data were pooled for all measurements over all subjects. This lack of correlation ($r=-0.13$, $P=0.19$) should not be interpreted to mean that autoregulation of CBF to changes in cerebral perfusion pressure was maintained over the wide range of arterial blood pressures (30–110 mmHg) during the CPB procedure. There was a 55% decrease in cerebral blood flow during CPB, with body temperature and $PaCO_2$ being significantly related to CBF. Variation of pump flow between 1.0 and 2.0 liters/min per square meter did not significantly affect regional CBF. This study employed a bubble oxygenator with nonpulsatile, hypothermic CPB. Patients studied were normotensive preoperatively and had no history of cerebrovascular disease.

In a series of experiments Lundar et al. (1982, 1983a, 1983b) found that the start of CPB was associated with a rapid fall in cerebral perfusion pressure which they ascribed at least in part to a rise in intracranial epidural pressure. More recently, his group has shown that middle cerebral artery flow velocity passively follows cerebral perfusion pressure during steady state nonpulsatile CPB. This suggests impaired autoregulation. CO_2 reactivity appeared to be preserved at cerebral perfusion pressure levels above 25 mmHg. However, actual CBF measurements were not made in these studies (Lundar et al. 1985a, 1985b, 1986).

Using Xe^{133} clearance Farrar et al. (1986) found that during normothermic CBP, CBF decreased in parallel with $CMRO_2$. During hypothermia, when CO_2 was added to the oxygenator, CBF exceeded the metabolic demands of the tissue.

Conclusions from Available Studies of CBF During CPB

Few studies have examined the effects of CPB on CBF and metabolism. Many previous studies have focused on global measurements of CBF and metabolism. Even regional techniques such as microspheres or ^{133}Xe clearance lack the high spatial detail of autoradiography and are likely to miss the highly heterogeneous disruptions of cerebral blood flow and metabolism associated with hypotension and hypoxia. Comparisons between available studies are difficult or impossible due to different measurement techniques: differences in CPB methodology such as type of oxygenator used and line filtration; failure to control such variables as arterial carbon dioxide tension, mean arterial pressure, or pump flow rates in some studies; the inclusion of nonhomogeneous patient populations; and the failure to document preanesthesia CBF. CBF changes during CPB appear complex and variable and their clinical significance is unknown. Mismatches between CBF and the metabolic demands of the brain compatible with ischemia ($CMRO_2$ exceeding CBF) during nonpulsatile CPB have not yet been demonstrated in any patient population.

Predicting, Detecting, and Preventing Brain Damage During Open Heart Surgery

Our experience and that of others indicates that there are few preoperative, intraoperative, or postoperative factors which can reliably predict the risk of stroke or encephalopathy during open heart surgery. Obviously, marked drops in blood pressure should be avoided, but many patients sustain relatively prolonged periods of hypotension without neurologic deficit. Potential embolic situations such as a brittle aorta, ventricular thrombus, air in the heart or bypass lines, and dysrhythmias should be watched for and dealt with appropriately.

The EEG may be a useful means of detecting the time of onset of focal or global brain ischemia intraoperatively and might provide clues to injury mechanisms (Salerno 1978; Kritikov 1977). However, it is impractical to monitor all surgical patients with EEG. The development of a preoperative rCBF stress test and autoregulation profile might allow identification of a subgroup of high-risk patients who could then be selectively monitored with EEG. For example, in patients with arteriolar disease, such as elderly hypertensive patients, the CBF autoregulation curve may shift to the right so that CBF begins to fall even with a mean arterial pressure exceeding 100 mmHg. Although most patients on cardiopulmonary bypass do well with a mean pressure greater than 50 mmHg, it would seem prudent to maintain a mean pressure of 60 mmHg or greater in patients with possible defective CBF autoregulation. Some cases of prolonged encephalopathy or unexplained coma may be due to relative hypotension in patients with defective autoregulation (Stockard 1974).

Regional CBF analysis might also allow a more rational approach to prophylactic endarterectomy in the patient with asymptomatic carotid stenosis. We do not routinely perform preoperative carotid noninvasive tests on all patients undergoing CABG, as others have recommended (Rosenthal 1984; Jones 1984). Nonetheless, an occasional patient undergoing CABG surgery probably harbors an asymptomatic ICA lesion which does increase the risk of ipsilateral stroke during sufficient hemodynamic stress. Presently there is no reliable way to identify such patients preoperatively. In most patients with ICA occlusion or severe stenosis CBF is matched to the metabolic demands of the tissue, and CBF changes cannot be predictably correlated with the degree of ICA obstruction (Powers 1985). However, recent positron emission tomography (PET) studies suggest that some patients with ICA disease have a decreased perfusion reserve. CBF ipsilateral to an ICA occlusion may be inappropriately low but compensated for by an increased oxygen extraction fraction (Gibbs 1984; Powers 1985). In some patients CBF and oxygen metabolism are normal but cerebral blood volume is increased, implying a compensatory vasodilatation. Possible defects in perfusion reserve may be elicitable only with 5% CO_2 inhalation or induced hypotension (Polcyn 1984; Vorstrup 1985). These early PET results may lead to the development of a reliable test of cerebral perfusion reserve, but have yet to be correlated with stroke risk during hemodynamic stress such as cardiopulmonary bypass, especially in patients with asymptomatic ICA lesions.

References

Addonizio VP, Smith JB, Strauss FJ III, Colman RW, Edmunds LH (1980) Thromboxane synthesis and platelet secretion during cardiopulmonary bypass with bubble oxygenator. J Thorac Cardiovasc Surg 79: 91–96

Aguilar MJ, Gerbode R, Hill JD (1971) Neuropathologic complications of cardiac surgery. J Thorac Cardiovasc Surg 61: 676–685

Becker R (1982) Neuropsychological considerations in the care and treatment of children undergoing cardiac surgery. In: Psychopathological and neurological dysfunctions following open heart surgery. Becker R, Katz J, Polonius MJ, Speidel H (eds) Springer, Berlin Heidelberg New York, p 185

Branthwaite MA (1972) Neurological damage related to open-heart surgery: a clinical study. Thorax 27: 748–753

Branthwaite MA (1974) Cerebral blood flow and metabolism during open-heart surgery. Thorax 29: 633–638

Branthwaite MA (1975) Prevention of neurological damage during open-heart surgery. Thorax 30: 258–261

Brennan RW, Patterson RH, Kessler J (1971) Cerebral blood flow and metabolism during cardiopulmonary bypass: evidence of microembolic encephalopathy. Neurology 21: 665–672

Breuer AC, Franco I, Marzewski D, Soto-Velasco J (1981) Left ventricular thrombi seen by ventriculography are a significant risk factor for stroke in open heart surgery. Ann Neurol 10: 103

Breuer AC, Furlan AJ, Hanson MR (1983) Central nervous system complications of coronary artery bypass graft surgery: prospective analysis of 421 patients. Stroke 14: 682–687

Buris L, Poczkodi S, Gomory A (1979) Embolism of heart tissue to the middle cerebral artery as a complication of heart surgery. Z Rechtsmedizin 83: 87–89

Cannon DS, Miller DC, Shumway NE, Fogarty TJ, Daily PO, Hu M, Brown B Jr, Harrison DC

(1974) The long-term follow-up of patients undergoing saphenous vein bypass surgery. Circulation 49: 77–85

Chendweth DE, Cooper SW, Hugli TE, Stewart RW, Blackstone EH, Kirklin JW (1981) Complement activation during cardiopulmonary bypass: evidence for generation of C3a and C5a anaphylatoxins. N Engl J Med 304: 497–503

Coffey CE, Massey EW, Roberts KB, Curtis S, Jones RH, Pryor DB (1983) Natural history of cerebral complications of coronary artery bypass graft surgery. Neurology 33: 1416–1421

Dawson DM, Fischer EG (1977) Neurologic complications of cardiac catheterization. Neurology 27: 496–497

Dorros G, Cawley MJ, Simpson J, Bentivoglio LG, Block PC, Bourassa M, Detre K, Gosselin AJ, Grunteig AR, Kelsey SF, Kent KM, Mock MB, Mullin SM, Meyer RK, Passamani ER, Stertzer SH, Williams DO (1983) Percutaneous transluminal coronary angioplasty: report of complications from the National Heart, Lung, and Blood Institute PTCA registry. Circulation 67: 723–730

Edmunds LH (1982) Pulseless cardiopulmonary bypass. J Thorac Cardiovasc Surg 84: 800–804

Fariello RG (1980) Epileptogenic properties of enflurane and their clinical interpretation. Electroenceph Clin Neurophysiol 48: 595–598

Fox LS, Blackstone EH, Kirklin JW, Bishop SP, Bergdahl LAL, Bradley EL (1984) Relationship of brain blood flow and oxygen consumption to perfusion flow rate during profoundly hypothermic cardiopulmonary bypass. J Thorac Cardiovasc Surg 87: 658–664

Cooper DM, Bazaral MG, Furlan AJ Seuilla E, Ghatias MA, Sheeler LR, Little JR, Hahn JF, Sheldon WC, Loop FO (1986) Pituitary apoplexy: a complication of cardiac surgery. Ann Thorac Surg 41: 547–550

Farrar JK, Murkin JM, Tweed WA, Guiraudon G, McKenzie EN (1986). Cerebral blood flow and metabolism during cardiopulmonary bypass. Stroke 17: 141

Furlan AJ, Breuer AC (1984) Central nervous system complications of open heart surgery. Stroke 15: 912–915

Furlan AJ, Cracium AR (1985) Risk of stroke during coronary artery bypass graft surgery in patients with internal carotid artery disease documented by angiography. Stroke 16: 797–799

Galbraith C, Salgado E, Furlan AJ, Holman J (to be published) Cerebrovascular complication of percutaneous transluminal coronary angioplasty. Stroke

Golding LR, Jacobs G, Murakam I, Takatani S, Valdes F, Harasaki H, Nose Y (1980) Chronic nonpulsatile flow in an alive awake animal: 34 day survival. Trans Am Soc Artif Intern Organs 26: 251–255

Gonzalez-Scarano F, Hurtig HI (1981) Neurologic complications of coronary artery bypass grafting: case-control study. Neurology 31: 1032–1035

Govier AV, Reves JG, McKay RD, Karp RB, Zorn GL, Morawetz R, Smith LR, Adams M, Freeman AM (1984) Factors and their influences on regional cerebral blood flow during nonpulsatile cardiopulmonary bypass. Ann Thorac Surg 38: 592–599

Gruntzig A, Hopff H (1974) Perkutane Rekanalisation chronischer artericeller Verschluss Nut Linem neuen Dilatation Satheter Modifikation der Dotter-Tecknik. Deutsch Med Wocchenschr 99: 2502–2511

Hansotia PL, Myers WO, Ray JF III, Greehling C, Sautter RD (1975) Prognostic value of electroencephalography in cardiac surgery. Ann Thoracic Surg 19: 127–134

Hart RG, Easton JD (1983) Management of cervical bruits and carotid stenosis in preoperative patients. Stroke 14: 290–297

Heller SS, Frank KA, Malm JR, Bowman FO, Harris PD, Charlton MH, Kornfeld DS (1970) Psychiatric complications of open-heart surgery. N Engl J Med 283: 1015–1020

Henriksen L, Hjelms E, Rygg IH, et al. (1981) Cerebral blood flow measured in patients during open heart surgery using intraarterially injected xenon-133: the effect of rewarming on cerebral blood flow. J Cereb Blood Flow Metab 1 [Suppl 1]: 432–433

Henriksen L, Hjelms E, Lindeburgh T (1983) Brain hyperperfusion during cardiac operations. J Thorac Cardiovasc Surg 86: 202–208

Henriksen L (1984) Evidence suggestive of diffuse brain damage following cardiac operations. Lancet 1: 316

Hill JD, Aguilor MJ, Baranco, DeLanerolle P, Gerbode F (1969) Neuropathological manifestations of cardiac surgery. Ann Thorac Surg 7: 409–419

Hinkley RE Jr (1976) Microtubule-macrotubule transformations induced by volatile anesthetics. Mechanism of microtubule assembly. J Ultrastruct Res 57: 237–250

Hodgman JR, Cosgrove DM (1976) Post-hospital course and complications following coronary bypass surgery. Cleve Clin Q 43: 125–129

Hotson JR, Pedley RA (1976) The neurological complications of cardiac transplantation. Brain 99: 673–694

Humphreys RP, Hoffman HJ, Mustard WT, Trusler GA (1975) Cerebral hemorrhage following heart surgery. J Neurosurg 43: 671–675

Hungxi S, Xiaoqin H, Kongsoon L, Jiaquiang G, Letien X (1982) Intracranial hemorrhage and hematoma following open heart surgery. In: Psychopathological and neurological dysfunctions following open-heart surgery. Becker R, Katz J, Polonius MJ, Speidel H (eds). Springer, Berlin Heidelberg New York, p 293–299

Hutchinson JE III, Green GE, Mekhjian HA, Kemp HG (1974) Coronary bypass grafting in 376 consecutive patients, with three operative deaths. J Thorac Cardiovasc Surg 67: 7–16

Jacobs HS, Craddock PR, Hammerschmidt DE, Moldon CF (1980) Complement-induced granulocyte aggregation, an unsuspected mechanism of disease. N Engl J Med 302: 789–794

Javid H, Tufo HM, Najafi H, Dye WS, Hunter JA, Julian OC (1969) Neurological abnormalities following open-heart surgery. J Thorac Cardiovasc Surg 58: 502–509

Jones EL, Craver JM, Michalik RA, Murphy DA, Guyton RA, Bone DK, Hatcher CR, Reichwald NA (1984) Combined carotid and coronary operations: when are they necessary? J Thorac Cardiovasc Surg 87: 7–16

Kolkka R, Hilberman M (1980) Neurologic dysfunction following cardiac operation with low-flow, low-pressure cardiopulmonary bypass. J Thorac Cardiovasc Surg 79: 432–437

Kritikov PE, Branthwaite MA (1977) Significance of changes in cerebral electrical activity at onset of cardiopulmonary bypass. Thorax 32: 534–538

Lee MC, Geiger J, Nicoloff D, Klassen AC, Resch JA (1979) Cerebrovascular complications associated with coronary artery bypass (CAB) procedure. Stroke 10: 13

Lockwood KI, Capraro J, Hanson M, Conomy J (1983) Neurologic complications of cardiac catheterization. Neurology 33 [Suppl 2]: 143

Loop FD, Cosgrove DM, Lytle BW, Thurer RL, Simpendorfer C, Taylor PC, Proudfit WL (1979) An 11-year evolution of coronary arterial surgery (1967–1978). Ann Surg 190: 444–455

Lundar T, Froysaker T, Nornes H, Lilleaasen P (1982) Aspects of cerebral perfusion in open heart surgery. Scand J Thorac Cardiovasc Surg 16: 217–222

Lundar T, Froysaker T, Nornes H, Lilleaasen P (1983a) Monitoring of intracranial pressure after open heart surgery. Scand J Thorac Cardiovasc Surg 17: 149–155

Lundar T, Froysaker T, Nornes H (1983b) The clinical significance of changes in cerebral perfusion pressure during open heart surgery. Scand J Thorac Cardiovasc Surg 17: 163–169

Lundar T, Froysaker T, Lindegaard K-F, Wiberg J, Lindberg H, Rostad H, Nornes H (1985b) Some observations on cerebral perfusion during cardiopulmonary bypass. Ann Thorac Surg 39: 318–323

Lundar T, Lindegaard K-F, Froysaker T, Aaslio R, Wiberg J, Nornes H (1985a). Cerebral perfusion during nonpulsatile cardiopulmonary bypass. Ann Thorac Surg 40: 144–150

Lundar T, Lindegaard K-F, Froysaker T, et al. (1986) Cerebral carbon dioxide reactivity during nonpulsatile cardiopulmonary bypass. Ann Thorac Surg 41: 525–530

Marvoudis C (1978) To pulse or not to pulse. Ann Thorac Surg 25: 259–271

McKibbin DW, Bulkley BH, Green WR, Gott VL, Hutchins GM (1976) Fatal cerebral atheromatous embolization after cariopulmonary bypass. J Thorac Cardiovasc Surg 71: 741–745

Montero CG, Martìnez AJ (1986) Neuropathology of heart transplantation: 23 cases. Neurology 36: 1149–1154

Muraoka R, Yokota M, Aoshima M, Kyoku I, Nomoto S, Kobayashi A, Nakano H, Ueda K, Saito A, Hojo H (1981) Subclinical changes in brain morphology following cardiac operations as reflected by computed tomographic scans of the brain. J Thorac Cardiovasc Surg 81: 364–369

O'Neill BJ, III, Furlan AJ, Hobbs RD (1983) Risk of stroke in patients with transient postoperative atrial fibrillation/flutter. Stroke 14: 133

Orenstein JM, Sato N, Aaron B, Buchholz B, Bloom S (1982) Microemboli observed in deaths following cardiopulmonary bypass surgery: silicone antifoam agents and polyvinyl chloride tubing as sources of emboli. Hum Pathol 13: 1082–1090

Pokar H, Bleese N, Fischer-Düsterhoff H, et al. (1982) Prevention of postoperative psychic and neurological disturbances after open heart surgery using prostacyclin: a clinical study. In: Becker R, Katz J, Polonius MJ, Speidel H (eds) Psychopathological and neurological dysfunctions following open heart surgery. Springer, Berlin Heidelberg New York, pp 312–319

Polcyn RE, Koeppe R, Hutchins GD, Nickles RJ, Gatley SJ, Rowe B (1984) Hypercapnia and cerebral blood flow: an approach to perfusion reserve. J Nucl Med 25: 110

Powers WJ, Raichle ME (1985) Positron emission tomography and its application to the study of cerebrovascular disease in man. Stroke 16: 361–376

Price DL, Harris J (1970) Cholesterol emboli in cerebral arterialis as a complication of retrograde aortic perfusion during cardiac surgery. Neurology 20: 1209–1214

Rosenthal D, Cavdill DR, Lamis PA, Logan W, Stanton PE (1984) Carotid and coronary arterial disease. A rational approach. Am Surg 50: 233–235

Salerno TA, Lince DP, White DN, Lynn RB, Charrette EJP (1978) Monitoring of electroencephalogram during open heart surgery: a prospective analysis of 118 cases. J Thorac Cardiovasc Surg 76: 97–100

Sanderson SM, Wright G, Sims FW (1972) Brain damage in dogs immediately following pulsatile and non-pulsatile blood flows in extracorporeal circulation. Thorax 27: 275

Sotaniemi KA, Mononen H, Hokkanen TE (1986) Long-term cerebral outcome after open-heart surgery. A five year neuropsychological follow-up study. Stroke 17: 410–416

Stockard JJ, Bickford RG, Schauble JF (1973) Pressure dependence cerebral ischemia during cardiopulmonry bypass, Neurology 23: 521–529

Stockard JJ, Bickford RG, Myers RR, Aung MH, Dilley RB, Schauble JF (1974) Hypotension-induced changes in cerebral function during cardiac surgery. Stroke 5: 730–746

Taylor KM, Devlin BJ, Mittra SM, Gillan JG, Brannan JJ, McKenna JM (1980) Assessment of cerebral damage during open-heart surgery. A new experimental model. Scand J Thorac Cardiovasc Surg 14: 197–203

Taylor KM (1982) Brain damage during open heart surgery. Thorax 37: 873–876

Thurlbeck WM, Castleman B (1957) Atheromatous emboli to the kidneys after aortic surgery. N Engl J Med 257: 442–447

Tufo HM, Ostfeld AM, Shekelle R (1970) Central nervous system dysfunction following open-heart surgery. JAMA 212: 1333–1340

Vorstrup S, Paulson OB, Lassen NA (1985) How to identify hemodynamic cases. In: Spetzler RF, Selman WR, Carter LP, Martin NA (eds) Cerebral revascularization for stroke. Thieme-Stratton, New York, pp 120–126

Wollam H, Stephen GW, Clement AJ, Danielson GK (1966) Cerebral blood flow in man during extracorporeal circulation. J Thorac Cardiovasc Surg 52: 558–564

Wright G, Sanderson JM (1972) Brain damage and mortality in dogs following pulsatile and non-pulsatile blood flow in extracorporeal circulation. Thorax 27: 738

Chapter 16

Management of Coexistent Carotid and Coronary Artery Disease: A Surgical Viewpoint

N. R. Hertzer, F. D. Loop, and E. G. Beven

Introduction

Perioperative stroke has been a potential risk of open heart surgery since the clinical introduction of extracorporeal pump oxygenation nearly 3 decades ago. Early studies confined to valve replacement and congenital heart disease identified neurologic deficits ranging in severity from mild intellectual impairment to diffuse encephalopathy in 19%–26% of all age groups, and autopsy examinations demonstrated that cerebral ischemia could be caused either by inadequate perfusion or by embolization of unvented air, fat, or calcium, and other particulate debris (Gilman 1965; Javid et al. 1969; Lee et al. 1971). Although patients who require simultaneous valve replacement or resection of ventricular aneurysms may still experience major embolic events, accumulated surgical experience and subsequent improvements in perfusion technology have produced a dramatic reduction in the incidence of neurolgic complications during the era of coronary artery bypass. In retrospective series comprising thousands of operations, Reul et al. (1972) and Loop et al. (1979) reported perioperative strokes in only 1%–2% of patients receiving direct myocardial revascularization.

Irrespective of the low overall stroke rate associated with pure coronary grafting, permanent strokes represent a devastating disability to individual patients and their families when they do occur. Considering the established safety of carotid endarterectomy at many cardiac surgical centers, it is reasonable that patients perceived to be at risk for stroke during coronary bypass because of coexistent carotid artery disease would be considered for extracranial reconstruction as well. This group includes those with a history of previous cerebrovascular symptoms or asymptomatic carotid bruits, both of which are concentrated among older patients who have generalized atherosclerosis. In an effort to protect every individual in whom neurologic complications seem especially predictable, staged or simultaneous carotid endarterectomy and myocardial revascularization have been performed at a number of centers for more than 10 years. While the number of cardiac patients having serious carotid disease confirmed by angiography is small and constitutes only 1.7% of those scheduled for myocardial revascularization at the Cleveland Clinic, recent recognition that many patients presenting primarily for extracranial operations may also warrant coronary bypass could eventually expand the total pool of patients with synchronous carotid and coronary atherosclerosis eligible for surgical management (Hertzer et al. 1983, 1985).

For a number of reasons, however, the merits of an aggressive surgical approach to associated carotid lesions have been difficult to prove. First, extracranial arterial disease is not the only plausible explanation for neurologic complications following myocardial revascularization. For example, cerebral embolization caused by the application of clamps to the ascending thoracic aorta during aortocoronary grafting is another likely source for stroke, particularly in older patients with advanced atherosclerosis. Furthermore, the group under consideration for surgical correction of coexistent carotid and coronary disease is so small that it is difficult to document the impact of this approach on the overall low stroke rate in large series of patients receiving coronary bypass. Finally, and perhaps most importantly, no prospective group of patients with extracranial carotid disease proven by angiography has yet undergone myocardial revascularization without the protection of carotid endarterectomy. Until such a study is undertaken, the virtue of staged or combined carotid endarterectomy in cardiac surgery patients must be judged in terms of late stroke prevention as well as within the more narrow context of perioperative prophylaxis. The most important consideration concerning selection of patients for either staged or combined carotid endarterectomy at the Cleveland Clinic has been whether extracranial reconstruction would be indicated even in the absence of surgical coronary disease.

Patient Selection

Previous Neurologic Symptoms

Patients with a history of transient ischemic attacks (TIAs) or previous strokes with good functional recovery are candidates for cerebral angiography to determine whether their symptoms are associated with significant carotid stenosis or an extracranial microembolic source. Although surgical treatment may be unnecessary for those with trivial angiographic findings, cardiac patients with recent neurologic symptoms in conjunction with ulcerated or preocclusive bifurcation disease deserve consideration for carotid endarterectomy in addition to myocardial revascularization.

The serious implications of TIA with respect to subsequent stroke risk are well recognized. It has been estimated that 20%–45% of symptomatic patients sustain completed strokes within 5 years following their original neurologic events and that many of these are concentrated during the first few months (Toole et al. 1978; Whisnant et al. 1978). Ziegler and Hassanein (1973) correlated angiographic stenosis with stroke risk in patients with TIA and uncorrected carotid lesions, and found that further neurologic complications occurred in half of their patients with advanced (>70%) carotid stenosis. Although carotid reconstruction has been widely accepted as an appropriate treatment for TIA in selected patients, its effectiveness has been questioned in those who already have sustained previous strokes. Bardin et al. (1982) suggested that the long-term benefit of carotid endarterectomy in patients with prior strokes was questionable because, in their experience, over 20% of this group eventually had additional deficits even after surgery. In contrast, McCullough et al. (1985) recently demonstrated that further complications occurred in 42% of their patients who were not evaluated for surgical management after presenting with stroke as an initial symptom. While the cumulative incidence of late cerebrovascular complications among patients with prior strokes chosen for carotid reconstruction at the Cleveland Clinic was 30% during a minimum follow-up of 10 years, only 6% experienced subsequent deficits referrable to the operated carotid artery (Hertzer and Arison 1985). This follow-up investigation showed that close surveillance of the contralateral carotid system is essential to continued protection after carotid procedures in all patients, including those with previous strokes.

Asymptomatic Carotid Stenosis

The presence of an asymptomatic carotid bruit is associated with significant (>75%) angiographic carotid stenosis in 46% of patients with peripheral vascular disease (Hertzer et al. 1984). The prevalence of high-grade asymptomatic carotid stenosis may be less impressive among patients evaluated primarily because of ischemic heart disease.

We prefer carotid cineangiography during cardiac catheterization or intravenous digital subtraction angiography for assessment of asymptomatic carotid bruits before myocardial revascularization, but noninvasive carotid testing (oculoplethysmography, carotid audiofrequency analysis, duplex scanning) has been found at other centers to be a dependable screening approach prior to selective angiography in patients with asymptomatic bruits (Brewster et al. 1978; Sumner et al. 1982; Long et al. 1985). Diagnostic methods notwithstanding, the management of carotid stenosis in asymptomatic patients is highly controversial especially within the limited perspective of perioperative stroke risk among patients scheduled for coronary bypass or other major vascular procedures. With the occasional exception of patients with contralateral internal carotid occlusion, prophylactic carotid endarterectomy usually is limited to asymptomatic patients found to have carotid stenosis exceeding 70% of lumen diameter by angiography. Provided the incidence of iatrogenic stroke approaches 1% under conventional circumstances, such lesions appear to warrant elective reconstruction if only for late protection for stroke (Cullen et al. 1983; Roederer et al. 1984).

It is virtually impossible to obtain data concerning perioperative stroke among patients who undergo coronary bypass in the presence of uncorrected carotid stenosis confirmed by angiography, but Table 16.1 presents information from three studies of coronary bypass which employed asymptomatic carotid bruits and noninvasive testing to define those at perceived risk (Turnipseed et al. 1980; Barnes et al. 1981; Kartchner and McCrae 1982). According to these reports, asymptomatic bruits are present in 6%–16% of cardiac patients, and abnormal noninvasive carotid testing in 12%–18%. Perioperative neurologic deficits occurred in 2%–5% of all patients in these studies, compared with the incidence

Table 16.1. Correlation of clinical indications of asymptomatic carotid disease with the incidence of perioperative neurologic deficits following coronary bypass procedures

Clinical features	Turnipseed et al. (1980)		Barnes et al. (1981)		Kartchner and McRae (1982)	
	No.	%	No.	%	No.	%
Patients	170	100	324	100	234[a]	100
A. Asymptomatic carotid bruits	28	16	21	6.5	NA	
B. Abnormal noninvasive testing (NIT)	20	12	40	12	42	18
C. Perioperative neurologic deficits	9	5.3	6	1.9	12	5.1
Bruit	2	7.1	2	9.5	NA	
No bruit	7	4.9	4	1.3	NA	
Abnormal NIT	2	10	1	2.5	10	24
Normal NIT	7	4.7	5	1.8	2	1.0

Abbreviation: NA, Data not available
[a] Includes 91 cardiac and 143 peripheral vascular patients

of 1%–2% expected among unselected patients receiving elective myocardial revascularization. Neurologic deficits occurred in 7%–9% of patients who had asymptomatic carotid bruits which were not otherwise investigated or treated, compared with 1%–5% of those who had no bruits. The incidence of perioperative deficits was comparable between groups of patients with abnormal noninvasive testing (2.5%) and with normal studies (1.8%) in the investigation reported by Barnes et al. In the other two studies neurologic complications occurred in 10%–24% of patients with abnormal noninvasive results, compared with 1%–5% of those who had no evidence of carotid stenosis.

Kartchner and McCrae interpreted their results to indicate that angiographic documentation and, if necessary, surgical correction of suspected carotid disease should be pursued in patients who have noninvasive indications of advanced carotid stenosis. Turnipseed et al. and Barnes et al. instead recommended that both asymptomatic bruits and abnormal noninvasive studies could be disregarded prior to coronary bypass because their observed differences in perioperative stroke rates failed to achieve statistical significance. Considering that only 1.7% of over 22000 coronary bypass patients were found to have severe coexistent carotid disease by angiography at the Cleveland Clinic (Hertzer et al. 1983), the fact that both Turnipseed et al. and Barnes et al. discovered abnormal noninvasive studies in 12% of their series could indicate that many of these patients were not at risk because they would not have been found to have high-grade carotid stenosis if angiograms had been obtained. Moreover, several apparent trends concerning perioperative stroke may not have gained statistical significance only because of the small sample size.

Table 16.2 contains data concerning the late implications of asymptomatic carotid stenosis discovered either on the basis of carotid bruits or abnormal noninvasive testing. Thompson et al. (1978) have demonstrated that carotid endarterectomy performed by experienced surgeons in asymptomatic patients is associated with late stroke in only 4%, whereas 17% of an unoperated control

Table 16.2. Late neurologic complications of uncorrected carotid stenosis suspected on the basis of asymptomatic bruits or noninvasive testing

Series and criteria	No.	years	Late complications					
			TIA No.	%	Strokes No.	%	Total No.	%
Asymptomatic carotid bruits								
Thompson et al. (1978)	138	4	37	27	24	17	61	44
Heyman et al. (1980)								
Bruit	72	6	NA		10	14	10	14
No bruit	1548	6	NA		52	3.4	52	3.4
Wolf et al. (1981)	171	2	2	1.2	19	11	21	12
Noninvasive carotid testing (NIT)								
Kartchner and McRae (1977)								
Abnormal NIT	147	2	7	4.8	17	12	24	16
Normal NIT	877	2	16	1.8	14	1.6	30	3.4
Barnes et al. (1981)								
Abnormal NIT	72	2	10	14	2	2.8	12	17
Normal NIT	254	2	2	0.8	0	–	2	0.8
Busuttil et al. (1981)								
Abnormal NIT	67	3	29	43	7	10	36	54
Normal NIT	71	3	6	8.4	2	2.8	8	11

Abbreviation: NA, data not available.

group with asymptomatic carotid bruits had strokes and another 27% experienced TIA within a mean follow-up interval of 4 years. Large population surveys from Evans County, Georgia (Heyman et al. 1980) and the Framingham Study (Wolf et al. 1981) also reported late strokes in 11%–14% of unstudied patients with asymptomatic bruits and suggested that stroke risk is especially high among men. Strokes occurred in 28% of men with asymptomatic bruits in Evans County and at a rate three times that in the normal male population in Framingham. Using noninvasive testing for screening of asymptomatic bruits, Kartchner and McCrae (1977) and Busuttil et al. (1981) have reported similar results for untreated patients within the first 3 years after evaluation. Strokes occurred in 10%–12% of patients with abnormal noninvasive findings, compared with 2%–3% of those with no indication of serious carotid stenosis. Continuing their investigation of the influence of asymptomatic carotid stenosis on perioperative results, Barnes et al. found that 17% of patients with abnormal noninvasive testing experienced neurologic events within 2 years of their examinations, compared with only 0.8% of those who had normal studies.

Surgical Management

Both staged and combined approaches to coexistent carotid and coronary artery disease require experienced surgeons and anesthesiologists whose success with either carotid reconstruction or coronary bypass alone is unquestioned. Anesthesia must be administered by personnel qualified in the care of patients with coronary disease when staged carotid endarterectomy is performed several days prior to myocardial revascularization. By the same token, the setting of combined procedures is quite unlike isolated carotid operations. Full systemic anticoagulation is continued immediately after endarterectomy, and the patient is placed under the controlled hypotension of cardiopulmonary bypass. For several postoperative hours, hemodynamic changes and volume requirements may be more dramatic than ordinarily is the case after simple carotid endarterectomy. Since sedation administered to control ventilation customarily interferes with an accurate neurologic evaluation until the following day, the absence of early technical complications at the site of endarterectomy must be a matter of course.

Staged Procedures

The choice of staged or combined operations is determined by strict assessment of the relative severity of carotid and cardiac risk factors. Although simultaneous procedures have been performed more often, staged operations are preferred at the Cleveland Clinic because the incidence of neurologic complications with this approach (1.5%) compares favorably with carotid endarterectomy in all other elective patients (Hertzer et al. 1978). Carotid reconstruction prior to coronary bypass should be restricted to patients who are free of cardiac symptoms or who are limited only by chronic stable angina. Critical coronary lesions, especially those involving the left main coronary artery, or severe multiple-vessel disease should not be present. Stable patients who require extensive or complicated myocardial revascularization, such as coronary artery reoperations, associated valve replacement, or ventricular aneurysm resection, are also candidates for staged operations.

Table 16.3 contains data concerning a total of 187 patients comprising several large studies of staged carotid and coronary procedures reported from 1972–1978. These results include scattered patients who underwent coronary bypass preceding carotid reconstruction, but most received the traditional approach with carotid endarterectomy as the initial operation. Seven patients (3.7%) sustained operative strokes, some of which required undesirable postponement of myocardial revascularization. Fourteen patients (7.5%) died, and most of

Table 16.3. Staged carotid endarterectomy and coronary bypass procedures: operative strokes and mortality

Series	No.	Strokes		Mortality	
		No.	%	No.	%
Bernhard et al. (1972)	22	2	9.1	5	23
Urschel et al. (1976)	25	1	4.0	0	–
Mehigan et al. (1977)	27	1	3.7	0	–
Morris et al. (1978)	48	2	2.1	8	17
Cleveland Clinic (Hertzer et al. 1978)	65	1	1.5	1	1.7
Total	187	7	3.7	14	7.5

these deaths were caused by myocardial infarction during the staging interval between operations. This particular liability of the staged approach to coexistent carotid and coronary disease encouraged Bernhard et al. to introduce combined reconstruction in 1972 and largely persuaded Morris et al. to abandon staged procedures by 1978.

Combined Procedures

Because of the risk for cardiac complications during any staging interval following carotid reconstruction, combined procedures should be considered for patients with left main coronary disease and for those having severe multiple-vessel lesions unassociated with adequate intercoronary collateral, as well as for any patient with unstable angina. Impaired ventricular function which is sufficiently severe to represent an additive risk during staged carotid endarterectomy may also be a relative indication for simultaneous operations. Table 16.4 contains the results for a composite series of 739 combined procedures reported since the initial experience of Bernhard et al. in 1972. The incidence of perioperative stroke ranged from 0% to 6.2% (mean, 3.2%), and operative mortality was 0%–12% (mean, 4.6%). Stroke risk was nearly identical for both staged and combined procedures, but fatal complications were more common with either approach than usually is anticipated following coronary bypass. It should be noted, however, that the mean age for 595 of the 739 tabulated patients for whom this information was available was 61 years, compared with a mean age of approximately 55 years for most patients who require myocardial revascularization (Loop et al. 1979). Several other studies have demonstrated that the mortality of coronary bypass in patients over 65 years of age is consistently in the range of 5% even in the absence of associated carotid disease (Ashor et al. 1973; Gersh et al. 1983; Hibler et al. 1983).

Table 16.4. Combined carotid endarterectomy and coronary bypass procedure: operative strokes and mortality

Series	No.	Strokes		Mortality	
		No.	%	No.	%
Bernhard et al. (1972)	16	1	6.2	0	–
Urschel et al. (1976)	8	0	–	0	–
Mehigan et al. (1977)	16	2	12	2	12
Okies et al. (1977)	16	1	6.2	1	6.2
Morris et al. (1978)	44	1	2.3	2	4.5
Ennix et al. (1979)	51	0	–	3	5.9
Rice et al. (1980)	54	1	1.9	0	–
Carver and Jones et al. (1982, 1984)	132	2	1.5	4	3.0
Emery et al. (1983)	42	0	–	2	4.8
Brener et al. (1984)	29	1	3.4	1	3.4
Cleveland Clinic (Hertzer et al. 1983)	331	15	4.5	19	5.7
Total	739	24	3.2	34	4.6

The Cleveland Clinic Experience

The management of patients with coexistent carotid and coronary disease at the Cleveland Clinic has been described in detail in previous reports (Hertzer et al. 1978, 1983). By the nature of their selection, 331 patients who received combined operations were older (mean age, 61 years) and had a higher incidence of left main coronary stenosis (21%), multiple-vessel coronary involvement (63%), and ventricular impairment (56%) than 22100 other patients who underwent coronary bypass alone during the same study period (1973–1981). All of these distinctions were statistically significant ($P<0.01$, chi-squared analysis).

Early Results

Postoperative neurologic complications occurred in 30 patients (9.0%), but only half of these either involved the cerebral hemisphere ipsilateral to simultaneous carotid reconstruction or were permanent. Sixteen patients (4.8%) had deficits appropriate to the ipsilateral carotid hemisphere, while ten others (3.0%)

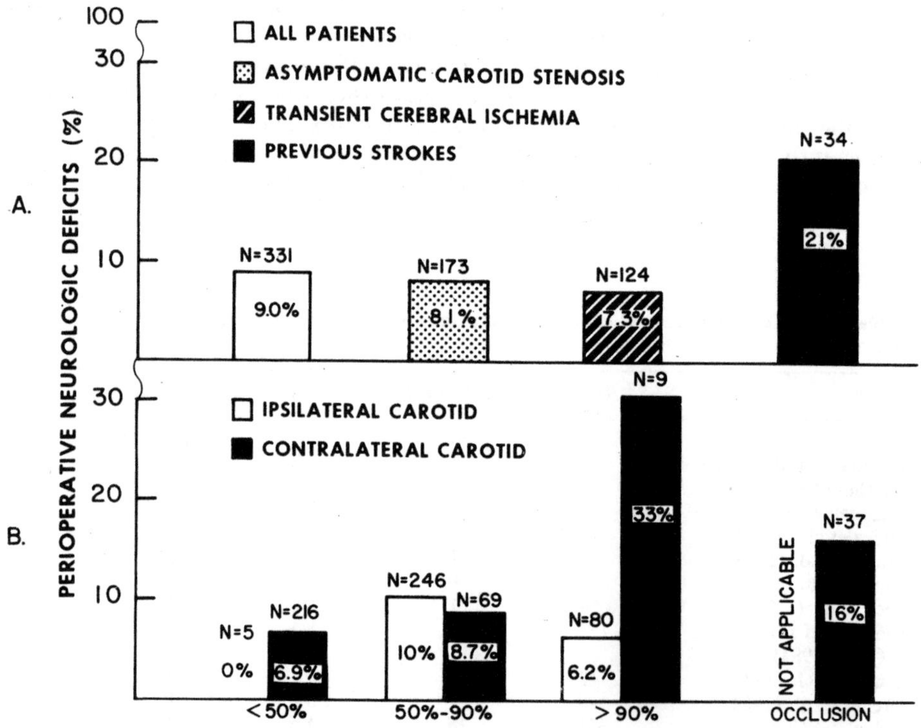

Fig. 16.1. Graphic correlation of (*A*) the preoperative neurologic status and (*B*) the angiographic severity of carotid stenosis with the incidence of perioperative neurologic deficits following 331 combined operations performed at the Cleveland Clinic (Hertzer et al. 1983).

occurred in the contralateral hemisphere and four (1.2%) involved the brain stem. A total of 15 deficits (4.5%) were temporary, including 13 that resolved within a few postoperative days and two completed strokes requiring a maximum of 2 months for complete recovery. Fifteen strokes (4.5%) produced some degree of permanent disability. Seven of these were associated with only mild impairment, but eight others were severe, including three (0.9%) which were fatal. There was a total of 19 deaths, for an operative mortality of 5.7%. Perioperative myocardial infarctions occurred in 6.3% of combined operations in comparison to 2.7% of all bypass procedures during the study interval, but multivariant analysis indicated that ventricular impairment was the only independent factor which influenced early mortality ($P < 0.05$).

Subsets of the series appearing to have particular risks for neurologic complications are illustrated in Fig. 16.1. Seven (21%) of 34 patients with a history of previous strokes sustained additional deficits after their simultaneous operations, compared with 7.3% of patients whose prior symptoms had been limited to TIA and 8.1% of those with asymptomatic carotid stenosis. This observation did not achieve statistical significance, but it is entirely consonant with previous experience with carotid endarterectomy at this center (Hertzer and Arison 1985). Other reports (Mehigan et al. 1977; Brenner et al. 1984) have suggested that the presence of bilateral carotid disease at the time of unilateral carotid endarterectomy and simultaneous coronary bypass is associated with a substantial risk for postoperative stroke, and we noted a similar trend (Fig. 16.1). Early neurologic deficits occurred in 6.9% of patients having insignificant contralateral disease, in 8.7% of those with 50%–90% stenosis, and in a total of 20% of those who had either subtotal stenosis or occlusion of the contralateral internal carotid artery ($P<0.02$).

Late Results

During a mean follow-up interval of 38 months, only 18 (5.8%) of 312 survivors of combined operations have experienced late strokes. Of the 15 patients for whom adequate clinical information was available, these events appeared to involve the cerebral cortex on the same side as simultaneous carotid endarterectomy in five (1.6%), the contralateral hemisphere in seven (2.4%), and the brain stem in three (1.0%). Four of these strokes were fatal.

Figure 16.2 illustrates 5-year actuarial survival for the same 312 patients in comparison to a number of other representative series collected at the Cleveland Clinic. Five-year survival for patients with coexistent carotid and coronary disease was 83%, compared with 90% for 757 patients aged 60–64 years who had successful coronary bypass at this center during approximately the same period of study (Cleveland Clinic Cardiovascular Registry, unpublished data). Late survival for the group receiving only coronary bypass is nearly identical to a normal population of the same general age. This comparison suggests that those in the combined group with coronary and cerebrovascular atherosclerosis have a steeper decline in late survival than most patients with coronary disease alone, despite the fact that their carotid lesions were corrected during simultaneous operations.

Life table survival for patients in the combined group was superior to 143 patients of similar age who only underwent carotid endarterectomy in the

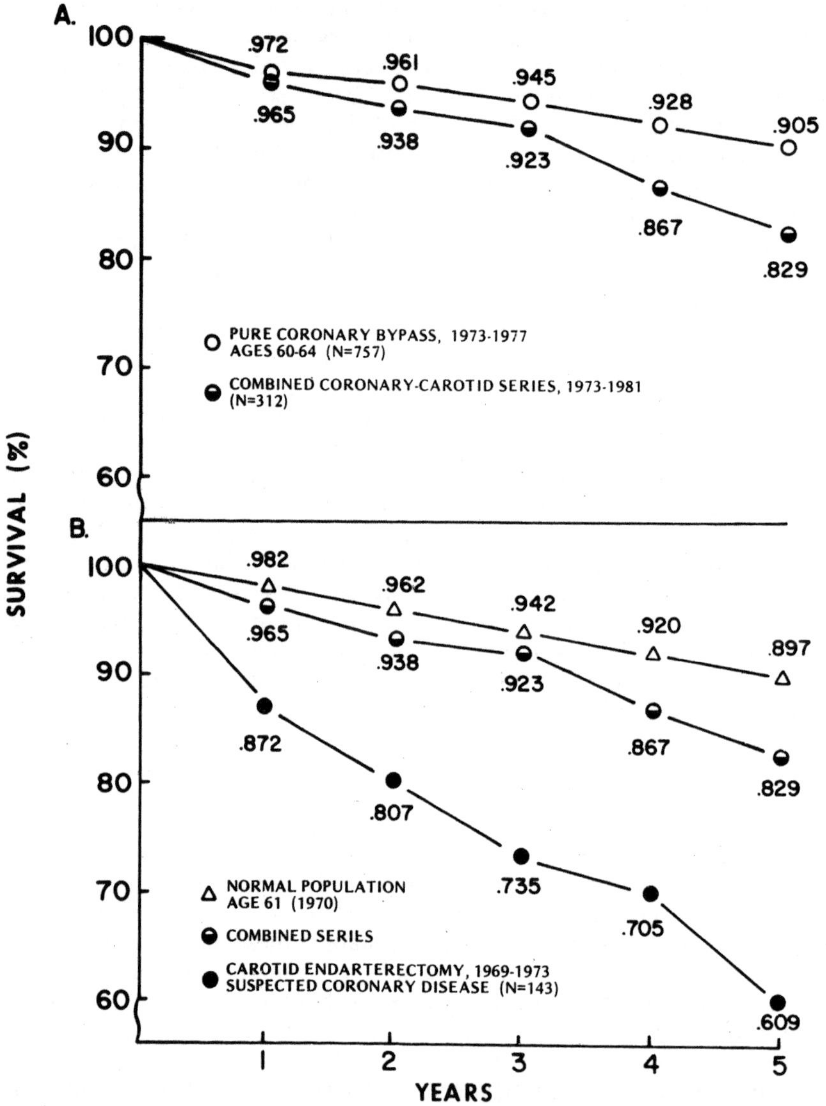

Fig. 16.2. Life table survival after successful simultaneous operations in 312 patients in comparison to other representative groups (Hertzer et al. 1983, 1985).

presence of suspected but undocumented coronary disease during an earlier study period (Hertzer and Arison 1985). Five-year survival in that group was 61%, and the difference in late mortality in comparison to patients who survived combined operations was statistically significant ($P<0.0005$) when analyzed using nonparametric methods (Lee and Desu 1972). The principles expressed by these and other data (Hertzer et al. 1984, 1985; Rokey et al. 1984) appear to be unmistakable. Severe carotid and coronary disease often occur in the same patient, and neither should be ignored.

A Prospective Study

Countless reports concerning coexistent carotid and coronary disease have encouraged a prospective, randomized study to address some of the unsettled issues regarding the management of these complicated patients. In 1983, such an investigation was begun at the Cleveland Clinic. On the basis of our previous experience, patients having recent neurologic symptoms or severe bilateral carotid stenosis were excluded from the initial phase of this study, and a few others with unilateral carotid lesions and stable cardiac disease continued to receive elective carotid endarterectomy preceding coronary bypass. All other asymptomatic patients documented by angiography to have advanced (≥70%) unilateral carotid stenosis have been prospectively randomized into two groups, one of which receives combined operations and the other coronary bypass followed by staged carotid endarterectomy.

A summary of results during the 1st year of this long-term project is presented in Table 16.5. Seventy-seven patients were evaluated, including 31 who underwent some type of staged approach and 46 who had combined procedures. Of 34 patients who were excluded from the randomization process, 7 with stable coronary disease underwent elective carotid endarterectomy as an initial procedure, while 27 others required combined operations because of previous neurologic symptoms or bilateral carotid lesions. Finally, the prospectively randomized group comprised 43 patients, including 24 who were scheduled for coronary bypass to be followed by carotid endarterectomy and 19 others who received simultaneous procedures.

Table 16.5. Preliminary results during the 1st year of the Cleveland Clinic randomized study of surgical staging among patients who require carotid endarterectomy and coronary bypass

Surgical approach	No.	Perioperative strokes					
		Ipsilateral hemisphere		Other sites		Total	
		No.	%	No.	%	No.	%
Staged procedure	31	3	9.7	0	–	3	9.7
Elective carotid endarterectomy first	7	0	–	0	–	0	–
Randomized to coronary bypass first	24	3	12	0	–	3	12
Combined procedure	46	1	2.2	4	8.7	5	11
Randomized subset	19	1	5.3	1	5.3	2	11
Study exclusions (previous symptoms or bilateral stenosis)	27	0	–	3	11	3	11
Total	77	4	5.2	4	5.2	8	10

In the staged group, three (12%) of 24 patients who underwent coronary bypass in the presence of unilateral carotid stenosis sustained perioperative strokes appropriate to the ipsilateral cerebral hemisphere. None of the seven patients receiving conventional staged management had neurologic complications. In the combined group, 1 (5.3%) of 19 randomized patients with unilateral carotid disease experienced an iatrogenic stroke in the appropriate hemisphere. This was the only neurologic complication involving the side of carotid endarterectomy. Four other patients had perioperative strokes at the time of combined operations, all of which involved the contralateral hemisphere or the posterior cerebral circulation. Strokes which were inappropriate to simultaneous carotid endarterectomy occurred in 3 (11%) of 27 patients excluded from the prospective study because of previous symptoms or bilateral carotid stenosis. These events could have been related either to uncorrected contralateral disease or to embolization during aortocoronary grafting.

While these preliminary results tend to support the early merit of combined operations in patients whose coronary disease precludes carotid endarterectomy prior to myocardial revascularization, at least 5 years will be necessary to accumulate sufficient data for analysis. By that time, the influence of each approach on the prevention of late stroke should also be apparent. Each of these considerations is indispensable for planning surgical strategy in patients who have synchronous carotid and coronary disease.

Conclusions

Despite the perpetual controversy concerning the fact that some patients who undergo carotid endarterectomy would never experience strokes even if no operations were performed, we believe that surgical management of associated carotid disease in cardiac patients with previous neurologic symptoms or severe asymptomatic stenosis is justified provided the operative risk is reduced to an absolute minimum. Using strict criteria, staged carotid endarterectomy several days prior to elective coronary bypass seems to be the safest and most logical approach for patients having stable cardiac symptoms and acceptable coronary anatomy. Although combined procedures may be necessary for those having active neurologic symptoms or bilateral carotid lesions in conjunction with diffuse or unstable coronary disease, the incidence of neurologic complications at the time of simultaneous operations may exceed the stroke risk for either carotid endarterectomy or coronary bypass alone in other patients whose clinical status is less desperate. In the final analysis, the asymptomatic patient presenting for coronary bypass who has unilateral carotid stenosis might best be managed by myocardial revascularization followed by elective carotid reconstruction.

References

Ashor GW, Meyer BW, Lindesmith GG, Stiles QR, Walker GH, Tucker BL (1973) Coronary artery disease. Arch Surg 107: 30–33

Bardin JA, Bernstein EF, Humber PB, Collins GM, Dilley RB, Devin JB, Stuart SH (1982) Is carotid endarterectomy beneficial in prevention of recurrent stroke? Arch Surch 117: 1401–1406

Barnes RW, Liebman PR, Marszalek PB, Kirk CL, Goldman MH (1981) The natural history of asymptomatic carotid disease in patients undergoing cardiovascular surgery. Surgery 90: 1075–1082

Bernhard VM, Johnson WD, Peterson JJ (1972) Carotid artery stenosis. Association with surgery for coronary artery disease. Arch Surg 105: 837–840

Brener BJ, Brief DK, Alpert J, Goldenkranz RJ, Parsonnet V, Feldman S, Gielchinsky I, Abel RM, Hochberg M. Hussain M (1984). A four-year experience with preoperative noninvasive carotid evaluation of two thousand and twenty-six patients undergoing cardiac surgery. J Vasc Surg 1: 326–338

Brewster DC, Schlaen HH, Raines JK, Abbott WM, Darling RC (1978) Rational management of the asymptomatic carotid bruit. Arch Surg 113: 927–930

Busuttil RW, Baker JD, Davidson RK, Machleder HI (1981) Carotid artery stenosis—hemodynamic significance and clinical course. JAMA 245: 1436–1445

Craver JM, Murphy DA, Jones EL, Curling PE, Bone DK, Smith RB III, Perdue GD, Hatcher CR Jr, Kandrach M (1982) Concomitant carotid and coronary artery reconstruction. Ann Surg 195: 712–720

Cullen SJ, Correa MC, Calderon-Ortiz M, Walburn FJ, Raines J (1983) Clinical sequelae in patients with asymptomatic carotid bruits. Circulation 68: 83–87

Emery RW, Cohn LH, Whittemore AD, Mannick JA, Couch NP, Collins JJ Jr (1983) Coexistent carotid and coronary artery disease. Arch Surg 118: 1035–1038

Ennix CL Jr, Lawrie GM, Morris GC Jr, Crawford ES, Howell JF, Reardon MJ, Weatherford SC (1979) Improved results of carotid endarterectomy in patients with symptomatic coronary disease: An analysis of 1546 consecutive carotid operations. Stroke 10: 122–125

Gersh BJ, Kronmal RA, Frye RL, Schaff HV, Ryan RJ, Gosselin AJ, Kaiser GC, Killip T III (1983) Coronary arteriography and coronary artery bypass surgery: morbidity and mortality in patients aged 65 or older. A report from the coronary artery surgery study. Circulation 67: 483–491

Gilman S (1965) Cerebral disorders after open-heart operations. N Engl J Med 272: 489–498

Hertzer NR, Arison R (1985) Cumulative stroke and survival ten years after carotid endarterectomy. J Vasc Surg 2: 661–668

Hertzer NR, Beven EG, Young JR, O'Hara PJ, Ruschhaupt WF III, Graor RA, deWolfe VG, Maljovec LC (1984) Coronary artery disease in peripheral vascular patients. A classification of 1000 coronary angiograms and results of surgical management. Ann Surg 199: 223–233

Hertzer NR, Beven EG, Young JR, O'Hara PJ, Graor RA, Ruschhaupt WF III (1984) Incidental asymptomatic carotid bruits in patients scheduled for peripheral vascular reconstruction: results of cerebral and coronary angiography. Surgery 96: 535–543

Hertzer NR, Loop FD, Taylor PC, Beven EG (1978) Staged and combined surgical approach to simultaneous carotid and coronary vascular disease. Surgery 84: 803–811

Hertzer NR, Loop FD, Taylor PC, Beven EG (1983) Combined myocardial revascularization and carotid endarterectomy. J Thorac Cardiovasc Surg 85: 577–589

Hertzer NR, Young JR, Beven EG, Graor RA, O'Hara PJ, Ruschhaupt WF III, deWolfe VG, Maljovec LC (1985) Coronary angiography in 506 patients with extracranial cerebrovascular disease. Arch Intern Med 145: 849–852

Heyman A, Wilkinson WE, Heyden S, Helms MJ, Bartel AG, Karp HR, Tyroler HA, Hames CG (1980) Risk of stroke in asymptomatic persons with cervical arterial bruits. A population study in Evans County, Georgia. N Engl J Med 302: 838–841

Hibler BA, Wright JO, Wright CG, Ehrenhaft JL, Doty DB, Rossi NP (1983) Coronary artery bypass surgery in the elderly. Arch Surg 118: 402–404

Javid H, Tufo HM, Najafi H, Dye WS, Hunter JA, Julian OC (1969) Neurological abnormalities following open-heart surgery. J Thorac Cardiovasc Surg 58: 502–509

Jones EL, Craver JM, Michalik RA, Murphy DA, Guyton RA, Bone DK, Hatcher CR, Reichwald NA (1984) Combined carotid and coronary operations: when are they necessary? J Thorac Cardiovasc Surg 87: 7–16

Kartchner MM, McRae LP (1977) Noninvasive evaluation and management of the "asymptomatic" carotid bruit. Surgery 82: 840–847

Kartchner MM, McRae LP (1982) Carotid occlusive disease as a risk factor in major cardiovascular surgery. Arch Surg 117: 1086–1088
Lee WH, Brady MP, Rowe JM, Miller WC Jr (1971) Effects of extracorporeal circulation upon behavior, personality and brain function: part II, hemodynamic, metabolic, and psychometric correlations. Ann Surg 173: 1013–1023
Lee ET, Desu MM (1972) A computer program for comparing K samples with right-censored data. Comput Programs Biomed 2: 315–321
Long JB, Lynch TG, Karafilian RG, Hobson RW III (1985) Asymptomatic carotid disease. Surg Gynecol Obstet 160: 89–98
Loop FD, Cosgrove DM, Lytle BW, Thurer RL, Simpfendorfer C, Taylor PC, Proudfit WL (1979) An 11 year evolution of coronary arterial surgery (1967–1978). Ann Surg 190: 444–455
McCullough JL, Mentzer RM Jr, Harman PK, Kaiser DL, Kron IL, Crosby IK (1985) Carotid endarterectomy after a completed stroke: Reduction in long-term neurologic deterioration. J Vasc Surg 1: 7–14
Mehigan JT, Buch WS, Pipkin RD, Fogarty TJ (1977) A planned approach to coexistent cerebrovascular disease in coronary artery bypass candidates. Arch Surg 112: 1403–1409
Morris GC Jr, Ennix CL Jr, Lawrie GM, Crawford ES, Howell JF (1977) Management of coexistent carotid and coronary artery occlusive atherosclerosis. Cleve Clin Q 45: 125–127
Okies JE, MacManus Q, Starr A (1977) Myocardial revascularization and carotid endarterectomy: a combined approach. Ann Thorac Surg 23: 560–563
Reul GJ, Morris GC Jr, Howell JF, Crawford ES, Stelter WJ (1972) Current concepts in coronary artery surgery. A critical analysis of 1287 patients. Ann Thorac Surg 14: 243–259
Rice PL, Pifarré R, Sullivan HJ, Montoya A, Bakhos M (1980) Experience with simultaneous myocardial revascularization and carotid endarterectomy. J Thorac Cardiovasc Surg 79: 922–925
Roederer GO, Langlois YE, Jager KA, Primozich JF, Beach KW, Phillips DJ, Standness DE Jr (1984) The natural history of carotid arterial disease in asymptomatic patients with cervical bruits. Stroke 15: 605–613
Rokey R, Rolak LA, Harati Y, Kutla N, Verani MS (1984) Coronary artery disease in patients with cerebrovascular disease: A prospective study. Ann Neurol 16: 50–53
Sumner DS, Russell JB, Miles RD (1982) Are noninvasive tests suffiiciently accurate to identify patients in need of carotid arteriography? Surgery 91: 700–706
Thompson JE, Patman RD, Talkington CM (1978) Asymptomatic carotid bruit: long-term outcome of patients having endarterectomy compared with unoperated controls. Ann Surg 188: 308–316
Toole JF, Yuson CP, Janeway R, Johnston F, Courtland D, Cordell AR, Howard G (1978) Transient ischemic attacks: a prospective study of 225 patients. Neurology 28: 746–753
Turnipseed WD, Berkhoff HA, Belzer FO (1980) Postoperative stroke in cardiac and peripheral vascular disease. Ann Surg 192: 365–368
Urschel HC, Razzuk MA, Gardner MA (1976) Management of concomitant occlusive disease of the carotid and coronary arteries. J Thorac Cardiovasc Surg 72: 829–834
Whisnant JP, Cartlidge NEF, Elveback LR (1978) Carotid and vertebral-basilar transient ischemic attacks: effect of anticoagulants, hypertension, and cardiac disorders on survival and stroke occurrence—a population study. Ann Neurol 3: 107–115
Wolf PA, Kannel WB, Sorlie P, McNamara P (1981) Asymptomatic carotid bruit and risk of stroke. The Framingham Study. JAMA 245: 1442–1445
Ziegler DK, Hassanein RS (1973) Prognosis in patients with transient ischemic attacks. Stroke 4: 666–673

Chapter 17

Asymptomatic Carotid Artery Disease in Patients Undergoing Open Heart Surgery: A Neurologic Viewpoint

J. D. Easton and R. G. Hart

Perioperative stroke, that is one which occurs intraoperatively or in the several days following an operation, is an infrequent, though often devastating, complication of surgical procedures. It occurs in 0.3% of general surgical patients, in about 1% of patients undergoing peripheral vascular reconstruction (PVR), and in 1%–5% of patients undergoing coronary artery bypass grafting (CABG) (Hart and Easton 1983). Patients undergoing PVR, including abdominal aorta surgery, and CABG are often considered to be at special risk of perioperative stroke if they have associated atherosclerotic carotid disease. An aggressive approach to the detection, evaluation, and treatment of asymptomatic cervical bruits and carotid stenosis in preoperative patients has been recommended in an effort to prevent perioperative stroke. This approach is based on the often unstated assumption that perioperative stroke is mediated by untreated carotid occlusive disease potentiated by intraoperative hypotension (Corman 1979; Hart and Hindman 1982).

Although this presumed sequence of events of perioperative stroke and its prevention is intuitively reasonable, justification for prophylatic carotid endarterectomy (CE) in preoperative patients requires critical review. Some of the important issues are: (1) what is the prevalence of asymptomatic carotid occlusive disease in preoperative patients, (2) can subgroups of preoperative patients at increased risk for perioperative stroke be effectively identified, (3) what are the mechanisms of perioperative stroke in these subgroups (and, consequently, is prophylactic CE likely to be effective), and (4) is the morbidity and mortality of prophylactic CE in these patients less than the perioperative stroke risk in patients who do not undergo prophylactic CE?

Although the primary issue here involves patients undergoing open heart surgery, the predictive value of cervical bruit and stenosis for perioperative stroke in CABG and PVR patients is reviewed. Potential differences in stroke prevalence and mechanism in these two groups necessitates their separate analysis, but the information derived from both groups is important to the final conclusion. Based on the available data, an approach to management is suggested and some of the specific issues requiring further study are defined.

Cervical Bruits and Carotid Occlusive Disease

Peripheral Vascular Reconstruction Patients

Asymptomatic cervical bruits occur in approximately 5% of the stroke-aged population and in 20% of patients undergoing PVR. These cervical bruits are not invariably associated with carotid occlusive disease as they may arise from several sources (David et al. 1973; Sandok et al. 1982). Further, cervical bruits may be present with hemodynamically insignificant degrees of carotid stenosis, only to disappear when the lumen is 1–2 mm or less in diameter (David et al. 1973).

The percentage of cervical bruits in preoperative PVR patients that is associated with carotid occlusive disease is difficult to determine since it varies with the method of investigation and criteria used to define abnormality. Noninvasive tests (NITs) of carotid occlusive disease, including oculoplethysmography, Doppler ultrasound, and carotid phonoangiography, are capable of detecting stenotic lesions compromising more than 50% of the lumen diameter with 90% sensitivity. When carotid arteries of PVR patients with asymptomatic cervical bruits are examined by NITs, only 40% show occlusive disease of the carotid bifurcation (Hart and Easton 1983). A single arteriographic study of 169 asymptomatic preoperative patients with cervical bruits (85% undergoing PVR or CABG) is available and it showed stenosis greater than 50% of the lumen diameter in nearly half of arteries with bruits. An additional 5% of arteries with bruits showed total occlusion.

Cervical bruits appear to be more common in preoperative PVR patients with a prior history of cerebral ischemia. This may reflect more careful auscultation of symptomatic patients. More likely it reflects the probability of cervical bruits being a marker, albeit unreliable, of cerebrovascular disease.

Prospective application of NIT to unselected, asymptomatic PVR patients reveals evidence of carotid stenosis in 15% (Hart and Easton 1983). One report includes a large number of PVR patients with prior cerebrovascular symptoms and demonstrates a higher prevalence of cervical bruits and carotid stenosis than do reports of asymptomatic patients. Of arteries with carotid occlusive disease demonstrated by NIT, only 45% have associated cervical bruits (Barnes et al. 1981).

All in all, cervical bruits appear to be an insensitive (about 50%) and nonspecific (about 50% false-positive rate) indicator of carotid occlusive disease in preoperative PVR patients.

Coronary Artery Bypass Graft Patients

Asymptomatic cervical bruits are present in about 10% of preoperative CABG patients and about half of such bruits are associated with carotid stenosis as demonstrated by NITs (Hart and Easton 1983). One arteriographic study of 100 CABG patients with cervical bruits, of whom one-third had prior cerebrovascular symptoms, showed carotid stenosis in nearly half (Mehigan et al. 1977).

Prospective evaluation of CABG patients with various noninvasive techniques has shown asymptomatic stenosis in about 9%, of which 30% had an associated bruit (Hart and Easton 1983).

The prevalence of both cervical bruits and carotid stenosis by NITs is consistently less in CABG patients than in PVR patients (Hennerici et al. 1981).

Perioperative Stroke Related to Cervical Bruits

Peripheral Vascular Reconstruction Patients

There are several studies describing the relationship of cervical bruits to perioperative stroke in PVR patients (Hart and Easton 1983). These reports conclude that cervical bruits do not effectively identify subgroups of asymptomatic PVR patients at risk for perioperative stroke (Mehigan et al. 1977). Perioperative stroke in these asymptomatic patients occurred in 1% of patients with bruits and in 1% of patients without bruits.

Because cervical bruits in preoperative PVR patients correlate poorly with carotid stenosis, and perhaps even more poorly with hemodynamically significant stenosis, this lack of correlation between asymptomatic cervical bruit and perioperative stroke is not surprising. However, three of these studies were retrospective and small numbers of patients in two studies were nonrandomly selected for prophylactic carotid endarterectomy. Nevertheless, in the two reports of consecutive patients with no prophylactic carotid endarterectomy, the perioperative stroke prevalence in asymptomatic PVR patients was 1% with bruits and 1% without bruits. Turnipseed et al.'s data on 16 perioperative stroke patients included 10 with nonfocal, "diffuse neurologic deficits," which are difficult to compare directly with studies reporting only focal deficits (Turnipseed et al. 1980).

The prevalence of perioperative stroke is increased in preoperative PVR patients with and without cervical bruits who have had prior cerebral ischemia (Hart and Easton 1983). These data further support the poor correlation between preoperative stroke and cervical bruit but suggest a subgroup of PVR patients at increased risk of perioperative stroke: no prior cerebrovascular symptoms—1% stroke rate; with prior symptoms—4%. In contrast, in 234 patients undergoing either PVR or CABG, Kartchner and McRae reported a 4% stroke rate in asymptomatic patients and a 4% stroke rate in patients with prior cerebrovascular symptoms (Kartchner and McRae 1981).

A single study purports to dispute the lack of relationship of cervical bruit to perioperative stroke (Thompson 1981). Thompson reported 4% perioperative strokes in 138 patients with asymptomatic bruits undergoing a variety of surgical procedures. It is not stated if the study was prospective or retrospective, whether the patients were consecutive, or what the prevalence of perioperative stroke was in age-matched controls without bruits.

In summary, cervical bruits do not identify a subset of PVR patients at special risk for perioperative stroke. On balance, the literature (Hart and Easton 1983; Ropper et al. 1982) supports Evans and Cooperman (1978), who state: "we can find no data to support the necessity for preoperative carotid arteriography and endarterectomy in the patient with an asymptomatic bruit prior to undergoing a major vascular procedure."

Coronary Artery Bypass Graft Patients

Data from several reports show an increase of perioperative stroke from about 3% in patients without bruits to about 7% in patients with bruits (Hart and Eastman 1983). In all asymptomatic patients, the perioperative stroke rate with CABG is 2% compared with 1% with asymptomatic PVR, despite a higher prevalence of cervical bruits and carotid stenosis in the latter group. Some studies report even lower stroke rates (Ivey et al. 1984; Ropper et al. 1982).

In summary, cervical bruits do not effectively identify subgroups of CABG patients with a clinically important increased risk of perioperative stroke.

Perioperative Stroke Related to Carotid Stenosis

Peripheral Vascular Reconstruction Patients

There are few studies relating perioperative stroke to carotid stenosis, as defined by NIT, in preoperative PVR patients (Hart and Easton 1983). One series prospectively evaluated 125 consecutive, asymptomatic PVR patients using Doppler ultrasound with spectral analysis (Barnes et al. 1981). Perioperative stroke occurred in 1 of 23 patients with severe carotid stenosis (but was contralateral to the side of senosis), and in 1 of 102 patients without carotid stenosis. Another study reported 7 perioperative strokes, 5 of which were nonfocal, in 160 PVR patients of whom one-third had prior cerebrovascular symptoms: 5% of patients with carotid stenosis experienced a stroke, and 4% of those without stenosis (Turnipseed et al. 1980).

In summary, data combining asymptomatic and symptomatic patients from these studies do not demonstrate an important increase in perioperative stroke in patients with carotid stenosis.

Conflicting data have been presented by Kartchner and McRae (1981) using oculoplethysmography (OPG). Of 234 patients undergoing PVR or CABG, the perioperative stroke rate was 1% in patients with normal OPG and 17% in those with moderate flow reduction (>30% flow reduction, >60% diameter stenosis). There were 31 patients who had an abnormal OPG and who were nonrandomly selected for prophylactic CE among the group with the 1% stroke rate. It was not stated how the patients were chosen for OPG or the relationship of the stroke to the side of OPG abnormality or timing of surgery, and 53% of the patients had experienced prior cerebrovascular symptoms.

The putative explanation for the reported differences in perioperative stroke rate associated with abnormal Doppler versus abnormal OPG is the relative specificity for high degrees of stenosis. If abnormal OPG reflects higher degrees of stenosis than abnormal Doppler, the reported differences would be compatible with a threshold phenomenon based on differences in technique.

However, the overall prevalence of abnormal OPG in Kartchner and McRae's series (31%) is higher than the prevalence of abnormal findings using Doppler. This suggests either that lesser degrees of stenosis were detected using OPG, or that a selected patient population was studied. The lack of correlation of abnormalities detected by NITs with perioperative stroke should be restricted to Doppler ultrasound techniques until further information is available for OPG, even though angiographic data on CABG patients does not lend support to the OPG data (see below). Ultimately, the use of angiography may offer the most useful data on the role of carotid occlusive disease in perioperative stroke in PVR patients.

Coronary Artery Bypass Graft Patients

Data from several reports using Doppler techniques show a slight increase (1.5% absolute) in perioperative stroke rate in CABG patients with carotid stenosis (more than 50% compromise of lumen diameter) (Hart and Easton 1983). As noted above, Kartchner and McRae's data using OPG in a combined population of CAGB and PVR patients showed a substantial increase in perioperative stroke in patients with abnormal OPG. But again, important details of the patient population were not provided.

Perioperative Stroke Related to Bilateral Stenosis

Some noninvasive techniques are often unreliable in predicting high degrees of stenosis or occlusion, stenosis in distal cerebral vessels, and the status of potential collateral vessels. Nevertheless, bilateral carotid stenosis detected by noninvasive testing does not appear to predict an increased risk of perioperative stroke. We and others have observed patients with perioperative stroke in the absence of carotid occlusive disease, proven angiographically or at postmortem examination, indicating that occult stenosis (false-negative NITs) is not a tenable explanation.

Based on these meager data, there is no obvious correlation between angiographic evidence of tight carotid stenosis or occlusion and perioperative stroke. Further, standard intraarterial angiography is associated with a morbidity-mortality rate which is at least 1%–2% in older patients with cardiovascular disease (Easton et al. 1983). The application of digital subtraction angiography may allow the safer definition of cerebrovascular anatomy in preoperative patients in future prospective studies.

Mechanisms of Perioperative Stroke

The mechanism of perioperative cerebral infarction is usually uncertain (Hart and Hindman 1982; Martin and Hashimoto 1982). A review of this complication in PVR patients reported in the literature shows the stroke onset to be postoperative, not intraoperative, in most patients (Hart and Easton 1983). Stroke is uncommon even in the presence of intraoperative hypotension. In CABG patients with focal perioperative stroke, half had the onset of their neurologic deficit postoperatively (Hart and Easton 1983). Thus mechanisms other than intraoperative hypotension potentiating carotid occlusive disease are probably etiologic in many perioperative stroke patients. The possibility that hypotension coupled with a diseased artery initiates a thrombotic event that eventuates in a stroke several hours later cannot be excluded.

Most reports of perioperative stroke do not define the temporal relationship of stroke to the surgery and do not consider the multiple possible mechanisms. It is possible that a subset of these patients exist in whom severe carotid occlusive disease combined with intraoperative hypotension are the crucial determinants of cerebral ischemia. However, most perioperative strokes occur in the absence of carotid occlusive disease or have their onset in the postoperative period (Hart and Easton 1983).

Correlation of occlusive disease with more subtle forms of perioperative cerebral ischemia has not been attempted but is of potential importance (Aberg et al. 1982).

Prevention of Perioperative Stroke by Endarterectomy

It cannot be assumed a priori that prophylactic removal of a carotid stenosis will be beneficial. Nevertheless, combined data concerning 63 patients undergoing PVR following successful prophylactic CE show no perioperative strokes while the predicted stroke rate in patients with carotid stenosis from other studies is 5% (Carney et al. 1977; Jain et al. 1980; Lefrak and Guinn 1974; Treiman et al. 1979). Additionally, Fields reported that perioperative stroke in patients with asymptomatic bruits was reduced from 3%–5% to an "almost negligible morbidity" after angiography and endarterectomy were routinely performed in such patients (Fields 1978).

In patients who underwent first prophylactic CE, then CABG, the combined data concerning 97 operations show one stroke following CABG (Hart and Easton 1983). The role of prophylactic CE in stroke prevention when performed simultaneously with CABG cannot be separately assessed from the overall neurologic morbidity of the combined CE/CABG procedure (5%–8%). Furlan and Craciun provide important data in this regard, leading them to conclude that asymptomatic unilateral stenosis of ⩾50% does not increase the risk of an ipsilateral brain infarct during CABG above the expected 5%. Hertzer et al. from the same institution state there is a "potential flaw" in several investigations, resulting in the conclusion that severe carotid stenoses in patients undergoing major vascular reconstruction operations can be ignored (Hertzer et al. 1984). These authors report on a large series of patients but their patients are nonconsecutive and nonrandomized and consequently no substantial scientific conclusions can be drawn.

Kartchner and McRae reported prophylactic CE in 31 patients with abnormal OPG (as part of a larger group noted above) with a perioperative stroke rate of

1% (the stroke rate in this subgroup of 31 patients could not be determined from published data) (Kartchner and McRae 1981). This compares with a 17% stroke rate in 41 patients with abnormal OPG who did not receive surgery. However, patient selection for OPG and surgery, and the relationship of perioperative stroke to the side of the OPG abnormality, were not defined.

In all of the published studies, nonconsecutive and nonrandom patients were selected for prophylactic CE.

Risk of Prophylactic Carotid Endarterectomy

The potential value of prophylactic CE in asymptomatic PVR patients requires consideration of the morbidity and mortality of the procedure in this patient population. Coexistent coronary artery disease is a major cause of perioperative morbidity in PVR and makes the risk of prophylactic CE in PVR patients higher than in the general population (Sundt et al. 1975). A review of four surgical series comprising 63 PVR patients undergoing CE, including some with prior TIA, shows a perioperative stroke rate of 5% (range 0%–10%) and a mortality rate of 2% (Carney et al. 1977; Jain et al. 1980; Lefrak and Guinn 1974; Treiman et al. 1979). Other reviews of CE in patients of all types show similar complication rates (Fields 1978; Hertzer et al. 1984). For prophylactic CE to be of value, a subgroup of PVR patients will have to be identified who have a natural history of perioperative stroke higher than the CE complication rate. This also assumes that CE will prevent most perioperative strokes. The long-term, potential benefit of CE in PVR patients may be considered but this is a separate issue, not involved in the decision to perform CE before other surgery.

Similarly, prophylactic CE in CABG shows a 5% (range 3%–11%) risk of perioperative cerebral ischemia and an additional 3% mortality in patients operated prior to their CABG, and a 5% (range 0%–12%) stroke rate in patients whose CE is performed simultaneously with their CABG (Hart and Easton 1983; Ivey et al. 1984). Patients undergoing simultaneous CE/CABG who have bilateral stenosis may be at special risk of complication. Except for the Ivey et al. study, these are aggregate data from reports of nonrandomized, nonconsecutive patients. It is possible that, on average, patients undergoing prophylactic CE have higher degrees of carotid stenosis than consecutive patients with carotid stenosis identified prospectively by NITs, confounding direct comparison.

A summary of the aggregate data, based on review of the literature (Fields 1978), is outlined in Table 17.1. It is emphasized that prophylactic CE patients were not chosen consecutively or randomly in these series and that the series consist of patients with and without prior cerebrovascular symptoms. Only the report of Kartchner and McRae demonstrating a 17% perioperative stroke rate in selected PVR and CABG patients with abnormal OPG suggests a subgroup that could potentially benefit from prophylactic CE. Their data conflict with consecutive series of other authors.

Table 17.1. Outcome for stroke in PVR and CABG surgery

	Ischemic stroke
Natural history	
PVR	
Bruit	2%
No bruit	1%
Stenosis[a]	5%
No stenosis[a]	3%
CABG	
Bruit	7%
No bruit	3%
Stenosis[a]	4%
No stenosis[a]	3%
Prophylactic CE	
PVR–before	5% (+2% mortality)
CABG–before	4% (+3% mortality)
CABG–simultaneous	5%

Abbreviations: PVR, peripheral vascular reconstruction; CABG, coronary artery bypass graft; CE, carotid endarterectomy
[a] Determined by Doppler studies.

Conclusions

1. Cervical bruits are common.
2. Bruits do not predict stroke, except minimally.
3. The stroke plus death rate in patients undergoing CABG is 1%–5%.
4. The stroke plus death rate in patients with bruit undergoing CABG is 2%–6%.
5. The stroke plus death rate in patients undergoing angiography plus CE is about 7%.
6. There is good evidence that cervical bruit and stenosis do not effectively identify patients at high risk for perioperative stroke and prophylactic CE has not been proven to be beneficial for patients undergoing open heart surgery.

References

Aberg T, Ronquist G, Tyden H, Ahlund P, Bergstrom K (1982) Release of adenylate kinase into cerebrospinal fluid during open-heart surgery and its relation to postoperative intellectual function. Lancet 1: 1139–1142

Balderman SC, Gutierrez IZ, Makula P, Bhayana JN, Gage AA (1983) Noninvasive screening for asymptomatic carotid artery disease prior to cardiac operation. Experience with 500 patients. J Thorac Cardiovasc Surg 85: 427–433

Barnes RW, Liebman PR, Marszalek PB, Kirk CL, Goldman MH (1981) The natural history of asymptomatic carotid disease in patients undergoing cardiovascular surgery. Surgery 90: 1075–1081

Breslau PJ, Fell G, Ivey TD, Bailey WW, Miller DW, Strandness DE Jr (1981) Carotid arterial disease in patients undergoing coronary artery bypass operations. J Thorac Cardiovasc Surg 82: 765–767

Carney WI, Stewart WB, DePinto DJ, Mucha SJ, Roberts B (1977) Carotid bruit as a risk factor in aortoiliac reconstruction. Surgery 81: 567–570

Corman LC (1979) The preoperative patient with an asymptomatic cervical bruit. Med Clin North Amer 63: 1335–1340

David TE, Humphries AW, Young FR, Beven EG (1973) A correlation of neck bruits and arteriosclerotic carotid arteries. Arch Surg 107: 729–731

Easton JD, Hart RG, Sherman DG, Kaste M (1983) Diagnosis and management of ischemic stroke. Part I. Threatened stroke and its management. Curr Probl Cardiol 8: 1–76

Evans WE, Cooperman M (1978) The significance of asymptomatic unilateral carotid bruits in preoperative patients. Surgery 83: 521–522

Fields WS (1978) The asymptomatic carotid bruit-operate or not? Stroke 9: 269–271

Furlan AJ, Cracium AR (1985) Risk of stroke during coronary artery bypass graft surgery in patients with internal carotid artery disease documented by angiography. Stroke 16: 797–799

Hart RG, Easton JD (1983) Management of cervical bruits and carotid stenosis in preoperative patients. Stroke 14: 290–297

Hart RG, Hindman BJ (1982) Mechanisms of perioperative cerebral infarction. Stroke 13: 766–773

Hennerici M, Aulich A, Sandmann W, Freund H-J (1981) Occurrence of asymptomatic extracranial arterial bruits. Stroke: 12: 750–758

Hertzer NR, Beven EG, Young JR, O'Hara PJ, Graor RA, Ruschhaupt WF III (1984) Incidental asymptomatic carotid bruits in patients scheduled for peripheral vascular reconstruction: results of cerebral and coronary angiography. Surgery 96: 535–544

Ivey TD, Straudness DE, Williams DB, Langlois Y, Misbach GA, Kruse AP (1984) Management of patients with carotid bruit undergoing cardiopulmonary bypass. J Thorac Cardiovasc Surg 87: 183–189

Jain KM, Hobson RW, Jamil Z, Marsters C, Berry SM (1980) Clinical screening of preoperative patients for carotid occlusive disease by oculoplethysmography. Am Surg 46: 679–685

Jones EL, Craver JM, Michalik RA, Murphy DA, Guyton RA, Bone DK, Hatcher CR, Reichwald NA (1984) Combined carotid and coronary operations: when are they necessary? J Thorac Cardiovasc Surg 87: 7–16

Kartchner MM, McRae LP (1981) Guidelines for noninvasive evaluation of asyptomatic carotid bruits. Clin Neurosurg 28: 418–428

Lefrak EA, Guinn GA (1974) Prophylactic carotid artery surgery in patients requiring a second operation. Southern Med J 67: 185–189

Martin WRW, Hashimoto SA (1982) Stroke in coronary bypass surgery. Can J Neurol Sci 9: 21–26

Mehigan JT, Buch WS, Pipkin RD, Fogarty TJ (1977) A planned approach to co-existent cerebrovascular disease in coronary artery bypass candidates. Arch Surg 112: 1403–1409

Ropper AH, Wechsler LR, Wilson LS (1982) Carotid bruit and the risk of stroke in elective surgery. N Engl J Med 307: 1388–1390

Sandok BA, Whisnant JP, Furlan AJ, Mickell JL (1982) Carotid artery bruits: prevalence survey and differential diagnosis. Mayo Clin Proc 57: 227–230

Sundt TM Jr, Sandok BA, Whisnant JP (1975) Carotid endarterectomy: complications and preoperative assessment of risk. Mayo Clin Proc 50: 301–306

Thompson J (1981) Discussant in Barnes RW et al. (1981) The natural history of asymptomatic carotid disease in patients undergoing cardiovascular surgery. Surgery 90: 1081

Treiman RL, Foran RF, Cohen JL (1979) Carotid bruit: a follow-up report on its significance in patients undergoing an abdominal operation. Arch Surg 114: 1138–1140

Turnipseed WD, Berkoff HA, Belzer FO (1980) Postoperative stroke in cardiac and peripheral vascular disease. Ann Surg 192: 365–368

Section E

EPIDEMIOLOGY AND RISK FACTORS

Chapter 18

Risk Factor Interaction in Cardiovascular and Cerebrovascular Disease*

P. A. Wolf, W. B. Kannel, L. A. Cupples, and R. B. D'Agostino

Introduction

Of the ten leading causes of death among adults in the United States, coronary heart disease (CHD) is number one and cerebrovascular disease ranks number three. The American Heart Association estimates that 554900 persons died of CHD and 159600 of stroke in the United States in 1982 (American Heart Association 1985). Furthermore, it is estimated there are 4670000 CHD and 1900000 stroke victims still living in 1982. These manifestations of atherosclerosis have been related to a number of host and environmental factors delineated over the past 4 decades chiefly through prospective epidemiologic study. The relative impact and evolution of these attributes into clinical atherosclerotic disease is not identical for coronary, cerebral, or limb arteries. The manifestions of these diseases and their precursors also differ in men and women, at different ages, and in different racial groups. Assessment of these differences may disclose important clues to pathogenesis and thereby provide strategies for prevention.

Utilizing data collected in the Heart Disease Epidemiology Study at Framingham, Massachusetts, it is possible to compare and contrast the determinants, incidence, and manifestations of stroke and CHD as they evolved in this general population sample over 30 years of follow-up. Assessment of risk factors measured systematically and prospectively, often many years prior to the appearance of clinical disease, provides the least distorted picture of the evolution of these host and environmental factors into clinical disease.

* Supported in part by grants numbers NIH-IPO-INS-16367 and 1-RO1-NS-17950-01 with Contract NO1-NS-2-2398 (Philip A. Wolf, M.D., National Institute of Neurological Communicative Disorders and Stroke); and Contracts number NIH-NO1-HV-92922 and NIH-NO1-HV-52971 (William B. Kannel, M.D., National Heart, Lung and Blood Institute).

Incidence of Atherosclerotic Cerebrovascular Disease and Coronary Heart Disease

The American Heart Association estimates that there were 500 000 new cases of stroke and 1 500 000 new cases of CHD in the United States in 1982 (American Heart Association 1985). The reported incidence of these events varies widely, depending on the source of the data (hospitalized cases or general population), its age composition, and whether initial and recurrent cases are included. It is estimated that approximately 400 000 stroke patients are discharged annually from acute-care hospitals in the United States, three-fourths after an initial stroke and the remainder following recurrence (Kurtzke 1976a; Robins and Buam 1981).

Analogous manifestions of CHD and stroke may be compared by examining these diseases as they have evolved in the general population sample at Framingham, Massachusetts. These Framingham data are derived from 30 years of follow-up of more than 5000 men and women age 30–62 and free of cardiovascular disease (CVD) at entry into the study in 1950. During the 30 years of follow-up 1334 instances of CHD and 478 cases of stroke and TIA have occurred.

The Framingham Heart Study population represents the respondents of a two-thirds sample of adults resident in the town in 1948 as well as their spouses and some volunteers. After the initial exam in 1950 those 5070 persons, 2252 men and 2818 women, found to be free of CVD have received biennial examination. Examination 18 was completed in 1985. Surveillance has been maintained at the only hospital in town for disease occurrence, and all deaths are monitored. Persons reporting neurologic symptoms or demonstrating signs consistent with stroke at the biennial exam have been evaluated by the study neurologist to document the event and findings. In recent years computerized tomographic scans of the brain have been available on virtually all stroke cases and arteriography has frequently been obtained by the subjects' personal physician. When autopsy was done, the neuropathologic examination findings at postmortem are taken into account in reaching a conclusion as to the presence and type of stroke.

Neurologic evaluation at the time of the stroke has been made for the past 20 years. This in-hospital assessment by the study neurologist has contributed to the documentation of stroke cases and in distinguishing stroke from other neurologic disease. Evaluation of subjects with stroke at the time of the event in the hospital has greatly facilitated identification of type of stroke, particularly during the years prior to CT scan. Utilizing all available information, it has often been possible to determine if the mechanism of stroke was subarachnoid or intraparenchymatous hemorrhage, infarction as a result of large vessel atherothrombosis, or due to lacunar disease, and to identify cases of stroke secondary to embolism from the heart. Follow-up of the population has been satisfactory, with 85% taking each exam and only 7% completely lost to follow-up for death after 30 years.

Relative frequency of CHD and stroke may be compared by examining age and sex-specific average annual incidence rates (per 1000) of myocardial infarction (MI) and atherothrombotic brain infarction (ABI) (Fig. 18.1). Both

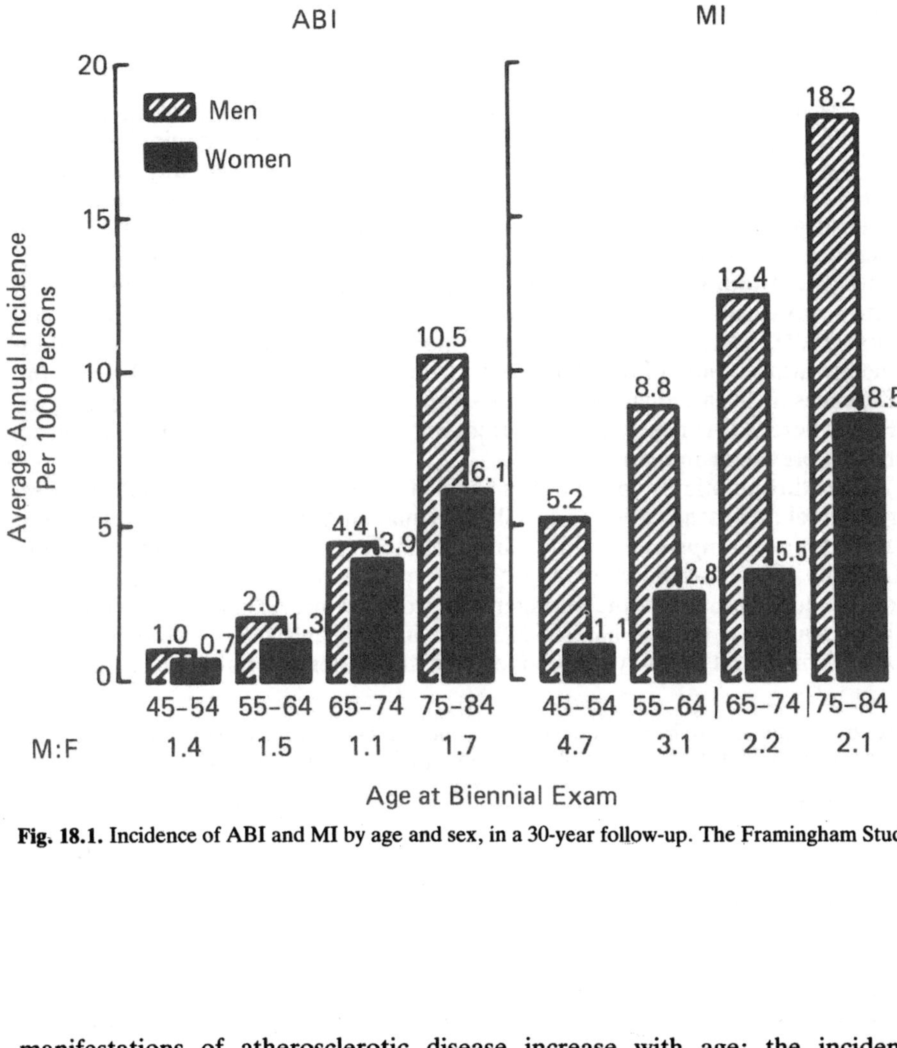

Fig. 18.1. Incidence of ABI and MI by age and sex, in a 30-year follow-up. The Framingham Study.

manifestations of atherosclerotic disease increase with age; the incidence doubles in each successive decade. In men, the age-adjusted average annual incidence rate of MI for ages 35–64 is 6/1000; for ages 65–94 it is 13/1000. In contrast, age-adjusted ABI rates are 1/1000 for ages 35–64 and 5/1000 at ages 65–94. Overall MI incidence is three times that of ABI. For women, age-adjusted average annual incidence rates for MI and ABI are less disparate at 2/1000 and 1/1000 for ages 35–64, and 7/1000 versus 4/1000 at 65–94 years respectively. In both sexes rates rise with age but the 20-year lag in MI incidence experienced by women does not occur for ABI, where age-specific rates are similar. Overall, the incidence rate of MI in men is 2.75 times the rate in women; while ABI is about 1.3 times more frequent in men. The rates for 30 years of follow-up are derived using a denominator that is different from that used in prior publications since the 30-year follow-up population at risk consists of subjects free of *all* cardiovascular disease.

Manifestations of Stroke and CHD

There is a greater variation in the manifestations of CHD than there is for stroke. Using the 30-year follow-up data derived from the Framingham Heart Study, it is apparent that manifestations of CHD differ substantially in men and women. At all ages, men have more MI and sudden death (SD) and women an excess of angina pectoris (AP) (Table 18.1). For stroke there is no substantial difference in stroke manifestation by sex; the major differences relate to age, with more stroke due to cerebral embolism (CE) in the older age group and slightly more subarachnoid hemorrhage (SAH) in younger men and women (Table 18.2). SAH and CE are slightly more frequent in women and transient ischemic attacks only (TIA Only) more frequent in younger men. Overall, the differences in disease manifestation by sex for stroke are far less striking than for CHD, where AP is nearly twice as frequent in women and MI and SD are 1.5 times as prevalent in men.

Atherothrombotic brain infarction, which includes infarction resulting from large vessel atherothrombosis as well as lacunar infarction, is the most frequent manifestation, comprising slightly more than half of all strokes regardless of age. TIA Only, which accounts for approximately 10% of all stroke events, may be more frequent in men in the younger age group, while CE, with a documented cardiac source, is the mechanism of stroke in 12% and 14% of younger stroke cases in men and women respectively. In the older age group CE incidence

Table 18.1. The relative frequency of clinical manifestations of coronary heart disease in men and women, ages 35–64, and 65–94, in a 30-year follow-up, The Framingham Study

CHD Manifestation	Ages 35–64		Ages 65–94	
	Men	Women	Men	Women
Myocardial infarction	43%	23%	43%	27%
Coronary insufficiency	8%	9%	5%	7%
Angina pectoris	31%	54%	20%	38%
Sudden death	10%	6%	15%	11%
CHD death nonsudden	8%	8%	17%	17%

Table 18.2. The relative frequency of clincial manifestations of stroke in men and women, ages 35–64, and 65–94, in a 30-year follow-up, The Framingham Study

Stroke type	Percentage of strokes by type			
	Ages 35–64		Ages 65–94	
	Men	Women	Men	Women
ABI	54%	54%	55%	52%
CE	12%	14%	20%	25%
IH	6%	4%	6%	3%
SAH	10%	13%	6%	8%
Other	2%	7%	3%	1%
TIA Only	16%	8%	10%	11%

doubles, with 20% of strokes in men and 25% of strokes in women attributable to embolism. Intracranial hemorrhage accounted for 14% of all stroke events; the hemorrhage was twice as frequently subarachnoid from a berry aneurysm as intraparenchymatous in type.

Risk Factors for Stroke and Coronary Heart Disease

Atherogenic Host Factors

Deposition of atheromatous material in the arterial wall leads to compromise of the arterial lumen and reduction of the blood supply to brain or heart muscle. This in turn results in the manifestations of CHD and in cerebral infarction, which accounts for approximately 85% of all strokes. Since the underlying process is similar, it is not surprising that the two diseases generally share common risk factors. However, the relative impact of the individual risk factors differs in the coronary and cerebral arteries, and certain of the precursors of stroke and CHD exert varying influences according to the sex and the age of the individual at risk. A knowledge of the importance of each of the precursors and of its interaction with other host and environmental factors may yield important clues to the understanding of disease development and thereby to disease prevention.

The relative importance of some of the major risk factors for cardiovascular disease may be examined in Table 18.3 for men and Table 18.4 for women. The impact of each risk factor may be deduced by comparing the size of the

Table 18.3. Comparison of risk factors for ABI and MI by means of standardized multivariate regression coefficients,[a] in men, ages 35–64 and 65–94, in a 30-year follow-up, The Framingham Study

Risk factor	Standardized multivariate regression coefficients			
	Atherothrombotic brain infarction		Myocardial infarction	
	Ages 35–64	Ages 65–94	Ages 35–64	Ages 65–94
Hypertension	0.823***	0.509***	0.292***	0.340***
Systolic BP	0.646***	0.470***	0.256***	0.342***
Diastolic BP	0.634***	0.226	0.257***	0.153
LVH by ECG	0.133*	0.104	0.049	0.173**
Cigarettes	0.422***	0.058	0.370***	−0.069
Total serum cholesterol	0.111	−0.140	0.225***	0.058
Glucose intolerance	0.050	0.113	0.122*	0.079
Metropolitan relative weight	0.158	−0.128	0.029	0.106
Hematocrit	0.320**	0.068	0.100	0.046

*$P<0.05$; **$P<0.01$; ***$P<0.001$

[a] Multivariate contains systolic blood pressure, LVH by ECG, cigarette smoking, glucose intolerance, total serum cholesterol, and the other appropriate variable

Table 18.4. Comparison of risk factors for ABI and MI by means of standardized multivariate regression coefficients,[a] in women, ages 35–64 and 65–94, in a 30-year follow-up, The Framingham Study

Risk factor	Standardized multivariate regression coefficients			
	Atherothrombotic brain infarction		Myocardial infarction	
	Ages 35–64	Ages 65–94	Ages 35–64	Ages 65–94
Hypertension	0.817***	0.647***	0.419***	0.256*
Systolic BP	0.624***	0.550***	0.416***	0.267**
Diastolic BP	0.665***	0.493***	0.395***	0.077
LVH by ECG	0.111	0.208***	0.036	0.151*
Cigarettes	0.019	0.235*	0.454***	0.047
Total serum cholesterol	0.124	−0.262*	0.276***	0.255**
Glucose intolerance	0.106	0.269**	0.221***	0.235**
Metropolitan relative weight	0.166	−0.117	0.044	0.135
Hematocrit	0.117	0.041	0.144	0.006

$^{*}P<0.05$; $^{**}P<0.01$; $^{***}P<0.001$

[a] Multivariate contains systolic blood pressure, LVH by ECG, cigarette smoking, glucose intolerance, total serum cholesterol, and the other appropriate variable

multivariate regression coefficients, standardized for the varied units and scales, and which take into account the contribution that other risk factors make to incidence of brain infarction (ABI) and to MI. The larger the standardized multivariate regression coefficient the greater the impact on disease incidence. The presence of a statistically significant coefficient indicates the risk factor makes a significant *independent* contribution to risk even after age and other pertinent risk factors are taken into account.

Hypertension. Hypertension is the dominant precursor of stroke. For ABI, the standardized multivariate regression coefficient for hypertension is large, denoting a powerful and independent contribution of definite hypertension, i.e., a blood pressure level of >160/95+ mmHg, to ABI risk. This is true in both sexes and in both age categories. Definite hypertension is also strongly and significantly related to MI.

Increasing severity of hypertension is related to increased incidence of ABI and MI (Fig. 18.2). It is clear that at all ages in the adult years, and in both sexes, there is a gradient of incidence for both ABI and MI from normotension (a blood pressure level of <140/90 mmHg), to borderline elevations of blood pressure (blood pressure levels greater than normortension but less than >160/95 mmHg), to definite hypertension. In every age group and in both sexes the *risk ratio* of definite hypertension to normotension is greater for ABI than for MI. There is no consistent differential in relative risk of hypertension for either MI or ABI according to sex.

Systolic Versus Diastolic Pressure Level. By comparing standardized coefficients (Tables 18.3, 18.4), it is apparent that systolic blood pressure coefficients are generally larger than diastolic ones in both men and women for both MI and

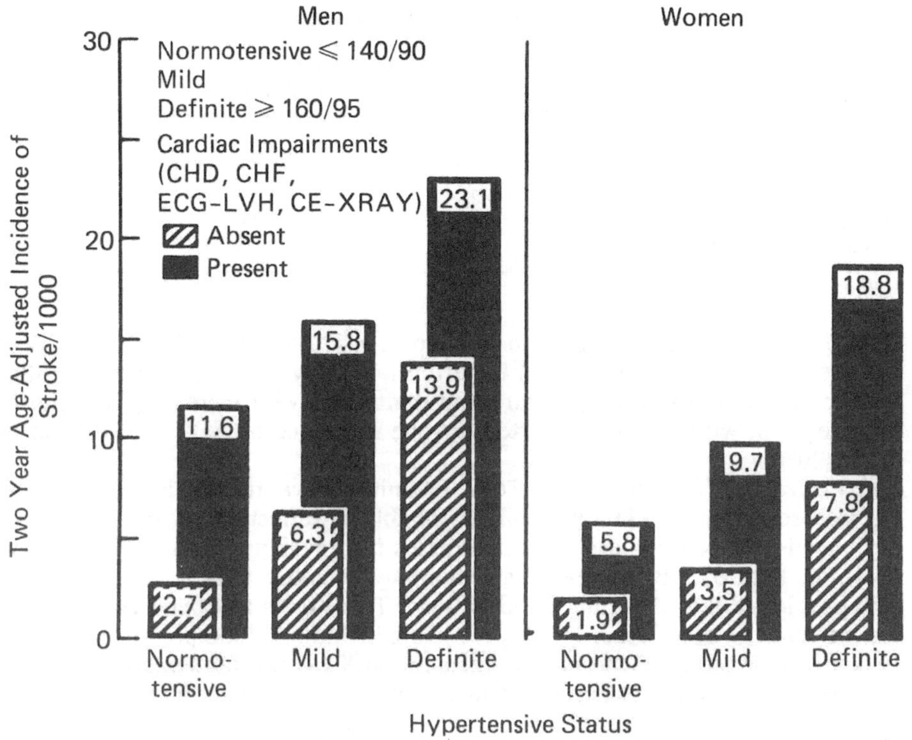

Fig. 18.2. Incidence of stroke according to hypertensive status and presence of cardiac impairments; The Framingham Study; subjects 35–84 years.

ABI. It is noteworthy that diastolic blood pressure coefficients do not reach statistical significance in the older age group in men for either MI or ABI or for older women for MI while systolic coefficients are both substantial and statistically significant in both diseases at all ages and in both sexes. Furthermore, by comparing standardized regression coefficients for systolic and diastolic pressure in each age group and by sex it is clear that systolic coefficients are generally larger than diastolic ones, that the coefficients are quite similar in men and women, and for stroke the coefficients do not decrease substantially with advancing age. These data contradict the notion that the effect of increased blood pressure on stroke incidence wanes with advancing age and that systolic elevations are innocuous, particularly in the elderly. There is no evidence that women tolerate hypertension better than men or that diastolic elevations are more important than systolic pressures.

Severity of Hypertension and Incidence of MI and ABI. It has been asserted that at borderline or mild levels of hypertension, CHD or MI is the major risk while at higher levels of pressure stroke or ABI is more likely. This impression was corroborated by determining the ratio of MI to ABI at three levels of hypertension, i.e., normotension, borderline, and definite hypertension, in the Framingham cohort (Table 18.5). The ratio of MI to ABI, in men, diminishes

Table 18.5. Ratio of MI to ABI according to hypertensive status, men and women, ages 35–94, in a 30-year follow-up, The Framingham Study

	Ratio of age-adjusted average annual incidence of MI and ABI	
Hypertensive status	Men	Women
Normotension	5.2	3.4
Borderline hypertension	4.8	2.0
Definite hypertension	2.2	1.1

from 5.2 to 4.8 to 2.2 going from nonhypertensive to borderline (or mild) to definite (or moderate and severe) hypertension. In women, the ratio is smaller for each category of blood pressure and diminishes with increasing severity of hypertension; with definite hypertension the incidence of ABI exceeds that of MI by 20%.

Left Ventricular Hypertrophy by ECG. Definite left ventricular hypertrophy by electrocardiogram (LVH by ECG), probably a reflection of the impact of prolonged or severe hypertension, increases in prevalence with age and blood pressure. Risk of ABI increased substantially by more than fourfold in those who developed this abnormal ECG pattern. This excess risk persists even after the influence of other atherogenic precursors including blood pressure and age. In contrast, generalized cardiac enlargement on X-ray was far less powerful than definite LVH by ECG, when other factors are taken into account.

Blood Lipids. Total serum cholesterol is significantly and independently related to the development of MI in women but only in younger men. The association is also quite strong for all other manifestations of CHD in both sexes but the impact seems to diminish beyond age 55, particularly in men. However, when blood cholesterol is partitioned into its components of high-, low-, and very low-density lipoproteins, a relationship with CHD in persons over age 55 reemerges. High-density lipoprotein-cholesterol (HDL) is inversely related to incidence of CHD, while low-density lipoprotein-cholesterol (LDL) is positively associated with CHD.

The association of total serum cholesterol and lipoprotein-cholesterol fractions with the occurrence of stroke or ABI is far less clear or consistent. The only significant correlation is in older women; an *inverse* relationship of higher serum cholesterol to lower ABI incidence. Six-year follow-up of the cohort after blood lipid fractionation showed no significant positive association of LDL cholesterol to ABI incidence and no protective effect of HDL cholesterol. The sole significant relationship of a lipoprotein-cholesterol fraction to stroke incidence is the *negative* association of LDL cholesterol to ABI in women, and there was no apparent relationship of triglyceride to ABI risk.

Diabetes. Clinical observation of diabetic patients has disclosed an increased susceptibility to atherosclerosis including cerebrovascular disease. From surveys of stroke and prospective study of stroke in defined populations it is clear that diabetics are at increased risk of developing symptomatic cerebrovascular disease. In the United States in 1976–1980, a medical history of stroke was 2.5–4 times more common in diabetics than in persons with normal glucose tolerance (Kuller et al. 1985).

In Framingham, peripheral arterial disease with intermittent claudication (IC) occurs more than four times more often in those with diabetes, and the coronary and cerebral arteries are also affected to a lesser extent. The impact of glucose intolerance, i.e., physician-diagnosed diabetes, glycosuria, or a blood sugar >150 mg/100 ml, is greater in women than men both for MI and ABI. The only instance where glucose intolerance makes a significant independent contribution to disease incidence in men is for MI and then only in the 35-to 64-year age group (Table 18.3). When the impact of diabetes on coronary, cerebral, and peripheral artery atherosclerotic disease is compared it is apparent that the relative risk for diabetes is greatest for IC than for ABI, with a lesser, but still substantial, effect on CHD (Table 18.6) (Kannel and McGee 1979).

Table 18.6. Average annual age-adjusted incidence per 1000 for specified cardiovascular events, men and women, aged 45–74 years, in a 20-year follow-up, The Framingham Study. (Kannel and McGee 1979)

Cardiovascular event	Men			Women		
	Diabetic	Nondiabetic	Relative risk	Diabetic	Nondiabetic	Relative risk
CHD	24.8	14.9	1.7	17.8	6.9	2.6
ABI	4.7	1.9	2.5	6.2	1.7	3.6
IC	12.6	3.3	3.8	8.4	1.3	6.5

Obesity. Obesity is clearly related to hypertension, impaired glucose tolerance, and elevated blood lipids. On this account alone overweight can be expected to be associated with increased stroke and CHD risk. However, when other relevant risk factors are taken into account there is no residual increase in risk from overweight, here represented as the Metropolitan Relative Weight (Tables 18.3, 18.4). That should not be taken to imply that obesity does not exert an adverse influence on health status, just that the mechanism of the increased disease occurrence is probably mediated through abnormal blood lipids, increased systolic blood pressure and hypertension, and impaired glucose tolerance and other mechanisms. Recent studies have suggested that the pattern of obesity is also important with abdominal deposition of fat associated with disease.

Hematocrit. Data from Framingham have demonstrated the relationship of high normal hematocrit level to increased incidence of cerebral infarction (Leonberg and Elliott 1981). Confirmation of this relationship has come from an autopsy study of Japanese stroke patients (Kannel et al. 1972) and from several clinical and radiologic studies of patients with stroke (Thomas et al. 1977; Tohgi et al. 1978; Pearson and Thomas 1979). In these 30-year follow-up data, elevated blood hematocrit, within the normal range, and generally not pathologically elevated red cell mass, is significantly and independently associated with ABI in men even after the confounding effects of cigarette smoking and hypertension are taken into account. The reason for the different impact in the two sexes is unclear. The influence of increments of concentration of red blood cells in concert with increasing blood fibrinogen levels on blood viscosity has recently been demonstrated (Kee and Wood 1984). This interplay may reach pathologic significance in narrowed small penetrating arteries (Tohgi et al. 1978), and in high-grade stenosis of a major cerebral artery (Grotta et al. 1982). Reduction of high normal hematocrit by venesection has decreased blood viscosity and correspondingly increased cerebral blood flow.

Fibrinogen. Serum fibrinogen has been implicated in atherogenesis and in arterial thrombus formation. In addition, laboratory and clinical studies have shown serum fibrinogen together with hematocrit to have important effects on blood viscosity and cerebral blood flow (Grotta et al. 1982). However, data from prospective epidemiologic study assessing the impact of fibrinogen and stroke incidence are quite sparse. A recent prospective study in Swedish men disclosed fibrinogen in concert with elevated systolic blood pressure to be a potent risk factor for stroke in sample of 54-year-olds followed for 13 years (Wilhelmsen et al. 1984).

On the 10th biennial exam fibrinogen was determined in Framingham in 1470 persons, approximately half of the surviving cohort. The 644 men and 826 women, then aged 47–79 and free of stroke, have been followed for the development of stroke, CHD, and CVD. Total CVD represents all cases of CHD, stroke, hypertensive cardiovascular disease, and congestive heart failure. After 12 years, 312 persons have developed CVD; 92 were stroke, 214 were CHD; half of the stroke cases were brain infarctions. Risk of stroke, CHD, and total CVD increased in proportion to fibrinogen level over the 180- to 450-mg/dl range in all age groups; the rise was steeper in men than women and in the 50–59 and 60–69 age groups. However, fibrinogen was also positively associated with most of the major risk factors for stroke, CHD, and total CVD incidence, including age, hypertensive status, hematocrit level, obesity, and diabetes. Fibrinogen levels increased with age in both sexes, with no significant difference between mean levels in men and women.

When a multivariate analysis of the pertinent risk factors was made including all the important risk factors, fibrinogen was significantly and independently related to total CVD ($P<0.01$), as was age, blood pressure, cholesterol, and diabetes. For either stroke or CHD, the coefficient for fibrinogen was not statistically significant in this limited number of cases. The 12-year age-adjusted incidence rates for total CVD, CHD, and stroke rise with increasing levels of fibrinogen. These trends are significant in both sexes for total CVD, and in men for stroke.

Race. The Japanese have been known to have low rates of CHD and a high prevalence of stroke (Omae et al. 1976). A recent survey of six mainland Chinese cities disclosed a high incidence and prevalence of stroke in Chinese at a level comparable to that in native Japanese in Japan (Li et al. 1985). The disparity between the stroke and CHD death rates, and presumably similar disparity in incidence rates, is usually attributed to the high prevalence of hypertension and the low levels of blood lipids in these racial groups (Takeya et al. 1984). Cerebrovascular disease was the most frequently certified cause of death in Japan during the decades following World War II, and the mechanism of stroke was most frequently thought to be intraparenchymatous hemorrhage. In the 1980s cancer has become the leading cause of death, with stroke falling to number 2 with CHD at number 3. In Japanese men in Hawaii and San Francisco deaths attributed to stroke are falling relative to CHD (and cancer) death rates (Kagan et al. 1985; Takeya et al. 1984; Tanaka et al. 1982).

In 1985 heart disease moved into second place as a cause of death in Japan at 114.8/100 000 following cancer (156.4/100 000), with stroke falling to number 3 with a mortality rate of 110.6/100 000 (Japanese Health and Welfare Ministry 1986).

Table 18.7. Leading causes of death in Japanese men, age 60+ years

Rank	Japan 1960s[a]	Japan 1981[b]	Hawaii 1981[c]	San Francisco 1981[c]
1.	Stroke	Cancer	Cancer	CHD
2.	Cancer	Stroke	CHD	Cancer
3.	CHD	CHD	Stroke	Stroke

[a] Omae et al. (1976)
[b] Takeya et al. 1984
[c] Kagan et al. 1985

Autopsy studies have disclosed the most frequent mechanism of stroke to be cerebral infarction not hemorrhage (Stemmerman et al. 1984). There is also a difference in the site of the arterial pathology with a predominance of intracranial arterial disease in native Japanese in contrast to the pattern in white Americans where the extracranial arteries are the focus of most of the atherosclerotic occlusive disease (EC/IC Bypass Study Group 1985). The Japanese migration to Hawaii and the western United States has created an experiment of nature where better nutrition, consisting of an increase in protein and fats in the diets of these Japanese, has been associated with an increase in serum cholesterol and in the development of CHD (Kagan et al. 1985). Recent clinical and angiographic studies in American blacks have suggested a predominance of intracranial arterial involvement similar to the pattern seen in the Japanese (Mohr et al. 1978).

Environmental Factors

Smoking. Cigarette smoking is significantly related to ABI and MI in men and women. A similar relationship between cigarette smoking and stroke has been seen in Hawaiian Japanese men after 12 years of follow-up in the Honolulu Heart Study, where cigarette smoking made a significant independent contribution to cerebral infarction and intracranial hemorrhage risk (Abbott et al. 1986).

In the Framingham cohort cigarette smoking is a significant independent contributor to ABI incidence in the older age category for women, but not in the younger group. This may be related to the relative rarity of women smokers in the Framingham cohort in the early years of the study and the small number of stroke events occurring to date in this younger age group of 35–64. The relationship of ABI to cigarette smoking in older women may represent an important and unique interaction between postmenopausal estrogen use, cigarette smoking, and cardiovascular disease development, particularly stroke (Wilson et al. 1985).

Oral Contraceptives. An increased risk of both myocardial infarction and stroke has been reported in users of oral contraceptives (OCs), particularly in older women, i.e., above age 35, and predominantly in those with other cardiovascular risk factors particularly hypertension and cigarette smoking (Stadel 1981). In a recent review it was estimated the relative risk of MI to be increased three- to fourfold above age 30 in OC users and of stroke to be increased fivefold for all types and all ages combined. For both diseases risk seemed to be concentrated in women above age 35 or 40 who smoked cigarettes (Longstreth et al. 1985).

The pathogenesis of cardiovascular disease and OC use is less clear for stroke than for MI. The pathology underlying MI in OC users, on the basis of postmortem examinations, was not coronary atherosclerosis but rather thrombotic occlusion (Mann and Inman 1975). Clotting is believed to be enhanced by the OC-induced increased platelet aggregability and by its alteration of clotting factors to promote thrombogenesis. In stroke, "thromboembolism" is often said to be increased (Stadel 1981), but series of cases often contain women with transient episodes of neurologic dysfunction ("TIAs"), and record reviews of cases for case-control studies are composed of a substantial number of strokes due to ill-defined and uncertain cause (Collaborative Group for the Study of Stroke in Young Women 1973, 1975). The risk seemed highest in women who took OCs containing higher levels of estrogen (Handin 1974), and the lower levels of estrogen in the newer OC formulations may have substantially reduced the risk (Stadel 1981).

Because of the relative rarity of stroke in the age group 15–45, most studies of the association of OCs to stroke have entailed a retrospective case-control methodology. There are data to suggest the relationship of OC to increased stroke incidence is not conclusively established. Death rates from stroke have fallen in this age group no less than in other ages and the rates have been nearly equal in men and women below age 45 both before and since the introduction of the pill (Wiseman and McRae 1981). Further, most large neurology centers encounter a small number of nonpuerperal strokes each year in otherwise healthy persons 15–45 years of age, with equal frequency in men and women (Schoenberg et al. 1970).

Prospective observation of over 40000 women half of whom were taking OCs showed an increased risk of fatal stroke in women taking OCs occurring mainly as a result of subarachnoid hemorrhage and not thromboembolism (Royal College of General Practitioners' Oral Contraception Study 1981). Risk was increased fourfold in cigarette smokers above age 35, with most cases confined to this group. The pathogenesis of increased risk of subarachnoid hemorrhage from berry aneurysm in older OC users who are cigarette smokers is unclear. Further study of this association may provide clues to the pathogenesis of stroke due to subarachnoid hemorrhage.

Alcohol Consumption. The impact of alcohol consumption on CHD and stroke risk is dependent on the amount of alcohol consumed. Heavy alcohol use, either habitual daily heavy alcohol consumption or binge drinking, seems to be related to an excess in CHD deaths and stroke (Hennekens 1983). Light or moderate alcohol consumption, on the other hand, is convincingly associated with a reduced incidence of CHD (Stason et al. 1976). Light and moderate alcohol use tends to raise the HDL cholesterol and may be associated with a reduction in

CHD incidence, while high levels of alcohol intake are linked to hypertension and hypertriglyceridemia and may in this way be associated with an increased rate of CHD and stroke.

The relationship of alcohol consumption to stroke occurrence is less clearly elucidated. Available evidence rather uniformly demonstrates an adverse effect of drinking alcohol on stroke. Stroke incidence has been positively associated with alcohol consumption in prospective studies in Yugoslavia and in Japanese men in Hawaii (Kozarevic et al. 1980; Blackwelder et al. 1980). Intracranial hemorrhage, but not thromboembolic stroke, was significantly associated with alcohol consumption in the Honolulu Heart Study of men of Japanese ancestry (Kagan et al. 1985). This association was attributed to the coexistent hypertension associated with alcohol intake. Data from the Framingham study also suggest an increased incidence of brain infarction and stroke with increased levels of alcohol use, but only in men.

Cigarette smoking is more frequent in heavy drinkers, and there is attendant hemoconcentration. Alcohol and cigarette smoking have been shown to increase blood hematocrit and viscosity (Dintenfass 1975) and rebound thrombocytosis during abstinence has been observed. Cardiac rhythm disturbances have been seen with alcohol intoxication (Ettinger et al. 1978) and acute intoxication has been suggested to be a precipitating factor in stroke in young people, in thrombotic stroke, and in subarachnoid hemorrhage (Hillbom and Kaste 1978 1982; Lee 1979; Taylor 1982).

Physical Activity. The relationship of job-related physical inactivity to increased CHD risk was demonstrated in studies of London busmen (Morris et al. 1966). Conductors with physically active duties had a lower level of CHD than the sedentary drivers. Longshoremen with duties demanding little physical work had a greater frequency of CHD than their more physically active coworkers (Paffenbarger et al. 1970). This association between high levels of physical activity on the job and lower CHD rates has not always been found, and no clear relationship has been shown for stroke. The more physically active longshoremen, with lower rates of myocardial infarction, had no reduction in stroke incidence (Paffenbarger et al. 1978).

Leisure-time vigorous physical activity has also been linked to lower CHD incidence. In a study of 17 000 former Harvard students, those who were more physically active had about half the risk and one-third the mortality rate of their least active fellow alumni (Paffenbarger et al. 1978). No such data are available demonstrating a reduction in stroke occurrence from vigorous habitual leisure-time physical activity.

Exercise may exert a beneficial influence on risk factors for atherosclerotic disease. Vigorous exercise may help to reduce elevated blood pressure by promoting weight loss. Physical activity acts to reduce the pulse rate, to raise the level of HDL-cholesterol and lower the LDL cholesterol, to improve glucose tolerance, and to promote a life style conducive to favorably changing detrimental health habits such as cigarette smoking (Leon and Blackburn 1983). These salutory effects have not been uniformly demonstrated to result in reducing stroke or CHD incidence. Furthermore, there are substantial limitations to studies of physical activity and disease, the principal potential pitfall being the self-selection of different levels of activity at work or leisure.

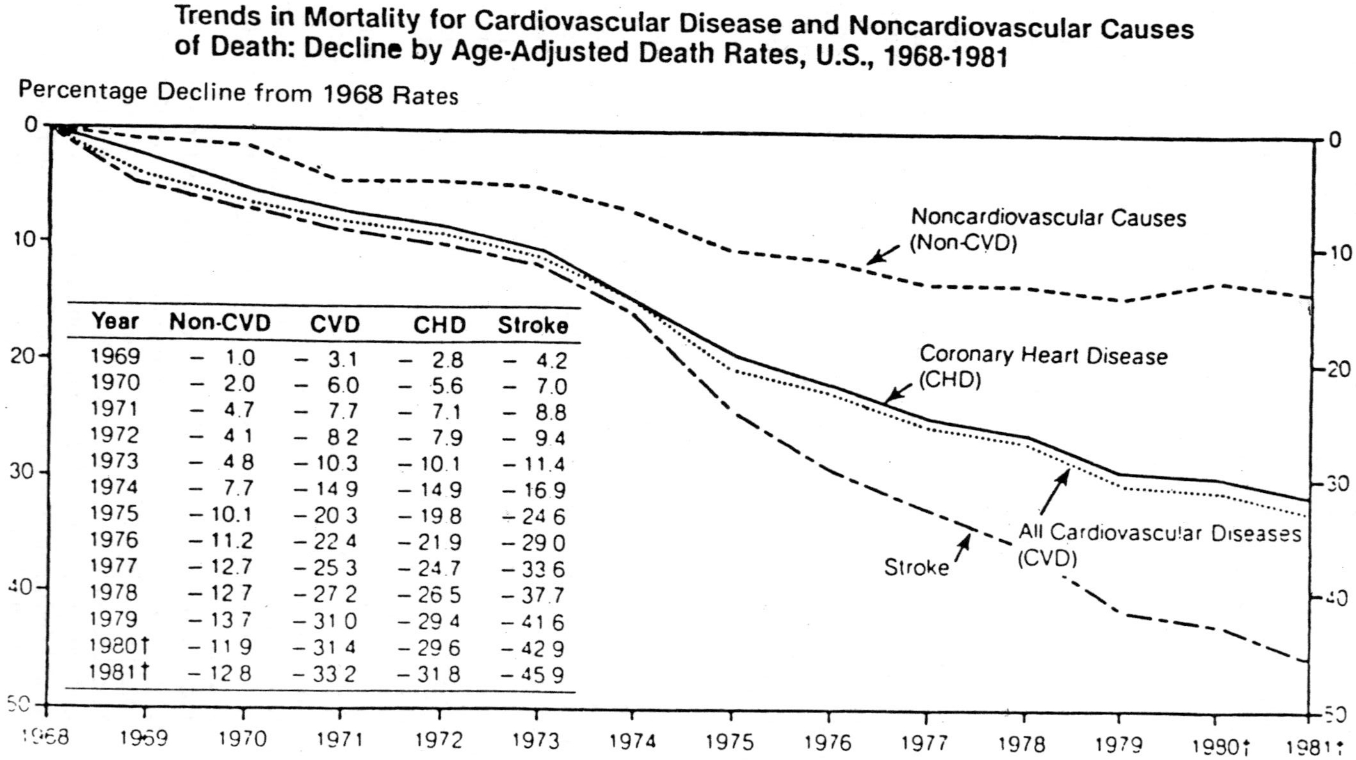

Year	Non-CVD	CVD	CHD	Stroke
1969	– 1.0	– 3.1	– 2.8	– 4.2
1970	– 2.0	– 6.0	– 5.6	– 7.0
1971	– 4.7	– 7.7	– 7.1	– 8.8
1972	– 4 1	– 8 2	– 7.9	– 9.4
1973	– 4 8	– 10 3	– 10.1	– 11.4
1974	– 7.7	– 14 9	– 14 9	– 16 9
1975	– 10.1	– 20 3	– 19 8	– 24 6
1976	– 11.2	– 22 4	– 21 9	– 29 0
1977	– 12.7	– 25 3	– 24.7	– 33 6
1978	– 12 7	– 27 2	– 26 5	– 37.7
1979	– 13 7	– 31 0	– 29 4	– 41 6
1980†	– 11 9	– 31 4	– 29 6	– 42 9
1981†	– 12 8	– 33 2	– 31 8	– 45 9

Fig. 18.3. Trends in mortality for cardiovascular disease and noncardiovascular causes of death: decline by age-adjusted death rates, United States, 1968–1981. From Wolf PA, Kannel WB, McGee DL (1986) Epidemiology of strokes in North American. In: Barnett HJM, Mohr JP, Stein B, Yatsu FM (eds) Stroke pathophysiology, diagnosis and management, vol 1. Churchill Livingstone.

Heart Disease as a Risk Factor for Stroke (a One-way Interaction)

Hypertension is the most potent and prevalent precursor of stroke, and its importance does not diminish with advancing age. However, while elevated blood pressure is the single most important risk factor for stroke, it is not uniformly so. At any level of blood pressure, those with other risk factor abnormalities, notably those with evidence of impaired cardiac function, are at increased risk of stroke (Fig. 18.3). Cardiac impairments include overt heart disease, congestive heart failure (CHF), coronary heart disease (CHD), or hypertensive heart disease (HHD), as well as occult or subclincal X-ray or electrocardiographic evidence of rhythm disturbance such as atrial fibrillation or impaired cardiac function. Cardiac impairment ranks third, following age and hypertension, as a risk factor for stroke in general and for ABI specifically. At any level of blood pressure, persons with cardiac disease, occult or overt, have more than twice the risk of stroke. Cardiac impairments include overt disease such as CHD and CHF, evidence of left ventricular hypertrophy (LVH) by ECG or X-ray, and rhythm abnormalities, particularly atrial fibrillation (AF).

Overt evidence of impaired cardiac function, prior CHD, and CHF are significantly related to stroke and ABI incidence. Risk of ABI is more than doubled in persons with CHD, and those with CHF have an even greater increase in risk. LVH by ECG, perhaps as a result of the impact of prolonged or severe hypertension, increases in prevalence with age and blood pressure. Risk of brain infarction is increased more than fourfold in those who develop this ECG abnormality, and this excess risk persists after adjustment for blood pressure and age. In contrast, generalized cardiac enlargement on X-ray is a less powerful precursor of ABI and makes no independent contribution to risk when LVH by ECG and other risk factors are taken into account. Nonspecific ST- and T-wave abnormalities, intraventricular block, and atrioventricular block are also associated with an increased ABI incidence.

Chronic AF, even in the absence of rheumatic valvular disease (NVAF), is a powerful precursor of stroke and is associated with more than a fivefold increased incidence of stroke even after age and hypertension are taken into account (Grotta et al. 1982; Wilhelmsen et al. 1984; Omae et al. 1976; Li et al. 1985). The increasing impact of NVAF on stroke risk with increasing age and NVAF-associated stroke was assessed in the Framingham Study cohort. After 30 years of follow-up, NVAF developed in 303 persons, and the proportion of strokes associated with NVAF represented 14.7% of the total 462 initial strokes. NVAF-associated stroke increased with increasing age from 6.7% at ages 50–59 to 36.2% at ages 80–89. In this elderly segment of the population, in whom the incidence of stroke is high, NVAF was associated with (and was probably responsible for) more than one-third of the strokes that occurred (Wolf et al. 1985).

Manifestations of CHD, notably MI and sudden death (SD), often develop unheralded by premonitory clinical symptoms, in persons who appear well, are without evidence of disease, and take no medication. Stroke, by contrast, usually develops on a background of hypertension and cardiac disease in persons receiving medications and already identified as being ill.

Secular Trends in Stroke and CHD

There has been a gradual decline in mortality rates from stroke in the United States dating back to 1915. The steady rate of decline of approximately 1%/year has accelerated rather dramatically, averaging 5%/year since 1968. This decrease in death rates from cerebrovascular disease seems to be quite real and is not an artifact of death certification practices. Despite an aging population of increasing size the total number of deaths attributed to cardiovascular disease recently fell to below one million for the first time in almost a decade (American Heart Association 1985). This decrease in stroke death rates has occurred in the presence of a steady decline in overall mortality and is part of the even more rapid decrease in deaths attributed to cardiovascular disease (Fig. 18.3). From 1968 to 1981 overall CHD deaths have fallen by 30% while cerebrovascular disease rates have dropped by 45%. These two major cardiovascular diseases, CHD and stroke, constitute the largest component of total mortality in older adults in the United States. The impact of these two diseases differs in men and women (Table 18.8). The male to female ratio for CHD mortality decreases with age while the male predominance in stroke death rates increases steadily from being only slightly higher in men at younger ages to a definite male excess above the age of 70.

Table 18.8. Death rates for coronary heart disease and stroke per 100 000, men and women aged 40–85, United States, 1980. (Wolf et al. 1986)

Age (years)	Coronary heart disease		Stroke	
	Men	Women	Men	Women
40–44	73.6	16.2	11.9	10.9
45–49	153.9	34.7	19.5	19.7
50–54	278.0	68.6	34.7	26.7
55–59	461.6	133.1	54.0	43.2
60–64	721.3	252.3	99.0	72.4
65–69	1114.0	448.0	184.7	132.1
70–74	1685.5	799.8	361.1	259.4
75–79	2486.5	1401.1	675.8	530.0
80–84	3800.6	2521.6	1217.4	1067.0
85+	6497.1	5279.1	2197.7	2327.5

While the steady *decline* in stroke death rates has accelerated in recent years the long-term *increase* in CHD death rates has ceased and rates have been falling. CHD deaths had climbed rapidly in the United States over 3 decades, reached a peak in 1968, and then began to decline. The 30% decline in CHD deaths has affected all segments of the adult population of the United States where CHD deaths have fallen more proportionally than in any other country, including those with equally sophisticated medical care. The United States now ranks *8th* instead of *2nd* in coronary mortality rates among 27 economically developed nations (Stamler 1984). Furthermore, in the United States proportional mortality from all cardiovascular diseases combined have fallen from 54% in

1968 to 49% in 1982 (Fig. 18.4). In 1982 stroke accounted for 8% of total mortality versus 11% in 1968 and CHD had fallen to 28% from 35% of all deaths.

There are three possible explanations for the declining mortality rates: (1) a significant change in death certification practices or diagnostic fashion, (2) a decline in case fatality rates either as a result of improved treatment of the disease or of associated conditions, and (3) a decline in the incidence of the disease.

1. The decline in CHD and stroke death rates has occurred at all ages, in both sexes, in blacks and whites, and in all regions of the United States and in many other developed western nations (Garraway et al. 1983). For this reason it is likely the decline is real and not an artifact of death certification, coding, or diagnostic practices (Table 18.9).

Table 18.9. Age-adjusted mortality rates for cerebrovascular diseases according to sex and race: United States, 1960–1975. (Adapted from Soltero 1978)

Years	White Male	White Female	Nonwhite Male	Nonwhite Female
1960	123	109	178	175
1968	112	97	171	155
1975	89	75	120	104
% Change 1960–1975	−28%	−31%	−33%	−41%

2. Case fatality rates for acute stroke have changed little over the years despite improvements in diagnostic techiques. In the residents of Rochester, Minnesota, where age and sex-adjusted average annual mortality rates have fallen from 91/100 000 in the period 1945–1949 to 30/100 000 in 1970–1974, a decline that is greater than that for United States whites during this period, 30-day case-fatality rates for cerebral infarction were substantially unchanged over this 30-year period (Garraway et al. 1979; Anderson and Whisnant 1982a).

Evidence that the decline in mortality rates for stroke is not due to improved medical treatment of stroke patients, or as a result of a decrease in the severity of the disease, comes from The Minnesota Heart Survey, which compared mortality, hospitalization, and case fatality rates for stroke in the Twin Cities metropolitan area at two time periods (Gillum et al. 1985). In the Twin Cities of Minneapolis and St. Paul, Minnesota age-adjusted mortality rates declined in the decade from 1970 to 1980 in both men and women. Age-adjusted mean length of hospital stay and severity of hospitalized cases did not change during these 10 years. Hospital case fatality rates were unchanged in women and in men aged 65–74 but did decline significantly in men aged 30–64 years. Overall, the findings were consistent with declining mortality not attributable to improved survival of hospitalized stroke patients.

Case fatality rates for CHD may have improved as a result of technological advances in: cardiopulmonary resuscitation; arrhythmia prevention, detection, and treatment; and more complete rational treatment of cardiac failure and shock following MI. Substantiating data for these contensions are sparse, but overall there is a suggestion that improved medical treatment of CHD victims

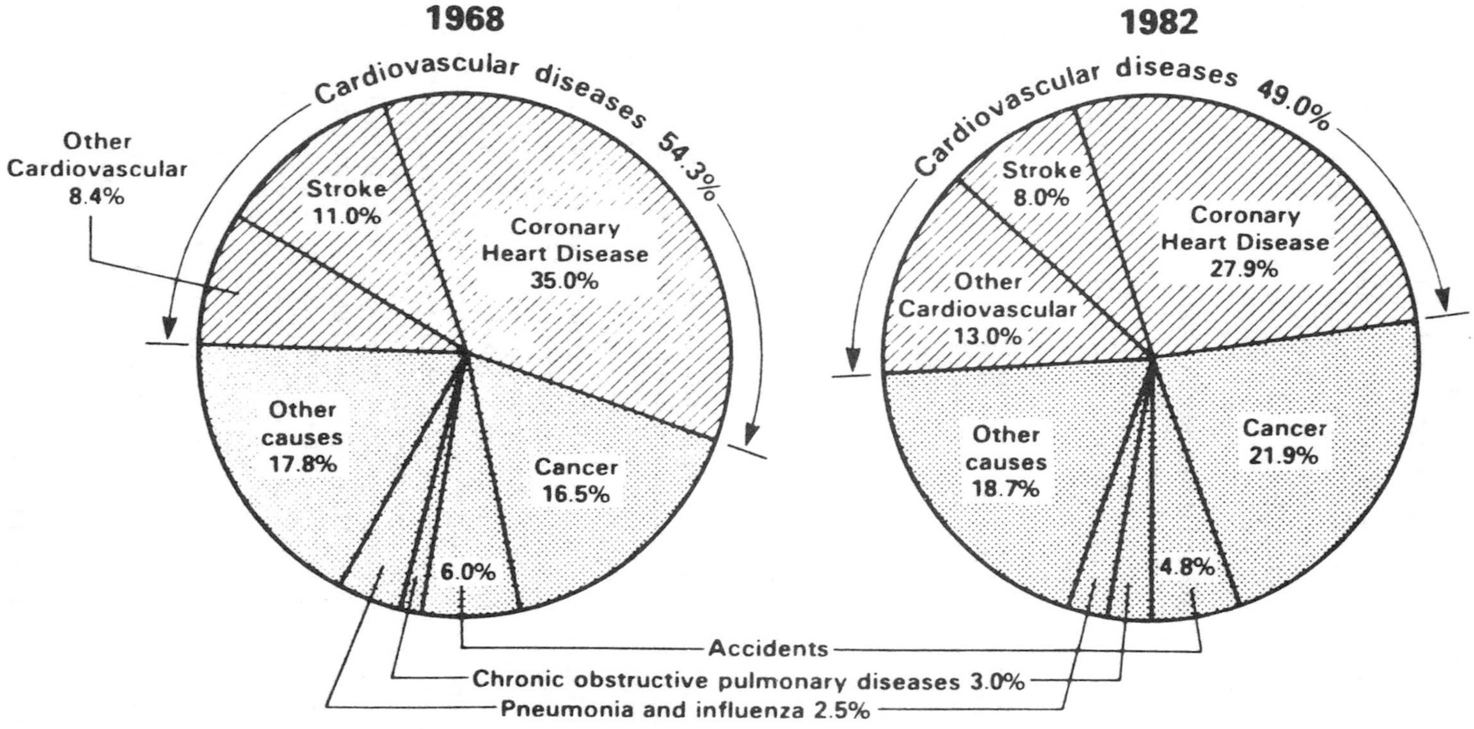

Fig. 18.4. Death by cause as percentage of total deaths in the United States, 1968 and 1982. Causes of death for 1968 classified by the Eighth Revision, and for 1982 by the Ninth Revision of the International Classification of Disease adapted for use in the United States. Data for 1982 are provisional; for 1968, final. From the National Center for Health Statistics, Division of Vital Statistics. (Feinlieb 1984)

including resuscitation of sudden unexpected deaths and arrhythmia prevention and treatment in coronary care units may have played a role in the decline in CHD mortality (Garraway et al. 1983a; Pell and Fairweather 1985; Mathewson et al. 1985; Elveback 1979; Gillum et al. 1984).

3. Is the fall in death rates from stroke the result of a decline in the incidence of the disease? Data to address this question are not easily obtained, but some information is available from the resident population of Rochester, Minnesota. These findings will need to be confirmed in other populations and in other geographic areas. A centralized population-based diagnostic index, the Mayo Clinic medical records linkage and indexing system, has been maintained and contains all diagnoses on persons who are residents of Rochester, Minnesota. There has been virtually complete case ascertainment for serious medical problems including stroke and CHD, and community rates have been reported from 1945 through 1979 (Garraway et al. 1983b). Diagnostic accuracy for Rochester, Minnesota, residents was excellent due to the high degree of neurologic expertise, the high autopsy rate of >50%, and the relatively uniform assignment of cause of death by Mayo Clinic pathologists for virtually all cases, autopsied or not.

Mortality rates for stroke have declined in Rochester, Minnesota, during the 3 decades 1945–1974 (Anderson and Whisnant 1982b). This decline occurred for all strokes combined and in all subtypes of stroke except subarachnoid hemorrhage. This trend in total stroke mortality in Rochester, Minnesota, was comparable to that of whites in the United States as a whole, although the decline was more rapid and death rates lower in Rochester. The decline in death rates was not due to increased survival following stroke from improved medical care (Garraway et al. 1983c) nor as a result of a diminution in the severity of the illness since 30-day case fatality rates were substantially unchanged over this 30-year period (Garraway et al. 1979).

The decline in mortality in Rochester, Minnesota, is clearly due to a decline in the incidence of stroke over the past 3 decades (Table 18.10). The age-adjusted average annual incidence rate of stroke, all types combined, has declined in every 5-year period since 1945–1949. The pattern of incidence has differed in the

Table 18.10. Average annual incidence rates for Rochester, Minnesota, per 100 000 population for specific stroke types, men and women over a 35-year time period. (Garraway et al. 1983b)

Diagnostic type	1945–1949	1950–1954	1955–1959	1960–1964	1965–1969	1970–1974	1975–1979
Cerebral infarction	143	157	145	125	117	92	75
Intracerebral hemorrhage	16	16	5	12	10	6	13
Subarachnoid hemorrhage	11	7	9	12	10	11	11
Stroke of uncertain type	17	9	16	8	7	8	4
All types	186	189	175	158	144	117	103
Adjusted for age and sex[a]	192	179	168	150	138	104	89

[a] Adjusted for age and sex to the 1950 United States white population.

two sexes (Fig. 18.5), with an earlier, more gradual and more substantial decline for women than men. For the 25 years prior to 1969, there was little change in the incidence rate of men but in the decade 1970–1979 incidence fell by 44%.

Utilizing 24 years of follow-up of the Framingham Heart Study cohort, temporal trends in stroke incidence were assessed (Kannel and Thom 1979). Incidence of stroke in each of the first seven biennial examination periods was determined for men and women age 50–61 at entry into the study in 1950, a 12-year follow-up period. Incidence was determined for all types of strokes combined, excluding those who had transient ischemic attacks only without stroke. For persons aged 50–61 at exam 7 in 1962, upon entering the second 12 years of the study, incidence of stroke was calculated in the same manner. These data are based upon 175 cases of stroke, all types combined (with TIA only cases excluded), in the earlier period and 72 cases in the second 12-year period. As in the Rochester data, temporal trends in the incidence of stroke in Framingham differ substantially by sex. Men had an incidence of stroke that was consistently higher in the later period and this trend continues rather smoothly over the 12 years. In women, quite the opposite occurred; stroke incidence was lower in the later period and the trend was toward a further decline in incidence with time.

There is a reason to believe that the decline in incidence of all cardiovascular disease including stroke and CHD is, at least in part, the result of some of the changes that have occurred in the dietary and lifestyle in the United States in the past 25 years. Surveys by the U.S. Department of Agriculture indicate that two-thirds of Americans have changed their eating habits and have decreased their dietary consumption of cholesterol and saturated fat substantially (Table 18.11). Concurrently, mean serum cholesterol levels have declined from the 235- to 245-mg/dl range in the 1940s to 1960s to the 210- to 215-mg/dl range in the 1970s and 1980s.

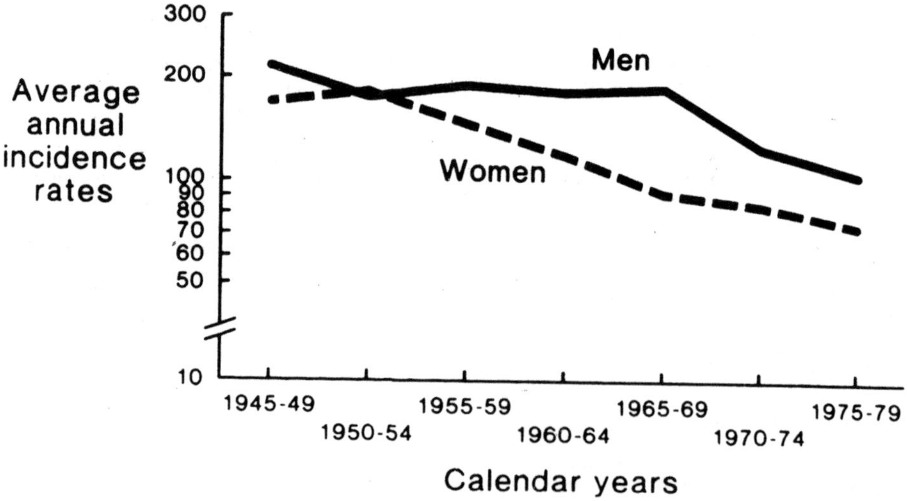

Fig. 18.5. Five-year average annual incidence rates per 100 000 population for all first episodes of stroke in men and women in Rochester, Minnesota, age adjusted to 1960 United States white population (Whisnant 1984).

Table 18.11. Change in per capita consumption in the United States, 1963–1980. (Adapted from Walker 1983)

Product	Change
Cigarette tobacco	27% Decline
Fluid milk and cream	24% Decline
Butter	33% Decline
Eggs	12% Decline
Animal fats and oils	39% Decline
Vegetable fats and oils	58% Increase
Fish	23% Increase

Preventive Implications

The appearance of overt symptoms of coronary or cerebrovascular disease should be considered a failure of prevention. Measures to diagnose and treat the already symptomatic patient with cardiovascular disease are often examples of too little too late. In the case of stroke, physicians must shift their efforts from the application of high-technology diagnostic and therapeutic maneuvers in the seriously impaired patient with advanced symptomatic cerebrovascular disease to the more mundane day-to-day business of modifying risk factors for disease prevention in the presymptomatic candidate for stroke. This requires attending to what are often considered medical trivia—modest elevation of the blood pressure, early signs of cardiac impairments, and the application of general hygienic measures to reduce obesity, cigarette smoking, and physical inactivity.

Prospects for prevention would be greatly enhanced by the demonstration of correctable environmental determinants of stroke. Unfortunately, there are few significant environmental contributors to stroke incidence or mortality. Acceleration in the decline in the incidence of stroke and mortality from cerebrovascular disease in recent years is a clear indication that stroke is not an inevitable consequence of aging or of genetic predisposition. Further evidence of the ability to modify risk factors for stroke is that decrease in stroke mortality has occurred at all ages, including the 8th and 9th decades of life.

The initial manifestation of symptomatic CHD is all too often sudden unexpected death, occurring in 18% of all coronary attacks in men and 24% in women in the Framingham cohort (Kannel and Thomas 1982). More than half of the huge annual toll of coronary mortality is in the form of sudden death and in a large percentage of these deaths it was the initial clinical manifestation of CHD. Clearly such a manifestation is most susceptible to a preventive remedy. Risk of sudden unexpected death in a previously asymptomatic and apparently well person varies substantially in relation to the major coronary risk factors and multivariate combination of these factors allows efficient prediction of sudden death in both men and women.

Prevention of stroke in hypertensive patients by reduction of blood pressure has been demonstrated in a series of randomized controlled clinical trials over the past 2 decades (Taguchi and Freis 1974; Management Committee 1980;

Hypertension Detection and Follow-up Program Cooperative Group 1979). Stroke rates have been reduced by about 50% by vigorous reduction of pressure in severe, moderate, and mild hypertensives with generally acceptable levels of adverse effects. Coronary attacks have been reduced by reduction in serum cholesterol levels with diet and drugs in persons with high serum lipid levels (Lipid Research Clinics Program 1984a,b; Arntzenius 1985). These dietary trials have not demonstrated a benefit in stroke prevention. It may be that the patient population was too young and the follow-up too short to demonstrate any benefit.

There is a wealth of evidence supporting a strong relationship between blood cholesterol levels and atherosclerotic coronary diseases; the link to cerebrovascular disease is less clear. However, risk of stroke must be related to nutritional and dietary factors; anything that promotes atherosclerosis or hypertension can be regarded as increasing the likelihood of stroke. Evidence is accumulating that dietary consumption of calories and total fats, particularly saturated fats and cholesterol, is related to increasing atherosclerosis whereas consumption of dietary fiber and certain minerals and trace elements is associated with reduction in hypertension and atherosclerotic lesions. Diet by means of its impact on hypertension and atherosclerosis is clearly related to the development of atherosclerotic cardiovascular disease including stroke. Direct evidence for stroke prevention by modification of nutritional and dietary components is lacking.

Control of blood pressure, particularly mild high blood pressure, by nutritional and other hygienic means is especially attractive in those with mild hypertension in view of the high prevalence of this condition in the stroke-age population, and the potential high cost and adverse effects of some anti-hypertensive medications.

References

Abbott RD, Yin Y, Reed DM, Yano K (1986) Risk of Stroke in Male Cigarette Smokers. N Engl J Med 315: 717–720

American Heart Association (1985) Heart facts 3

Anderson GL, Whisnant JP (1982a) A comparison of trends in mortality from stroke in the United States and Rochester, Minnesota. Stroke 13: 804

Anderson GL, Whisnant JP (1982b) A comparison of trends in mortality from stroke in the United States and Rochester, Minnesota. Stroke 13: 804–809

Arntzenius AC, Kromhout D, Barth JD, Reiber JH, Vruschke AV, Buis B, van Gent CM, Kempen-Boogd N, Strikwerda S, van der Velde EA (1985) Diet, lipoproteins, and the progression of coronary atherosclerosis. The Leiden Intervention Trial. N Engl J Med 312: 13: 805–811

Blackwelder WC, Yano K, Rhoads GG, Kagan A, Gordon T, Palesch Y (1980) Alcohol and mortality. The Honolulu Study. Am J Med 68: 164–169

Collaborative Group for the Study of Stroke in Young Women (1973) Oral contraception and increased risk of cerebral ischemia or thrombosis. New Engl J Med 288: 871–878

Collaborative Group for the Study of Stroke in Young Women (1975) Oral contraceptives and stroke in young women: associated risk factors. JAMA 231: 718–722

Dintenfass L (1975) Elevation of blood viscosity, aggregation of red cells, haematocrit values and fibrinogen levels in cigarette smokers. Med J Aust 1: 617

EC/IC Bypass Study Group (1985) The International Cooperative Study of Extracranial/Intracranial Arterial Anastomosis (EC/IC Bypass Study): methodology and entry characteristics. Stroke 16 (3): 397–406

Elveback LR (1979) Coronary heart disease in Rochester, Minnesota. 1950–1975: incidence and survivorship. In: Havlik RJ, Feinleib M (eds) Proceedings of the conference on decline in coronary heart disease mortality. Washington, DC: Government Printing Office. (NIH Publication No. 79–1610, pp 116–118

Ettinger PO, Wu CF, DeLaCruz C Jr, Weisse AB, Ahmed SS, Regan TJ (1978) Arrythmias and the "holiday heart": alcohol-associated cardiac rhythm disorders. Am Heart J 95: 55

Feinleib M (1984) The magnitude and nature of the decrease in coronary heart disease mortality rate. Am J Cardiol 54: 2C–6C

Garraway WM, Whisnant JP, Kurland LT, O'Fallon WM (1979) Changing pattern of cerebral infarction: 1945–1974. Stroke 10: 657–662

Garraway WM, Whisnant JP, Drury I (1983c) The changing pattern of survival following stroke. Stroke 14: 699–703

Garraway WM, Whisnant JP, Drury I (1983b) The continuing decline in the incidence of stroke. Mayo Clin Proc 58: 520–523

Garraway WM, Connolly DC, Elveback LR, Whisnant JP (1983a) The dichotomy of myocardial and cerebral infarction. Lancet: 1332–1335

Gillum RF, Folsom AR, Blackburn H (1984) Decline in coronary heart disease mortality: old questions and new facts. Am J Med 76: 1055–1065

Gillum RF, Gomez-Marin O, Kottke TE, Jacobs DR Jr, Prineas RJ, Folsom AR, Luepker RV, Blackburn H (1985) Acute stroke in a metropolitan area, 1970 and 1980, The Minnesota Heart Survey. J Chron Dis 38: 11: 891–898

Grotta J, Ackerman R, Correia J, Fallick G, Chang J (1982) Whole blood viscosity parameters and cerebral blood flow. Stroke 13: 296–301

Handin R (1974) Thromboembolic complications of pregnancy and oral contraceptives. Prog Cardiovasc Dis 16: 395

Hennekens CH (1983) Alcohol. In: Kaplan NM, Stamler J (eds) Prevention of coronary heart disease, practical management of the risk factors (eds) Saunders, Philadelphia 11: 130–138

Hillbom M, Kaste M (1978) Does ethanol intoxication promote brain infarction in young adults? Lancet 2: 1181

Hillbom M, Kaste M (1982) Alcohol intoxication: a risk factor for primary subarachnoid hemorrhage. Neurology 32: 706

Hypertension Detection and Follow-up Program Cooperative Group (1979) Five-year findings of the hypertension detection and follow-up programs. I. Reduction in mortality of persons with high blood pressure, including mild hypertension. JAMA 242: 2562–2571

Japanese Health & Welfare Ministry (1986) AMA Medical News, January 17: 12

Kagan A, Popper JS, Rhoads GG, Yano K (1985) Dietary and other risk factors for stroke in Hawaiian Japanese men. Stroke 16 (3): 390–396

Kannel WB, McGee DL (1979) Diabetes and cardiovascular disease, The Framingham Study. JAMA 241: 2035–2038

Kannel WB, Thom TJ (1979) Implications of the recent decline in cardiovascular mortality. Cardiovascular Medicine 4: 983–997

Kannel WB, Thomas HE Jr (1982) Sudden coronary death: The Framingham Study. Ann NY Acad Sci 382: 3–20

Kannel WB, Gordon T, Wolf PA, McNamara P (1972) Hemoglobin and the risk of cerebral infarction: The Framingham Study. Stroke 3: 409–419

Kee DB Jr, Wood JH (1984) Rheology of the cerebral circulation. Neurosurgery 15 (1): 135–131

Kozarevic DJ, McGee D, Vojvodic N, Racic Z, Dawber T, Gordon T, Zukel W (1980) Frequency of alcohol consumption and morbidity and mortality: The Yugoslavia Cardiovascular Disease Study. Lancet 1: 613–616

Kuller LH, Dorman JS, Wolf PA (1985) Cerebrovascular diseases and diabetes. In: Diabetes in America, Diabetes Data compiled 1984. National Diabetes Data Group, U.S. Dept. of Health and Human Services, NIH Publication No. 85–1468, August 1985; XVIII: 1–18

Kurtzke JF (1976a) Epidemiology of cerebrovascular disease. In: Cerebrovascular survey report for Joint Council Subcommittee on Cerebrovascular Disease. National Institute of Neurological and Communicative Disorders and Stroke, and National Heart and Lung Institute, Rochester, Minnesota. Whiting, Minnesota, p 213

Lee K (1979) Alcoholism and cerebrovascular thrombosis in the young. Acta Neurol Scand 59: 270

Leon AS, Blackburn H (1983) Physical inactivity. In: Kaplan NM, Stamler J (eds) Prevention of coronary heart disease, practical management of the risk factors. Saunders, Philadelphia 7: 86–97

Leonberg SC Jr, Elliott FA (1981) Prevention of recurrent stroke. Stroke 12: 731–735

Li S, Schoenberg S, Wang C, Cheng X, Bolis CL, Wang K (1985) Cerebrovascular disease in the People's Republic of China: epidemiologic and clinical features. Neurology 35: 1708–1713
Lipid Research Clinics Program (1984a) The Lipid Research Clinics coronary primary prevention trial results. I. Reduction in incidence of coronary heart disease. JAMA 251: 351–364
Lipid Research Clinics Program (1984b) The Lipid Research Clinics coronary primary prevention trial results. II. The relationship of reduction in incidence of coronary heart disease to cholesterol lowering. JAMA 251: 365–374
Longstreth WT, Koepsell TD, Yerby MS, van Belle G (1985) Risk factors for subarachnoid hemorrhage. Stroke 16 (3): 377–385
Management Committee (1980) The Australian Therapeutic Trial in Mild Hypertension. Lancet: 1261–1267
Mann JI, Inman WHW (1975) Oral contraceptives and death from myocardial infarction. Br Med J 2: 245–248
Mathewson ZM, Evans AE, McCloskey BG, Russell CJ (1985) Mobile coronary care and community mortality from myocardial infarction. Lancet: 441–444
Mohr JP, Caplan LR, Melski JW, Goldstein RJ, Duncan GW, Kistler JP, Pessin MS, Bleich HL (1978) The Harvard Cooperative Stroke Registry: a prospective registry. Neurology 28: 754–762
Morris JN, Hagan A, Patteson DC, Gardner MJ (1966) Incidence and prediction of ischemic heart disease in London Busmen. Lancet 2: 553–559
Omae T, Takeshita M, Hirota Y (1976) The Hisayama Study and Joint Study on Cerebrovascular Disease in Japan. In: Scheinberg P (ed) Cerebrovascular diseases. Raven, New York, pp 255–265
Paffenbarger RS Jr, Laughlin ME, Gina AS, Black RA (1970) Work activity of longshoremen as related to death from coronary heart disease and stroke. N Engl J Med 282: 1109
Paffenbarger RS, Wing AL, Hyde RT (1978) Physical activity as an index of heart attack risk in college alumni. Am J Epidemiol 108: 161–175
Pearson TC, Thomas DJ (1979) Physiological and pharmacological factors influencing blood viscosity and cerebral blood flow. In: Tognoni G, Gerattinin S (eds) Drug treatment and prevention in cerebrovascular disorders. Elsevier North-Holland, Amsterdam, p 33
Pell S, Fayerweather WE (1985) Trends in the incidence of myocardial infarction and in associated mortality and morbidity in a large employed population, 1957–1983. N Engl J Med 312: 1005–1011
Robins M, Buam HM (1981) Incidence: the National Survey of Stroke. Stroke [Suppl 1] 12: 145–147
Royal College of General Practitioners' Oral Contraception Study: Further Analyses of Mortality in Oral Contraceptive Users. Lancet 1: 541–546
Schoenberg BS, Whisnant JP, Taylor WF, Kempers RO (1970) Strokes in women of childbearing age: a population study. Neurology 20: 181
Soltero I, Liu K, Cooper R, Stamler J, Garside D (1978) Trends in mortality from cerebrovascular disease in the United States, 1960 to 1975. Stroke 9: 549–555
Stadel BV (1981) Oral contraceptives and cardiovascular disease. N Engl J Med 30: 612–618, 672–677
Stamler J (1984) Coronary heart disease: doing the "right things." Editorial. N Engl J Med 312: 1053–1055
Stason WB, Neff RK, Miettinen OS, Jick H (1976) Alcohol consumption and nonfatal myocardial infarction. Am J Epidemiol 104: 603–608
Stemmerman GN, Hyashi T, Resch JA, Chung CS, Reed DM, Rhoads GG (1984) Risk factors related to ischemic and hemorrhagic cerebrovascular disease at autopsy: the Honolulu Heart Study. Stroke 15 (1): 23–28
Taguchi J, Freis ED (1974) Partial reduction of blood pressure and prevention of complications in hypertension. N Engl J Med 291: 329
Takeya Y, Popper JS, Shimizu Y, Kato H, Rhoads GG, Kagan A (1984) Epidemiologic studies of coronary heart disease and stroke in Japanese Men living in Japan, Hawaii and California: incidence of stroke in Japan and Hawaii. Stroke 15 (1): 15–23
Tanaka H, Tanaka Y, Hayashi M, Ueda Y, Date C, Baba T, Shoji H, Horimoto T, Owada K (1982) Secular trends in mortality for cerebrovascular disease in Japan, 1960 to 1979. Stroke 13 (5): 574–581
Taylor JR (1982) Alcohol and strokes. N Engl J Med 306: 1111
Thomas DJ, DuBoulay GH, Marshall J, Wetherley-Mein G, Pearson TC, Ross Russell RW, Symon L, Zilkha E (1977) Effect of haematocrit on cerebral blood-flow in man. Lancet 2: 941
Tohgi J, Yamanouchi H, Murakami M, Kameyama M (1978) Importance of the Haematocrit as a risk factor in cerebral infarction. Stroke 9: 369–374
Walker WJ (1983) Change in per capita consumption in the United States 1963–1980. N Engl J Med 308: 650
Whisnant JP (1984) The decline of stroke. Stroke 15: 160–168

Wilhelmsen L, Svarsdudd K, Korban-Bengsten K, Larsson B, Welin L, Tibblin G (1980) Fibrinogen as a risk factor for stroke and myocardial infarction. N Engl J Med 311: 501–505
Wilson PWF, Garrison RJ, Castelli WP (1985) Postmenopausal estrogen use, cigarette smoking and cardiovascular morbidity in women over 50. The Framingham Study. N Engl J Med 313: 1038–1043
Wiseman RA, MacRae KD (1981) Oral contraceptives and the decline in mortality from circulatory disease. Fertil Steril 35: 277
Wolf PA, Kannel WB, Abbott RD (1985) Atrial fibrillation and stroke in the elderly: The Framingham Study. Stroke 16: 138
Wolf PA, Kannel WB, McGee DL (1986) Epidemiology of strokes in North America. In: Barnett HJM, Mohr JP, Stein B, Yatsu FM (eds) Stroke pathophysiology, diagnosis and management, vol. 1. Churchill Livingstone, New York

References

Chapter 19

Detection of Coronary Artery Disease in Patients with Cerebrovascular Disease

R. E. Hobbs and A. J. Furlan

Relationship Between Atherosclerotic Cerebrovascular Disease and Cardiovascular Disease

Postmortem studies suggest that atherosclerosis is often a generalized process which develops sequentially and in parallel severity in the abdominal aorta, peripheral arteries, coronary arteries, extracranial cerebral arteries, and, finally, the intracranial vessels (Fisher 1965; Young 1980; Solberg 1968; Mitchell 1962). Hence, when a patient manifests symptoms or signs of cerebrovascular atherosclerosis an assumption could be made that coronary atherosclerosis is probably present as well. Recent clinical and epidemiologic studies indicate that this assumption would be correct in many cases.

Based on population studies and large stroke prevention trials such as the Canadian and American aspirin studies, about 33% of patients presenting with transient ischemic attacks (TIAs) or stroke will have a prior history of myocardial infarction or angina pectoris (Kannel 1983; Furlan 1979; Whisnant 1979; Canadian Cooperative Study Group 1978; Fields 1977). The prevalence of symptomatic coronary artery disease appears similar in patients presenting with an asymptomatic carotid bruit (Kroener 1980; Moore 1978).

Cardiac disease is the major cause of death in virtually every cerebrovascular patient population studied. The rate of cardiac death is about 5%/year for patients with asymptomatic carotid bruits, TIAs, or stroke (Heyman 1980; Wolf 1981; Moore 1985). Coronary deaths are also frequent among patients with intracranial cerebral atherosclerosis (Marzewski 1982; Craig 1982), vertebral basilar atherosclerosis (Moufarrij 1984), and internal carotid artery occlusion (Furlan 1980). Cardiovascular deaths were twice as common as stroke-related deaths in patients with TIA treated with aspirin in the American and Canadian trials (Canadian Cooperative Study Group 1978; Fields 1977). Toole (1978) reported a 25% incidence of cardiovascular deaths among 225 patients with TIA managed either medically or surgically during a 5.5-year follow-up. The Joint Study of Extracranial Arterial Occlusion (Fields 1970) also found that cardiac deaths were the leading cause of late mortality in patients with TIA managed medically or surgically.

Coronary Disease in Cerebrovascular Surgery Patients

Coronary artery disease is the major cause of early postoperative mortality as well as late deaths among patients undergoing carotid endarterectomy. Ennix (1979) reported an 18.2% mortality rate for carotid endarterectomy in patients with angina pectoris compared with a 1.5% mortality rate in patients with no symptoms of coronary artery disease. Debakey (1965) reported a 9.5% operative mortality rate in patients with a history of heart disease. Lye and Downs (1980) found a 2.3% incidence of postendarterectomy myocardial infarction, which was the second leading cause of perioperative death in patients undergoing carotid surgery. Thus, the risk of carotid endarterectomy is increased in the presence of coronary artery disease, and myocardial infarction is one of the major causes of postoperative mortality and morbidity.

Myocardial infarction is also the leading cause of late deaths following carotid endarterectomy (Hertzer 1981). The annual mortality rate from heart disease following carotid surgery is approximately 5%. Fatal myocardial infarction also appears to be the major long-term cause of death in patients undergoing extracranial-intracranial arterial anastomosis (Sundt 1985). Most studies indicate that cardiac deaths exceed deaths from stroke by twofold in patients undergoing cerebrovascular surgery, and that at least 50% of late deaths are due to heart disease (Adams 1984).

Silent Coronary Disease in Cerebrovascular Patients

How prevalent is silent coronary artery disease in patients presenting with cerebrovascular disease? Whisnant (1978) found that prior clinical evidence of cardiac disorders had no effect on survival rates among patients presenting with their first TIA (Fig. 19.1). However, the most common cause of death, regardless of prior cardiac history, was heart disease. This suggested a high prevalence of clinically silent coronary artery disease among patients with TIA. Rokey (1984) performed rest and exercise radionuclide ventriculography as well as thallium-201 scintigraphy on 34 patients with TIA or mild stroke, but no clinical evidence of coronary artery disease. One or both tests were abnormal in 41% of patients (Table 19.1). Nine patients underwent cardiac catheterization and eight of these had severe coronary artery disease. In our institution, Hertzer (1985) performed cardiac catheterizations on 200 patients presenting with asymptomatic carotid bruit, TIA, or prior stroke but without clinical manifestations of coronary artery disease. Eighty-six percent had angiographic evidence of coronary artery disease, which was advanced in 40% (Table 19.2). The nature of the cerebrovascular presentation (asymptomatic bruit versus symptomatic) was not related to the probability of detecting severe coronary artery disease with catheterization. These studies suggest that there is a high prevalence of asymptomatic coronary artery disease in patients presenting with a variety of cerebrovascular problems.

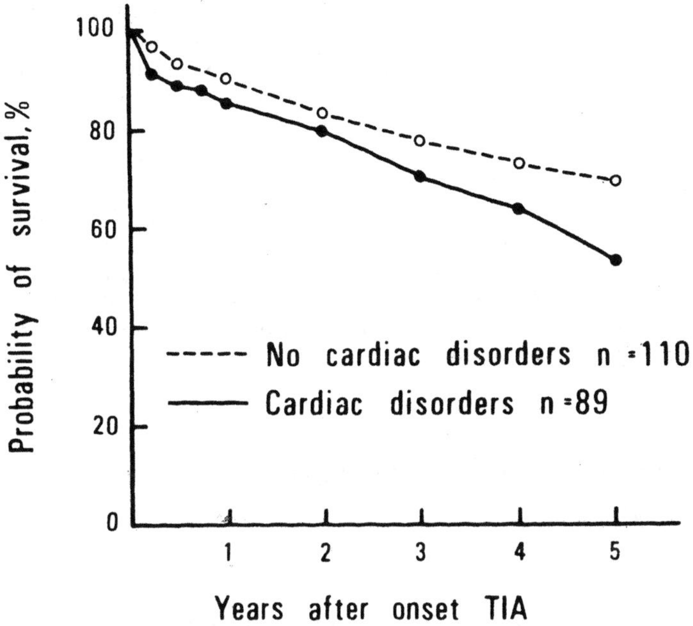

Fig. 19.1. Survival following onset of TIA related to the presence of clinical history of cardiac disease (Whisnant 1978).

Table 19.1. Results of testing for coronary artery disease (CAD) in 34 patients with cerebrovascular disease but no clinical evidence of CAD. (Modified from Rokey et al. 1984)

	No.
Abnormal radionuclide tests (total)	14
Abnormal radionuclide ventriculogram only	4
Abnormal thallium scintigram only	3
Both radionuclide tests abnormal	7
Abnormal exercise ECG	5
Abnormal cardiac catheterization	8/9

Table 19.2. Results of coronary angiography among 200 patients presenting with cerebrovascular disease but without clinical evidence of coronary artery disease (CAD). (Modified from Hertzer et al. 1985)

	No.	%
Normal coronary arteries	27	14
Mild to moderate[a] CAD	93	46
Advanced but compensated CAD	45	22
Severe[b] operable CAD	32	16
Severe inoperable CAD	3	2

[a] Moderate = $\leq$70% stenosis of $\geq$1 coronary artery
[b] Severe = >70% stenosis of $\geq$1 coronary artery

Adams et al. (1984) have pointed out that the 5% annual mortality rate for heart disease among patients with cerebrovascular disease exceeds the 4% annual mortality rate of patients with angina pectoris. Cardiac mortality in patients with symptomatic cerebrovascular disease is similar to that in patients with angiographically confirmed triple vessel coronary artery disease. Nevertheless, despite the overwhelming evidence that cerebrovascular disease is a major marker of coronary atherosclerosis, a cardiovascular evaluation is often neglected and seldom integrated into the management of this group of patients. Medical or surgical therapy directed only at the cerebrovascular system may not address the major risk factor affecting long-term mortality in this population. If long-term benefits are to be achieved by medical or surgical treatment of cerebrovascular disease, underlying coronary artery disease must be identified and aggressively managed in these patients.

Screening for Coronary Artery Disease in Cerebrovascular Patients

Since coronary artery disease is often asymptomatic, evaluating these patients can be a challenging and difficult task for the clinician. The high prevalence of coronary artery disease and cardiac morbidity and mortality in cerebrovascular disease patients makes screening a mandatory process. The major goals of screening for coronary artery disease are detection of myocardial ischemia and documentation of coronary artery obstructions so that appropriate management can be instituted.

Traditional methods for detecting coronary artery disease such as the history, physical examination, and the electrocardiogram are useful if abnormal, but lack sensitivity when coronary artery disease is subclinical. Noninvasive methods of screening for coronary artery disease include the electrocardiographic exercise test, radionuclide imaging, and digital subtraction imaging. These methods vary in their diagnostic accuracy, cost, ease of application, and availability. Noninvasive tests record physiologic abnormalities, electrocardiographic changes, perfusion abnormalities, or impairment of mechanical function produced by myocardial ischemia.

Cardiac catheterization with angiography is the most accurate means of detecting and quantitating coronary artery disease and recording left ventricular function. However, the cost and invasive nature of this technique make it an unacceptable screening tool for many cerebrovascular patients.

History and Physical Examination

Most patients presenting with cerebrovascular disease have no symptoms suggestive of coronary artery disease. In these patients, coronary disease may be absent, mild, or severe but preclinical. Asymptomatic, severe coronary artery disease has been recognized more frequently due to routine noninvasive screening techniques. The mechanism whereby severe coronary artery disease produces silent myocardial ischemia remains unclear. Forty percent of patients with coronary artery disease experience an acute myocardial infarction as the first clinical manifestation of their disease. More importantly, 15%–25% of patients with coronary artery disease experience sudden death as their first and last manifestation (Kannel 1974). Thus, a catastrophic event is the first clinical manifestation of coronary artery disease in two-thirds of patients.

Symptomatic coronary artery disease appears to be less common than asymptomatic disease in patients undergoing cerebrovascular evaluation. A history of typical angina pectoris has high predictive accuracy for the presence of severe coronary artery disease (Proudfit 1966). Angina pectoris is a specific indicator of coronary artery disease and is its first manifestation in 35% of patients (Kannel 1976). However, angina pectoris is not pathognomonic for coronary arterial lesions since it may occur with valvular or myocardial disease. A small percentage of patients with a history of angina pectoris have normal coronary arteriograms. Atypical chest discomfort decreases the predictive accuracy of the history by approximately half. The absence of angina pectoris does not exclude coronary artery disease nor does the severity of symptoms correlate with the severity of coronary artery disease (Proudfit 1978). That is, mild symptoms do not imply mild coronary artery disease.

The presence of other cardiovascular risk factors such as diabetes mellitus, hypertension, hyperlipidemia, cigarette smoking, and familial coronary artery disease increase the likelihood of coronary artery disease. Diabetes mellitus also increases the chances of discovering diffuse inoperable coronary artery lesions (Hertzer 1985).

The physical examination has limited usefulness in detecting coronary artery disease. The corneal arcus and ear lobe creases have little if any correlation with coronary artery anatomy. On auscultation, the atrial gallop (S4) indicates a noncompliant left ventricle which may be caused by coronary artery disease or hypertension. Signs of atherosclerosis in peripheral vessels (carotid and femoral bruits, abdominal aortic aneurysm, or absent lower extremity pulses) also increase the likelihood of coronary artery disease. Auscultation during an episode of chest discomfort may provide several clues suggesting that the pain is cardiac in origin. These include atrial or ventricular gallop sounds, a new or increased apical systolic murmur, paradoxical splitting of the second heart sound, and transient bibasilar rales. It is unlikely, however, that the examiner will witness an episode of chest pain during routine evaluation.

Electrocardiogram, Chest Radiograph and Cardiac Fluoroscopy

Generally the ECG is not a useful diagnostic tool in the asymptomatic patient since it is usually normal or nonspecific. In symptomatic patients with chronic stable angina pectoris, the resting ECG is normal in 70% of cases (Hurst 1982). This test lacks sensitivity and specificity since ST segment depression or elevation may not occur if the myocardial oxygen supply-demand ratio is not stressed. A normal resting ECG therefore does not exclude coronary artery disease and, likewise, an abnormal electrocardiogram does not necessarily signify coronary artery disease.

Electrocardiogram abnormalities increase with age. ST segment depression is nonspecific because it is associated with a variety of cardiac and noncardiac conditions. Occasionally, stroke produces marked ST-T changes in the absence of coronary artery disease. ST segment elevation may occur with early repolarization, acute myocardial infarction, acute pericarditis, or chronic left ventricular aneurysm.

Q waves are highly predictive of coronary artery disease and indicate the presence of myocardial scar (Bodenheimer 1975). However, Q waves are absent in one-third of patients with previous myocardial infarction. ST segment depression or elevation during episodes of chest pain is highly predictive of fixed or vasospastic coronary artery lesions.

The chest radiograph provides little information about the status of the coronary arteries in most cases. Very rarely coronary artery calcifications are visible on the routine chest roentgenogram. Since coronary calcifications are extremely difficult to detect on a routine chest roentgenogram, their presence indicates heavy deposition of calcium and a high likelihood of coronary artery disease. Occasionally, patients with a remote myocardial infarction have a characteristic bulge in the cardiac silhouette resulting from chronic left ventricular aneurysm, and rarely calcification of a scar is seen.

Cardiac fluoroscopy utilizing a conventional image intensifier is also relatively insensitive in detecting coronary artery calcifications unless the calcium deposition is heavy (Aldrich 1979). Coronary calcifications in young individuals correlate well with the presence of at least moderate coronary artery obstructions, but specificity decreases with age.

Exercise Testing

Exercise electrographic testing is a safe procedure with a mortality rate of approximately 1 per 10000 tests. It has a low predictive accuracy when utilized for screening asymptomatic patients in the general population. The predictive value of the test, however, increases when the prevalence of coronary artery disease reaches at least moderate levels. Hence patients with cerebrovascular disease represent a reasonable population for exercise testing.

Despite a high frequency of false-positive and false-negative tests, exercise electrocardiographic testing represents the most useful and widely employed noninvasive screening method presently available for detecting severe coronary artery disease. Stress electrocardiographic testing is performed with a variety of exercise protocols using either treadmills or stationary bicycle ergometer systems. Ideally multiple-lead systems are monitored, since the sensitivity of the procedure increases as more leads are applied. Graded exercise is performed under supervision and the electrocardiographic response is recorded. Symptoms, blood pressure response, and the duration of exercise are other important parameters observed during the test. In order to insure reliability, the patient must be physically able and motivated to achieve maximal exercise. Eighty-five percent of the age-estimated maximal heart rate must be achieved in order to insure that a negative test truly supports the absence of disease. Patients who are unable to exercise because of obesity, intermittent claudication, debilitation, or neurologic deficits should not be subjected to standard exercise testing.

ST segment displacement is the ECG hallmark of myocardial ischemia. An abnormal ECG response to exercise is characterized by 1 mm or greater ST segment depression 80 ms after the J point of the QRS complex. If the ST segments are already abnormal at rest, then 1 mm additional ST segment depression is required for an abnormal test. In general, the greater the ST segment depression, the greater the probability of coronary artery disease (Hamby 1984). ST segment depression which occurs early in exercise or persists long into the recovery period is likely to be a truly positive abnormal response and also suggests more severe disease. ST segment elevation is rare and indicates coronary artery spasm or fixed obstructive coronary disease with resulting transmural ischemia. However, ST segment elevation in the presence of pathologic Q waves is secondary to wall motion abnormalities from previous myocardial infarction. Frequent premature ventricular complexes or ventricular tachycardia during exercise may be a marker for severe coronary disease, but the specificity is much lower than ST segment deviation (Weiner 1984). Progressive hypotension during exercise is an indicator of left ventricular dysfunction.

A negative submaximal exercise test is nondiagnostic and does not exclude severe coronary artery obstruction. Therefore a patient who is unable to achieve maximum exercise has not been effectively screened by the test. This limits the usefulness of exercise testing in many patients who have suffered a prior stroke.

Even with maximal effort, exercise testing has limited predictive accuracy because of a high frequency of false-positive and false-negative studies. In symptomatic patients with arteriographically proven coronary artery disease, the incidence of true-positive tests ranges from 60% to 80% and the false-negative rate varies between 15% and 40% (Chaitman 1978). The more severe the coronary artery disease, the greater the sensitivity of the test. Downsloping ST segment depression has the lowest likelihood of false positivity whereas upsloping ST segment depression has the highest. False-negative stress tests may be secondary to concomitant use of nitrates, beta blockers, or calcium channel blockers. False-positive tests may occur with drugs such as digitalis, tricyclic antidepressants, estrogens, diuretics, lithium carbonate, and phenothiazines. Cardiomyopathies, valvular heart disease, mitral valve prolapse, and preexcitation syndromes may produce false-positive studies in the absence of coronary disease.

Nuclear Imaging

Cardiac nuclear imaging has gained increasing popularity in the past 5 years and has become more readily available for screening patients suspected of having coronary artery disease. The two major radionuclide imaging techniques currently utilized are thallium perfusion imaging and radionuclide exercise ventriculography. The reliability of radionuclide studies is dependent upon availability and skill in interpretation.

Thallium-201 Imaging

Thallium-201 is a radionuclide analog of potassium which achieves reasonably high myocardial concentrations after passing through the circulation. Thallium

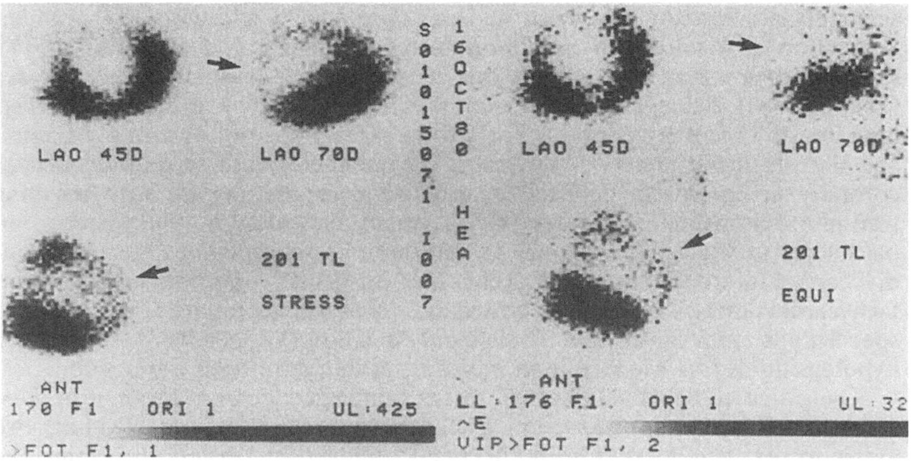

Fig. 19.2. Exercise and redistribution planar thallium images demonstrating a persistent anterior wall perfusion defect consistent with myocardial scar (*arrow*).

distribution to the myocardium is directly related to myocardial blood flow. Areas with impaired blood flow receive relatively smaller amounts of thallium and have lower radioactivity levels. The patient undergoing thallium imaging exercises according to a standard protocol on a treadmill or stationary bicycle. The ECG blood pressure response and heart rate are monitored throughout the test. At maximum exercise, 1.5–2 mCi thallium-201 is injected intravenously. Cardiac radioactivity is then imaged by a gamma camera in at least three views (anterior, left anterior oblique, left lateral). Immediate postexercise images are acquired and processed by a computer. Redistribution images are obtained in the same fashion 2–4 h after exercise. The immediate postexercise images and the redistribution images are examined for defects or "cold spots" in the myocardium corresponding to areas of impaired flow (Fig. 19.2). Thallium perfusion defects which occur with exercise, but which resolve in the redistribution phase, are indicative of myocardial hypoperfusion or "ischemia." Thallium defects in the postexercise scan as well as the redistribution scan indicate myocardial scar.

Interpretation is made either by visual inspection of the gamma camera display or by computerized techniques. The images have a doughnut or horseshoe appearance with a central lucency representing the left ventricular cavity. Decreased activity is normally seen in the region of the aortic and mitral valves and occasionally at the apex. The right ventricle is faintly visualized, but has considerably less uptake than the left ventricle.

Maximal exercise is a prerequisite for accurate scanning. The myocardial to lung ratio of thallium distribution, corresponding to the intensity of exercise, should be greater than 2.5:1 (resting ratio is 2:1). The information obtained from thallium imaging is based on regional differences of myocardial uptake, and does not provide accurate data on the exact number of diseased coronary vessels (Bodenheimer 1980b). Thus, triple vessel coronary artery disease may cause global ischemia and only small differences in regional perfusion. Decreased regional perfusion usually precedes mechanical, ECG, and metabolic manifestations of myocardial ischemia, and theoretically should be the most sensitive means of detecting coronary artery disease. However, the sensitivity of planar thallium imaging in patients without previous myocardial infarction ranges between 65% and 100% (average 75%) (Becker 1980). False-positive scans may occur with left ventricular hypertrophy, cardiomyopathies, obesity, prominent pectoral muscles, breast tissue, and diaphragmatic overlap (Schiavone 1984). Thallium imaging is of little additional assistance in assessing the patient with typical angina who has an abnormal ECG response to exercise.

Tomographic thallium imaging enhances the accuracy of radionuclide scanning (MacIntyre 1982). Tomographic images are obtained by a gamma camera mounted on a gantry which rotates in a 360° axis around the patient. Multiple images are obtained and reconstructed into tomographic slices (Fig. 19.3). This technique eliminates superimposed myocardial segments and provides a more accurate estimate of the extent of ischemia. The effects of soft tissue attenuation on radioactivity are also minimized, reducing false positivity. Limited availability and the need for major computer support are drawbacks to tomographic thallium imaging at this time.

Dipyridamole-Induced Thallium Imaging. Dipyridamole-induced thallium imaging is an alternative means of assessing myocardial perfusion in patients who are unable to exercise (Josephson 1982). Dipyridamole pharmacologically produces coronary vasodilatation similar to that of dynamic exercise. This increases blood flow to normal myocardium and minimally changes blood flow to areas supplied

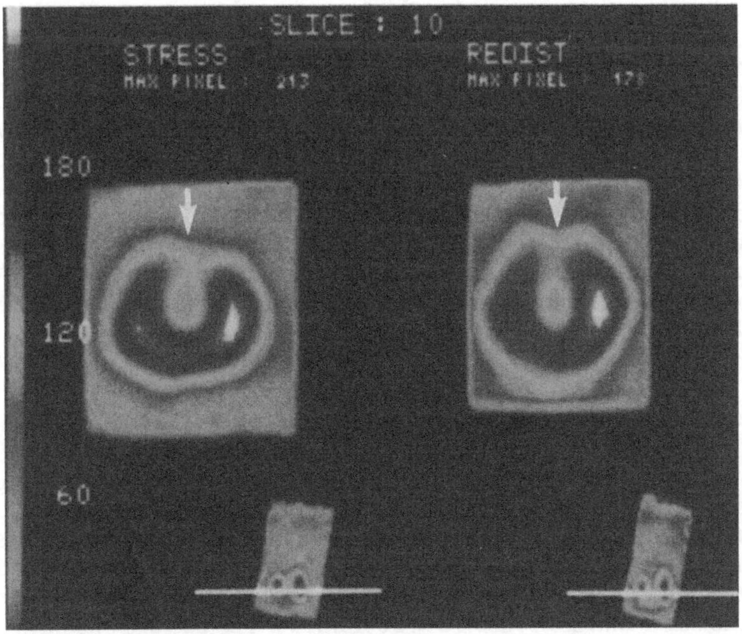

Fig. 19.3. Tomographic thallium images after exercise and at rest demonstrating a persistent anterior wall defect consistent with myocardial scar (*arrow*).

by an obstructed vessel. The test is performed by administering dipyridamole intravenously over 4 min. Thallium-201 is then injected intravenously and images are obtained within 5 min and 4 h later. Thallium images are reconstructed in a planar or tomographic format. The sensitivity, specificity, and accuracy of dipyridamole thallium imaging appears to be similar to that of conventional thallium studies (Albro 1978). Peripheral vasodilatation induced by dipyridamole causes increased heart rate and slightly decreased blood pressure. Common side effects include chest distress, headache, nausea, vomiting, and dizziness. Serious morbidity has not occurred.

Radionuclide Ventriculography

Exercise radionuclide ventriculography records left ventricular wall motion and estimates ejection fraction at rest and during exercise. Technetium-99 is injected intravenously and the heart is imaged at rest and during bicycle exercise. Two techniques currently are utilized: first-pass studies (using rapid acquisition multiple crystal gamma cameras) and gated blood studies (MUGA scans). The advantages of first-pass studies are rapid acquisition time, decreased patient motion, and increased quantification of right ventricular function. However, first-pass studies require specialized equipment and expertise. Gated blood pool studies, which are more commonly performed, utilize a standard gamma camera and conventional computer software. Images are obtained over several hundred heartbeats producing composite time-activity curves of the cardiac cycle. Sixteen or more images are constructed, with emphasis placed on the end-diastolic and end-systolic frames.

Normally, left ventricular ejection fraction increases during exercise. With severe coronary artery disease, the ejection fraction may not increase and frequently decreases (Bodenheimer 1980a). Myocardial ischemia causes regional or global loss of left ventricular function which may be manifested as wall motion abnormalities at rest or during exercise. These changes usually occur before the development of angina pectoris or ST segment depression, and are observed in 60%–70% of patients with coronary disease during testing (Fig. 19.4). The reliability of exercise radionuclide ventriculography versus thallium imaging varies among institutions. The sensitivity for coronary artery disease is similar, but thallium specificity is somewhat higher. The major limiting factor of exercise radionuclide ventriculography is the dependence on maximal exercise which cannot be accomplished by some individuals requiring screening.

Digital Subtraction Ventriculography

Digital subtraction ventriculography may be performed at rest and during exercise to assess left ventricular function in a manner similar to radionuclide imaging (Detrano 1984). Thirty to 40 ml of iodinated contrast medium is injected through a large-bore catheter inserted in the antecubital vein and positioned in the superior vena cava. The heart is imaged in the right anterior oblique projection and data are collected at 30 frames/s. The passage of contrast is followed throughout the cardiac chambers allowing assessment of right ventricular as well as left ventricular function. The patient then performs supine

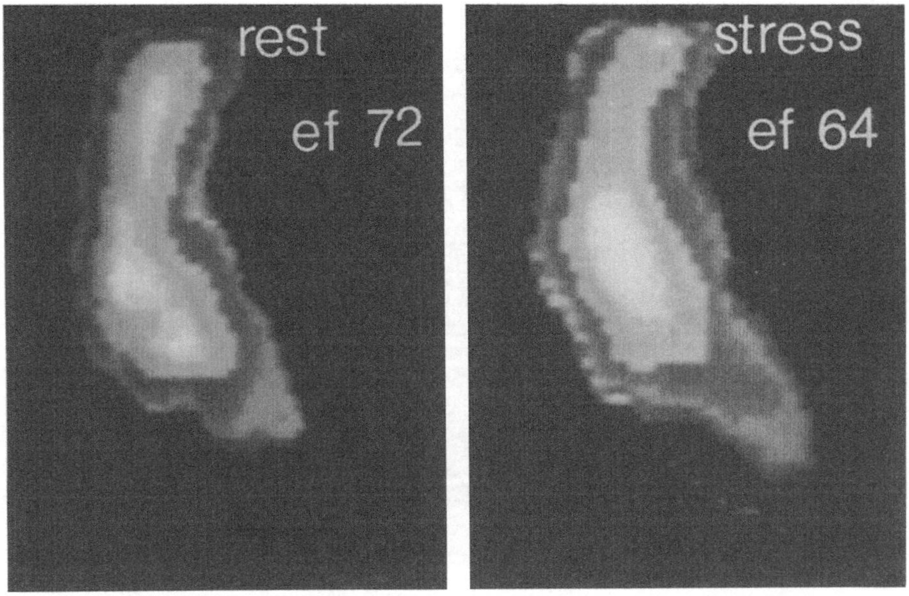

Fig. 19.4. Resting and stress radionuclide left ventriculography documenting a fall in ejection fraction from 72% to 64% with exercise.

bicycle exercise until maximal exertion is achieved. Contrast medium is injected intravenously once again and images are obtained immediately following exercise. Wall motion is assessed after exercise and compared with wall motion previously recorded at rest (Fig. 19.5). Exercise digital subtraction ventriculography appears to be superior to echocardiography or radionuclide ventriculography in defining ventricular structures. Its predictive accuracy is similar to exercise thallium imaging. Digital subtraction ventriculography utilizes low-radiation exposure, but requires maximal supine bicycle exercise. Iodinated contrast agents have been associated with a low incidence of adverse reactions.

Digital Subtraction Fluorography

Digital subtraction fluorography is a new technique for detecting coronary artery calcifications in a manner similar to conventional fluoroscopic imaging. The presence of coronary artery calcifications on digital fluorography usually corresponds with at least moderate coronary artery disease detected angiographically. Digital subtraction fluorography is performed in the cardiac catheterization laboratory with a conventional image intensifier coupled to a digital subtraction unit. Images are obtained in the right anterior oblique and left anterior oblique projections. Mask subtraction eliminates background structures such as spine, ribs, sternum, and great vessels. Cardiac motion allows coronary calcifications to escape subtraction. Digital mask subtraction enhances images of radiodense objects making coronary calcifications more visible to the viewer (Fig. 19.6). In our institution, digital fluorography has an 88% sensitivity and 64% specificity for detecting coronary artery disease when at least one calcified

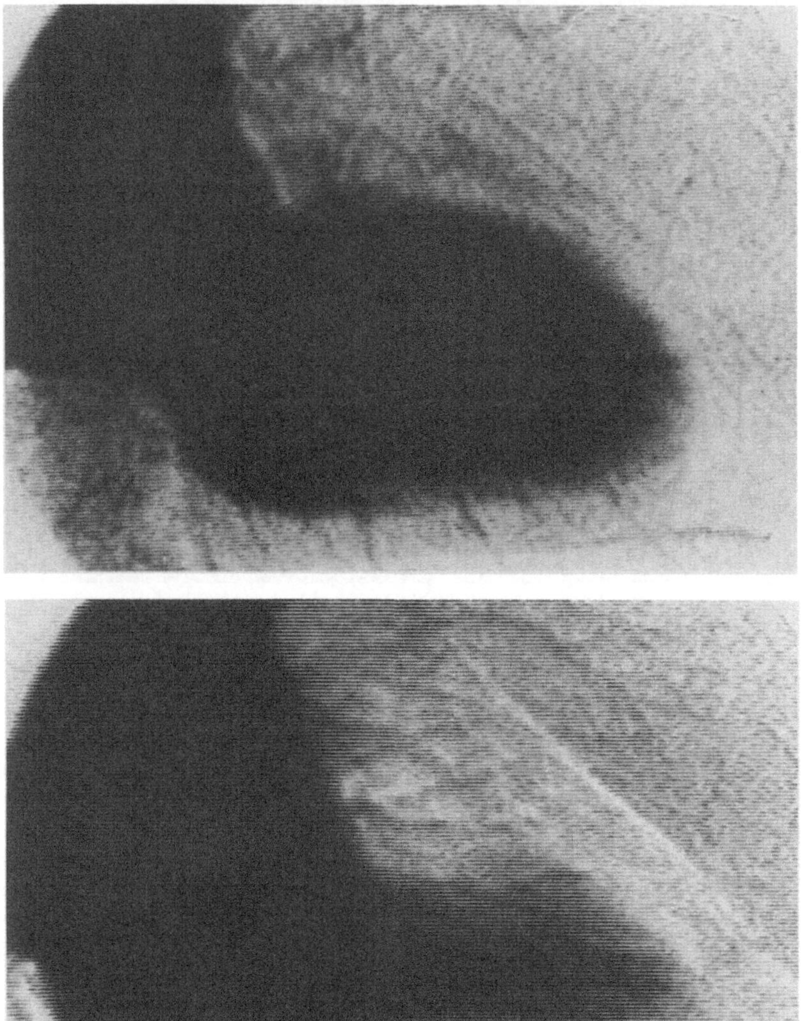

a

b

Fig. 19.5a,b. Intravenous digital subtraction left ventriculogram (RAO projection) demonstrating anterior and apical hypokinesis during exercise. **a** End diastole; **b** end systole.

coronary artery is visualized (Detrano 1985). Since coronary artery calcification increase with age, this technique loses specificity after age 55. Digital subtraction fluorography is inexpensive, safe, and involves low radiation exposure. It does not require exercise or the injection of contrast agents. Its major drawback at present is limited availability.

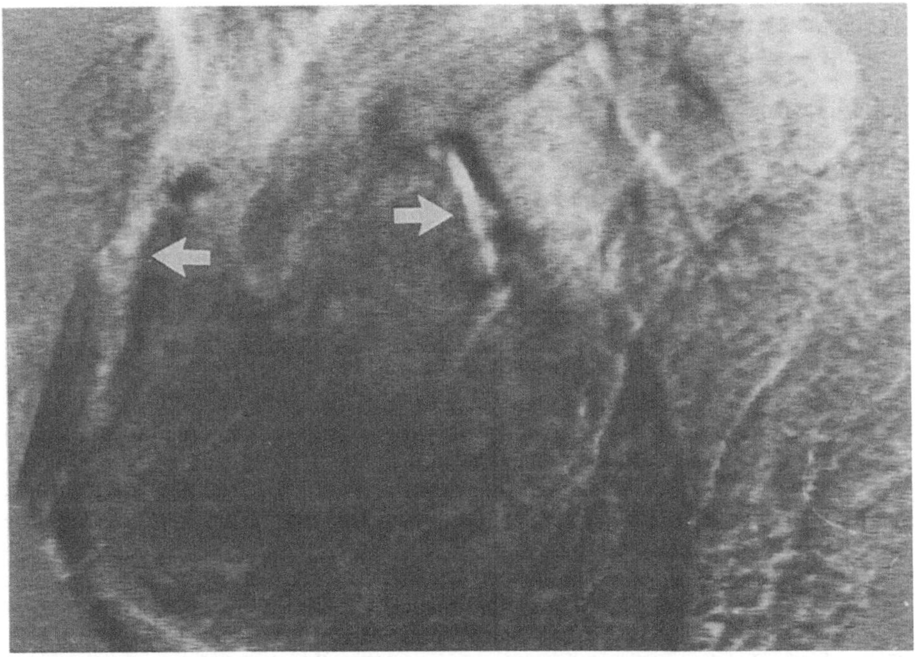

Fig. 19.6. Digital subtraction fluorography (LAO projection) enhances visualization of heavy calcification in the proximal portions of the right and left coronary arteries (*arrows*).

Coronary Arteriography

Coronary arteriography is currently the most accurate means of diagnosing coronary artery disease. This technique localizes coronary artery obstructions, defines the severity of specific lesions, visualizes collateral vessels, and documents coronary artery spasm. Left ventriculography defines overall and segmental left ventricular function. Coronary arteriography may be performed utilizing the brachial or femoral approach. The technique requires the use of contrast agents and is somewhat uncomfortable for the patient. It is relatively expensive and is usually performed in a hospital setting. In most instances, the information obtained from coronary arteriography justifies the small risk and the cost of the procedure. Minor complications occur in approximately 1% of cases and major complications are seen in less than 0.1% (Kennedy 1982a,b).

The prognosis of patients with coronary artery disease is primarily dependent upon the number of diseased coronary vessels as well as left ventricular function (Proudfit 1966). Since cardiac angiography defines both parameters, this test should provide the most useful data for predicting survival in groups of patients. Coronary arteriography should be performed when there is a need to know the coronary anatomy, when noninvasive tests are abnormal, or as a guide to planning therapy.

Recommended Approach to Coronary Artery Disease in Patients with Cerebrovascular Disease

Patients with symptomatic atherosclerotic cerebrovascular disease or asymptomatic carotid stenosis who are in good neurologic and medical condition and who are less than 70 years old should be screened for asymptomatic coronary artery disease. The best means of screening for coronary artery disease in asymptomatic patients is uncertain at the present time. Standard exercise ECG stress tests with or without thallium scanning represent the most widely utilized noninvasive means for screening. A negative maximal stress test is fairly reliable in ruling out major coronary lesions, but a negative submaximal test does not exclude severe coronary artery disease. An abnormal stress test or thallium scan is an indication for coronary arteriography.

Patients with typical angina pectoris should proceed directly to coronary arteriography without undergoing noninvasive studies. Patients with atypical symptoms could be evaluated either noninvasively or by coronary arteriography based on the likelihood of detecting coronary artery disease. A patient who is unable to achieve maximal exercise should undergo coronary arteriography or dipyridamole thallium imaging.

Many factors about coronary artery disease are unknown. The pathophysiology of silent myocardial ischemia, the natural history of coronary disease, and the prognosis in patients without symptoms have been incompletely defined. Thus, the optimal management of coronary artery disease is often uncertain and the treatment of both symptomatic and asymptomatic coronary disease must always be individualized. Nevertheless, certain guidelines can be recommended based on available data (Borhani 1985).

Multiple large clinical studies have shown that the prognosis of patients with coronary artery disease is related to the number of diseased vessels and to left ventricular function rather than severity of symptoms (Proudfit 1978). Prognosis is uncertain for individual patients, but can be predicted for groups of patients with similar clinical and anatomic characteristics. Prognosis is also directly related to progression of arterial lesions. If anatomic progression could be prevented, then death from coronary artery disease would be unlikely. Unfortunately, incomplete knowledge of the cause of coronary atherosclerosis limits our ability to estimate and prevent its progression.

Noninvasive testing is used to select candidates for cardiac angiography. Risk stratification and management are determined by cardiac angiography and not by noninvasive testing. Most patients with single vessel disease have a relatively good 5-year survival rate (approximately 90%) (Proudfit 1978). Prognosis seems to be determined mainly by progression of disease in the other arteries. Traditionally, asymptomatic patients with single vessel disease have been managed medically. If the affected coronary artery is large and supplies extensive myocardium, coronary angioplasty (PTCA) or bypass surgery may be recommended. However, all three forms of therapy (medical, PTCA, bypass) have similar 5- year survival rates. Although single vessel disease is considered to be relatively benign, approximately 15% of the cases of sudden death are associated with one vessel involvement (Loop 1983).

Patients with two vessel disease have a more uncertain prognosis and the management is more controversial. Medical management of asymptomatic or symptomatic double vessel disease can be supported by the conclusions of several large clinical trials (Loop 1983). However, many centers with surgical expertise and low operative complication rates favor myocardial revascularization. Coronary angioplasty represents an alternative form of therapy in selected patients.

Triple vessel disease and left main trunk obstruction have a relatively poor 5-year survival rate (Proudfit 1978). Left ventricular dysfunction decreases survival rates by half. Severe multivessel or left main disease, especially in the presence of left ventricular dysfunction, is best managed surgically whether or not symptoms are prominent. Surgical management of these high-risk patients is supported by many large clinical trials (Loop 1983).

References

Adams HP, Kassell NF, Mazuz H (1984) The patient with transient ischemic attacks—Is this the time for a new therapeutic approach? Stroke 15: 371–375

Albro PC, Gould KL, Westcott RJ (1978) Noninvasive assessment of coronary stenosis by myocardial imaging during pharmacologic coronary vasodilatation III, clinical trial. Am J Cardiol 42: 751–760

Aldrich RF, Brensike JF, Battaglini JW (1979) Coronary calcifications in the detection of coronary artery disease and comparison with electrocardiographic exercise testing. Circulation 59: 1113–1124

Becker LC (1980) Diagnosis of coronary artery disease with exercise radionuclide imaging: state of the art. Am J Cardiol 45: 1301–1304

Bodenheimer MM, Bank VS, Helfant RH (1975) Q waves and ventricular asynergy: predictive value and hemodynamic significance of anatomic localization. Am J Cardiol 35: 615–618

Bodenheimer MM, Banka VS, Helfant RH (1980a) Nuclear cardiology I. Radionuclide angiographic assessment of left ventricular contraction: uses, limitations and future directions. Am J Cardiol 45: 661–673

Bodenheimer MM, Banka VS, Helfant RH (1980b) Nuclear cardiology II. The role of myocardial perfusion imaging using thallium-201 in diagnosis of coronary heart disease 45: 674–684

Borhani NO (1985) Prevention of coronary heart disease in practice: implications of the results of recent clinical trials. JAMA 254: 253–262

Canadian Cooperative Study Group (1978) A randomized trial of aspirin and sulfinpyrazone in threatened stroke. N Engl J Med 299: 53–59 (also see NAPS document 03284)

Chaitman BR, Bourassa MG, Wagniart P (1978) Improved efficiency of treadmill exercise testing using a multiple lead ECG system and basic hemodynamic exercise response. Circulation 57: 71–79

Craig DR, Meguro K, Watridge C, Robertson JT, Barnett HJM, Fox AJ (1982) Intracranial internal carotid artery stenosis. Stroke 13: 825–828

DeBakey ME, Crawford ES, Cooley DA, Morris GC, Garrett HE, Fields WS (1965) Cerebral arterial insufficiency: one to 11-year results following reconstructive operation. Ann Surg 161: 921–945

Detrano R, Simpfendorfer C, O'Donnell J (1984) Comparison of stress digital ventriculography, stress thallium scintigraphy, and digital fluorography in screening for coronary artery disease. Circulation 70: II–31

Detrano R, Markovic D, Simpfendorfer C (1985) Digital subtraction fluoroscopy: a new method of detecting coronary calcifications with improved sensitivity for the prediction of coronary disease. Circulation 71: 725–732

Ennix CL Jr, Lawrie GM, Morris GC Jr, Crawford ES, Howell JF, Reardon MJ, Weathorford SC (1979) Improved results of carotid endarterectomy in patients with symptomatic coronary disease. An analysis of 1546 consecutive carotid operations. Stroke 10: 122–125

Fields WS, Maslenikov V, Meyer JS, Hass, WK, Remington RD, Macdonald M (1970) Progress report of prognosis following surgery or nonsurgical treatment for transient cerebral ischemic attacks and cervical carotid artery lesions. JAMA 211: 1993–2003

Fields WS, Lemak NA, Frankowski NA, Hardy RJ (1977) Controlled trial of aspirin in cerebral ischemia. Stroke 8: 301–316

Fisher CM, Gore I, Okabe N, White PD (1965) Atherosclerosis of the carotid and vertebral arteries— extracranial and intracranial. J Neuropathol Exp Neurol 24: 455–476

Furlan AJ, Whisnant JP, Elveback LR (1979) The decreasing incidence of primary intracerebral hemorrhage: a population study. Ann Neurol 5: 367–373

Furlan AJ, Whisnant JP, Baker HL Jr (1980) Long-term prognosis after carotid artery occlusion. Neurol 30: 986–988

Hamby RI, Davison ET, Hilsenrath J (1984) Functional and anatomic correlates of markedly abnormal stress tests. JACC 3: 1375–1381

Hertzer NR, Lees CD (1981) Fatal myocardial infarction following carotid endarterectomy. Three hundred and thirty-five cases followed 6–11 years after operation. Ann Surg 194: 212–218

Hertzer NR, Young JR, Beven EG (1985) Coronary angiography in 506 patients with extracranial cerebrovascular disease. Arch Int Med 145: 849–852

Heyman A, Wilkinson WE, Heyden S, Helms MJ, Bartel AG, Karp HR, Tryoler HA, Hames CG (1980) Risks of stroke in asymptomatic persons with cervical arterial bruits. N Engl J Med 302: 838– 841

Hurst JW, King SB III, Walter PF (1982) Atheroscloerotic coronary heart disease: angina pectoris, myocardial infarction, and other manifestations of myocardial ischemia. In: Hurst JW (ed) The heart. McGraw-Hill, New York, pp 1009–1149

Josephson MA, Brown BG, Hecht HS (1982) Noninvasive detection and localization of coronary stenoses in patients: comparison of resting dipyridamole and exercise thallium-201 myocardial perfusion imaging. Am Heart J 103: 1008–1018

Kannel WB (1976) Some lessons in cardiovascular epidemiology from Framingham. Am J Cardiol 37: 269–282

Kannel WB, Doyle JT, McNamara PM)1974) Precursors of sudden coronary death: factors related to the incidence of sudden death. Circulation 51: 606–613

Kannel WB, Wolf PA, Verter J (1983) Manifestations of coronary disease predisposing to stroke. The Framingham Study. JAMA 250: 2942–2946

Kennedy JW (1982a) Complications associated with catheterization and angiography. Cathet Cardiovasc Diagn 8: 5–11

Kennedy JW, Baxley WA, Bunnel IL (1982b) Mortality related to cardiac catheterization and angiography. Cathet Cardiovasc Diagn 8: 323–350

Kroener JM, Dorn PL, Shoor PM, Wickbom IG, Bernstein EF (1980) Prognosis of asymptomatic ulcerating carotid lesions. Arch Surg 115: 1387–1391

Loop FD (1983) Progress in surgical treatment of coronary atherosclerosis, parts 1, 2. Chest 84: 611–624, 740–755

Lye CR, Downs AR (1980) Carotid endarterectomy. Early and late results in 161 patients. Can J Surg 23: 536–540

MacIntyre WJ, Go RT, Cook SA, et al. (1982) Comparison of stress and redistribution 201-thallium planar imaging with a single photon transaxial tomographic technique. Proceedings: Third world congress of nuclear medicine and biology II: 1281–1284

Marzewski DJ, Furlan AJ, St. Louis P, Little JR, Modic MT, Williams G (1982) Intracranial internal carotid artery stenosis: long-term prognosis. Stroke 13: 821–824

Mitchell JRA, Schwartz CJ (1982) Relationship between arterial disease in different sites. A study of the aorta and coronary, carotid, and iliac arteries. Br Med J 1: 1293–1301

Moore WS, Boren C, Malone JM, Roon AJ, Eisenberg R, Goldstone J, Mani R (1978) Natural history of nonstenotic, asymptomatic ulcerative lesions of the carotid artery. Arch Surg 113: 1352–1358

Moufarrij NA, Little JR, Furlan AJ, Williams G, Marzewski DJ (1984) Vertebral artery stenosis: long-term follow-up. Stroke 15: 260–263

Proudfit WL, Shirey EK, Sones FM Jr (1966) Selective cine coronary arteriography. Correlation with clinical findings in 1000 patients. Circulation 33: 901–910

Proudfit WL, Bruschke AVG, Sones FM Jr (1978) Natural history of obstructive coronary artery disease: ten-year study of 601 nonsurgical cases. Prog Cardiovasc Dis 21: 53–78

Rokey R, Rolak LA, Harati Y, Kutkan N, Verani MS (1984) Coronary artery disease in patients with cerebrovascular disease: a prospective study. Ann Neurol 16: 50–53

Schiavone WA, Underwood DA, Go RT (1984) Causes of false-positive thallium-201 images in the diagnosis of coronary artery disease. Cleve Clin Q 51: 13–18

Solberg LA, McGarry PA, Moossy J, Strong JP, Tejada C, Loken AC (1968) Severity of atherosclerosis in cerebral arteries, coronary arteries, and aortas. NY Acad Sci 149: 956–973
Sundt TM Jr, Whisnant JP, Fode NC, Piepgras DG, Houser OW (1985) Results, complications, and follow-up of 415 bypass operations for occlusive disease of the carotid system. Mayo Clin Proc 60: 230–240
Toole JF, Yuson CP, Janeway R, Johnston F, Davis C, Cordell R, Howard G (1978) Transient ischemic attacks: a prospective study of 225 patients. Neurol (Minneap) 28: 746–753
Underwood DA, Rincon G, Yiannikas J (1982) Clinical usefulness of thallium 201 scintigraphy in the study of coronary artery disease: a comparison of two exercise systems. Cleve Clin Q 49: 73–78
Weiner DA, Levine SR, Klein MD (1984) Ventricular arrhythmias during exercise testing: mechanism, response to coronary bypass surgery and prognostic significance. Am J Cardiol 53: 1553–1557
Whisnant JP, Cartlidge NEF, Elveback LR (1978) Carotid and vertebral-basilar transient ischemic attacks: effect of anticoagulants, hypertension, and cardiac disorders on survival and stroke occurrence—a population study. Ann Neurol 3: 107–115
Wolf PA, Kannel WB, Sorlie P, McNamara P (1981) Asymptomatic carotid bruit and risk of stroke. The Framingham Study. JAMA 245: 1442–1445
Yatsu FM, Fields WS (1985) Asymptomatic carotid bruit. Stenosis or ulceration, a conservative approach. Arch Neurol 42: 383–385
Young W, Gofman JW, Tandy M (1960) The quantitation of atherosclerosis. The extent of correlation of degree of atherosclerosis within and between the coronary and cerebral vascular beds. Am J Cardiol 6: 300–308

Subject Index

GPSR Compliance

The European Union's (EU) General Product Safety Regulation (GPSR) is a set of rules that requires consumer products to be safe and our obligations to ensure this.

If you have any concerns about our products, you can contact us on ProductSafety@springernature.com

In case Publisher is established outside the EU, the EU authorized representative is:

Springer Nature Customer Service Center GmbH
Europaplatz 3
69115 Heidelberg, Germany

Batch number: 10838062

Printed by Printforce, the Netherlands